Second Edition

Appleton & Lange's Review for the
ULTRASONOGRAPHY
EXAMINATION

Charles S. Odwin, RT, RDMS
Supervisor of Ultrasound
Department of Radiology
Bronx-Lebanon Hospital Center
Bronx, New York

Trudy Dubinsky,† MA, RDMS
Program Director
Diagnostic Ultrasound Technology Program
New York University Medical Center
New York, New York

Arthur C. Fleischer, MD
Professor of Radiology and Radiological Sciences
Professor of Obstetrics and Gynecology
Chief of Diagnostic Sonography
Vanderbilt University Medical Center
Nashville, Tennessee

†Deceased.

Appleton & Lange Reviews/McGraw-Hill
Medical Publishing Division

New York St. Louis San Francisco Auckland Bogotá Caracas Lisbon London
Madrid Mexico City Milan Montreal New Delhi San Juan
Singapore Sydney Tokyo Toronto

McGraw-Hill

A Division of The McGraw·Hill Companies

Appleton & Lange's Review for the Ultrasonography Examination, Second Edition

11 12 13 14 15   CCI/CCI   0 9 8 7 6 5 4 3 2

ISBN: 0-8385-9073-X

Notice

Medicine is an ever-changing science. As new research and clinical experience broaden our knowledge, changes in treatment and drug therapy are required. The authors and the publisher of this work have checked with sources believed to be reliable in their efforts to provide information that is complete and generally in accord with the standards accepted at the time of publication. However, in view of the possibility of human error or changes in medical sciences, neither the authors nor the publisher nor any other party who has been involved in the preparation or publication of this work warrants that the information contained herein is in every respect accurate or complete, and they disclaim all responsibility for any errors or omissions or for the results obtained from use of the information contained in this work. Readers are encouraged to confirm the information contained herein with other sources. For example and in particular, readers are advised to check the product information sheet included in the package of each drug they plan to administer to be certain that the information contained in this work is accurate and that changes have not been made in the recommended dose or in the contraindications for administration. This recommendation is of particular importance in connection with new or infrequently used drugs.

Library of Congress Cataloging-in-Publication Data

Odwin, Charles S.
Appleton & Lange's Review for the ultrasonography examination / Charles S.
  Odwin, Trudy Dubinsky, Arthur C. Fleischer. — 2nd ed.
      p.   cm.
    ISBN 0-8385-9073-X
    1. Diagnosis, Ultrasonic—Examinations, questions, etc.
  I. Dubinsky, Trudy.   II. Fleischer, Arthur C.   III. Odwin, Charles S.
  Ultrasonography examination and review.   IV. Title: Appleton & Lange's review
  for the ultrasonography examination.
    [DNLM: 1. Ultrasonography—examination questions. WB 18 027u]
  RC78.7.U4038   1993
  616.07′543′076—dc20
  DNLM/DLC   92-49035
  for Library of Congress   CIP

Acquisitions Editor: Jane Licht
Production Editor: Karen W. Davis
Designer: Penny Kindzierski

This book is dedicated to the memory of Trudy Dubinsky, MA, RDMS, the founder and Program Director of the New York University Medical Center School of Diagnostic Medical Sonography. Trudy was a well-known, superb teacher whose dedication and contribution to her profession will always be remembered. She will be sadly missed.

Contributors

Dunstan Abraham, MPH, RDMS
Adjunct Instructor, Diagnostic Medical Imaging
  Program, College of Health Related Professions
SUNY/Health Sciences Center at Brooklyn
Clinical and Adjunct Instructor
Diagnostic Ultrasound Technology Program
New York University Medical Center
Supervisor of Ultrasound
Bronx-Municipal Hospital Center
Bronx, New York

Mark N. Allen, BS, RDCS
Administrator and Chief Cardiac Sonographer
University of Rochester Medical Center
Rochester, New York

Dale R. Cyr, BS, RDMS
Chief Sonographer
University of Washington Medical Center
Seattle, Washington

Rena Dubinsky, BS, RDMS
Adjunct Instructor
Diagnostic Ultrasound Technology Program
New York University Medical Center
New York, New York

Trudy Dubinsky, MA, RDMS
Program Director
Diagnostic Ultrasound Technology Program
New York University Medical Center
New York, New York

Arthur C. Fleischer, MD
Professor of Radiology and Radiological Sciences
Professor of Obstetrics and Gynecology
Chief of Diagnostic Sonography
Vanderbilt University Medical Center
Nashville, Tennessee

Pamela M. Foy, BS, RDMS
Clinical Coordinator of Ultrasound Services
Department of Obstetrics and Gynecology
The Ohio State University
Columbus, Ohio

Milagros Garay, RDMS
Adjunct Instructor
Diagnostic Ultrasound Technology Program
New York University Medical Center
New York, New York

Thomas G. Hoffman, BS, RDMS, RVT
Adjunct Instructor, Diagnostic Medical Imaging
  Program, College of Health Related Professions
SUNY/Health Sciences Center at Brooklyn
Clinical and Adjunct Instructor
Diagnostic Ultrasound Technology Program
New York University Medical Center
Supervisor of Ultrasound
Weiler Hospital of the Albert Einstein College of
  Medicine
Bronx, New York

Steven Horii, MD
Associate Professor of Georgetown University Hospital
Georgetown University Hospital
Washington, D.C.

Sandra Katanick, RN, RVT
Former Field Applications Specialist–Peripheral
  Vascular
Acuson Computed Sonography
Mountain View, California
Executive Director of ICAVL
Rockville, Maryland

Charles S. Odwin, RT, RDMS
Clinical Instructor, Diagnostic Medical Imaging
  Program, College of Health Related Professions
SUNY/Health Sciences Center at Brooklyn
Clinical and Adjunct Instructor
Diagnostic Ultrasound Technology Program
New York University Medical Center
Supervisor of Ultrasound
Department of Radiology
Bronx-Lebanon Hospital Center
Bronx, New York

Chandrowti Devi Persaud, RT, RDMS
Clinical Instructor
New York University Medical Center
Diagnostic Ultrasound Technology Program
   Sonographer
Bronx-Lebanon Hospital Center
Bronx, New York

Raymond L. Powis, PhD
Clinical Science and Communications Manager
Quantum Medical Systems
Issaguah, Washington

Ronald R. Price, PhD
Director, Division of Radiological Sciences
Professor of Radiology and Radiological Sciences
Vanderbilt University Hospital
Professor of Physics and Astronomy
Vanderbilt University
Nashville, Tennessee

David L. Rollins, MD
Director of Surgery
St. Vincent's Charity Hospital
Cleveland, Ohio

Henny Wasser Rudansky, BS, RDCS
Adjunct and Clinical Instructor, Diagnostic Medical
   Imaging Program, College of Health Related
   Professions
SUNY/Health Sciences Center at Brooklyn
Supervisor of Echocardiography
Department of Cardiology
Maimonides Hospital
Brooklyn, New York

Carolyn M. Semrow, BS, EE
Director of Vascular Research
St. Vincent's Charity Hospital
Cleveland, Ohio

Diana Kawai Yankowitz, BS, RDCS
Pediatric Echocardiographer
University of California San Francisco Medical Center
San Francisco, California

Contents

Preface

The clinical application of Diagnostic Medical Ultrasound has expanded considerably since the first edition was published. Accordingly, we have developed a comprehensive up-to-date self-examination and study guide which incorporates these new applications. This single multispecialty, comprehensive examination review has long been anticipated.

This edition is comprised of ten examination specialties with each specialty containing a study guide followed by numerous questions and explanations.

Over 3000 questions with accompanying answers and explanations and over 600 sonograms and illustrations are organized into a single textbook. Color images have also been added in order to cover the most current applications of diagnostic ultrasound. Candidates seeking RDMS, RDCS, and RVT certifications will find this edition informative and invaluable. In addition, this review guide was carefully revised for sonography students as a supplement to classroom lectures.

It is our desire that you will find this new edition not only a means to study for the Registry but a useful tool to enhance your professional growth and clinical effectiveness.

We applaud you in your search for knowledge and we thank you for the opportunity of sharing our experience with you.

Charles S. Odwin
Trudy Dubinsky
Arthur C. Fleischer

Acknowledgments

The creation of this textbook has been hard work, and without support it would not have been achieved. We wish to extend our thanks to all the Radiologists at the Bronx-Lebanon Hospital Center. I am deeply grateful to Richard A. Rosen, MD, Director of the Department of Radiology, Harvey Stern, MD, Associate Director of the Department of Radiology, and Walter McKoy, Administrator of the Department of Radiology, who were kind enough to allow me the time and flexibility to complete this text, and special thanks to David P. Neumann, MD, Chief Resident, for his constructive criticism of the first edition. I would especially like to thank Mrs. La Rosa Pinder for her secretarial assistance. To conclude, I wish to thank my ultrasound colleagues and students for their support and encouragement.

How to Use This Book

This book has been written as a study guide for review and self-examination and serves as a useful tool for preparation for the American Registry of Diagnostic Medical Sonography Examination and the ultrasound portions of the American Board of Radiology Examination.

To get the most from this book, first read the Study Guide then go through the Questions answering them all regardless of difficulty, just as you would take the actual test. The Questions are either multiple choice or matching, and many are accompanied by a sonogram or illustration.

At the end of each set of Questions, there is an An-swer and Explanation section. In this section the answer is explained, and a reference is given for each answer. The first number of the reference indicates a book or journal, as numbered in the References section. The second number or numbers indicate the page or pages on which the relevant material can be found. If only one number is given, the reference is to the entire book.

Do not be discouraged if you are unable to answer all of the questions on the first try. We encourage you to try again.

Best wishes for success in your study of ultrasound.

CHAPTER 1

ULTRASONIC PHYSICS AND INSTRUMENTATION

*Trudy Dubinsky, Steven Horii, Charles S. Odwin,
Ronald R. Price, Arthur C. Fleischer, and Milagros Garay*

Study Guide

WHAT IS ULTRASOUND?

Ultrasound is a mechanical, longitudinal wave that carries variations of quantities referred to as *acoustic variables*. Ultrasound is above the range of human hearing (20,000 hertz [or cycles per second] or greater).

Ultrasound waves are produced by oscillatory motion of the particles in a medium, creating regions of compression and rarefaction. The continued movement of particles propagating through a medium is the result of collision between particles that make up the medium.

Ultrasound can be continuous or pulsed. In the *continuous* mode the vibratory motions are produced by the source in an uninterrupted stream, whereas in the *pulsed* mode the sound is delivered in a series of packets, or pulses. In almost all of the diagnostic applications of ultrasound, *pulsed ultrasound* is used.

The following terms are commonly used in diagnostic medical sonography:

Mechanical wave. A wave that requires a medium in which to travel and therefore cannot propagate in a vacuum.

Longitudinal wave. A wave in which the particle motion travels parallel to the energy source (as opposed to shear or transverse waves, which travel perpendicular).

Acoustic variable. Each of the following is considered an acoustic variable: *pressure, temperature, density, particle motion.* Note that all of these variables change as an acoustic wave passes through the medium.

Parameters of a wave (Fig. 1–1A).

The following terms are common to all waves:

Cycle. A cycle is composed of one compression and one rarefaction, or a complete positive and negative change in an acoustic variable.

Frequency (*f*). The number of cycles per second. Frequency describes how many times the acoustic variable (whether it be pressure, density, particle motion, or temperature) changes in one second. *Units:* hertz (Hz), megahertz (MHz).

$$\text{frequency } (f) = \frac{\text{propagation speed}}{\text{wavelength}}, \qquad f = \frac{c}{\lambda}$$

Period. The time it takes for 1 cycle to occur; the inverse of frequency. *Units:* seconds (s), microseconds (μs).

$$\text{period} = \frac{1}{\text{frequency}}, \qquad p = \frac{1}{f}$$

As the frequency increases, the period decreases. Conversely, as the frequency decreases, the period increases.

Wavelength (λ). The distance that the wave must travel in 1 cycle. Wavelength is determined by both the source of the wave and the medium in which it is propagating (Fig. 1–1B). *Units:* meters (m), millimeters (mm).

$$\text{wavelength } (\lambda) = \frac{\text{propagation speed } (c)}{\text{frequency } (f)}, \qquad \lambda = \frac{c}{f}$$

With a velocity or propagation speed (*c*) of 1540 m/s, the wavelength of 1 MHz is 1.54 mm, of 2 MHz is 0.77 mm, and of 3 MHz is 0.51 mm.

Propagation speed. The maximum speed with which an

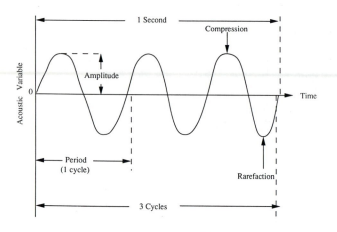

Figure 1–1A. The parameters of a wave. The frequency of this wave variable is 3 Hz (or cycles per second). A period is 1 complete cycle; therefore this wave consists of 3 periods. *Note:* The vertical direction is compression and downward direction is rarefaction and both represent pressure and density. Otherwise, it represents a positive (upward) or negative (downward) change in the acoustic variable.

acoustic wave can move through a medium, determined by the density and stiffness of the medium. Propagation speed increases proportionally with the stiffness (ie, the more stiff the medium the faster the variable will travel). Density is the concentration of mass per unit volume, and propagation speed is inversely proportional to density. *Units:* meters/second (m/s), millimeters/microsecond (mm/μs).

$$\text{propagation speed} \approx \sqrt{\frac{\text{elasticity (stiffness)}}{\text{density}}}, \qquad c \approx \frac{e}{p}$$

It should be emphasized that *compressibility* is the opposite of stiffness. If compressibility increases, then the propagation speed decreases.

Propagation speed is greater in solids > liquids > gases. Propagation speed (*c*) is equal to frequency (*f*) times wavelength (λ) {$c = f \times \lambda$}. Since the propagation speed is constant for a given medium, if the frequency increases the wavelength will decrease. Conversely, if the frequency decreases the wavelength will increase.

Example

If the frequency of an ultrasound wave traveling through soft tissue is increased from 5 to 10 MHz, what happens to the wavelength?
Steps to Solution:

$$\text{propagation speed} = 1540 \text{ m/s or } 1.54 \text{ mm/μs}$$

$$\text{frequency} = 5 \text{ MHz}$$

$$\frac{\text{propagation speed}}{\text{frequency}} = \text{wavelength}$$

$$1.54 \text{ mm/μs/5 MHz} = 0.31 \text{ (mm)}$$

$$\text{frequency} = 10 \text{ MHz}$$

$$1.54 \text{ mm/μs/10 MHz} = 0.154 \text{ (mm)}$$

Doubling the frequency halves the wavelength in a given medium. Note how the wavelength gets smaller.

PARAMETERS USED TO DESCRIBE PULSED WAVES

Pulse repetition frequency (PRF). The number of pulses per second. *Units:* hertz (Hz), kilohertz (kHz).

The PRF used depends on imaging depth: As the imaging depth increases, the PRF must decrease. This phenomenon is characteristic of the pulse–listening period–receiving cycle of the transducer. The longer it takes the returning signals (echoes) to come back to the transducer, the greater the interval between pulses. Therefore, the farther away a target, the longer the return trip, and the greater the interval between transmissions of the pulsed wave.

Pulse repetition period (PRP). The time from the beginning of one pulse to the beginning of the next (Fig. 1–2A). *Units:* seconds (s), milliseconds (ms).

$$\text{PRP} = \frac{1}{\text{PRF}}$$

The PRP increases as imaging depth increases. When depth decreases the PRP decreases.

Pulse duration (PD). The time it takes for a pulse to occur: the period of the ultrasound in the pulse multiplied by the number of cycles in the pulse (see Fig. 1–2A). *Units:* seconds (s), milliseconds (ms).

$$\text{pulse duration} = \text{number of cycles } (n) \times \text{period } (p)$$

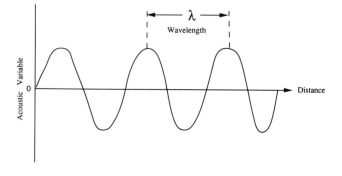

Figure 1–1B. A wavelength represents the distance between two adjacent wave peaks.

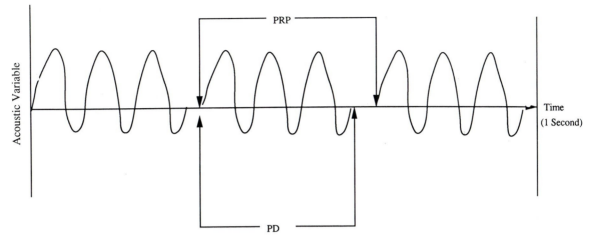

Figure 1–2A. Pulse repetition period (PRP).

Duty factor. The fraction of time that the transducer is generating a pulse. *Maximum value:* 1.0. In continuous wave the transducer is always generating a pulse. A second transducer acts as the listening device. *Minimum value:* 0.0. The transducer is *not* being excited (therefore no pulse will be generated). In clinical imaging, using pulse echo system the duty factor ranges from 0.001 to 0.01. *Units:* unitless.

$$\text{duty factor} = \frac{\text{PD } (\mu s)}{\text{PRP (ms)} \times 1000}$$

Note: Since the duty factor is unitless and PD is usually in microseconds, it is necessary to divide by 1000 to cancel out the units in the formula. In using this formula, the units must match (PD and PRP both must be in seconds, milliseconds, or microseconds). If not, a correction factor, such as the 1000 in the denominator, must be used.

The duty factor can also be computed by the following formula:

$$\text{duty factor} = \frac{\text{PD} \times \text{PRF}}{1000}$$

Spatial pulse length (SPL). The distance over which a pulse occurs (Fig. 1–2B). *Unit:* millimeters (mm).

$$\text{spatial pulse length (SPL)} = \text{wavelength } (\lambda) \times \text{number of cycles in a pulse } (n)$$

Amplitude. The maximum variation that occurs in an acoustic variable. It indicates the strength of the sound wave. To arrive at this variation, the undisturbed value is subtracted from the maximum value and the unit for the acoustic variable is applied (Fig. 1–3). Peak-to-peak amplitude (P–P) is the maximum to minimum value.

Power. The rate of energy transferred. The power is proportional to the wave amplitude squared. *Unit:* watts (W).

$$\text{power} \approx \text{amplitude}^2$$

Intensity. The power in a wave divided by the area of the beam. *Unit:* Watts per centimeter squared (W/cm^2).

$$\text{intensity} = \frac{\text{power (W)}}{\text{area (cm}^2)}$$

Note: The intensity is proportional to the amplitude squared. If the amplitude doubles, then the intensity quadruples.

Figure 1–2B. Spatial pulse length (SPL).

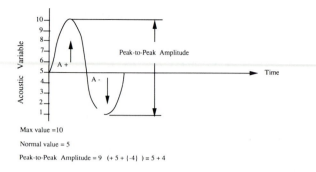

Figure 1–3. A wave amplitude. Amplitude is equal to the maximum value minus the normal value. Peak-to-peak amplitude (P–P) is equal to the maximum plus absolute value of the minimum.

POWER AND INTENSITY

The ultrasound power and the intensity of the ultrasound beam are not identical, although the two terms are sometimes used interchangeably. The *ultrasound power* is the rate at which work is done; it is equal to the work done divided by the time required to do the work. The intensity is the power per unit area and represents the strength of the ultrasound beam. The intensities used in diagnostic medical sonography applications range from 1 to 50 mW/cm^2. Understanding of the ultrasound intensity is important when studying the biologic effects of ultrasound in tissue (discussed later in this chapter).

Intensities have both a peak value and an average value. The intensity of the sound beam as it travels through a medium varies across the beam (*spatial intensity*) and with time (*temporal intensity*).

Spatial peak (SP). Intensity at the center of the beam.

Spatial average (SA). Intensity averaged throughout the beam.

Temporal peak (TP). Maximum intensity in the pulse, (measured when the pulse is on).

Temporal average (TA). Intensity averaged over one on–off beam cycle (takes into account the intensity from the beginning of one pulse to the beginning of next).

Pulse average (PA). Intensity averaged over the duration of the single pulse.

Six intensities result when spatial and temporal considerations are combined:

spatial peak–temporal peak	SPTP (highest)
spatial average–temporal peak	SATP
spatial peak–temporal average	SPTA
spatial average–temporal average	SATA (lowest)

spatial average–pulse average	SAPA
spatial peak–pulse average	SPPA

In pulsed ultrasound, the TP is greater than the PA, which is greater than the TA. When using continuous wave ultrasound, however, TP and TA intensities are the same.

Spatial peak intensity is related to SA by the beam uniformity ratio (BUR).

Beam uniformity ratio (BUR) is a unitless coefficient that describes the distribution of ultrasound beam intensity in space. The higher the SP, the more concentrated and the higher the SA, the less concentrated the intensity. *Units:* unitless.

$$\text{spatial average} = \frac{\text{spatial peak intensity (W/cm}^2)}{\text{beam uniformity ratio}},$$

$$SA = \frac{SP}{BUR}$$

$$\text{spatial peak} = \text{beam uniformity ratio} \times \text{spatial average}$$

$$(SP) = BUR \times SA$$

Temporal average intensity is related to TP by the duty factor (DF). *Units:* unitless.

$$\text{duty factor} = \frac{\text{temporal average}}{\text{temporal peak}},$$

$$DF = \frac{TA}{TP}$$

Attenuation
Attenuation is the reduction of the sound beam's amplitude and intensity as it travels through a medium. It is the reason why the echoes from deep structures are weaker than those from more superficial structures. The factors that contribute to attenuation are:

Absorption. The conversion of sound energy into heat. Absorption is the major source of attenuation in soft tissues.

Scattering. *Diffuse scattering* is the redirection of the sound beam after it strikes rough or small boundaries, when the wavelength is larger than the reflecting surface. Liver parenchyma and red blood cells represent diffuse scattering.

Reflection. The return of a portion of the ultrasound beam back toward the transducer (an echo). Of interest in diagnostic sonography is *specular reflection,* which occurs when the wavelength of the pulse is much smaller than the boundary it is striking and the surface is smooth. The best examples of specular reflectors are the diaphragm, liver capsule, and gallbladder walls. Reflection of the ultrasound beam depends on the *acoustic impedance mismatch* at the boundary between two media (discussed in detail later in this chapter).

The unit in which attenuation is given is the decibel (dB). *The decibel is the unit of intensity ratio, or power; it is the quantity obtained by taking 10 times the log of the ratio of two intensities.*

$$\text{decibels (dB)} = 10 \log \frac{\text{final intensity}}{\text{initial intensity}}$$

Attenuation coefficient is the attenuation per unit length of sound wave travel. For soft tissue, it is approximately half of the operating frequency of the transducer; that is, for every centimeter per megahertz (MHz) there is approximately 0.5 dB of attenuation. For example, if the operating frequency of a transducer is 5 MHz, then the attenuation coefficient is approximately 2.5 dB/cm.

$$\text{attenuation (dB)} = \text{attenuation coefficient (dB/cm)} \times \text{pathlength (cm)}$$

Note: Pathlength is the distance the sound beam travels in a medium. The actual calculation of decibel values is complex and need not be part of the sonographer's bank of common knowledge, but the sonographer should understand that since decibels are exponents, a small change in decibels can mean a large change in resulting values. The most useful way to handle these values is to memorize the commonly encountered ones (Table 1–1).

Example 1

The ultrasound beam produced by a 4-MHz transducer has an initial intensity of 20 mW/cm² after traveling through 3 cm of tissue. What is the intensity of the beam at the end of this path?

> *Given:* Frequency is 4 MHz; original intensity is 20 mW/cm²; pathlength is 3 cm; attenuation coefficient is ½ frequency, ie, ½(4 MHz) = 2 dB/cm.
>
> *Then:* If attenuation is attenuation coefficient × pathlength, then attenuation is 2 dB/cm × 3 cm = 6 dB.
> If attenuation is 0.25, then the decibel value is −6 dB.
> (See Table 1–1.)

TABLE 1–1. DECIBEL VALUES OF ATTENUATION

Decibels (dB)	Value	
−3 dB	(1/2)	0.5
−6 dB	(1/4)	0.25
−9 dB	(1/8)	0.13
−10 dB	(1/10)	0.10
−20 dB	(1/100)	0.01
−30 dB	(1/1000)	0.001

To obtain the final intensity, multiply the intensity ratio by the original intensity:

$$\text{mW/cm}^2 \times 0.25 = 5 \text{ mW/cm}^2$$

The intensity was therefore reduced to 25% of its original value. Another way to do this example is to note that a 3-dB reduction means halving a value. Since 6 dB = 3 dB + 3 dB, an attenuation of 6 dB reduces the power by one-half (20 W → 10 W), then by one-half again (10 W → 5 W).

Example 2

After passing through soft tissue media, an ultrasound beam with an initial intensity of 100 mW/cm² has a remaining intensity of 0.01 mW/cm². Calculate the amount of attenuation.

> *Given:* Initial intensity is 100 mW/cm²; final intensity is 0.01 mW/cm².
>
> *Then:* If decibels = $10 \log \frac{0.01}{100} = 10 \log \frac{1}{10,000}$
>
> $$= 10 \ (-4) = 40 \text{ dB}$$

Note: In strict mathematical terms the 40 dB should be negative, but for our purpose it can be simply stated as 40 dB of attenuation.
The attenuation, therefore, was 40 dB (−40 dB).

The *half-intensity depth* is the distance at which the intensity will be half that of the original; the distance the sound beam will travel through a medium before its intensity is reduced by 50%. It is calculated by the formula:

$$\text{half-intensity depth} = \frac{3}{\text{attenuation coefficient (dB/cm)}}$$

The half-intensity depth can also be calculated from the frequency:

$$\text{half-intensity depth} = \frac{6}{\text{frequency (MHz)}}$$

The half-intensity depth is a good indicator of the frequency that should be selected to view different structures in the body. For example, if 50% of the intensity is gone before one reaches a certain depth, then it is obvious that deeper structures will receive less of the sound beam and thus generate weaker echoes. To visualize deep structures it therefore is necessary to use a lower frequency.

Time gain compensation (TGC). An electronic compensation for tissue attenuation.

Echoes

Echoes are the reflections of the sound beam as it travels through the media. An echo is generated each time the beam encounters an acoustic impedance mismatch, but its strength depends on a number of factors. One very impor-

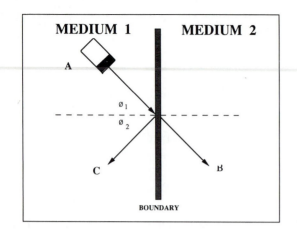

Figure 1–4A. (A) An oblique incidence striking a boundary; **(B)** refraction of the sound beam; **(C)** reflection of the sound beam. *Note:* An oblique incidence is *not* a normal incidence. A normal incidence is 90° (perpendicular). An incidence beam can be

1. Perpendicular (normal)
2. Oblique incidence (an incidence beam at an oblique angle) *not* perpendicular

The angle of incidence is the angle of any of the incidence beams.

tant factor, the *angle of incidence,* is the angle at which the incident beam strikes a boundary. The angle of incidence is equal to the angle of reflection (Fig. 1–4A).

Perpendicular Incidence. A beam traveling through a medium perpendicular to a boundary and encountering the boundary at a 90° angle (Fig. 1–4B). Perpendicular incidence is also known as *normal incidence.*[1] The portion of the beam that is not reflected continues in a straight line; this is called *transmission.*

Perpendicular incidence will produce a reflection when the acoustic impedance changes at the boundary. *Acoustic*

Figure 1–4B. The transmission of the perpendicular incidence sound beam, also called *normal incidence.* **(A)** Normal incidence striking a boundary perpendicularly; **(B)** the intensity transmitted; **(C)** reflection of energy at the boundary of medium 1 and medium 2. *Note:* Beam **(C)** actually travels back along the beam coming from **(A)**, but it is depicted separately.

impedance is the product of the density of a medium and the velocity of sound in that medium.

Acoustic impedance (rayls) = density (kg/m)
$$\times \text{ propagation speed (m/s)}$$
$$Z = p \times c$$

At an acoustic impedance mismatch the sound beam will proceed (transmission), be reflected, or both.

The relationship between *perpendicular incidence* and the *intensity* of the echoes can be characterized by the following formulas:

$$\frac{\text{intensity reflection}}{\text{coefficient (IRC)}} = \left(\frac{z_2 - z_1}{z_2 + z_1}\right)^2$$

$$\frac{\text{intensity reflection}}{\text{coefficient (IRC)}} = \frac{\text{reflected intensity}}{\text{incident intensity}}$$

$$\frac{\text{intensity transmission}}{\text{coefficient (ITC)}} = \frac{\text{transmitted intensity}}{\text{incident intensity}}$$

The ITC can also be calculated by the formula:

$$ITC = 1 - IRC$$

Incident intensity = IRC × incident intensity + ITC
$$\times \text{ incident intensity}$$

Example

Given two media, one with an acoustic impedance of 20 rayls and the other with an acoustic impedance of 40 rayls, calculate the intensity reflection coefficient (IRC), the intensity transmission coefficient (ITC), the reflected intensity and the transmitted intensity. (Assume that the incident intensity is 10 mW/cm².)

$$Z_1 = 20 \text{ rayls}; Z_2 = 40 \text{ rayls}$$

$$IRC = \left(\frac{40 - 20}{40 + 20}\right)^2 = \left(\frac{20}{60}\right)^2 = \left(\frac{1}{3}\right)^2 = \frac{1}{9} = 0.11$$

Given: The IRC is 0.11.

Then: ITC = 1 − IRC

ITC = 1 − 0.11 = 0.89

If the reflected intensity is equal to the IRC times the original intensity, then reflected intensity = 0.11 × 10 mW/cm² = 1.1 mW/cm².

If the transmitted intensity is equal to the ITC times the original intensity, then transmitted intensity = 0.89 × 10 mW/cm² = 8.9 mW/cm².

Oblique incidence. An angle of incidence that is not 90° perpendicular to a boundary. The angle of transmission will be equal to the angle of incidence as long as the propagation speeds of the media on each side of the boundary are equal. If the propagation speeds are different, however, then the angle of incidence will not be equal to the angle of transmission. The change in direction, the difference in the angle of incidence and the angle of transmission (Fig. 1–5A, B, and C), is called *refraction* (Snell's law).

The angle of incidence is equal to the angle of reflection, but the angle transmission is variable and can be calculated as follows:

angle of transmission = angle of incidence

$$\times \frac{\text{propagation speed (medium 2)}}{\text{propagation speed (medium 1)}}$$

ϕ_2 = angle of transmission

ϕ_1 = angle of incidence

$$\phi_2 = \phi_1 \times \frac{C_2}{C_1}$$

Note: The above equation is only an approximation; at larger angles it is subject to larger error. To obtain true accuracy use the full form of Snell's law.

$$\sin \phi_2 = \sin \phi_1 \times \frac{C_2}{C_1}$$

The *range equation* is the relationship between the round-trip travel time of the pulse and the distance to a reflector. This equation determines the position a reflector will have in depth on the display monitor.

$$\text{distance to the reflector (mm)} = \frac{1}{2} \times \text{propagation speed (mm/}\mu\text{s)}$$

$$\times \text{ pulse round-trip time (}\mu\text{s)}$$

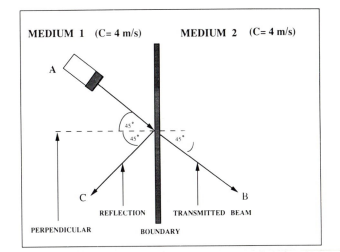

Figure 1–5B. In medium 1, the propagation speed is 4 m/s; in medium 2, the propagation speed is 4 m/s, therefore the angle incidence will be equal to the angle of transmission with *no* refraction. **(A)** Incidence striking a boundary; **(B)** transmitted beam; **(C)** reflected beam.

If we assume the propagation speed to be constant at 1540 m/s or 1.54 mm/μs, then one-half the propagation speed is equal to 0.77 mm/μs and the formula can be simplified:

$$\text{distance to the reflector (}d\text{)} = 0.77 \times \text{pulse round-trip time (}t\text{)}$$

If we assume that for every 13 μs the pulse travels 1 cm, then $d = t/13$. The value of (t) must be given in microseconds if the propagation speed is in millimeters per microseconds. The range equation defines the position a reflector will have in depth on the display monitor.

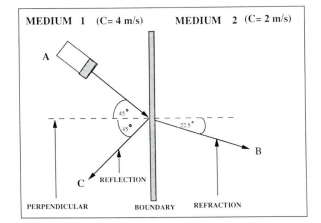

Figure 1–5A. In medium 1, the propagation speed is 4 m/s; in medium 2, the propagation speed is 2 m/s, therefore the beam bends towards the normal plane. **(A)** Incidence striking a boundary; **(B)** refraction of the sound beam; **(C)** reflected beam.

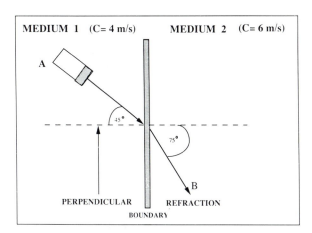

Figure 1–5C. In medium 1, the propagation speed is 4 m/s; in medium 2, the propagation speed is 6 m/s, therefore the beam bends away from the normal angle. **(A)** Incidence striking a boundary; **(B)** refraction of the sound beam; **(C)** reflected beam.

TRANSDUCERS

A *transducer* is a device that converts one form of energy to another. In diagnostic sonography the transducer converts electrical energy to pressure energy (acoustic energy) and vice versa.

1. *Active element*

    A. *Piezoelectric principle.* The conversion of electrical energy to pressure energy and vice versa. Ultrasound (pressure energy) is generated by electric stimulation of the piezoelectric element causing expansions and contractions of the element that in turn generate the ultrasound pulse. The resultant ultrasound pulse produces a similar distortion of the element and then converts back to an electric signal (Fig. 1–6).

    B. *Material.* The active element can be *natural* (eg, quartz, tourmaline, Rochelle salt) or *synthetic* (eg, lead zirconate titanate (PZT), barium titanate, lithium sulfate). Synthetic elements are most commonly used in today's diagnostic equipment because of their availability and low cost. To turn one of these manufactured substances into a piezoelectric element, it is heated to its Curie point, or the temperature at which a ferroelectric material, such as many piezoelectric materials, loses its magnetic properties. The dipoles within the material are then polarized with an electric current. When the element cools the dipoles are fixed (Fig. 1–7). The material is cut and shaped, then housed in the transducer.

    C. *Properties of elements (crystals).* The frequency of the acoustic wave produced by a standard pulsed-wave imaging system is determined by the *thickness* of the piezoelectric element and the *propagation speed* of the crystal. The propagation speed of the crystal is approximately three to five times greater than the speed of ultrasound in soft tissue, namely, 4 to 8 mm/μs. The thinner the crystal, the greater the frequency.

$$\text{frequency (MHz)} = \frac{\text{propagation speed of the crystal (mm/μs)}}{2 \times \text{thickness (mm)}}$$

Figure 1–6. Applied electrical voltage. **(A)** Physical compression on the crystal will generate a potential difference across the faces of the crystal. The effect is called *piezoelectric effect.* **(B)** Voltage applied on the crystal will generate mechanical energy (ultrasound). The effect is called *reverse piezoelectric effect.*

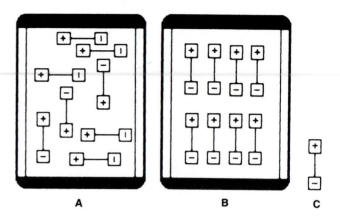

Figure 1–7. Synthetic material with dipoles. **(A)** nonpolarized; **(B)** polarized; **(C)** dipole.

The diameter of the crystal does not affect the pulse frequency; it does, however, determine the *lateral resolution.* Neither the impedance of the matching layer nor the thickness of the backing material is a primary determinant of ultrasound pulse frequency.

In contrast to pulse wave, *the frequency of continuous wave ultrasound is equal to the frequency of the electric voltage that drives the piezoelectric crystal.* In simpler terms, when the pulser of a continuous wave system produces an electric signal with a frequency of 6 MHz, the frequency of the emitted acoustic signal will also be 6 MHz.

2. *Damping material (backing material).* An epoxy resin attached to the back of the element that absorbs the vibrations and reduces the number of cycles in a pulse (Fig. 1–8). By reducing the number of cycles the following are accomplished:

    A. Pulse duration (PD) and spatial pulse length (SPL) are reduced.

$$\text{pulse duration (PD)} = \text{number of cycles } (n) \times \text{time } (t)$$

where t = period of ultrasound in pulse.

$$\text{spatial pulse length (SPL)} = \text{number of cycles } (n) \times \text{wavelength } (\lambda)$$

By reducing these two factors the axial resolution will be improved.

$$\text{axial resolution } (R_A) = \frac{\text{SPL}}{2}$$

    B. *Bandwidth* (the width of the frequency spectrum) is increased by increasing the damping. When the bandwidth increases, the quality factor (Q factor) of the transducer decreases.

ELECTRICAL CONNECTOR

SHIELD

TUNING COIL

BACKING MATERIAL

HOUSING

DAMPING MATERIAL

FACE MATERIAL

MATCHING LAYER

PIEZOELECTRIC CERAMIC MATERIAL

Figure 1–8. Components of a transducer.

$$\text{quality factor} = \frac{\text{operating frequency}}{\text{bandwidth}}$$

C. The duty factor is decreased.

3. *Matching layer.* A substance placed in front of the transducer element's face material to decrease the reflection at the transducer–tissue interface. The matching layer is necessary because the impedance difference between the transducer crystal and the soft tissue is so large that most of the energy will be reflected back at the skin surface. The matching layer provides an intermediate impedance, allowing transmission of the ultrasound beam into the body.

The thickness of the matching layer is usually equal to one-quarter of the wavelength.[1] Multiple layers are often used to avoid reflections caused by the variety of frequencies and wavelengths present in short pulses. In addition to the matching layer of the transducer, a *coupling gel* is used to form a transducer surface–skin contact that will eliminate air and prevent reflection at this boundary.

Bandwidth and Quality Factor

The transducer produces more than one frequency. For example, the operating frequency may be 3.5 MHz, but a spectrum of other frequencies are also generated known as the bandwidth. The shorter the pulse the more of these other frequencies are generated. Therefore, the bandwidth and the pulse length are inversely proportional; as the pulse length decreases, the bandwidth increases (Fig. 1–9). Continuous-wave ultrasound has a very narrow bandwidth.

If the bandwidth increases, the Q factor decreases. If, however, the operating frequency increases, the Q factor increases. A low Q factor indicates:

1. broad bandwidth
2. low operating frequency
3. shortened pulse length
4. uniform near field (Many frequencies in a pulse result in a more uniform intensity distribution.)

Types of Transducers

There are several ways to classify transducers; one is the way the sound beam is swept (or steered). This process can be either mechanical or electrical.

A *mechanical transducer* (Fig. 1–10) has a scan head that contains a single disk-shaped active element. One type of mechanical transducer is the *oscillatory or rotary type,* which has an element that is physically attached to a mechanical device to move it through a pathway (see Fig. 1–10A). A second type has an *oscillatory mirror* that mechanically moves while the element remains stationary (see Fig. 1–10B).

Focusing the beam produced by a mechanical transducer is achieved by curvature of the crystal, a curved lens on the crystal, or the reflecting mirror. Focusing occurs at a *specific depth* on both the horizontal and vertical planes. To change the focal depth the operator must select another transducer with the desired focal zone. The mechanical transducer produces a sector-shaped image (see Fig. 1–10C). *Mechanical transducers are mechanically steered (MS) and mechanically focused (MF).*

The *annular array* is a mechanical transducer. The transducer element consists of 5 to 11 rings of transducer elements mounted on a mechanically moved (steered) arm (Fig. 1–11). The advantage of the annular array over the single element transducer is the presence of many elements, allowing for electronic focusing. By focusing trans-

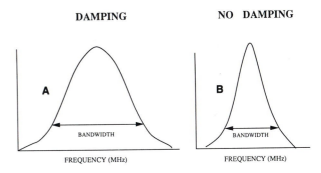

DAMPING

NO DAMPING

A

B

BANDWIDTH

BANDWIDTH

FREQUENCY (MHz)

FREQUENCY (MHz)

Figure 1–9. Bandwidth (**A**) with damping, (**B**) without damping. *Note:* Damping increases bandwidth.

Figure 1–10 (A) mechanical sector real-time transducer that is mechanically steered and mechanically focused. **(B)** A mechanical sector real-time transducer that moves a mirror instead of the transducer. **(C)** Image presentation from a mechanical sector.

Figure 1–11. Annular array real-time transducer probe that contains four transducer rings (multi-element) on a mechanically steered shaft.

A

B

C

Figure 1–12. Linear sequential array. (**A**) A real-time linear-array transducer. (**B**) Design of a linear segmental phased-array transducer. These transducers consist of a long strip of piezoelectric crystals divided into elements, which are arranged next to each other; (**C**) Operation of a linear segmental phased-array transducer. The crystal elements are pulsed in groups of four in this example, with each group sending and receiving in succession.

mission and reception of the ultrasound energy, greater depth resolution is achieved. The image produced by an annular array is also a sector. *Annular arrays are mechanically steered (MS) and electronically focused (EF).*

An *electronic transducer* is an assembly of multiple elements called an *array*. There are many types of arrays, each with a particular set of characteristics:

Linear sequential array (linear array). Shown in Fig. 1–12. This type of transducer produces a rectangular image (Fig. 1–13B).

Curved array (radial array, convex array). The array of transducer elements are arranged with specific curvature (Fig. 1–14). Focusing the beam is achieved by internal and electronic focusing; there is no beam steering. The curved design of the transducer head creates a *sector or trapezoid image.*

Sector phased array (phased array). The voltage pulses are applied to the entire groups of elements with varying time delays. The beam can be electronically focused (EF) and steered (ES). The image format is sector (Fig. 1–15).

Focusing Techniques

Transducers can be either mechanically or electronically focused. *Mechanical focusing* is accomplished by using a curved crystal or an acoustic lens for each element. This type of focusing is usually applied to mechanical transducers and will improve lateral resolution by limiting the beam width.

There are two types of electronic focusing: transmit focusing and receive focusing.

Transmit focusing. Electronic focusing during transmission. It is accomplished by firing a group of elements with a small time delay (nanoseconds) between various elements in the group. The wavefront generated by each element in the group will arrive at a specific point in space, resulting in a focused beam. Using transmit focus will improve lateral resolutions and create several possible focal zones. Multizone transmit focusing will result in a slower frame rate. If, for example, there are three focal zones, then the frame rate will be reduced compared to a single focus zone. If the rate is very slow, then the image will flicker causing a "perceived" distortion of the image.

Receive focusing. Electronic focusing of the received echoes; by electronically delaying the return of the

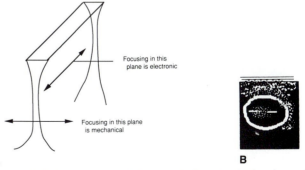

Focusing in this plane is electronic

Focusing in this plane is mechanical

A

B

Figure 1–13. Linear sequential array. (**A**) Focusing in the plane of the long axis of the transducer is electronic; focusing in the plane perpendicular to the long axis is mechanical. (**B**) Image presentation from a linear phased array transducer. Note the rectangular image.

Figure 1–14. Curved linear array. The array of transducer elements are arranged with a specific curvature. There is no beam steering; focusing of the beam is achieved internally by mechanical and electronic means.

Figure 1–16. The ultrasound beam from an unfocused transducer.

signals to the processing system within the diagnostic unit, the optimum range of the focal zone can be extended. This process will enhance image clarity.

Note: Many phased arrays are capable of both transmit and receive focusing. Both transmit and receive electronic focusing are sometimes called *dynamic focusing* because focusing is done as the beam is being generated or received.

Sound Beam

A *sound beam* is the acoustic energy emitted by the transducer. The beam can be pulsed or continuous wave. *Pulsed waves follow Huygens' principle, which states that the resultant beam is a combination of all sound arising from different sources (wavelets) on the transducer crystal face. Focusing is the superimposition (algebraic summation) of all sound waves in the beam.*[1–3] As the various wavelets within a beam collide, interference (constructive and destructive) results in the formation of a sound beam (Fig. 1–16).

Constructive interference. The waves are in phase, producing an increase in amplitude.

Destructive interference. The waves are not in phase, producing a decrease in amplitude or even zero amplitude. Zero amplitude occurs if the out-of-phase waves completely cancel each other.

The beam is composed of a near zone, a focal point, and a far zone.

1. *Near zone (near field, fresnel zone).* The portion of the sound beam in which the beam diameter narrows as the distance from the transducer increases until it reaches its narrowest diameter. This distance is the *near zone length* (NZL). At the far end of the NZL the diameter of the beam is equal to

Figure 1–15. Sector phased array real-time transducer. This diagram illustrates how electronic pulses are used to steer the ultrasound beam.

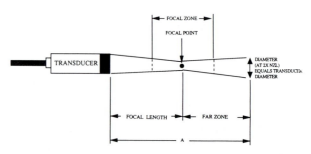

Figure 1–17. The components of the ultrasound beam in a focused transducer. (A) Note that the diameter of the beam is equal to the diameter of the transducer face.

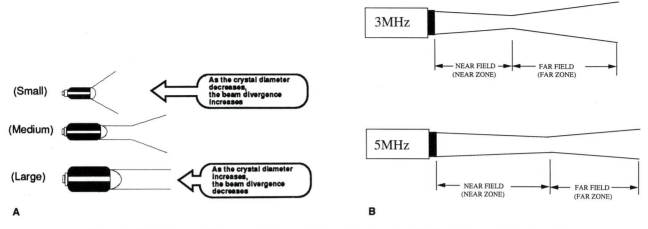

Figure 1–18 (A) Beam diversion with increasing crystal diameter. **(B)** Transducer crystal size shown in relationship to frequency. *Note:* The higher the frequency of the transducer, the smaller the beam diameter and the longer the near-zone. The angle of beam divergence in the far field is smaller with a higher frequency transducer.

one-half the diameter of the transducer. The NZL is also related to the frequency: Increasing the frequency increases the NZL, and vice versa. Components of the beam of a focused transducer are shown in Fig. 1–17.

2. *Focal point.* The point at which the beam reaches its narrowest diameter. As the diameter narrows the beam width resolution improves, becoming the best at the focal point. The *focal zone* is the distance between equal beam diameters that are some multiple of the diameter of the focal point (often two times the diameter of the focal point). The focal zone extends toward the transducer from the focal point, and toward the far zone. The *focal*

length is the region of the beam from the transducer to the focal point.

3. *Far field (far zone, Fraunhofer zone).* The portion of the sound beam (after the NZL) in which the diameter of the beam increases as the distance from the transducer increases. At a distance of two times the NZL, the beam diameter once again equals the diameter of the transducer. The divergence of the beam in the far field is inversely proportional to the crystal diameter and frequency. The larger the transducer element and the higher the frequency, the smaller the angle of divergence in the far field (Fig. 1–18A and B).

Figure 1–19 (A) *Lateral Resolution:* the ability of the ultrasound beam to separate two structures lying at a right angle (perpendicular) to the beam direction. Lateral resolution is also referred to as azimuthal, transverse, angular, or horizontal. **(B)** *Axial Resolution:* The ability of the ultrasound beam to separate two structures lying along the path of (parallel to) the beam direction. Axial resolution is also referred to as linear, longitudinal, depth, or range.

Resolution

There are two types of resolution, lateral and axial (Figs. 1–19A and B).

Lateral resolution (azimuthal, transverse, or angular resolution). Equal to the beam diameter (see Fig. 1–19A). The distance between two interfaces has to be greater than the beam diameter (width) for the two interfaces to be resolved as separate entities. Lateral resolution applies to interfaces perpendicular to the direction of the sound beam. With an unfocused transducer, lateral resolution is best in the near field; with a focused transducer, the lateral resolution is best at the focal point. A transducer with a smaller diameter will improve lateral resolution in the near zone, but will decrease the lateral resolution as the beam diverges in the far zone.

Axial resolution (linear, range longitudinal, or depth resolution). Related to the spatial pulse length (SPL). Two interfaces at different depths will be distinguished from each other only if the distance between them is equal to or greater than one-half the SPL (see Fig. 1–19B).

$$\text{axial resolution} = \frac{\text{spatial pulse length (SPL)}}{2}$$

To obtain maximum image quality, axial resolution (R_A) should be as small as possible. Axial resolution improves when wavelength or the number of cycles per second decreases (both of these factors are related to SPL). Frequency also affects the axial resolution. As the frequency increases the wavelength decreases, thus the axial resolution improves. However, as the frequency increases the depth of penetration decreases, creating a need to compromise resolution for adequate penetration into the tissues. This compromise is the reason why the frequency range for diagnostic procedures is usually between 2 and 10 MHz.

IMAGING PROCESS

The components of a pulsed-echo diagnostic ultrasound system are the pulser, receiver, scan converter, and display (Fig. 1–20).

Pulser

The *pulser* produces an electric voltage that activates the piezoelectric element, causing it to contract and expand to produce the longitudinal compression wave (sound beam). A second function of the pulser is to signal the receiver and scan converter that the transducer has been activated. Each electric pulse generates an ultrasonic pulse. The number of ultrasonic pulses per second is defined as the *pulse repetition frequency* (PRF). With array transducers, the pulser is responsible for the delay and variations in pulse amplitude needed for electronic control of beam scanning, steering, and shaping. In improving the dynamic

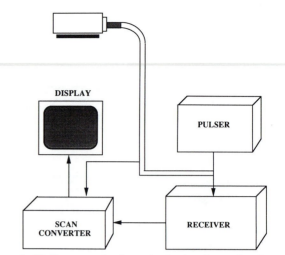

Figure 1–20. Components of a pulsed-echo diagnostic ultrasound system.

range of multi-element transducers the pulser suppresses grating lobes, a process termed *dynamic apodization*.[1]

Increasing the power output control of a system will raise the intensity by signaling the pulser to put out more voltage. To reduce the potential for harmful bioeffects, it is desirable to keep the power low. Therefore, to increase the number of echoes displayed it is recommended that the operator increase the gain control, not the power.

Receiver

The receiver processes electric signals returned from the transducer (ie, ultrasonic reflections converted into electric signals by the transducer). Processing involves amplification, compensation, compression, demodulation, and rejection (Fig. 1–21).

Amplification. The process that increases small electric voltages received from the transducer to a level suitable for further processing. This process is sometimes referred to as "over-all-gain" enhancement or increase. Gain is the ratio of output electric power to input electric power and is measured in decibels (dB). *Dynamic range* is the range of values between the minimum and maximum echo amplitudes. It is the ratio of the largest power to the smallest power in the working range of the diagnostic unit. Dynamic range is also expressed in decibels.

Compensation. Also referred to as gain compensation, swept gain, or time gain compensation. It is the mechanism that compensates for the loss of echo strength caused by the depth of the reflector. It allows reflectors with equal reflection coefficients to appear on the screen with equal brightness and to compensate, to a certain extent, for the effects of attenuation caused by greater depth. For the average soft tissues, the attenuation coefficient is equal to one-half the frequency (expressed in decibels per centimeter).

Compression. The internal process in which larger echoes are equalized with smaller echoes. Compression decreases dynamic range.

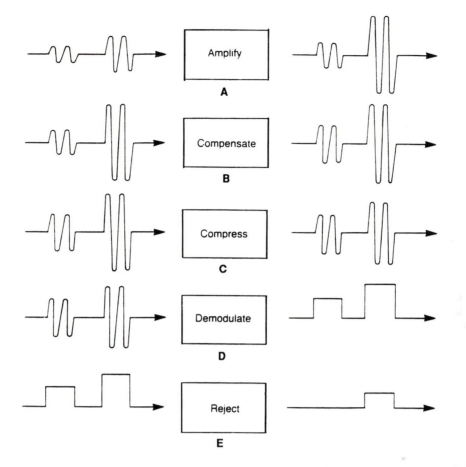

Input to each process   Output from each process

Figure 1–21. The five functions of the receiver. **(A)** Amplification of both pulses. **(B)** Amplification of the weaker pulses. **(C)** The difference between the pulse amplitudes is reduced. **(D)** The pulses are converted to another form. **(E)** The weaker pulse is rejected. *(Kremkaw FW. Diagnostic Ultrasound: Principles, Instruments, and Exercises, 3rd ed. Philadelphia: WB Saunders, 1989.)*

Demodulation. The process of converting voltages delivered to the receiver to a more useful form. Demodulation is done by rectification (removal of negative components, replacement with positive values) and smoothing (averaging of the new wave form).

Rejection. Also termed suppression or threshold. Rejection is the elimination of smaller amplitude voltage pulses produced by weaker reflections. This mechanism helps to reduce noise by removing low-level signals that do not contribute to meaningful information in the image.

Scan Converter (Memory)

The *scan converter, or memory,* transforms the incoming echo data into a suitable format for the display, storing all of the necessary information for the two-dimensional image. As the tissue is scanned, several images (frames) are acquired per second. Memory allows for a single scan consisting of one or more frames to be displayed. Most instruments have enough memory to store the last several frames scanned (cine loop). There are two types of scan converters (memories): analog and digital.

Analog scan converters. Found in older machines, these consist of semiconductors arranged in square matrices. As the ultrasound pulse transverses the tissues, an electronic beam scans the square matrix. It is swept in the same direction as the beam in the body. The current within the electronic beam corresponds to the intensity of the returning echoes. If the echoes are weak the current in the electronic beam is decreased, and vice versa. The strengths of the electrical charges are precisely what are stored in the individual insulators of the matrix. These electronic charges have values that correspond to brightness levels. To read the stored images, the electronic beam is scanned across the stored matrix. The stored charge in each element affects the current in the electronic beam, and together these charges are used to vary the brightness of display.

Digital scan converters. Store image brightness values as numbers instead as of electrical charges. A digital scan converter consists of three components: an analog-to-digital (A–D) converter, which changes the voltages of received signals into numeric values; a

Figure 1–22. A 10 × 10 pixel, 4-bit-deep digital memory. *(Kremkau FW. Diagnostic Ultrasound: Principles, Instruments, and Exercises. 3rd ed. Philadelphia: WB Saunders, 1989.)*

digital memory, which stores these image echo values; and a circuit, which translates these stored numbers back into analog (voltage) values when needed (a digital-to-analog, or D–A, converter).

The digital memory component is the same as computer memory. Modern computers use circuits that have only two states: off and on. Within the computer, these states may be represented, for example, by the absence or presence of electrical current, the open or closed condition of switches, or the direction of magnetization on a magnetic disk or tape. Each of these examples has two states, which the computer considers zero (0) or one (1). At first, it seems that this system, called the *binary number system,* or binary,[4] is not very useful for computing, but it can represent any number that the more common decimal system can. Instead of using increasing powers of 10, as the decimal system does, the binary system uses increasing powers of 2. In the decimal system, the right-most digit represents units, the next to the left tens, the next hundreds, etc. In the binary system, the right-most binary digit or bit is ones, the next left twos, the next fours, the next eights, etc[1] (Fig. 1–22).

Display

How is this system used to represent ultrasound images? Imagine that the image is divided into many small squares similar to a checkerboard. Each square is assigned a number that represents the ultrasound echo amplitude. For example, for white-on-black displays, the highest echo value is white, and the lowest is black (the reverse is true for black-on-white displays).[2] A square located in a part of the image that has the highest echo values (eg, echoes in a gallstone) would be assigned a high number value, while a square in the surrounding bile would receive a small number value. In color flow imaging, each square would be assigned a number that represents the Doppler shift value. If the squares are made small enough, then the eye will not be able to see them as separate. Typically, ultrasound images are divided into 512 by 512 of these little squares.[1]

The squares are called picture elements, or pixels. The number 512 is a power of two (two to the ninth power) and also happens to fit well in a standard television frame. This number yields an image containing 262,144 pixels.

If each of these pixels could store only one binary value, then the results would be very much like an old bistable image, having only black and white values. Each pixel could be either black or white, with no gray values. To store gray scale images each pixel must have more than one binary digit (or bit). For example, with three bits per pixel each pixel could represent eight different shades of gray. To calculate how many different shades of gray can be represented by a pixel containing a set number (n) of data bits, the following formula can be applied:

$$\text{number of shades} = 2^n$$

The largest value that can be represented by a given number of bits is calculated by the formula:

$$\text{largest value for } n \text{ bits} = 2^n - 1$$

If, for example, we are considering 3 bits, we could represent eight different shades of gray with the largest gray value equal to seven.

Most ultrasound machines generate images with 4 to 8 bits of gray scale (16 to 256 shades of gray). Color-flow Doppler machines need more bits to represent the various colors. Since the machine makes no distinction of color (to the machine the image is only an array of numbers), the color values are stored as a number value for each of three primary colors. Combinations of these three primaries (usually red, green, and blue) can yield almost any color.

Fig. 1–22 is an example of a 10 × 10 pixel matrix with 4 bits/pixel. To calculate how many bits an ultrasound image contains, the following formula can be applied:

$$\text{number of bits/image} = \text{number of image rows}$$
$$\times \text{ number of image columns}$$
$$\times \text{ number of bits/pixel}$$

or

$$\text{number of bits/image} = \text{total number of pixels}$$
$$\times \text{ number of bits/pixel}$$

In computer terminology, 8 binary digits or 8 bits equals 1 *byte.* To determine the number of bytes of memory an image requires, divide the number of bits per image by eight:

$$\text{number of bytes/image} = \frac{\text{number of bits per image}}{8}$$

Examples

If an image has 10 pixel columns and rows with 2 bits/pixel, then:

$$\text{number of bits/image} = 10 \times 10 \times 2 = 200 \text{ bits}$$

TABLE 1–2. UNIT OF MEASUREMENT IN COMPUTER TERMINOLOGY

Unit	Prefix	Symbol	Quantity
byte[a]	kilo-	K	1000[a]
byte	mega-	M	1,000,000
byte	giga-	G	1,000,000,000

[a] 1 kilobyte equals 1024 characters, but can be rounded off to 1000.

$$\text{number of bytes/image} = \frac{200 \text{ bits/image}}{8} = 25 \text{ bytes}$$

If a 512×512 pixel image has 8 bits/pixel, then:

$$\text{number of bits/image} = 512 \times 512 \times 8 = 2{,}097{,}152 \text{ bits}$$

$$\text{number of bytes/image} = \frac{2{,}097{,}152}{8} = 262{,}144 \text{ bytes}$$

A single image can thus contain over 2 million bits or more than ¼ million bytes. To reduce the number of digits used to describe these values, multipliers are applied, such as kilo-, mega-, giga- (Table 1–2). These multipliers are not identical to their counterparts in the metric system, however. For example, 1 kilobit is not 1000 bits, but 1024 bits or 2 to the 10th power. For convenience, large numbers may be rounded (eg, 262,144 bytes may be rounded to 260 kilobytes).

The image can be stored in the digital memory as numbers, but it cannot be viewed unless the numbers are converted back to an image. Otherwise, a large list of numbers is all that would be displayed. The third part of the digital scan converter does this conversion: It takes the number values stored in the memory and changes them back into an analog voltage. The voltage varies the brightness of a spot on the cathode ray tube, generating an image that the human eye can interpret. The hardware that performs this function is the digital-to-analog (D–A) converter.

DYNAMIC IMAGING

Dynamic imaging is simply the process of viewing an image in motion. The dynamic image is displayed on a *cathode-ray tube* (CRT), the unit of visual display that receives electrical impulses and translates them into the picture on the screen by varying the brightness of the trace or lines displayed. The CRT in Fig. 1–23 is an electrostatic deflection CRT; another type, the magnetic deflection CRT, substitutes a magnetic coil to serve the same function as the deflection plates (ie, to move the electron beam). The front face of the CRT, the screen, is phosphor coated and displays the product of the aforementioned process in the form of a recognizable image.

A *frame* is a single image composed of multiple scan lines. To produce a dynamic or moving image, numerous

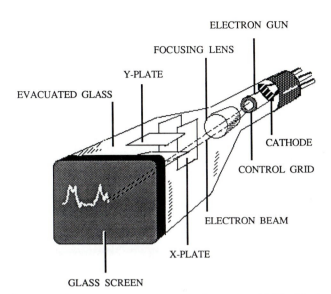

Figure 1–23. Basic structure of a cathode ray tube (CRT). *(Modified from McDicken W: Diagnostic Ultrasonics: Principles and Use of Instruments, 2nd ed. New York, Wiley, 1981, p 15).*

frames are required. To freeze a frame, or stop the image to record or view it, the memory of the system is activated. The *frame rate* (FR) is the number of frames displayed or scanned per second. In most diagnostic medical sonography or echocardiography systems, the frame rate is usually 10 to 60 frames/s. If the display frame rate is below 20/s, then the real-time image appears to flicker, preventing the eye from integrating the images.

The pulse repetition frequency (PRF) is the number of pulses produced by the transducer in a given time period. It is related to the number of lines per frame and the frame rate by the formula:

$$\text{pulse repetition frequency (PRF)} = \text{lines per frame (LPF)}$$
$$\times \text{ frame rate (FR)}$$

The PRF, LPF, and FR are directly related to the propagation speed. The maximum effective velocity is 77,000 cm/s, or one-half the propagation speed of ultrasound in soft tissues (1540 m/s or 154,000 cm/s). The one-half value results from the pulse having to make a round-trip to be received.

$$\text{depth} \times \text{LPF} \times \text{FR} = 77{,}000$$

Note: LPF $\times$ FR = PRF. Hence the equation can also be stated

$$\text{depth} \times \text{PRF} = 77{,}000$$

Improving image quality by increasing the lines per frame will reduce the frame rate if the depth remains constant. Increasing the depth of penetration while maintaining a constant number of lines per frame also reduces the frame rate. The frame rate can be increased if the depth of penetration is decreased, assuming the LPF is constant.

The *display format* refers to how the image appears on the screen, as either a rectangular display or a sector display. A *rectangular display* image appears in the form of a rectangle. The width of the display is given in centimeters; the *line density* is expressed as the number of lines per centimeter. To determine the line density for a rectangular display the lines per frame are divided by the display width in centimeters:

$$\text{line density (lines/cm)} = \frac{\text{lines per frame (LPF)}}{\text{display width (cm)}}$$

A *sector display* yields a pie-shaped image. The scans form an angle so that the line density is expressed as lines per degree.

$$\text{line density (lines/degree)} = \frac{\text{lines per frame (LPF)}}{\text{sector angle (degrees)}}$$

The *scan converter,* electronic circuitry in the machine's display, transforms a rectangular or arc-shaped image into a rectangular video frame, and adds the text and graphics (such as depth markers).

Modes of Display

The *A-mode,* or amplitude mode, is a one-dimensional graphic display with vertical deflections of the baseline. The height of the deflection represents the amplitude, or strength, of the echo; the distance in time is a function of where on the baseline the deflection occurs.

The *B-mode,* or brightness mode, displays the echoes as variations in the brightness of a line of spots on the CRT. The position of the spot on the baseline is related to the depth of the reflecting structure; the brightness is proportional to the strength of the echo. Each row of spots represents information obtained from a single position of the transducer or scanning beam. When successive rows of these spots are integrated into an image, a B-scan is produced.

The *M-mode,* or motion mode, is a two-dimensional recording of the reflector's change in position, or motion, against time. Most M-modes display the brightness of the signal in proportion to the strength of the echo. This mode is most commonly used for the study of dynamic structures such as the heart.

ARTIFACTS

Unlike the Grecian urn, which is an *artifact* from a past culture, the term in diagnostic medical sonography has a very different implication. It refers to something seen on an image that does not, in reality, exist in the anatomy studied. An artifact can be beneficial to the interpretation of the image, or it can detract from this process. For exam-

ple, certain artifacts are known to occur in cystic structures and are notably absent from a solid mass, and this information can therefore be used in a beneficial way when determining the nature of a mass. Conversely, there are artifacts that can appear similar to the placenta, making delineation of the limits of the placenta more difficult. Artifacts can be subdivided by the physical principles that produce them, namely: resolution artifacts, propagation artifacts, attenuation artifacts, or miscellaneous artifacts.

Resolution Artifacts

Axial resolution. The failure to resolve two separate reflectors parallel to the beam.

Lateral resolution. The failure to resolve two separate reflectors perpendicular to the beam.

Speckle. Scatter in tissues, causing interference effects referred to as noise.

Section thickness. The finite width of the beam producing extraneous echoes, or debris, in normally anechoic, or echo-free, structures.

Propagation Artifacts

Reverberation. Repetitive reflections between two highly reflective layers. The bouncing back and forth increases travel time, causing the signals to be displayed at different depths. The reverberations are seen on the image as equally spaced bands of diminishing amplitude.

Refraction. The change in direction of the sound beam as it passes from one medium to another. This phenomenon will cause a reflection to appear improperly positioned on the image.

Multipath. Because the returning signal does not necessarily follow the same path as the incident beam, the time required for some parts of the signal to return to the transducer will vary, causing reflections to appear at incorrect depths.

Mirror image. Generated when objects present on one side of a strong reflector are also shown on the other side of the reflector. Such artifacts are commonly seen around the diaphragm.

Attenuation Artifacts

Shadowing. The reduction in echo strength of signals arising from behind a strong reflector or attenuating structure. Structures such as gallstones, renal calculi, and bone will produce shadowing.

Enhancement. An increase in the amplitude of echoes located behind a weakly attenuating structure. The increase pertains to the relative strength of the signals as compared with neighboring signals passing through more highly attenuating media. For example, stronger reflections may be seen behind a fluid-filled structure than behind a solid structure (eg, the urine-filled bladder versus a solid tumor of the uterus).

Refraction or edge shadowing. The beam may bend at a curved surface and lose intensity, producing a shadow. If the beam is traveling from a higher velocity medium (less dense) to a low-velocity medium, a narrower shadow will be generated. Conversely, a sound beam traveling from a low-velocity medium to a higher one will project a wider shadow.

Miscellaneous Artifacts

Comet tail. Produced by a strong reflector; similar in appearance to reverberation. The comet tail, however, is composed of thin lines of closely spaced discrete echoes.

Ring down. Thought to be caused by a resonance phenomenon and is associated with gas bubble. It also appears very similar to reverberation, producing numerous parallel echoes. Sometimes discrete echoes cannot be differentiated, giving the appearance of a continuous emission of sound.

Propagation speed error. Most diagnostic ultrasound equipment operates on the assumption that the speed of sound in the body is 1540 m/s. This is not always true, as different tissues do have different propagation speeds. If the beam passes from a medium of one speed into a medium of a greater speed, then the calculated distance will be less than the actual distance, causing the echo to be erroneously displayed too close to the transducer. If the propagation speed decreases, then the echo will appear farther from the transducer than it actually is.

Side lobes. The result of the transducer element being finite in size. The difference in vibration at the center and edge results in acoustic energy emitted by the transducer flowing along the main axis of the sound beam. The energy that diverts from the main path is the cause of the side lobes, which will generate reflections at improper, off-axis locations in the image.

Grating lobes. Seen with linear array transducers, which also produce off-axis acoustic waves as a result of the regular spacing of the active elements. All grating lobes will cause reflections to appear at improper, off-axis locations in the image.

QUALITY OF PERFORMANCE

To guarantee efficiency of performance, all ultrasound diagnostic equipment is tested under a quality assurance (QA) program. To ensure that the instrument is operating correctly and consistently, it is checked for

1. imaging performance
2. equipment performance and safety

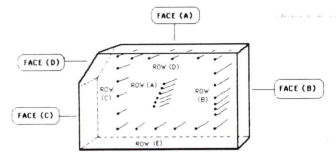

Figure 1–24. AIUM 100-mm test object.

3. beam measurements
4. acoustic output
5. preventative maintenance

AIUM Test Object

The American Institute of Ultrasound in Medicine (AIUM) has designed a test object specifically to measure imaging performance of an ultrasound system (Fig. 1–24). The AIUM test object is a "tank" consisting of a series of stainless steel rods, 0.75 mm in diameter, arranged in a specific pattern between two transparent plastic sides, with the other boundaries formed by thin, acrylic plastic sheets.[1,4] The tank is filled with a mixture of alcohol, an algae inhibitor, and water, which allows the propagation speed to approximate the speed of sound in soft tissues (1540 m/s). The results obtained are not affected by normal fluctuations in room temperature; the speed varies less than 1% for a temperature variation of 5° Celsius (5° C).

The following factors are measured by the AIUM test object (Table 1–3):

System sensitivity. Measured by determining the weakest signal that the system will display.

Axial resolution. Determined by placing the transducer on face A and scanning rod group (a). The six rods are separated by 4, 3, 2, and 1 mm, respectively. The system's axial resolution in millimeters is equal to the distance between the two closest yet distinguishable echoes.

Lateral resolution. Measured by placing the transducer on face B and scanning rod group (b). The lateral resolution is equal to the distance between the two closest rods in this group.

Dead zone. The region of the sound beam in which imaging cannot be performed; the area closest to the transducer. To determine the extent of the dead zone, the transducer is placed on face A and rod group (d) is scanned. The distance from the transducer to the first rod imaged is equal to the length of the dead zone.

Range accuracy (depth accuracy). Measured by placing the transducer on face A and scanning rod group (e). For the system to be operating properly, the echoes should appear at their actual depths and spacings within 1 mm (The rods in this group are 2 cm apart).

TABLE 1–3. PERFORMANCE MEASUREMENTS FOR THE AIUM TEST OBJECT

Measurement	Row	Test Object Face	Parameter Tested
Dead zone	D	Face (A)	The distance measured between the transducer face and the first rod depicted
Lateral resolution	B	Face (B)	Linear measurement of the echoes produced by Row D
Depth calibration	C or E	Face (A) or (B)	The distance measured between the first and the last line in Row E
Registration	E	Face (A), (B), (C), and (D)	—✕—Good ⊥▷ Poor
Axial resolution	A	Face (A)	5 mm to 1 mm pins spaced at decreasing intervals of 1 mm in Row A
Digital calipers	E	Face (C)	A distance of 10 cm or 100 mm measured on the horizontal pins in Row E, indicating the digital calipers are functioning correctly
Liquid velocity	E	Face (C)	The cursors are positioned at the leading edge echo to the other end leading edge echo, on the horizontal pins in Row E. A 100 mm measurement indicates the liquid medium velocity is correct

Checking the range accuracy ensures the accuracy of the internal calipers of the system.

In addition to the AIUM test object, other devices have been designed to measure different parameters of imaging performance. The *beam profiler* is designed to record three-dimensional reflection amplitude information. It consists of a pulser, receiver, transducer, and tank equipped with rods placed at different distances from the transducer.[1]

The transducer is pulsed and scanned across the rods. The fluctuation in amplitude of each reflection returning to the transducer is recorded in an A-mode pattern. The *hydrophone* is one of several devices that measure acoustic output; it consists of a small transducer element mounted on a narrow tube.[1] When used with an oscilloscope, the voltages produced in response to variations in pressure can be displaced and evaluated. The output produced by the hydrophone permits calculation of the period, pulse repetition period, and pulse duration. The hydrophone can also be used as a beam profiler.

Tissue/Cyst Phantom

This test device contains a medium that simulates soft tissue (Fig. 1–25). Enclosed in the phantom are structures that mimic cysts and solid masses and a series of 0.375-mm targets, in two groups. Each group measures depth and angular resolution. The phantom is used to evaluate the ultrasound system and transducer performance. Sonographic equipment can be evaluated for depth and angular resolution, vertical and horizontal distance calibration, and ring down.[5]

Bioeffects

To date, there is no concrete evidence to support any truly detrimental bioeffects from the application of diagnostic ultrasound to human tissues.[1] The study of possible effects is ongoing, however, and the definitive answer has not been found. It is generally agreed that the potential value of the information obtained from the procedure far outweighs the possibility of deleterious effects. Greater study of the microscopic effects of sound on tissue will have to take place before additional conclusions can be reached. To clarify what is known to date, the potential bioeffects are categorized in three groups: mechanical effects, thermal effects, and cavitation.

Mechanical effects include all types of damage not categorized as thermal or cavitational. There is very little information on this type of effect.

Thermal effects are produced primarily by the mechanisms of attenuation. As a major component of attenuation, absorption by the tissue leads to a rise in tissue temperature. Increased temperatures can cause irreversible damage, depending on the extent of the exposure. It is generally agreed that *exposure producing a maximum temperature of 1° C can be used without any effects. A rise*

Figure 1–25. Multi-purpose tissue/cyst phantom. *(Courtesy of Nuclear Associates, Carle Place, NY. Printed with permission.)*

in temperature of the tissues to 41° C or above is considered dangerous to a fetus. The longer that this temperature is maintained, the greater the potential risk for damage.[1]

Cavitation is the result of pressure changes in the medium causing gas bubbles to form; it can produce severe tissue damage. The two types of cavitation are stable cavitation and transient cavitation. *Stable cavitation* involves microbubbles already present in tissue that respond by expanding and contracting when pressure is applied. These bubbles can intercept and absorb a large amount of the acoustic energy. Stable cavitation can result in shear stresses and microstreaming in the surrounding tissues.

Transient cavitation is dependent on the pressure of the ultrasound pulses. The tissue bubbles expand and collapse violently. This type of cavitation can cause highly localized, violent effects involving enormous pressures, markedly elevated temperatures, shock waves, and mechanical stress. Cavitation may occur with short pulses. It has been shown that pulses with peak intensities of greater than 3300 W/cm^2 can induce cavitation in mammals.[1] Precise determination of when cavitation will occur is not currently within our capabilities. For specific conditions of homogeneous media, it is possible to estimate an index for the cavitation threshold.

The following guidelines are adapted from an official statement by the American Institute of Ultrasound in Medicine (AIUM): *Bioeffects Considerations for the Safety of Diagnostic Ultrasound.* Bethesda, MD, American Institute of Ultrasound Medicine, 1988. The reader is urged to read the full AIUM text.

Intensity. No independently confirmed significant biological effects in mammalian tissues exposed in vivo with unfocused transducers with intensities below 100 mW/cm^2 and below 1 W/cm^2 for focused transducers.

Exposure. Exposure times can be > 1 s and < 500 s for an unfocused transducer; and < 50 s/pulse for a focused transducer. No significant bioeffects have been observed even at higher intensities than noted above (as long as the intensity × time product is < 50 J/cm^2).

Thermal. A maximum temperature rise of 1° C is acceptable, but an increase in the in situ temperature to 41° C or greater is hazardous to fetuses.

Cavitation. Can result if pressure peaks are greater than 3300 W/cm^2. However, it is not possible to specify a threshold at which cavitation will occur.

Randomized studies are the best method for assessing potential effects. *There are no independent confirmed biologic effects on patients or operators.*[1]

COMPUTERS AND ULTRASOUND

The majority of modern ultrasound equipment is computerized or has some computer capabilities. Today's ultrasound equipment can calculate gestational age, store

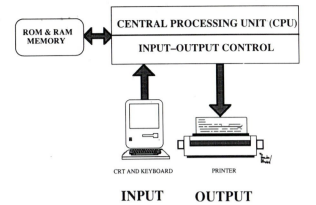

Figure 1–26. Computer organization.

nomograms, store patient data, and transfer sonographic images from one hospital to another via a modem (modulator/demodulator).

What Is a Computer?

A computer is a device that contains a microprocessor and can perform high-speed mathematical calculations, assemble and store data, and perform logic operations. The graphics in this book, for example, were processed and stored by a computer.

The Computer Brain. The "brain" of the computer (Fig. 1–26) comprises three general parts:

1. the central processing unit (CPU)
2. the memory unit
3. the input–output unit

The *main computer storage* (MCS) is the memory of the computer. There are two kinds of computer memory[6]:

ROM (Read-only memory). ROM is permanent and unchangeable. It is installed by the computer manufacturer and contains instructions needed by the CPU when the computer is turned on.

RAM (Random-access memory, or read and write). RAM is temporary and changeable. It is usable memory for the operator to change depending on needs. This is temporary memory because when the computer is turned off, the RAM is lost. However, data can be extracted from the RAM before the computer is turned off to be stored permanently on a floppy disk or hard disk for use at a later time.

When the sonographer looks at the contents of the memory, he or she is *reading.* When the sonographer is entering or changing information, he or she is *writing* (read and write memory).

REFERENCES

1. Kremkau FW. *Diagnostic Ultrasound: Principles, Instruments and Exercises,* 3rd ed. Philadelphia: WB Saunders, 1989.

2. Edelman SK. *Understanding Ultrasound Physics: Fundamentals and Exam Review.* Houston: EPS Publishers, 1990.

3. Pinkney N. *A Review of the Concepts of Ultrasound Physics and Instrumentation,* 4th ed. Philadelphia: Sonior, 1983.

4. Bushong SC, Archer RB. *Diagnostic Ultrasound: Physics, Biology, and Instrumentation.* St. Louis: Mosby–Year Book, 1991.

5. *Diagnostic Ultrasound: Test Equipment and Accessories.* New York: Nuclear Associates, Catalog U-2, 1991, pp. 2–3.

6. Shelly G, Cashman T. *Computer Fundamentals for an Information Age.* Brea, CA: Anaheim Publishing, 1984.

Questions

1. An example of a nonspecular reflector is

   (A) the liver surface
   (B) the diaphragm
   (C) red blood cells
   (D) any structure that does *not* produce a strong echo

2. The spatial pulse length

   (A) determines penetration depth
   (B) usually decreases with frequency
   (C) is improved with rectification
   (D) determines lateral resolution

3. Axial resolution

   (A) is improved in the focal zone
   (B) depends on the TGC slope
   (C) is improved by digital scan converters
   (D) depends on the wavelength

4. Lateral resolution

   (A) and ring-down are the same
   (B) depends on the beam diameter
   (C) improves with frequency
   (D) cannot be measured in the far zone

5. The beam of an unfocused transducer diverges

   (A) because of inadequate damping
   (B) in the Fresnel zone
   (C) in the Fraunhofer zone
   (D) when the pulse length is long

6. Reverberation artifacts are a result of

   (A) electronic noise
   (B) improper TGC settings
   (C) the presence of two or more strong reflecting surfaces
   (D) an angle of incidence that is too small

7. Grating lobes are essential for the proper operation of a linear phased array.

   (A) true
   (B) false

8. Electronically steered scanners always produce higher resolution images than do mechanically steered scanners.

   (A) true
   (B) false

9. An annular array scanner uses mechanical beam steering.

   (A) true
   (B) false

10. A linear sequenced array cannot be dynamically focused.

    (A) true
    (B) false

Questions 11 through 15: Match the following group of wires with its function for the AIUM test object (Fig. 1–27).

11. registration or B-mode alignment _____

12. axial resolution _____

13. lateral resolution _____

14. dead zone _____

15. depth calibration _____

16. Decreasing the spatial pulse length

    (A) reduces the field of view
    (B) reduces lateral resolution
    (C) improves axial resolution
    (D) improves lateral resolution

Figure 1–27. AIUM 100-mm test object.

17. How much will a 3.5-MHz pulse be attenuated after passing through 2 cm of soft tissue?

    (A) 7 dB
    (B) 3.5 dB
    (C) 17 dB
    (D) 1.75 dB

18. Propagation speed errors result in

    (A) reverberation
    (B) improper axial position
    (C) shadowing
    (D) a Doppler shift

19. Enhancement is caused by

    (A) strongly reflecting structures
    (B) propagation speed errors
    (C) Snell's law
    (D) weakly attenuating structures

20. The Doppler shift frequency is

    (A) directly proportional to the velocity of the reflector
    (B) greater in pulsed Doppler systems
    (C) greater at high intensity levels
    (D) dependent on the number of transducer elements being used

21. The number of frames per second necessary for a real-time image to be flicker free is

    (A) more than 15
    (B) less than 10
    (C) between 6 and 10
    (D) between 3 and 6

22. The SPTA intensity will always be larger than the SATA intensity.

    (A) true
    (B) false

23. The intensity of the ultrasound beam is usually greater at the focal zone because of

    (A) decreased attenuation
    (B) the smaller beam diameter
    (C) diffraction effects
    (D) a shorter duty factor

24. If the amplitude is doubled, the intensity is

    (A) doubled
    (B) cut in half
    (C) increased by four times
    (D) unchanged

25. The attenuation for soft tissue is

    (A) increased with tissue thickness
    (B) determined by the scope of the TGC curve
    (C) increased with decreasing wavelength
    (D) unimportant when using digital scan converters

26. The acoustic impedance of the matching layer

    (A) can be chosen to improve transmission into the body
    (B) must be much larger than the transducer material to reduce attenuation
    (C) is not necessary with real-time scanners
    (D) must be made with the same material as the damping material

27. In a pulse–echo system, the quality factor should be made as large as possible.

    (A) true
    (B) false

28. The beam diameter is constant in the near zone.

    (A) true
    (B) false

29. The operating frequency

    (A) depends on the transducer's ring-down time
    (B) depends on the thickness of the crystal
    (C) is increased as the crystal diameter is decreased
    (D) depends on the strength of the pulser

30. The period of an ultrasound wave is

    (A) the time at which it is no longer detectable
    (B) determined by the duty factor
    (C) the time of one wavelength
    (D) independent of the frequency

31. The dynamic range of a system

    (A) is increased when specular reflectors are scanned
    (B) is decreased when shadowing is present
    (C) can be increased through the use of coupling gel
    (D) is the ratio of smallest to largest power level that the system can handle

32. The intensity of an ultrasonic beam can be measured with radiation force balance.

    (A) true
    (B) false

33. Increasing the pulse repetition period

    (A) improves resolution
    (B) increases the maximum depth that can be imaged
    (C) decreases the maximum depth that can be imaged
    (D) increases refraction

34. Ultrasound bioeffects

    (A) do not occur
    (B) do not occur with diagnostic instruments
    (C) are not confirmed below 100 mW/cm^2 SPTA
    (D) are not confirmed below 1 W/cm^2 SPTA

35. No refraction can occur at an interface if the media impedances are equal.

    (A) true
    (B) false

36. Smaller transducers always produce smaller beam diameters.

    (A) true
    (B) false

37. The ultrasound beam profile can be measured with a hydrophone.

    (A) true
    (B) false

38. The pulsed-Doppler system yields better depth resolution than the continuous wave (CW) system.

    (A) true
    (B) false

39. The gray-scale display was made possible when digital scan converters replaced analog scan converters.

    (A) true
    (B) false

40. Videotape recorders operating at 30 frames per second cannot be used with mechanical real-time units because the frame rate is too slow.

    (A) true
    (B) false

41. Linear phased array scanners need no form of mechanical focusing since focusing is performed electronically.

    (A) true
    (B) false

42. The frame rate of real-time scanners depends on the number of lines used to form the image.

    (A) true
    (B) false

43. It is *not* possible to steer an annular phased array electronically.

    (A) true
    (B) false

44. The near zone length should be kept as short as possible.

    (A) true
    (B) false

45. What percentage of intensity of an ultrasound pulse incident on an interface of 0.25 and 0.75 rayls is reflected?

    (A) 50%
    (B) 100%
    (C) 25%
    (D) 75%

46. Axial resolution can be improved by using

    (A) higher frequency transducers
    (B) lower frequency transducers
    (C) larger transducers
    (D) poorly damped transducers

47. When particle motion of a medium is parallel to the direction of a wave propagation, the wave being transmitted is called a

    (A) longitudinal wave
    (B) shear wave
    (C) surface wave
    (D) lamb wave

48. The wavelength in a material having a wave velocity of 1500 m/s employing a transducer frequency of 5 MHz is

    (A) 0.3 mm
    (B) 0.3 cm
    (C) 0.6 mm

49. The factor that determines the amount of reflection at the interface of two dissimilar materials is

    (A) the index of refraction
    (B) the frequency of the ultrasonic wave
    (C) Young's modulus
    (D) the specific acoustic impedance

50. The equation that describes the relationship among propagation, wavelength, and frequency is

    (A) $V = f\lambda$
    (B) wavelength = 2(frequency × velocity)
    (C) $Z = pV$
    (D) wavelength = frequency + velocity

51. Which of the following can occur when an ultrasonic beam reaches the interface of two dissimilar materials?

    (A) reflection
    (B) refraction
    (C) mode conversion
    (D) all of the above

52. The acoustic impedance of a material is

    (A) directly proportional to density and inversely proportional to velocity
    (B) directly proportional to velocity and inversely proportional to density
    (C) inversely proportional to density and velocity
    (D) equal to the product of density and velocity

53. The average velocity of ultrasonic waves in soft tissue is

    (A) 1540 ft/s
    (B) 3300 m/s
    (C) 1540 m/s
    (D) 300×10^6 m/s

54. Receiver-angle values in CW Doppler analysis do *not* influence the final Doppler shift.

    (A) true
    (B) false

55. Refraction occurs due to difference in _____ across an interface between two materials.

    (A) acoustic impedance
    (B) wave velocity
    (C) density
    (D) none of the above

56. Reflection factor at an interface between two materials depends primarily on the change in _____ across the interface.

    (A) acoustic impedance
    (B) wave velocity
    (C) density
    (D) none of the above

57. The velocity of sound waves is primarily dependent on

    (A) angulation
    (B) reflection
    (C) the material through which the sound is being transmitted and the mode of vibration
    (D) none of the above

58. Increasing the frequency of an ultrasonic longitudinal wave will result in _____ in the velocity of that wave.

    (A) an increase
    (B) a decrease
    (C) no change
    (D) a reversal

59. The change in direction of an ultrasonic beam, when it passes from one medium to another, in which elasticity and density differ from those of the first medium is called

    (A) refraction
    (B) rarefaction
    (C) angulation
    (D) reflection

60. A long near zone can be obtained by

    (A) using a higher frequency transducer
    (B) adding a convex lens to the transducer
    (C) decreasing the diameter of the transducer
    (D) increasing the damping

61. If a 2-MHz frequency is used in human soft tissue, the wavelength is approximately

    (A) 0.75 mm
    (B) 0.15 mm
    (C) 0.21 mm
    (D) 0.44 mm

62. The ratio of particle pressure to particle velocity at a given point within the ultrasonic field is

    (A) interference
    (B) impedance
    (C) incidence
    (D) noise

63. What is the following formula used to determine?

    $$\frac{2 \times \text{velocity of reflector} \times \text{original frequency}}{\text{velocity of sound}}$$

    (A) shift in frequency due to the Doppler effect
    (B) degree of attenuation
    (C) distance a wave front travels
    (D) amount of amplification necessary to produce diagnostic ultrasound

64. The principle which states that all points on a wave-front can be considered as point sources for the production of spherical secondary wavelets was postulated by

(A) Doppler
(B) Young
(C) Huygens
(D) Langevin

65. A 10-dB difference in signal intensity is equivalent to a _____ difference.

(A) twofold
(B) tenfold
(C) hundredfold
(D) thousandfold

66. The level below which signals are *not* transmitted through an ultrasound receiver system is the

(A) sensitivity level
(B) threshold or negative level
(C) impedance level
(D) dynamic range level

67. Gray-scale systems typically use _____ as a means of signal dynamic range reduction.

(A) rejection
(B) compression
(C) relaxation
(D) elimination

68. The strength of the echo is related to the height of the deflection on the oscilloscope for the _____ display.

(A) A-mode
(B) B-mode
(C) B-scan
(D) M-mode

69. Which of the following is *not* a method for restricting the dynamic range of the signal?

(A) suppression
(B) rejection
(C) compression
(D) relaxation

70. Most of the scan converters currently in use are of the _____ type.

(A) analog
(B) digital
(C) bistable
(D) static

71. The fraction of time that pulsed ultrasound is actually on is the

(A) duty factor
(B) frame rate
(C) cavitation
(D) intensity transmission coefficient

72. The ability of an imaging system to detect weak reflections is called

(A) compression
(B) demodulation
(C) gain
(D) sensitivity

73. Which of the following image shapes is produced by a linear sequenced array real-time transducer?

A   B   C   D

74. The major factor in determining the acoustic power output of the transducer is the

(A) size of the transducer
(B) magnitude of the voltage spike
(C) amount of amplification at the receiver
(D) amount of gain

75. Two primary mechanisms that produce sound changes in cells or tissues are

(A) oscillations and radiation
(B) absorption and reflection
(C) direct and indirect
(D) thermal and cavitational

76. The _____ relates bandwidth to operating frequency.

(A) near zone
(B) piezoelectric crystal
(C) quality factor
(D) far zone

77. The extraneous beams of ultrasound generated from the edges of individual transducer elements and not in the direction of the main ultrasonic beam are called

(A) a phased array
(B) impedance artifacts
(C) side lobes
(D) acoustic errors

78. The product of the period and the number of cycles in the pulse is the

    (A) pulse repetition frequency
    (B) continuous wave
    (C) pulse repetition period
    (D) pulse duration

79. The substance typically used as a matrix on the imaging surface of an analog scan converter tube is

    (A) mercurous chloride
    (B) silicon oxide
    (C) manganese sulfide
    (D) lithium fluoride

80. Specular reflection occurs when

    (A) the frequency is small compared with the wavelength
    (B) the object that causes the reflection is small
    (C) the reflector surface is smooth as compared with the wavelength
    (D) the angle of incidence and the angle of reflection differ by at least 45°

81. The refractive index of water is slightly altered when a sound beam passes through it, thus causing compression and rarefaction of the water molecules. The phenomenon is the basis for the _____ technique of beam measurement.

    (A) isoamplitude
    (B) Schlieren
    (C) relative echo
    (D) attenuator calibration

82. Artifacts appearing as parallel, equally spaced lines are characteristic of

    (A) acoustic shadowing
    (B) off-normal incidence
    (C) specular reflection
    (D) reverberation

83. An increase in reflection amplitude from reflectors that lie behind a weakly attenuating structure is called

    (A) the incidence angle
    (B) enhancement
    (C) the intensity reflection coefficient
    (D) the effective reflecting area

84. The amount of dispersion in the far field of an ultrasound beam can be decreased by

    (A) using a transducer with a convex face
    (B) using a larger diameter transducer
    (C) decreasing the intensity of the beam in the near field
    (D) using a lower frequency transducer

85. Longitudinal or axial resolution is directly dependent on

    (A) depth of penetration
    (B) spatial pulse length
    (C) damping
    (D) the angle of incidence

86. The transducer _____ is equal to the ratio of the operating frequency to the frequency bandwidth.

    (A) frequency
    (B) Q factor
    (C) resolution
    (D) polarity

87. The technique that uses an optical system to produce a visible image of an ultrasonic beam is the _____ technique.

    (A) M-mode
    (B) B-scan
    (C) Schlieren
    (D) kinetic scanning

88. Which of the following is the least obstacle to the transmission of ultrasound?

    (A) muscle
    (B) fat
    (C) bone
    (D) blood

89. The ratio of the largest power to the smallest power that the ultrasound system can handle is the

    (A) dynamic range
    (B) gain
    (C) rejection
    (D) amplification factor

90. Ultrasound waves in tissue are called _____ waves.

    (A) shear
    (B) lateral displacement
    (C) rotational vibration
    (D) longitudinal

Questions 91 through 99 refer to Fig. 1–28.

91. The row of wires in the middle are used to check

    (A) lateral resolution
    (B) axial resolution

Scan A   Scan B   Scan C

Figure 1–28. Diagram of the AIUM 100-mm test object.

(C) dead zone
(D) horizontal distance calibration
(E) all of the above

92. Which of the diagrams shows correct arm registration?

(A) scan A
(B) scan B
(C) scan C
(D) all the above
(E) none of the above

93. The row of wires on top is used to check

(A) dead zone
(B) vertical distance calibration
(C) horizontal distance calibration
(D) axial resolution
(E) none of the above

94. While using the AIUM test object to test an articulated-arm scanner you obtain an image similar to scan A. You should

(A) call for service
(B) increase the contrast setting
(C) switch to another type of transducer
(D) try another test object

95. The row of wires on the bottom is used to check for

(A) axial resolution
(B) lateral resolution
(C) horizontal caliper check
(D) vertical distance calibration
(E) dead zone

96. All except the following can be checked when the test object is scanned from the top only.

(A) axial resolution
(B) lateral resolution
(C) vertical distance calibration
(D) horizontal distance calibration

97. Which of the following parameters cannot be evaluated by the AIUM test object?

(A) gray scale
(B) dynamic range
(C) azimuthal resolution
(D) depth resolution
(E) both A and B
(F) all of the above

98. Scanning a test object from three sides without erasing would be used to check

(A) gray scale
(B) depth resolution
(C) horizontal distance calibration

(D) registration
(E) all of the above

99. When using the AIUM test object, which of the following should be kept constant for comparisons?

(A) output power
(B) TGC
(C) reject
(D) transducer, MHz, and focus
(E) all of the above

100. Which type of ultrasound machine can be used with the AIUM test object?

(A) linear array
(B) static scanner
(C) phased array
(D) annular array
(E) sector scanner
(F) all of the above
(G) A and C only

101. There are many types of natural and synthetic crystals that possess and exhibit piezoelectric properties. Which of the following are not natural?

(A) tourmaline
(B) quartz
(C) lead zirconate titanate (PZT-4 or PZT-5)
(D) barium titanate
(E) rochelle salt
(F) lithium sulfate
(G) lead metaniobate
(H) ammonium dihydrogen phosphate

102. Which of the following materials would not be suitable as acoustic insulators for transducer backing?

(A) cork
(B) rubber
(C) oil
(D) araldite loaded with tungsten powder
(E) epoxy resin
(F) B and E only
(G) all of the above

103. Ultrasound can be described as a(an)

(A) mechanical vibration that can be transmitted through matter
(B) mechanical vibration that can be transmitted through a vacuum
(C) electromagnetic wave that can be transmitted through tissues
(D) x-ray that can be transmitted through soft tissues

104. If the frequency of sound is below 16 Hz it is called

   (A) infrasound (subsonic)
   (B) audible sound
   (C) ultrasound
   (D) x-rays

105. If the frequency of sound is above 20 kHz it is called

   (A) infrasound (subsonic)
   (B) ultrasound
   (C) audible sound
   (D) x-rays

106. If the frequency of sound is between 16 Hz and 20 kHz it is called

   (A) x-rays
   (B) audible sound
   (C) ultrasound
   (D) infrasound (subsonic)

107. Which of the following is not among the spectrum of electromagnetic waves?

   (A) x-rays
   (B) ultrasound
   (C) ultraviolet
   (D) infrared
   (E) visible light

108. The term Hertz denotes

   (A) density
   (B) milliwatts per centimeter square (mW/cm²)
   (C) kilogram
   (D) cycle per second

109. An ultrasound transducer converts

   (A) electrical energy into light and heat
   (B) electrical energy into mechanical energy and vice versa
   (C) mechanical energy into radiation
   (D) sound into ultrasound

110. Which of the following is(are) an example(s) of a transducer?

   (A) battery
   (B) loudspeaker
   (C) light bulb
   (D) human being
   (E) all of the above
   (F) none of the above
   (G) A and B only

111. When electric voltage is applied on both faces of a piezoelectric crystal, the crystal will

   (A) increase in size
   (B) decrease in size
   (C) lose its polarization

   (D) increase or decrease in size depending on the voltage polarity

112. The abbreviation 5 MHz denotes

   (A) 5 hundred thousand cycles per second
   (B) 5 hundred million cycles per second
   (C) 5000 cycles per second
   (D) 5 million cycles per second

113. The function of the damping material in the transducer housing is to

   (A) reduce pulse duration
   (B) improve axial resolution
   (C) reduce spatial pulse length
   (D) improve lateral resolution
   (E) A and B only
   (F) A and D only
   (G) A, B, and C only

114. What is the velocity of ultrasound in human soft tissue at 37°C?

   (A) 1540 meters per second
   (B) 1540 miles per second
   (C) 741 miles per hour
   (D) 1087 meters per second

115. In physical science, the word period denotes

   (A) the pressure or height of a wave
   (B) the speed of a wave
   (C) the time it takes to complete a single cycle
   (D) propagation

116. Longitudinal waves are characterized by

   (A) motion of particles parallel to the axis of wave propagation
   (B) motion of particles perpendicular to the axis of wave propagation
   (C) twisting action of the particles in motion
   (D) surface vibrating particles

117. Transverse waves are characterized by

   (A) motion of particles parallel to the axis of wave propagation
   (B) surface vibrating particles
   (C) motion of particles perpendicular to the axis of wave propagation
   (D) twisting action of the particles in motion

118. Ultrasound wave propagation causes displacement of particles in a medium. The regions of greatest particle concentration are called

   (A) acoustic impedance
   (B) condensations
   (C) rarefactions
   (D) attenuation

119. Ultrasound wave propagation causes displacement of particles in a medium. The regions of lowest particle concentration are called

    (A) acoustic impedance
    (B) condensations
    (C) rarefactions
    (D) attenuation

120. The prefix piezo- is derived from a Greek word that denotes

    (A) electric
    (B) transducer
    (C) crystal
    (D) pressure

121. Axial resolution is

    (A) the ability to distinguish two objects parallel to the ultrasound beam
    (B) the ability to distinguish two objects perpendicular to the ultrasound beam
    (C) the same as depth, longitudinal, and range resolution
    (D) the same as azimuthal, angular, and transverse resolution
    (E) both A and D
    (F) both A and C

122. Lateral resolution is

    (A) the same as depth, longitudinal, and range resolution
    (B) the ability to distinguish two objects perpendicular to the ultrasound beam
    (C) the ability to distinguish two objects parallel to the ultrasound beam
    (D) the same as azimuthal, angular, and transverse resolution
    (E) both A and B
    (F) both B and D

Questions 123 through 131: Match the structures in Fig. 1–29 with the list of parts given.

123. _____
124. _____
125. _____
126. _____
127. _____
128. _____
129. _____
130. _____
131. _____

    (A) tuning coil
    (B) damping material
    (C) electrical connector
    (D) piezoelectric ceramic material
    (E) housing
    (F) shield
    (G) matching layer
    (H) backing material
    (I) face material

Questions 132 through 140: Match the structures in Fig. 1–30 with the list of parts given.

132. _____
133. _____
134. _____
135. _____
136. _____
137. _____
138. _____
139. _____
140. _____

    (A) cathode
    (B) Y-plate
    (C) glass screen
    (D) electron gun
    (E) evacuated glass
    (F) X-plate
    (G) control grid
    (H) electron beam
    (I) focusing lens

141. If frequency increases, the wavelength will

    (A) decrease
    (B) increase
    (C) increase 10 times
    (D) remain the same

Figure 1–29. Components of a transducer.

Figure 1–30. Basic structure of a cathode ray tube (CRT).

142. If frequency decreases, the wavelength will

(A) decrease
(B) increase
(C) increase 10 times
(D) remain the same

143. As frequency increases, the penetration will

(A) decrease
(B) increase
(C) increase 10 times
(D) remain the same

144. As frequency increases, the resolution will

(A) decrease
(B) increase
(C) increase 10 times
(D) remain the same

145. As frequency increases, the beam width will

(A) decrease
(B) increase
(C) increase 10 times
(D) remain the same

146. Ultrasound has difficulty in propagating through

(A) air
(B) bone
(C) $BaSO_4$
(D) IVP contrast
(E) all of the above
(F) A, B, and C only
(G) A and B only

147. Which of the following *cannot* be used as a coupling medium?

(A) water
(B) saline
(C) barium sulfate
(D) aqueous gels

148. Attenuation denotes

(A) progressive weakening of the sound beam as it travels
(B) density of tissue and the speed of sound in the tissues
(C) the redirection of the ultrasound back to the transducer
(D) bending of the transmitted wave after crossing an interface

149. The piezoelectric effect can be best described as

(A) density of tissue and the speed of sound in the tissues
(B) mechanical deformation that results from

high voltage applied on faces of the crystal, and in turn generates ultrasound
(C) piezoelectric crystals subjected to pressure resulting in electrical charge appearing on their surfaces
(D) having a damaging effect on crystal due to high voltage

150. The reverse piezoelectric effect can be best described as

(A) density of tissue and the speed of sound in the tissues
(B) mechanical deformation that results from high voltage applied on faces of the crystal, and as a result generate ultrasound
(C) piezoelectric crystals subjected to pressures resulting in electrical charges appearing on their surfaces
(D) having a damaging effect on crystal due to high voltage

151. The parameter used to express attenuation is

(A) $\left(\dfrac{Z_2 - Z_1}{Z_2 + Z_1} \right)^2 \times 100$

(B) $dB = 10 \log_{10} \dfrac{l_2}{l_1}$

(C) $Z = pV$

(D) $\dfrac{\sin i}{\sin r} = \dfrac{V_1}{V_2}$

152. A waveform transfers _____ from one point in space to another point in space.

(A) particles
(B) matter
(C) energy
(D) mass

153. In a mechanical wave, there are material particles that

(A) oscillate around an equilibrium point
(B) move forward at a set rate
(C) move away from an equilibrium point
(D) move backward at a set rate

154. Wavelength is a measure of

(A) time
(B) voltage
(C) distance
(D) pulse duration

155. Ultrasonic waves are

(A) mechanical
(B) x-ray

(C) electromagnetic
(D) solar

156. Acoustic impedance is

(A) the amount of tissue × the speed of sound in tissue
(B) the density of tissue × the speed of sound in tissue
(C) the transducer frequency × the speed of sound in tissue
(D) the distance from one interface to the next

157. Amplitude is measured in

(A) W/cm^2
(B) $A = pV$
(C) $\dfrac{\sin i}{\sin r} = \dfrac{V_1}{V_2}$
(D) dB

158. The spectrum of ultrasonic frequency is

(A) less than 20 Hz
(B) above 20,000 Hz
(C) 20–20,000 Hz
(D) 1–3 million Hz

159. Period is inversely proportional to

(A) velocity
(B) watts
(C) hertz
(D) frequency

160. As the ultrasound beam becomes more perpendicular to the organ interface

(A) scattering becomes greater
(B) there are more refracted echoes
(C) there are fewer specular echoes
(D) there are more specular echoes

161. A decibel (dB) describes the

(A) ratio of two sound intensities
(B) sum of two sound intensities
(C) amount of scattering
(D) velocity of the sound wave

162. Axial resolution is also known as all of the following except

(A) depth
(B) range
(C) azimuthal
(D) longitudinal

163. Which of the following has the highest sound velocity?

(A) soft tissue
(B) bone

(C) air
(D) water

164. According to the AIUM, no significant biologic effects have been proven in mammals exposed to

(A) SPTA intensities above $100\ mW/cm^2$
(B) SPTA intensities below $100\ mW/cm^2$
(C) SPTP intensities below $10\ mW/cm^2$
(D) SATP intensities below $2\ mW/cm^2$

165. Temporal peak intensity is measured at

(A) the time the pulse is present
(B) the center of the beam
(C) the time cavitation occurs
(D) none of the above

166. Which of the following has the lowest intensity?

(A) SPTP
(B) SATP
(C) SPTA
(D) SATA

167. What is the definition of the beam uniformity ratio?

(A) the spatial average intensity divided by the spatial intensity
(B) the spatial peak intensity divided by the spatial average intensity
(C) the temporal average intensity divided by the spatial average intensity
(D) the temporal peak intensity divided by the spatial peak intensity

168. The duty factor of a pulsed echo system is normally less than

(A) 10%
(B) 100%
(C) 1%
(D) 25%

169. A shortened spatial pulse length results in

(A) better lateral resolution
(B) low frequency
(C) poor resolution
(D) better axial resolution

170. The equation for measuring the relationship among velocity, frequency, and wavelength is

(A) $\left(\dfrac{Z_2 - Z_1}{Z_2 + Z_1}\right)^2 \times 100$
(B) $V = f\lambda$
(C) $Z = pV$
(D) $\dfrac{\sin i}{\sin r} = \dfrac{V_1}{V_2}$

171. Attenuation of an ultrasound beam can occur by

(A) divergence of a beam
(B) scattering
(C) reflection
(D) all of the above

172. Attenuation coefficient of sound can be defined by which of the following units?

(A) dB/cm/MHz
(B) dB/cm²/Hz
(C) cm/Hz/dB
(D) m/dB/cm³

173. If the transducer Q factor is low, the bandwidth will be

(A) narrow
(B) high
(C) wide
(D) low

174. Axial resolution can be improved by

(A) reducing the spatial pulse length
(B) increasing the spatial pulse length
(C) lowering the transducer frequency
(D) all of the above

175. Axial resolution is primarily affected by

(A) beam width
(B) spatial pulse length
(C) strength of the echo
(D) velocity of the medium

176. Which of the following will improve both axial and lateral resolution?

(A) short pulse length
(B) narrow beam width
(C) increase beam diameter
(D) increase transducer frequency

177. All of the following are also known as lateral resolution except

(A) azimuthal
(B) transverse
(C) range
(D) angular

178. Continous wave Doppler has a duty factor of

(A) less than 1%
(B) 100%
(C) greater than 100%
(D) 50%

179. Acoustic impedance is defined as

(A) density × propagation speed
(B) frequency × propagation

(C) elasticity + propagation
(D) density × elasticity

180. Acoustic impedance is defined by which of the following?

(A) rayons
(B) meters/dB
(C) mW/cm²
(D) rayls

181. Acoustic impedance is not dependent on which of the following?

(A) frequency
(B) density
(C) stiffness
(D) none of the above

182. The height of the vertical spike on the A-mode display corresponds to

(A) the strength of the echo
(B) the distance to the reflector
(C) round-trip time of the echo
(D) the pulse repetition frequency

183. B-mode ultrasound includes all of the following except

(A) static scans
(B) M-mode scans
(C) real-time scans
(D) all of the above are B-mode

184. The correct equation for calculating the percentage of reflection is

(A) $R = \left(\dfrac{Z_2 - Z_1}{Z_2 + Z_1} \right)^2 \times 100$

(B) $R = \dfrac{Z_1 \times Z_2}{2}$

(C) $R = \sqrt{Z_1 + Z_2 \times \pi}$

185. The reflection coefficient between water and air is

(A) 1%
(B) 50%
(C) 75%
(D) nearly 100%

186. What happens to the ultrasound beam beyond the critical angle?

(A) 100% is transmitted
(B) 100% is reflected
(C) 75% is transmitted, 25% is reflected
(D) 75% is reflected, 25% is transmitted

187. Rayleigh scattering occurs if the particle dimensions are

(A) less than the wavelength
(B) greater than 3 mm
(C) greater than the wavelength
(D) none of the above

188. One of the acoustic parameters that determines the intensity of an ultrasound wave is

(A) waveform
(B) particle displacement
(C) period
(D) power

189. Power is defined as energy per unit

(A) mass
(B) distance
(C) time
(D) force

190. The ability to resolve structures lying perpendicular to the axis of the ultrasound beam is called

(A) lateral resolution
(B) axial resolution
(C) depth resolution
(D) longitudinal resolution

191. In most soft tissue the attenuation coefficient varies approximately

(A) inversely with frequency
(B) with the square of the frequency
(C) logarithmically with frequency
(D) directly with frequency

192. Ultrasound absorption in a medium results in

(A) conversion of ultrasound into heat
(B) dissipation of ultrasound into x-rays
(C) conversion of ultrasound into visible light
(D) dissipation of ultrasound into gamma rays

193. The typical value of attenuation in soft tissue is

(A) 2 dB/cm²/Hz
(B) 1 dB/cm/Hz
(C) 2 dB/cm²/MHz
(D) 0.5 dB/cm/MHz

194. False echoes are produced by

(A) reflection
(B) rarefaction
(C) reverberation
(D) diffraction

195. Approximately what percentage of the ultrasound beam will be transmitted between fat and muscle?

(A) 1%
(B) 10%
(C) 50%
(D) 99%

196. Huygens' principle describes

(A) multiple point sources
(B) refraction
(C) velocity
(D) cathode ray tubes

197. Enhancement occurs posterior to

(A) strong attenuations
(B) weak attenuations
(C) strong diffractors
(D) weak diffractors

198. The role of sound attenuation in tissue is expressed in terms of

(A) half-value layer
(B) Huygens' principle
(C) duty cycle
(D) spatial peak

199. Improper location of an echo may be due to

(A) shadowing
(B) Huygens' principle
(C) density error
(D) propagation speed error

200. The range equation explains

(A) side lobes
(B) distance to reflector
(C) attenuation
(D) calibration

201. For a specular reflector

(A) the angle of incidence is equal to the angle of reflection
(B) the angle of incidence is greater than the angle of reflection
(C) there is no dependence on beam angle
(D) the angle of incidence is equal to the angle of transmission

202. Which of the following is determined by the medium?

(A) intensity
(B) period
(C) propagation speed
(D) amplitude

203. Which of the following is not an acoustic variable?

(A) density
(B) pressure
(C) temperature
(D) force

204. The acronym TGC denotes

(A) tissue gain characteristic
(B) time gain compensation
(C) transducer generator control
(D) temperature generator control

205. The propagation speed for fat is

(A) higher than 1540 m/s
(B) lower than 1540 m/s
(C) equal to 1540 m/s
(D) cannot be measured

206. Which of the following has a propagation speed closest to the average soft tissue?

(A) bone
(B) air
(C) fat
(D) muscle

207. Arrange the following media in terms of propagation velocity, from lowest to highest.

(A) air, fat, muscle, bone
(B) bone, fat, air, muscle
(C) bone, muscle, fat, air
(D) muscle, air, fat, bone

208. As frequency increases, backscatter

(A) decreases
(B) is not affected
(C) increases
(D) is reflected

209. The angle at which total reflection occurs is called

(A) critical angle
(B) warp angle
(C) reflectivity angle
(D) diffraction angle

210. The pulse repetition frequency is the number of pulses occurring per

(A) wave
(B) returning echo
(C) microsecond
(D) second

211. The unit(s) used for the duty factor is (are)

(A) rayls
(B) m/s/Hz

(C) m/μs/MHz
(D) unitless

212. The typical value for attenuation coefficient for 6 MHz ultrasound in soft tissue is

(A) 3 dB/cm
(B) 1 dB/cm/Hz
(C) 3 dB/cm²
(D) 2 dB

213. Normal incidence occurs when the ultrasound beam travels _____ to the boundary between the two media

(A) parallel
(B) perpendicular
(C) obliquely
(D) at 1540 m/s

214. The amount of energy transmitted and/or reflected at the boundary between two media depends on

(A) acoustic impedance mismatch
(B) the frequency of the beam
(C) the propagation speed of the first medium
(D) the propagation speed of the second medium

215. Which of the following has a higher acoustic impedance coefficient?

(A) solid
(B) liquid
(C) gas
(D) all the above have an equal acoustic impedance coefficient

216. According to Snell's law, the transmission angle is greater than the incidence angle if the propagation speed

(A) of medium 2 is greater than that of medium 1
(B) of medium 1 is greater than that of medium 2
(C) of the two media are equal
(D) is calculated at 3 dB down

217. According to the range equation, which of the following are necessary to calculate the distance to the reflector?

(A) attenuation coefficient and type of reflector
(B) density and type of reflector
(C) propagation speed and pulse round-trip time
(D) density and pulse round-trip time

218. The mirror image artifact is commonly seen around which of the following structures?

(A) kidney
(B) pancreas

(C) spleen

(D) diaphragm

219. The comet tail artifact can be seen posterior to an object that has

(A) a much lower acoustic impedance than its surroundings

(B) a much higher acoustic impedance than its surroundings

(C) either a much lower or a much higher acoustic impedance than its surroundings

(D) the same acoustic impedance as its surroundings

220. Which of the following may produce the comet tail artifact?

(A) liver-kidney interface

(B) spleen-kidney interface

(C) tissue-gas interface

(D) gas-fluid interface

221. If the ultrasound beam passes through a mass in the liver that contains fat, how might the diaphragmatic echo posterior to it appear?

(A) closer than it really is

(B) farther than it really is

(C) will not be affected

(D) will not be visualized

222. Bandwidth can be increased by

(A) increasing the quality factor

(B) increasing frequency

(C) increasing pulse length

(D) increasing damping

223. Which of the following is not a control affecting the amplification of echoes?

(A) output

(B) compression

(C) time gain curve

(D) balance

224. On some sonographic equipment, adjusting the compression will affect which of the following processes?

(A) slope position

(B) dynamic range

(C) output

(D) balance

225. Generally, ultrasound transducers have

(A) better axial resolution than lateral resolution

(B) better lateral resolution than axial resolution

(C) better azimuthal resolution than radial resolution

(D) equal axial resolution and lateral resolution

226. The pulse repetition frequency of an ultrasound unit is typically

(A) 1 Hz

(B) 10 Hz

(C) 100 Hz

(D) 1000 Hz

227. B-mode display denotes

(A) basic modulator

(B) beam motion

(C) beam modulator

(D) brightness modulation

228. What percentage of the time is a typical pulsed ultrasound system capable of receiving echoes?

(A) 100%

(B) 99.9%

(C) 75%

(D) 50%

229. If the frequency doubles, what happens to the wavelength?

(A) increases fourfold

(B) increases twofold

(C) decreases by one-half

(D) no relationship to wavelength

230. Which of the following does not display a sector format?

(A) linear-sequenced array

(B) electronic-phased array

(C) mechanical rotating wheel

(D) mechanical wobbler

231. The equation for measuring acoustic impedance is

(A) $\left(\dfrac{Z_2 - Z_1}{Z_2 + Z_1} \right)^2 \times 100$

(B) $V = f\lambda$

(C) $Z = pV$

(D) $\dfrac{\sin i}{\sin r} = \dfrac{V_1}{V_2}$

232. Which of the following are most commonly used in ultrasound transducers?

(A) lead zirconate titanate (PZT)

(B) barium sulfate

(C) metaniobate

(D) quartz

233. Transmit–delay focusing in a linear array transducer will

(A) improve axial resolution

(B) improve lateral resolution

(C) improve the frequency

(D) decrease the depth of penetration

234. For real-time systems, which of the following is not related to the others?

(A) frame rate
(B) lines per frame
(C) pulse repetition frequency
(D) frequency

235. The pulse repetition frequency is

(A) pulses emitted per second
(B) time from the beginning of one pulse to the beginning of the next
(C) the time during which the pulse actually occurs
(D) cannot be defined

236. Which of the following is not a role of the pulser?

(A) driving the transducer
(B) telling the receiver when the ultrasound pulses are produced
(C) telling the memory when ultrasound pulses are produced
(D) beam steering

237. Demodulation is a process of

(A) converting the voltage delivered to the receiver from one form to another
(B) decreasing the differences between the smallest and largest amplitudes
(C) eliminating the smaller amplitude voltage produced by electronic noise
(D) rejecting weak echoes to reduce noise

238. Which of the following are not operator adjustable?

(A) compensation and rejection
(B) amplification and compensation
(C) demodulation and compression
(D) rejection and amplification

239. Which of the following varies with distance from the transducer?

(A) lateral resolution
(B) frequency
(C) axial resolution
(D) spatial pulse length

240. A period can be described by which number on the following diagram?

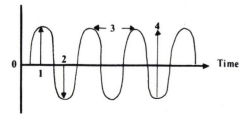

(A) #2
(B) #1
(C) #3
(D) #4

241. Increasing axial resolution by increasing frequency also results in

(A) increasing penetration
(B) decreasing half-intensity depth
(C) decreasing the pulse repetition frequency
(D) none of the above

242. Reflection refers to

(A) the bending of the ultrasound beam as it crosses a boundary
(B) conversion of ultrasound to heat
(C) redirection of a portion of the ultrasound beam from a boundary
(D) the scattering of the ultrasound beam in many directions

243. Digital computers use a special number system called

(A) digital number system
(B) alphanumeric system
(C) chronologic system
(D) binary number system

244. The term *bit* in computer science denotes

(A) binary digit
(B) buffer
(C) baud rate
(D) BASIC programming

245. An 8-bit binary number is referred to as

(A) byte
(B) baud rate
(C) buffer register
(D) BUS

246. Which of the following is not an example of computer hardware?

(A) monitor
(B) program
(C) disk drive
(D) printer

247. The acronym RAM denotes

(A) reset-auxiliary memory
(B) random-access memory
(C) retailing American microcomputers
(D) retailing American machines

248. The acronym ROM denotes

(A) read-only memory
(B) read-only modem

(C) retailing only microcomputers

(D) run-output machine

249. Which of the following is not an input device?

(A) keyboard
(B) printer
(C) disk drive
(D) magnetic disk

250. The type of permanent memory that is produced at the time of manufacture and cannot be changed by the computer user is called

(A) RAM
(B) ROM
(C) PROM
(D) EPROM

251. The type of programmable memory that allows the user to write, store, or erase data is called

(A) PLA
(B) ROM
(C) PROM
(D) EPROM

252. The acronym CPU denotes

(A) computer program update
(B) central processing unit
(C) capacitor power unit
(D) computer portable unit

253. The most common binary word length in microprocessors is

(A) 8, 16, or 32 bits
(B) 12 or 24 bits
(C) 128K bytes
(D) 64K bytes

254. An 8-bit word microcomputer with 128K words of memory can store how many bits of data?

(A) 1000
(B) 128,000
(C) 1,048,576
(D) 128

255. The contents of EPROM can be completely erased by which of the following applications?

(A) light waves
(B) infrared
(C) ultrasound
(D) ultraviolet light

256. A sonographic image can be transferred from one computer to another by way of

(A) fixed disk drive
(B) modem

(C) printer
(D) keyboard

257. The most commonly used programming language for personal computers is

(A) COBOL
(B) FORTRAN
(C) BASIC
(D) LOGO

258. The unit for measuring the speed of data communication is called

(A) buffer
(B) booting
(C) output unit
(D) baud rate

259. Which of the following disks has the highest storage capacity and fastest access time?

(A) $3\frac{1}{2}$-in microfloppy double density
(B) Hard disk
(C) $5\frac{1}{4}$-in minifloppy
(D) $3\frac{1}{2}$-in microfloppy high density

260. The acronym BASIC denotes

(A) basic American scientific instructional code
(B) basic American scientific information center
(C) beginner's all-purpose symbolic instruction code
(D) business application software information center

261. A modem is an electronic device that

(A) simulates human voice
(B) prints data
(C) translates signals from digital into analog and analog into digital
(D) senses data from a card inserted into it

262. Each binary digit in a binary number is represented in memory by a memory element, which at any time is in one of _____ states.

(A) many
(B) two
(C) none of the above

263. In binary numbers, how many values are used for each digit?

(A) 10
(B) multiples of 10
(C) 2
(D) 5

264. The number 30 in binary is

(A) 0110
(B) 1110
(C) 1001
(D) 1111
(E) none of the above

265. How many gray levels (echo amplitude levels) can a 4-bit deep digital scan converter store?

(A) 2
(B) 4
(C) 8
(D) 16
(E) 32

266. An ultrasound instrument that could represent 64 shades of gray would require a(n) _____ bit memory

(A) 8
(B) 6
(C) 4
(D) 16

267. Which of the following are effects seen in tissue at high ultrasound intensities?

(A) fusion, ionization
(B) heating, cavitation
(C) expansion, encrustation
(D) reabsorption, dehydration

268. Which of the following is the correct list of functions performed by the receiver system in the ultrasound machine (B-scanner)?

(A) inspection, detection, correction, rejection, depression
(B) randomization, amplification, modulation, rectification, limitation
(C) amplification, compensation, compression, rejection
(D) expansion, contraction, band limitation, sonification

269. A large amplitude pulse from the pulser results in

(A) a long duration pulse from the transducer
(B) a short duration pulse from the transducer
(C) shutdown of the receiver
(D) a large amplitude pulse from the transducer
(E) a large amplitude pulse from the display

270. Voltage pulses from the pulser go to the

(A) transducer and display
(B) transducer and receiver
(C) transducer and TGC control
(D) display and image memory
(E) amplifier and receiver

271. The five major components of a pulse–echo ultrasound system are

(A) flux capacitor, image memory, transducer, scan arm, amplifier
(B) interrossitor, pulser, receiver, display, power supply
(C) image memory, display, scan arm, TGC control, foot switch
(D) transducer, receiver, image memory, pulser, display

272. Transducers are focused by two major methods: internal focusing and external focusing. These methods can be accomplished by

(A) thickening the crystal and adding a water path
(B) cutting a curved transducer element and/or using an acoustic lens
(C) "doping" the crystal with metal ions and damping
(D) using a crystal pulse and a bandwidth limiter
(E) all of the above will focus a transducer element

273. The unit applied to the Q factor (quality factor) that describes the ratio of operating frequency to bandwidth is called

(A) megahertz (MHz)
(B) percent
(C) millimeter per microsecond
(D) Fresnel
(E) none of the above; Q factor is unitless

Questions 274 through 282: Match the terms in Column A with the correct definition in Column B.

COLUMN A	COLUMN B
274. acoustic shadow _____	(A) without echoes
275. acoustic enhancement _____	(B) echoes of lower amplitude than the normal surrounding tissues
276. anechoic _____	(C) the surface forming the boundary between two media having different acoustic impedances
277. artifact _____	
278. echogenic _____	
279. hyperechoic _____	
280. hypoechoic _____	
281. interface _____	(D) an echo that does not correspond to the real target
282. sonolucent _____	(E) reduction in echoes from a region distal to an attenuating structure
	(F) a tissue or structure that does not have internal echoes (echo-free)

(G) an increase in echoes from a region distal to a weakly attenuating structure or tissue

(H) echoes of higher amplitude than the normal surrounding tissues

(I) a structure that possesses echoes

283. The backing material that is usually constructed in a continuous-wave Doppler transducer is

(A) epoxy resin
(B) cork
(C) air
(D) tungsten powder

284. Transducers with continuous-wave operation are commonly used in which of the following applications?

(A) diagnostic, surgical, therapeutic, and Doppler
(B) diagnostic and surgical
(C) diagnostic and Doppler
(D) surgical, therapeutic, and Doppler

285. Which of the following waves are visible under normal conditions?

(A) water waves
(B) x-ray waves
(C) radio waves
(D) sound waves

286. Ultrasound can travel in all of the following *except*

(A) IVP contrast
(B) solid tissue
(C) vacuum
(D) blood

287. The Greek letter lambda (λ) represents

(A) period
(B) wavelength
(C) frequency
(D) velocity

288. The time it takes to complete a single cycle is called

(A) period
(B) wavelength
(C) frequency
(D) velocity

289. A wave vibration at 20 cycles per second has a frequency of

(A) 20 MHz
(B) 20 Hz

(C) 20 kHz
(D) 120 kHz

290. A wave vibrating at 1 million cycles per second has a frequency of

(A) 1 GHz
(B) 1 kHz
(C) 1 MHz
(D) 100 MHz

291. The device that produces the ultrasound beam is commonly called a

(A) cathode-ray tube (CRT)
(B) scan converter
(C) transducer
(D) mechanical arm

Questions 292 through 294: Match the questions in Column A with the correct answer in Column B.

COLUMN A

292. Which statement best describes A-mode? _____

293. Which statement best describes B-mode? _____

294. Which statement best describes M-mode? _____

COLUMN B

(A) a graphical presentation with vertical spikes arising from a horizontal baseline; the height of the vertical spikes represents the amplitude of the deflected echo

(B) a two-dimensional image of internal body structures displayed as dots; the brightness of the dots is proportional to the amplitude of the echo; the image is applicable to both real-time and static scanners

(C) a graphical presentation of moving structures in a waveform; the display is presented as a group of lines representing the motion of moving interfaces versus time

(D) unidimensional presentation of moving structures displayed in a pie-shaped or rectangular image; the image is applicable only to real-time scanners

295. Which of the following is *not* an essential part of the cathode-ray tube (CRT)?

    (A) electron gun
    (B) fluorescent screen
    (C) silicon
    (D) deflection system (horizontal and vertical plates)

296. The CRT used in ultrasound usually encloses

    (A) air
    (B) vacuum
    (C) oil
    (D) gas

297. The positively (+) charged CRT terminal is called the

    (A) anode
    (B) cathode
    (C) both anode and cathode

298. The negatively (−) charged CRT terminal is called the

    (A) anode
    (B) cathode
    (C) both anode and cathode

299. The intensity of the ultrasound beam

    (A) is measured in watts
    (B) is always constant
    (C) depends on the beam diameter
    (D) is measured with the AIUM phantom

300. Whose principle states, "All points on an ultrasound waveform can be considered as point sources for the production of secondary spherical wavelets"?

    (A) Doppler's
    (B) Curie's
    (C) Huygens'
    (D) Young's

301. The fraction of time that a pulsed ultrasound system is actually producing ultrasound is called the

    (A) duty factor
    (B) curie factor
    (C) frame rate
    (D) transmission factor

302. Real-time ultrasound instrumentation can be classified as

    (A) annular, sector, linear, and static scanners
    (B) sector scanners only
    (C) sector, linear, and annular scanners
    (D) static scanners only

303. The speed at which ultrasound propagates within a medium depends primarily on

    (A) its frequency
    (B) the compressibility of the medium
    (C) its intensity
    (D) the thickness of the medium

304. An artifact that results from a pulse that has traveled two or more round-trip distances between the transducer and the interface is called

    (A) a multipath
    (B) a side lobe
    (C) reverberation
    (D) scattering

305. The ratio of output electric power to input electric power is termed

    (A) power
    (B) intensity
    (C) gain
    (D) voltage

306. Multipath artifacts result from

    (A) echoes that return directly to the transducer
    (B) shotgun pellets
    (C) echoes that take an indirect path back to the transducer
    (D) none of the above

307. A scan converter will accept echo signals from the receiver and store them in the "memory" of the instrument. Identify the types of memory used in scan converters.

    (A) gray scale and bistable
    (B) analog and digital
    (C) static and real-time
    (D) none of the above

308. To achieve the best possible digital representation of an analog system, the echo signals should undergo

    (A) postprocessing
    (B) preprocessing
    (C) rectification
    (D) amplification

309. Near zone length may be increased by increasing

    (A) wavelength
    (B) wavelength and bandwidth
    (C) transducer diameter
    (D) frequency and transducer diameter

Questions 310 through 319: Match the terms in Column A with the correct definition in Column B.

COLUMN A

310. density _____
311. propagation _____
312. frequency _____
313. power _____
314. duty factor _____
315. bandwidth _____
316. acoustic impedance
     _____
317. absorption _____
318. quality factor
     _____
319. intensity _____

COLUMN B

(A) rate at which work is done
(B) mass divided by volume
(C) conversion of sound to heat
(D) number of cycles per unit time
(E) density multiplied by sound propagation speed
(F) range of frequencies contained in the ultrasound pulse
(G) the product of pulse duration and pulse repetition rate
(H) progression or travel
(I) operating frequency divided by bandwidth
(J) power divided by area

320. Which of the following is a true definition for a highly damped transducer?

(A) increased efficiency, sensitivity, and spatial pulse length
(B) decreased efficiency, sensitivity, and spatial pulse length
(C) increased efficiency and sensitivity, but decreased spatial pulse length
(D) decreased efficiency, but increased sensitivity and spatial pulse length

321. Gain compensation is necessary due to

(A) reflector motion
(B) gray scale
(C) attenuation
(D) resolution

322. The frequency bandwidth may be determined by which of the following?

(A) spectral analysis
(B) Schlieren system
(C) hydrophone analysis
(D) cathode analysis

323. Analog scan converters

(A) function perfectly as peak deflectors
(B) have greater image sharpness than digital scan converters
(C) store any increment of signal amplitude
(D) have better image uniformity than digital scan converters

324. The gray-scale resolution for a 5-bit digital instrument that has a dynamic range of 42 dB is

(A) 1.9 dB
(B) 3 dB
(C) 1.3 dB
(D) 0.07 dB

325. If it takes 0.01 second for a pulse emitted by the transducer to reach an echo source of soft tissue, what distance must the pulse travel in order to be recorded?

(A) 1540 cm
(B) 30.8 m
(C) 15.4 m
(D) both A and C

326. An artifact that is produced from interaction of the incident beam with a curved surface and results in an acoustic shadow is referred to as

(A) a ghost artifact
(B) an edge artifact
(C) a comet tail artifact
(D) a ring down artifact

327. An artifact that results from refraction of the ultrasound beam at a muscle–fat interface and gives rise to double images is called

(A) a split image artifact
(B) an edge artifact
(C) a comet tail artifact
(D) a ring down artifact

328. An artifact that would *least* likely produce a pseudomass is

(A) a comet tail artifact
(B) a multipath artifact
(C) a mirror image artifact
(D) a slide lobe artifact

329. Split image artifact is more noticeable in

(A) athletic patients and mesomorphic habitus patients
(B) patients with underdeveloped rectus muscle
(C) mesomorphic habitus patients and patients with underdeveloped rectus muscle
(D) all of the above

330. Select the least likely cause or causes for a split image artifact:

(A) abdominal scar
(B) lateral margins of the rectus muscles
(C) gas bubble
(D) refraction of the sound beam at a muscle–fat interface

331. The most likely cause for a beam thickness artifact is

(A) metallic surgical clips
(B) gas bubble
(C) partial volume effect
(D) shotgun pellets

332. Beam thickness artifact is primarily dependent on

(A) position of the patient
(B) gas bubble
(C) beam angulation
(D) gravity

333. Which of the following is not true for side lobe artifact?

(A) caused by multiple side lobes of the transducer
(B) apparent in real-time image
(C) may be diffuse or specular in appearance
(D) not visible on real-time image

334. Which of the following is least likely to produce an acoustic shadow?

(A) bone interface
(B) metallic surgical clips
(C) gallstones
(D) gas interface

335. The most common type of artifact encountered in patients with shotgun wounds is

(A) comet tail artifact
(B) multipath artifact
(C) mirror image artifact
(D) side lobe artifact

336. The type of reverberation echo that usually results from a small gas bubble and appears as a high-amplitude echo occurring at regular intervals is called a

(A) multipath artifact
(B) mirror image artifact
(C) side lobe artifact
(D) ring-down artifact

337. The amount of splitting that occurs in a split image artifact for a given structure

(A) can be calculated using Snell's law
(B) cannot be calculated because it is an artifact
(C) can be calculated using the equation $Z = pV$
(D) can be calculated using a 5-MHz transducer with the equation: split (m/s) = $D\pi/T$

338. The first vertical deflection on the A-mode that corresponds to the transducer face is called

(A) bistable
(B) side lobe

(C) main bang
(D) gain

339. The type of real-time system that employs a combination of electronic and mechanical means is called

(A) wobbler sector real-time
(B) rotating wheel real-time
(C) annular-array real-time
(D) linear-sequenced array

340. If the amount of acoustic coupling medium is insufficient, what changes could result?

(A) decrease in amplitude of the returning echo
(B) increase in amplitude of the returning echo
(C) the transducer will slide on the skin easier
(D) no effect on the image

341. Which of the following is not a hard copy?

(A) x-ray film
(B) Polaroid film
(C) floppy disk
(D) videotape recorder

Questions 342 through 344: Each diagram represents modes of operation used in diagnostic ultrasound.

342. Identify the type of mode displayed in the following diagram.

(A) B-mode
(B) A-mode
(C) M-mode
(D) R-mode

343. Identify the type of mode displayed in the following diagram.

(A) B-mode
(B) A-mode
(C) M-mode
(D) R-mode

344. Identify the type of mode displayed in the following diagram.

(A) B-mode
(B) A-mode
(C) M-mode
(D) R-mode

345. The effects of diagnostic ultrasound on human soft tissue are called

(A) sensitivity effects
(B) biologic effects
(C) neurologic effects
(D) pressure effect

346. The average propagation speed of ultrasound in soft tissue is

(A) 1.54 mm/μs
(B) 741 mph
(C) 1560 m/s
(D) 331 mm/s

Questions 347 through 350: Identify the regions on the diagram below by filling in the blanks to the right of each term given.

347. slope _____
348. delay _____
349. far gain _____
350. near gain _____

DIAGRAM OF TGC CURVE

Questions 351 through 360: Match the terms in Column A with the correct definition in Column B.

COLUMN A
351. attenuation _____
352. bistable _____
353. bit _____
354. cavitation _____
355. coupling medium
    _____
356. damping _____
357. gray scale _____
358. matching layer
    _____
359. pixel _____
360. static imaging
    _____

COLUMN B
(A) picture element
(B) the production and behavior of bubbles in sound
(C) progressive weakening of the sound beam as it travels through a medium
(D) a liquid placed between the transducer and the skin
(E) the number of intensity levels between black and white
(F) having two stages
(G) binary digit
(H) a method of reducing pulse duration by electrical or mechanical means
(I) single-frame imaging
(J) plastic material placed in front of the transducer face to reduce the reflection at the transducer surface

361. The intensity of ultrasound is measured in

(A) kg/m³
(B) N/m²
(C) Hz
(D) W/cm²

362. There is no known adverse biologic effect in tissue at intensities below

(A) 100 mW/cm² SPTA
(B) 1000 mW/cm² SAPA
(C) 10 W/cm² SPTP
(D) 500 m/Wcm² SATA

363. The acronym SPTA denotes

(A) static probe transmission amplitude
(B) static probe transmission absorption
(C) spatial peak temporal average
(D) sound propagation temperature artifact

Questions 364 through 370: Match the quantity in Column A with the correct unit in Column B.

COLUMN A	COLUMN B
364. density _____	(A) W/cm²
365. speed _____	(B) kg/m³
366. frequency _____	(C) m
367. work _____	(D) m/s
368. intensity _____	(E) J
369. wavelength _____	(F) Hz
370. attenuation _____	(G) dB

371. The general range of intensities in diagnostic ultrasound is

(A) 0.5 W/cm²–2.0 W/cm² SPTA
(B) 0.002 W/cm²–0.5 W/cm² SPTA
(C) 50 W/cm²–100 W/cm² SPTA
(D) the general range of intensities in diagnostic ultrasound is unknown

372. The general range of intensities in therapeutic ultrasound is

(A) 0.5 W/cm²–2.0 W/cm² SPTA
(B) 0.002 W/cm²–0.5 W/cm² SPTA
(C) 50 W/cm²–100 W/cm² SPTA
(D) the general range of intensities in therapeutic ultrasound is unknown

373. Which of the following characteristics does *not* apply to diagnostic ultrasound at normal diagnostic intensity levels?

(A) noninvasive
(B) atraumatic
(C) ionizing
(D) nontoxic

374. The most common result of high intensity ultrasound is

(A) cavitation
(B) brain damage
(C) fetal developmental anomalies
(D) heat

375. In the study of bioeffects, cavitation denotes

(A) production and behavior of gas bubbles
(B) necrosis
(C) cell membrane rupture
(D) chromosome breakage

376. The two types of cavitation are

(A) silent and noisy
(B) micro and macro
(C) membrane and nonmembrane
(D) stable and transient

377. An instrument used to detect frequency shift is called

(A) Doppler
(B) real-time
(C) A-mode
(D) static scanner

378. Specular reflections

(A) occur when the interface is larger than the wavelength
(B) occur when the interface is smaller than the wavelength
(C) arise from interfaces smaller than 3 mm
(D) are not dependent on the angle of incidence

379. Nonspecular reflections

(A) occur when the interface is larger than the wavelength
(B) occur when the interface is smaller than the wavelength
(C) arise from mirror-like surfaces
(D) are beam-angle dependent

380. The acronym SATA denotes

(A) static amplitude transmission average
(B) spatial average temporal average
(C) spatial average tissue absorption
(D) sound attenuation transmission average

381. The acronym SPPA denotes

(A) static probe power average
(B) static probe transmission absorption
(C) spatial peak pulse average
(D) sound propagation performance average

382. The mode not applicable to a Doppler instrument is

(A) static
(B) pulsed
(C) continuous
(D) audible

383. Which of the following transducers would be most useful for imaging superficial structures?

(A) 5-MHz, short-focus
(B) 3-MHz, long-focus
(C) 5-MHz, long-focus
(D) 2.5-MHz, short-focus

384. Which of the following transducers would be most useful for good penetration on an obese patient?

(A) 5-MHz, short-focus
(B) 3-MHz, long-focus
(C) 5-MHz, long-focus
(D) 2.5-MHz, short-focus

385. The digital memory represents a picture element called a

(A) pixel
(B) bistable
(C) real-time
(D) matrix

386. How many shades of gray can the human eye distinguish?

(A) about 16 shades
(B) between 16 and 32 shades
(C) more than 64 shades
(D) more than 124 shades

387. The most recent digital storage employs what size memory?

(A) $512 \times 512 \times 6$-bit deep
(B) $64 \times 64 \times 2$-bit deep
(C) $128 \times 128 \times 4$-bit deep
(D) $16 \times 16 \times 2$-bit deep

388. A disadvantage of pulsed-wave Doppler (PW) relative to continuous-wave Doppler (CW) is that

(A) it is unidirectional
(B) the Doppler shift depends on frequency
(C) it is subject to "aliasing"
(D) it does not provide in-depth information

389. Which of the following is (are) essential to a TGC display?

(A) static system
(B) real-time system
(C) bistable system
(D) all of the above

390. What is the effect of ultrasound absorption on tissues at normal intensity levels?

(A) dissipation of heat by conduction
(B) significant temperature elevations
(C) significantly lowered temperature
(D) necrosis

391. CRT monitors normally have how many horizontal lines?

(A) 16
(B) 64
(C) 100
(D) 525

392. How many frames per second are displayed by a CRT monitor?

(A) 525
(B) 30
(C) 16
(D) 60

393. How many times each second does the electron beam scan each field on a CRT monitor in order to produce a flicker-free display?

(A) 30
(B) 60
(C) 40
(D) 10

394. The dynamic range of the dots on the average oscilloscope or CRT monitor is

(A) 50–60 dB
(B) 20–25 dB
(C) 125 dB
(D) 525 dB

395. The term matrix, when referring to digital memory, denotes

(A) number of rows and columns
(B) analog
(C) pixel
(D) buffer

396. Digital memory resembles

(A) squares on a checkerboard
(B) a transducer
(C) an electron beam
(D) a hydrophone

397. A region that is anechoic is displayed as

(A) echo-free
(B) echogenic
(C) hyperechoic
(D) hypoechoic

398. A region that is hyperechoic is

(A) anechoic
(B) echogenic
(C) echo-free
(D) transsonic

399. Which of the following cannot be measured by a hydrophone?

(A) pressure amplitude
(B) spatial pulse length
(C) impedance
(D) intensity

400. The hydrophone is made up of

(A) x-rays
(B) transducer elements
(C) ultraviolet lights
(D) all of the above

401. Bioeffects at medium intensity levels on laboratory animals have resulted in

(A) cancer
(B) death
(C) growth retardation
(D) no effects

402. Which of the following is the least likely cause for attenuation?

(A) absorption
(B) reflection
(C) refraction
(D) scattering

403. Absorption refers to

(A) bending of the sound beam crossing a boundary
(B) conversion of sound to heat
(C) redirection of a portion of the sound from a boundary beam
(D) redirection of the sound beam in several directions

404. Diffraction refers to

(A) spreading-out of the ultrasound beam
(B) conversion of sound to heat
(C) redirection of a portion of the sound from a boundary beam
(D) bending of the sound beam crossing a boundary

405. Scattering refers to

(A) bending of the sound beam crossing a boundary
(B) conversion of sound to heat
(C) redirection of a portion of the sound from a boundary beam
(D) redirection of the sound beam in several directions

406. The method for sterilizing transducers is

(A) heat sterilization
(B) steam
(C) recommended by the transducer manufacturer
(D) autoclave

407. An example of an acoustic window is

(A) liver interface
(B) rib interface
(C) tissue/air interface
(D) tissue/bone interface

408. The binary number 1010 equals the decimal number

(A) 10
(B) 11
(C) 110
(D) 200

409. Real-time imaging is similar to

(A) static scanning
(B) fluoroscopy
(C) MRI
(D) all of the above

410. When attempting to identify fetal heart motion, the frame rate of the real-time system should be

(A) turned off to avoid confusion
(B) set at a slow rate
(C) set at a fast rate
(D) set at five frames per second

411. Select the recommended orientation for a transverse scan.

(A) all transverse scans should be viewed from the patient's feet
(B) all transverse scans should be viewed from the patient's head
(C) all transverse scans should be viewed lateral from the patient's right side
(D) all transverse scans should be viewed lateral from the patient's left side

412. The recommended orientation for longitudinal scans is

(A) the patient's head to the right of the image and feet to the left of the image
(B) the patient's head to the left of the image and feet to the right of the image
(C) the patient's head to the top (anterior) of the image and feet to the bottom (posterior) of the image
(D) none of the above

413. Demodulation is a function performed by the

(A) pulser
(B) amplifier
(C) receiver
(D) transmitter

414. Which of the following statements about ultrasound waves is not true?

(A) ultrasound waves are mechanical vibrating energy
(B) ultrasound waves can be polarized
(C) ultrasound waves are not part of the electromagnetic spectrum
(D) ultrasound waves cannot travel in a vacuum

415. The transducer crystal most likely to be employed in high-frequency work, above 18 MHz, is

(A) lithium sulfate
(B) PZT-5
(C) Rochelle salt
(D) quartz

416. The advantage that PZT-5 has over other ceramic material is that it is

(A) easy to shape
(B) effective at low voltage
(C) inexpensive
(D) all of the above

417. The trade name for lead zirconate titanate is

(A) $BaSO_4$
(B) quartz
(C) PZT-5
(D) synthetic-P

418. How many shades of gray can be displayed using a scan converter with 8 bits per memory element?

(A) 8
(B) 16
(C) 128
(D) 256

419. The transducer that would be best suited for intercostal scanning is

(A) linear-sequenced array real-time
(B) mechanical sector real-time transducer

(C) static with large diameter

(D) no type of transducer can scan between the intercostal space

420. The difference between real-time and fluoroscopy is

(A) ultrasound does not need contrast media

(B) fluoroscopy has potential biologic effects, whereas ultrasound has no known biologic effects at normal intensity level

(C) ultrasound is nonionizing

(D) a movie-like image is displayed, whereas real-time displays a single frame image

(E) all of the above

(F) A and D

(G) A, B, and C

421. Which of the following contrast media used in x-ray do *not* obscure the propagation of ultrasound?

(A) barium sulfate ($BaSO_4$) for upper GI examination

(B) hypaque for IVP examination

(C) air for lower GI examination

(D) telepaque for oral cholecystogram

(E) C and D

(F) B and D

(G) none of the above

(H) all of the above

Questions 422 through 430: Match each term in Column A with the correct definition in Column B.

COLUMN A

422. acoustic lens _____

423. pixel _____

424. sector _____

425. acousto-optical converter _____

426. side lobe _____

427. wavefront _____

428. rayl _____

429. Snell's law _____

430. Doppler effect _____

COLUMN B

(A) unit of impedance

(B) the portion of the sound beam outside of the main beam

(C) picture element

(D) pie shaped

(E) a change in frequency as a result of reflector motion between the transducer and the reflector

(F) a device that changes sound waves into visible light patterns

(G) the ratio between the angle of incidence and the refraction

(H) imaginary surface passing through particles of the same vibration as an ultrasound wave

(I) a device used to focus sound beams

431. Lateral resolution is equal to

(A) the wavelength

(B) the beam diameter

(C) the near-zone length

(D) the wave number

432. Which of the following materials are used to make acoustic lenses?

(A) aluminum

(B) Perspex (acrylic plastic)

(C) polystyrene

(D) ethylene oxide

(E) all of the above

(F) A, B, and C

(G) B and D

433. Ultrasound beams can be focused and defocused with the use of

(A) a concave or convex mirror

(B) acoustic lenses

(C) both A and B

(D) ultrasound beam cannot be focused, only light can

434. The normal range of wavelength in medical application is

(A) 0.1–1.5 mm

(B) 1.5–2 mm

(C) 2–5 mm

(D) 5.5–15 mm

435. Which of the following cannot be distinguished on diagnostic ultrasound?

(A) tissue

(B) solid mass

(C) individual cells

(D) male and female genitalia

436. Density is defined as

(A) unit of impedance

(B) force divided by area

(C) force multiplied by displacement

(D) mass per unit volume

437. Ultrasound absorption is directly proportional to

(A) viscosity

(B) frequency

(C) distance

(D) all of the above

438. The confirmed bioeffect(s) on pregnant women with the use of real-time diagnostic instruments is (are)

(A) brain damage

(B) fetal developmental anomalies

(C) growth retardation

(D) no known effect

439. The confirmed bioeffects on pregnant mice exposed to continuous wave ultrasound in a laboratory setting have resulted in

(A) cancer
(B) death
(C) neurocranial damage
(D) no known effect

440. Which of the following combinations of frequency and intensity would *most* likely result in cavitation?

(A) high frequency and low intensity
(B) low frequency and high intensity
(C) high frequency and high intensity
(D) intensity has no effect on cavitation

Questions 441 through 448: Match each term in Column A with the correct definition in Column B.

COLUMN A
441. in vivo _____
442. in vitro _____
443. spectral analysis
_____
444. viscoelasticity
_____
445. rejection _____
446. relaxation _____
447. red cell stasis
_____
448. acoustic power
_____

COLUMN B
(A) an in vivo phenomenon characterized by erythrocytes within small vessels stopping the flow and collecting in the low pressure regions of the standing wave field
(B) elimination of small amplitude echo
(C) a process of acoustic energy absorption
(D) energy transported per unit time
(E) tissue cultures in a test tube
(F) a method of analyzing a waveform
(G) the property of a medium characterized by energy distortion in the medium and irreversibly converted to heat
(H) living human tissue

449. Which of the following statements about bioeffects is (are) unconfirmed?

(A) ultrasound exposure in humans is accumulative
(B) most harmful bioeffects that occurred in experimental conditions have been confirmed in humans in a clinical setting
(C) intensity, frequency, and exposure time used on experimental animals were compatible to those used in a clinical setting

(D) continuous wave used in experimental studies gives the same tissue exposure as pulsed ultrasound used in a clinical setting
(E) the exposure of pregnant women to high intensity levels resulted in growth retardation of their offspring
(F) A and E
(G) all of the above are false or unconfirmed
(H) all of the above are true

450. The number of known human injuries resulting from diagnostic medical ultrasound exposure is

(A) 2500 in England
(B) 115 in the United States
(C) 1500 in Japan
(D) no exposure injuries in humans have been reported

451. What is the distinction between real-time scans and B-scans?

(A) no distinction; real-time scans are B-scans
(B) real-time scans display gray-scale images, whereas B-scans display bistable images
(C) real-time scans exhibit motion images, whereas B-scans exhibit static images
(D) B-scans are specific for static scanners; real-time scans are not

452. Transonic regions are always

(A) echo-free
(B) anechoic
(C) echogenic
(D) uninhibited to propagation

453. Which of the following is not related to real-time?

(A) A-mode
(B) static imaging
(C) dynamic imaging
(D) M-mode

454. Which of the following is *not* a component of the time-gain compensation (TGC) curve?

(A) gray scale
(B) far gain
(C) knee
(D) delay

455. The range of pulse repetition frequencies used in diagnostic ultrasound is

(A) 0.5–4 kHz
(B) 1–10 MHz
(C) 1–7 kHz
(D) 10–15 MHz

456. The spatial pulse length is defined as the product of the _____ multiplied by the number of _____ in a pulse.

(A) cycles, frequency
(B) frequency, velocity
(C) wavelength, cycles
(D) frequency, wavelength

457. Which of the following is (are) one-dimensional?

(A) B-mode and A-mode
(B) A-mode and M-mode
(C) B-mode
(D) static imaging

458. Continuous wave ultrasound is

(A) applicable to real-time instruments only
(B) used in all Doppler instruments
(C) used in some Doppler instruments
(D) applicable only to static scanners

459. Which imaging modality is audible?

(A) x-ray
(B) ultrasound
(C) Doppler
(D) computed tomography (CT)

460. Which mode requires two crystals: one for transmitting and one for receiving?

(A) A-mode
(B) M-mode
(C) continuous wave mode
(D) pulse-echo mode

Questions 461 through 464: Identify the components in Fig. 1–31 by correlating them with the list of terms given.

461. _____
462. _____
463. _____
464. _____

(A) motor
(B) acoustic mirror
(C) scanner head
(D) piezoelectric crystal

465. The normal range of intensities used in Doppler instruments is

Figure 1–31. Diagram of a mechanical sector real-time transducer.

(A) 0.2–400 W/cm²
(B) 0.2–400 mW/cm²
(C) 400–800 mW/cm²
(D) 800–900 mW/cm²

466. If the media boundary is moving toward the source, the reflected sound wave will have

(A) a higher frequency than the incident frequency
(B) a lower frequency than the incident frequency
(C) no change in frequency
(D) be delayed

467. If the media boundary is moving away from the source, the result will be

(A) a higher frequency than the incident frequency
(B) a lower frequency than the incident frequency
(C) no change in frequency
(D) be delayed

468. A Doppler instrument that can distinguish between positive and negative shifts is called

(A) bistable
(B) a modulator–demodulator
(C) bidirectional
(D) a polarized shifter

469. Which statement about Doppler application is not true?

(A) color Doppler is not beneficial
(B) Doppler can produce audible sound
(C) Doppler instruments use both pulsed and continuous wave
(D) Doppler can display an image

Questions 470 through 474: Match the time gain compensation (TGC) controls in Column A with the control functions in Column B.

COLUMN A

470. near gain _____
471. far gain _____
472. slope _____
473. delay _____
474. knee _____

COLUMN B

(A) control used to suppress or increase echoes in the far field
(B) control used to suppress or increase echoes in the near field
(C) control used to delay the start of the slope
(D) control the upward incline of the TGC, used to display an even texture throughout an organ
(E) controls the point where the slope ends

475. The range of frequencies contained in an ultrasound pulse is called

(A) propagation
(B) bandwidth
(C) refraction
(D) rejection

476. Which quantity is unitless?

(A) Q-factor
(B) volume
(C) intensity
(D) force

477. Which of the following would *most* likely cause acoustic enhancement?

(A) a solid mass
(B) a fluid-filled mass
(C) a calcified mass
(D) a gallstone

478. Which of the following would *most* likely cause acoustic shadowing?

(A) gallbladder
(B) a fluid-filled mass
(C) a calcified mass
(D) urinary bladder

479. Continuous-wave Doppler uses how many piezoelectric element(s)?

(A) 1
(B) 2
(C) 64
(D) none

480. The greatest Doppler angle is achieved

(A) when the beam strikes a vessel at a sharp angle
(B) when the beam strikes a vessel perpendicular
(C) when the beam strikes a vessel at a 30° angle
(D) when the beam strikes a vessel at a 70° angle

481. If the power output of an amplifier is 100 times the power at the input, the gain is

(A) 10 dB
(B) 20 dB
(C) 30 dB
(D) 40 dB

482. Which control is used to minimize the effects of attenuation?

(A) reject
(B) field-of-view
(C) frame rate
(D) depth-gain compensation

483. When an ultrasound beam passes obliquely across the boundary between two materials, _____ will occur if there is a difference in _____ in the two materials.

(A) reflection, impedance
(B) reflection, density
(C) refraction, impedance
(D) refraction, propagation speed

484. A decreased pulse duration leads to

(A) better axial resolution
(B) decreased spatial resolution
(C) decreased longitudinal resolution
(D) better lateral resolution

485. What is the reflected intensity from a boundary between two materials if the incident intensity is 1 mW/cm² and the impedances are 25 and 75?

(A) 0.25 mW/cm²
(B) 0.33 mW/cm²
(C) 0.50 mW/cm²
(D) 1.00 mW/cm²

486. The near zone length of an unfocused transducer depends on

(A) frequency and thickness
(B) frequency and diameter
(C) resolution and field of view
(D) diameter and field of view

487. The frequency of a transducer depends primarily on

(A) overall gain
(B) the speed of ultrasound
(C) the element diameter
(D) the element thickness

488. An ultrasound beam that is normally incident on an interface will experience no

(A) attenuation
(B) refraction
(C) reflection
(D) absorption

489. The average speed of propagation of ultrasound in soft tissue is

(A) 1540 ft/s
(B) 1.54 dB/cm
(C) 1.54 mm/μs
(D) 1540 mW/cm²

490. The duty factor for a system with a pulse duration (PD) of 5 μs and a pulse repetition period (PRP) of 500 μs is

(A) 0.1%
(B) 0.5%

(C) 1.0%
(D) 10.0%

491. Ultrasound is defined as sound with frequencies above

(A) 20 Hz
(B) 20 kHz
(C) 20 MHz
(D) 20 GHz

492. Frequency is a significant factor in

(A) propagation speed
(B) tissue compressibility
(C) tissue attenuation
(D) transducer diameter

493. In a pulse-echo system, a 3.5 MHz beam in 2 cm of tissue will be attenuated by

(A) 3.5 dB/cm
(B) 7.0 dB/cm
(C) 3.5 dB
(D) 7.0 dB

494. The characteristic acoustic impedance of a material is equal to the product of the material density and

(A) path length
(B) wavelength
(C) frequency
(D) propagation speed

495. For a focused transducer, the beam intensity will remain constant through the scan field.

(A) true
(B) false

496. For normal incidence, if the intensity reflection coefficient is 30%, the intensity transmission coefficient will be

(A) 30%
(B) 60%
(C) 70%
(D) 100%

497. A Fourier transform of a returning echo will result in a presentation of the ＿＿＿＿ contained within the echo

(A) frequencies
(B) wavelength
(C) intensity
(D) power

498. The range equation relates

(A) frequency, velocity, and wavelength
(B) frequency, velocity, and time
(C) distance, velocity, and time
(D) distance, frequency, and time

499. The axial resolution of a system is determined by

(A) spatial pulse length
(B) beam intensity
(C) beam diameter
(D) spatial resolution

500. The Doppler shift frequency is zero when the angle between the receiving transducer and the flow direction is

(A) 0°
(B) 45°
(C) 90°
(D) 180°

501. The frame rate of real-time scanner that uses an electronic array will be limited only by the speed of the scan converter memory.

(A) true
(B) false

502. The dynamic range of a pulse-echo ultrasound system is defined as

(A) the ratio of the maximum to the minimum intensity that can be processed
(B) the range of propagation speeds
(C) the range of gain settings allowed
(D) none of the above

503. The digital scan converter will generally have a dynamic range that is ＿＿＿＿ than other components of the system.

(A) larger
(B) smaller

504. The time-gain or depth-gain compensation control

(A) compensates for attenuation effects
(B) compensates for increased patient scan time
(C) compensates for machine malfunctions
(D) compensates for video-image drifts

505. A digital scan converter is essentially a

(A) radio receiver
(B) video monitor
(C) television set
(D) computer memory

506. A mechanical real-time scanner will always produce images at a slower frame rate than does an electronic realtime scanner.

(A) true
(B) false

507. Acoustic enhancement can be observed when scanning

(A) highly attenuating structures
(B) weakly attenuating structures
(C) highly reflective structures
(D) structures with large speed differences

508. Changes in the preprocessing controls will not affect the numbers stored in the scan converter.

(A) true
(B) false

509. The lateral resolution of a system

(A) is equal to the beam diameter
(B) is better at higher frequencies
(C) is constant throughout the image
(D) changes with gain settings

510. If the lines per degree in a mechanical sector scanner remain constant, a decreased sector angle can result in

(A) decreased resolution
(B) increased frame rate
(C) decreased frame rate
(D) increased resolution

511. The threshold control is equivalent to the

(A) TGC control
(B) DGC control
(C) modulation control
(D) reject control

512. If the actual propagation speed in soft tissue is 1700 m/s, current diagnostic scanners will display a reflector at a location _____ the transducer.

(A) too close to
(B) too far from
(C) displaced to the left of
(D) displaced to the right of

513. Continuous-wave (CW) ultrasound is used in

(A) static B-scanners
(B) bistable systems
(C) most modern B-scan systems
(D) some Doppler systems

514. If the gain of an amplifier is 18 dB, what will the new gain setting be if one reduces the gain setting by one-half?

(A) 9 dB
(B) 36 dB
(C) 15 dB
(D) 0.5 dB

515. Decreasing the pulse repetition period

(A) decreases spatial resolution
(B) decreases axial resolution
(C) decreases the maximum depth imaged
(D) increases the maximum depth imaged

516. The AIUM 100-mm test object

(A) measures power output
(B) measures beam intensity
(C) measures frequency
(D) measures spatial resolution

517. Real-time imaging is impossible without electronic arrays.

(A) true
(B) false

518. Grating lobes in electronic array systems

(A) increase with increased steering angle
(B) decrease with increased steering angle
(C) are eliminated at high frame rates
(D) are not likely to produce artifacts

519. The attenuation coefficient is expressed in units of

(A) mW/cm²
(B) dB
(C) dB/cm
(D) mW

520. The wave equation relates

(A) time, mass, and distance
(B) time, velocity, and frequency
(C) wavelength, velocity, and frequency
(D) wavelength, distance, and frequency

521. The ability of a system to detect low-amplitude echoes accurately is referred to as

(A) resolution
(B) sensitivity
(C) accuracy
(D) dynamic range

522. The primary mechanisms whereby ultrasound can produce biologic effects are

(A) thermal and cavitation
(B) absorption and reflection
(C) reflection and transmission
(D) heat and cold

523. The near-zone length of a transducer depends on

(A) propagation speed and frequency
(B) frequency and transducer diameter
(C) field of view and transducer diameter
(D) path length

524. The AIUM Committee on Biological Effects (1982) stated that _____ biologic effects have been observed for ultrasound intensities below 100 mW/cm².

(A) no
(B) no confirmed
(C) few
(D) many

525. The intensity of a focused beam is generally

(A) constant
(B) highest at the transducer surface
(C) highest at the focal zone
(D) lowest at the transducer surface

526. The wavelength of a 5 MHz wave passing through soft tissue is approximately

(A) 0.1 mm
(B) 0.3 mm
(C) 0.5 mm
(D) 1.0 mm

527. An echo that has undergone an attenuation of 3 dB will have an intensity that is _____ than its initial intensity.

(A) three times smaller
(B) three times larger
(C) two times smaller
(D) two times larger

528. A pulse–echo system should have a high Q factor (quality-factor).

(A) true
(B) false

529. A 5 MHz transducer used in a pulse-echo system will generally produce

(A) a wide band of frequencies centered at 5 MHz
(B) frequencies only at 5 MHz
(C) frequencies only at 5 MHz or multiples of 5 MHz
(D) a wide band of frequencies above 5 MHz

530. The transducer _____ determines its _____.

(A) diameter, intensity
(B) damping, lateral resolution
(C) thickness, sensitivity
(D) thickness, resonance frequency

531. The axial resolution of a transducer can be improved with _____ but at the expense of _____.

(A) increased damping, sensitivity
(B) frequency, lateral resolution
(C) focusing, sensitivity
(D) focusing, lateral resolution

532. A material that changes its dimensions when an electric field is applied is called a _____ material.

(A) piezoelectric
(B) elastic
(C) inelastic
(D) compressible

533. The process of making the impedance values on either side of a boundary as close as possible to reduce reflections is called

(A) damping
(B) refracting
(C) matching
(D) compensating

534. When the pressure peaks of two waves coincide at a point to produce a new pressure that is larger than either of the two initial waves, the effect is called

(A) phase cancellation
(B) destructive interference
(C) enhancement
(D) constructive interference

535. Shadowing occurs with

(A) highly attenuating structures
(B) large changes in propagation speed
(C) low frequencies more often than with high frequencies
(D) weak reflectors

536. Reverberation artifacts

(A) occur most often at high frequencies
(B) occur with multiple strong reflecting structures
(C) occur only with real-time arrays
(D) cannot occur in color Doppler systems

537. A transducer with a large bandwidth is likely to have

(A) good axial resolution
(B) a large ring-down time
(C) poor resolution
(D) a high Q factor

538. The near zone is also referred to as the

(A) Fraunhofer zone
(B) Fresnel zone
(C) focal zone
(D) divergence zone

539. Refraction will not occur at an interface

  (A) when high frequencies are used
  (B) if the acoustic impedances are equal
  (C) if the propagation speeds are significantly different
  (D) with normal incidence of the ultrasound beam

540. Acoustic power output is determined primarily by

  (A) the diameter of the transducer
  (B) the thickness of the transducer
  (C) the pulser voltage spike
  (D) focusing

541. Specular reflections occur when

  (A) the reflecting object is small with respect to the wavelength
  (B) the reflecting surface is large and smooth with respect to the wavelength
  (C) the reflecting objects are moving
  (D) the angle of incidence and angle of reflection are unequal

542. The angle at which an ultrasound beam is bent as it passes through a boundary between two different materials is described mathematically by

  (A) Huygen's principle
  (B) Curie's principle
  (C) Snell's law
  (D) Doppler's law

543. An annular array real-time scanner

  (A) is steered electronically
  (B) is steered mechanically
  (C) is not capable of electronic focusing
  (D) is not used with digital-scan converters

544. The percentage of an ultrasound beam reflected at an interface between gas and soft tissue is approximately

  (A) 90–100%
  (B) 40–50%
  (C) 1–10%
  (D) < 1%

545. The percentage of an ultrasound beam reflected at an interface between fat and muscle is approximately

  (A) 90–100%
  (B) 40–50%
  (C) 1–10%
  (D) 0%

546. By using a waterpath offset,

  (A) tissue attenuation can be reduced
  (B) the focal zone can be moved to the skin surface
  (C) lower frequencies can be used
  (D) no reflections will occur at the skin surface

547. Ultrasound waves in tissue are referred to as

  (A) shear waves
  (B) transverse waves
  (C) vibrational waves
  (D) longitudinal compression waves

548. High-frequency transducers have

  (A) shorter wavelengths and less penetration
  (B) longer wavelengths and greater penetration
  (C) shorter wavelengths and greater penetration
  (D) longer wavelengths and less penetration

549. When the piezoelectric crystal continues to vibrate after the initial voltage pulse, this is referred to as

  (A) ring-down time
  (B) pulse delay
  (C) pulse retardation
  (D) overdamping

550. Annular phased arrays unlike linear phased arrays

  (A) can be dynamically focused
  (B) electronically focus in two dimensions rather than one
  (C) can be used in Doppler systems
  (D) can achieve high frame rates

551. Which group is arranged in the correct order of increasing propagation speed?

  (A) gas, bone, muscle
  (B) bone, muscle, gas
  (C) gas, muscle, bone
  (D) muscle, bone, gas

552. The lower useful range of diagnostic ultrasound is determined primarily by _____, whereas the upper useful range is determined by _____.

  (A) resolution, penetration
  (B) scattering, propagation speed
  (C) cost, resolution
  (D) scattering, resolution

553. Color Doppler systems are not subject to aliasing.

  (A) true
  (B) false

554. Which of the following is true?

  (A) SPTA is always equal to or greater than SPTP

(B) SPTP is always equal to or greater than SPTA

(C) SATA is always equal to or greater than SATP

(D) SPTA is always equal to or greater than SATP

555. A beam-intensity profile is often mapped with

(A) a radiation force balance
(B) a SUAR phantom
(C) a hydrophone
(D) AIUM phantom

556. Real-time scanners are generally classified as either

(A) electronic or mechanical
(B) dynamic or fixed
(C) programmable or fixed
(D) static or electronic

557. The technique of passing an ultrasound beam through water so that compression and rarefaction of the water molecules allow the beam pattern to be measured is referred to as the

(A) Doppler method
(B) Schlieren method
(C) hydrostatic method
(D) water-density method

558. Pulse duration is the _____ for a pulse to occur.

(A) space
(B) range
(C) intensity
(D) time

559. The frame rate of a real-time scanner will not depend on

(A) the depth of view
(B) the line density
(C) the frequency
(D) the propagation speed

560. The unit of measure of SPTA is

(A) dB
(B) W/cm²
(C) W
(D) Hz

561. The piezoelectric properties of a transducer will be lost if the crystal is heated above the

(A) dew point
(B) dynamic range
(C) Curie point
(D) linear range

562. If the amplitude of a wave is increased threefold, the intensity will

(A) decrease threefold
(B) increase threefold
(C) increase ninefold
(D) increase sixfold

563. A videotape recorder records at a rate of 30 frames/s and therefore cannot be used to record images from a mechanical scanner operating at lower frame rates.

(A) true
(B) false

564. If the frequency is increased, the _____ will be _____.

(A) velocity, increased
(B) attenuation, decreased
(C) velocity, decreased
(D) velocity, unchanged

565. Beam steering is achieved in a linear phased array by

(A) mechanical motion
(B) electronic time-delay pulsing
(C) an acoustic lens
(D) dynamic focusing

566. Dynamic focusing

(A) is made possible by array-based systems
(B) is made possible by acoustic lens
(C) is not possible in a linear-switched array
(D) is often used in single-element systems

567. Quality assurance measurements are not required with electronic scanners with digital scan converters.

(A) true
(B) false

568. Sound will travel _____ in 1 μs in soft tissue.

(A) 1540 m
(B) 1.54 cm
(C) 1.54 mm
(D) 0.75 mm

569. The arrow in Fig. 1–32 points to a

(A) ring-down artifact
(B) mirror image artifact
(C) side lobe artifact
(D) ghost artifact

Figure 1–32. Sonogram of an artifact.

Figure 1–33. Image from a tissue-equivalent phantom.

570. In the image in Fig. 1–33, which represents a tissue-equivalent phantom, the small open arrows point to

(A) rods for measuring "ring down"
(B) parallel rods used for horizontal calibration
(C) rods used for axial resolution
(D) rods used for measure registration

571. In the image in Fig. 1–33, which represents a tissue-equivalent phantom, the curved open arrow points to

(A) a dead zone
(B) a simulated solid lesion
(C) a ghost artifact
(D) a side lobe artifact

572. In the image in Fig. 1–33, which represents a tissue-equivalent phantom, the solid black arrow points to

(A) a ghost artifact
(B) a dead zone
(C) a simulated cyst
(D) a side lobe artifact

Answers and Explanations

At the end of each explained answer there is a number combination in parentheses. The first number identifies the reference source; the second number or set of numbers indicates the page or pages on which the relevant information can be found.

1. **(C)** Red blood cells. Structures smaller than a wavelength will scatter sound in all directions and are sometimes called diffuse reflectors. *(2:42)*

2. **(B)** Spatial pulse length is defined as the product of the number of cycles in the pulse and its wavelength. This is generally shorter for higher frequencies since the wavelength is shorter. *(2:64)*

3. **(D)** Axial resolution, also called longitudinal, range, or depth resolution, is determined by the wavelength, damping, and frequency. Axial resolution improves with increased frequency. *(2:64)*

4. **(B)** Lateral resolution is defined as being equal to the beam diameter. *(2:65)*

5. **(C)** The beam of an unfocused transducer diverges in the Fraunhofer (far) zone. *(1:360)*

6. **(C)** Reverberation artifacts are present when two or more strong reflectors are located within the beam. One of these may be the transducer itself. *(2:142)*

7. **(B)** False. Grating lobes are an undesirable property of multi-element array transducers. *(4:31)*

8. **(B)** False. Resolution is a function of the focusing characteristics of any scanner and cannot be assumed to be better for any particular scanner configuration. *(1:390–399)*

9. **(A)** True. Annular arrays may be used for creating variable focusing in two dimensions but are not capable of electronic steering of the beam. *(5:233)*

10. **(B)** False. The focusing of a linear array is controlled by timing and is thus capable of dynamic focusing. *(4:29)*

11. **(A, B, C, D, E)** All rods must be used to check registration accuracy. *(2:158)*

12. **(A)** See Fig. 1–24 and Table 1–3, Study Guide. *(2:156)*

13. **(B)** See Fig. 1–24 and Table 1–3, Study Guide. *(2:156)*

14. **(D)** See Fig. 1–24 and Table 1–3, Study Guide. *(2:156)*

15. **(C or E)** See Fig. 1–24 and Table 1–3, Study Guide. *(2:156)*

16. **(C)** Decreasing the spatial pulse length improves axial resolution. Axial resolution is equal to one-half of the spatial pulse length. *(2:64)*

17. **(B)** A rule of thumb approximating the attenuation coefficient of a reflected echo in soft tissue is 0.5 dB/cm/MHz. Thus the attenuation coefficient will be one-half the operating frequency.

    attenuation (dB) = attenuation coefficient (dB/cm)
    × path length (cm)
    dB = 1.75 dB/cm × 2 cm = 3.5 dB
    (2:23)

18. **(B)** Improper axial (along-the-beam) position. *(2:139)*

19. **(D)** Weakly attenuating structures. *(2:139)*

20. **(A)** Directly proportional to the velocity of the reflector. *(1:386)*

21. **(A)** More than 15 frames per second. *Note:* The scan converter in most modern systems turns the scanning frame rate (which is the subject of this question) into a display frame rate (or video frame rate) which is usually faster (30 video frames/s). This is done by displaying the same scan frame more than once if the scan frame is less than the video rate. *(4:34)*

22. **(A)** True. Spatial peak (SP) values will always be greater than spatial average (SA) intensity values.   *(2:21)*

23. **(B)** Smaller beam diameter. Intensity is defined as power per unit beam area; as the beam area decreases the intensity increases.   *(2:18)*

24. **(C)** Increased by four times. Intensity equals the square of the amplitude.   *(2:18)*

25. **(A)** Increased with tissue thickness. Attenuation is the product of the attenuation coefficient and path length.   *(2:23)*

26. **(A)** Should be chosen to be at a value approximately equal to the mean of impedances of the material on either side of it.   *(1:370)*

27. **(B)** False. The Q factor, or quality factor, of a transducer refers to the length of time that the sound persists. High-Q transducers tend to ring for a long time, whereas low-Q transducers ring for a shorter time. A low Q produces a short pulse length, which is necessary to provide good images.   *(1:359)*

28. **(B)** False. The beam diameter reduces to one-half of the transducer diameter from the face of the transducer to the focal point.   *(2:58)*

29. **(B)** Depends on crystal thickness. Thickness equals one-half the wavelength.   *(2:50)*

30. **(C)** The time of one wavelength.   *(2:6)*

31. **(D)** Ratio of smallest to largest power level.   *(2:84)*

32. **(A)** True. Radiation pressure can be measured with a sensitive balance and converted to intensity.   *(5:89)*

33. **(B)** Increases the maximum depth that can be imaged.   *(4:36)*

34. **(C)** Are not confirmed below 100 mW/cm² SPTA.   *(3:9)*

35. **(B)** False. Refraction comes as a result of changes in sound velocity across a boundary, not impedance.   *(4:7)*

36. **(B)** False. Beam diameter depends on whether or not the transducer is focused, the distance from the transducer, and whether one is in the near field or far field. Small transducers produce greatly diverging beams in the far field.   *(1:364)*

37. **(A)** True. A hydrophone is usually a very small piezoelectric crystal that can be moved in front of the transmitting crystal to map its beam characteristics.   *(5:85)*

38. **(A)** True. Pulsed Doppler utilizes range gating to localize the signals to specific depths.   *(5:385)*

39. **(B)** False. Gray-scale ultrasound images were also possible with analog storage devices.   *(5:198)*

40. **(B)** False. If the imaging rate is slower than the video framing rate, frames are duplicated to fill in.   *(4:44)*

41. **(B)** False. Linear arrays must also be focused in the direction perpendicular to the array axis to reduce the slice thickness. This is usually accomplished by mechanical focusing.   *(1:394)*

42. **(A)** True. Real-time scanners display 15 to 60 images per second, called the frame rate. This rate must be greater than 15 frames per second to produce a flicker-free image. Each frame is made of scan lines, the number of lines per frame, and the number of frames per second are related to one another.   *(4:35, 2:105)*

43. **(A)** True. Annular phased arrays must be steered mechanically, most frequently through the use of an oscillating acoustic mirror.   *(3:4)*

44. **(B)** False. Images produced in the near zone have the best lateral resolution; therefore, the near zone length should be long enough to include all time regions-of-interest.   *(1:362)*

45. **(C)** Twenty-five percent. The reflection coefficient (*r*) is equal to:

$$r = \left(\frac{Z_2 - Z_1}{Z_2 + Z_1} \right)^2 = \left(\frac{0.75 - 0.25}{0.75 + 0.25} \right)^2 = 0.25$$

where Z_1 and Z_2 are the acoustic impedances of each material.   *(1:366)*

46. **(A)** Higher frequency transducers usually produce shorter spatial pulse lengths and thus improve axial resolution.   *(2:64)*

47. **(A)** Longitudinal wave.   *(4:2)*

48. **(A)** 0.3 mm.

$$\text{wavelength (mm)} = \frac{\text{velocity (mm/}\mu\text{s)}}{\text{frequency (MHz)}} = \frac{1.5}{5} = 0.3 \text{ mm}$$

(4:2)

49. **(D)** The specific acoustic impedance. The fraction of sound reflected at an interface (r) is given by:

$$r = \left(\frac{Z_2 - Z_1}{Z_2 + Z_1} \right)^2$$

where Z_1 and Z_2 are the acoustic impedance of the boundary material.   *(1:366)*

50. **(A)** V or C = propagation velocity (cm/s)
    f = frequency (cycles/s)
    λ = wavelength (cm)
    $V = f\lambda$ *(31:9; 12:2)*

51. **(D)** All of the above. Reflection refers to echoes; refraction refers to the bending of the beam; and mode conversion refers to a change in the propagation mode transverse, shear, surface, or longitudinal waves.   *(5:15–19)*

52. **(D)** Equal to the product of density and velocity for longitudinal waves.   *(1:365)*

53. **(C)** 1540 meters per second.   *(1:353)*

54. **(B)** False. The magnitude of the Doppler shift frequency is directly related to the cosine of the angle between the direction of the blood flow and the receiver angle. The maximum shift frequency is therefore observed when the flow is along the receiver line-of-sight.   *(1:386)*

55. **(B)** Wave velocity. Refraction is described by Snell's law, which relates the incident angle (θ_i) to the transmitted angle (θ_t) to the relative velocities of the two media making up the interface:

$$\frac{\sin \theta_i}{\sin \theta_t} = \frac{V_1}{V_2}$$

          (1:367)

56. **(A)** Acoustic impedance.   *(1:366)*

57. **(C)** The material through which the sound is being transmitted and the mode of vibration.   *(1:353)*

58. **(C)** No change. The velocity of sound propagation depends on the material through which it is being transmitted and is independent of frequency. *(1:353)*

59. **(A)** Refraction.   *(1:367)*

60. **(A)** Using a higher frequency transducer. The near zone length (x) is given by:

$$x = \frac{r^2}{\lambda}$$

where r is the radius of the transducer and λ is the wavelength. Thus, a longer near zone length is achieved by increasing the transducer diameter or increasing the frequency.   *(1:367)*

61. **(A)** 0.75 mm. The wavelength can be determined by using the following equation:

$$\lambda = \frac{v}{f}$$

    v = propagation velocity (m/s)
    f = frequency (Hz)
    λ = wavelength (m)

For example: $\lambda = \dfrac{1500 \text{ meters per second}}{2 \text{ MHz}}$

$$\lambda = \frac{1.5 \times 10^3 \text{ meters per second}}{2 \times 10^6 \text{ cycles per second}}$$

$$\lambda = 0.75 \times 10^{-3} \text{ meters}$$

$$\lambda = 0.75 \text{ mm}$$

          (2:8; 12:2)

62. **(B)**

$$\begin{array}{l} Z \text{ (impedance)} \\ \text{for longitudinal waves} \end{array} = \frac{\text{particle pressure}}{\text{particle velocity}}$$

          (5:13)

63. **(A)** Doppler-shift formula.   *(2:125)*

64. **(C)** Huygens.   *(1:362; 5:26)*

65. **(B)** Tenfold difference in intensity or power. *(2:255)*

66. **(B)** Threshold, negative, or reject level.   *(1:376)*

67. **(B)** Compression.   *(2:84)*

68. **(A)** A-mode.   *(1:370)*

69. **(D)** Relaxation processes are modes by which ultrasound may be attenuated in passing through a material. Suppression is another name for rejection.   *(2:79–85)*

70. **(B)** Digital scan converter.   *(3:31)*

71. **(A)** Duty factor.   *(2:55)*

72. **(D)** Sensitivity.   *(2:155)*

73. **(B)** Linear array transducers produce a rectangular image. (Sector scanners produce a pie-shaped image.)   *(3:18–26)*

74. **(B)** Magnitude of the voltage spike applied to the transducer by the pulser.   *(2:77)*

75. **(D)** Thermal and cavitational.   *(2:171)*

76. **(C)** Quality factor, or Q factor, is equal to the operating frequency divided by the bandwidth.   *(1:36)*

77. **(C)** Side lobes.   *(5:29)*

78. **(D)** Pulse duration.   *(2:15)*

79. **(B)** The silicon oxide matrix is charged by a scanning electron beam, producing an image pattern that can be displayed on a video monitor.   *(5:198)*

80. **(C)** Reflectors whose boundaries are smooth relative to a wavelength behave as mirrors and are called specular reflectors.   *(2:42)*

81. **(B)** Schlieren technique of measurement.   *(1:362)*

82. **(D)** Reverberation.   *(2:140)*

83. **(B)** Enhancement.   *(2:146)*

84. **(B)** Using a larger diameter transducer. The dispersion angle in the far field (θ) is given as: $\sin \theta = 1.22\, \lambda/d$, where λ is the wavelength and d is the diameter of the transducer. The angle can be reduced by using either a larger transducer or a higher frequency (smaller wavelength).   *(1:364)*

85. **(B)** Spatial pulse length.

$$\text{axial resolution (mm)} = \frac{\text{spatial pulse length (mm)}}{2}$$

(2:64)

86. **(B)** Quality factor (Q factor).

$$Q = \frac{f_0}{f_2 - f_1}$$

where f_0 is the central resonance frequency and ($f_2 - f_1$) is the frequency bandwidth.   *(2:53; 1:360)*

87. **(C)** Schlieren technique.   *(1:362)*

88. **(D)** Blood.   *(1:369)*

89. **(A)** Dynamic range.   *(2:84)*

90. **(D)** Longitudinal waves.   *(1:352)*

91. **(B)** Axial resolution.   *(2:156)*

92. **(C)** Scan C.   *(2:158)*

93. **(A)** Dead zone.   *(2:156)*

94. **(A)** Call for service.   *(6:23–24)*

95. **(C)** Horizontal caliper check.   *(6:15)*

96. **(B)** Lateral resolution.   *(6:19–26)*

97. **(E)** Gray scale and dynamic range.   *(2:158; 6:19–24)*

98. **(D)** Registration.   *(6:18)*

99. **(E)** All of the answers given are correct.   *(6:10–24)*

100. **(F)** All of the answers given are correct.   *(6:10–24)*

101. **(C, D, F, G, H)** Lead zirconate titanate, barium titanate, lithium sulfate, lead metaniobate, and ammonium dihydrogen phosphate are not natural.   *(7:85–87; 8:28)*

102. **(C)** Cork, rubber, epoxy resin, and tungsten powder in araldite are good acoustic insulators. Water and oil are not.   *(8:38–39)*

103. **(A)** Sound and ultrasound are mechanical vibrations that can propagate in matter, such as liquid and solid. However, sound or ultrasound cannot travel in a vacuum.   *(10:1)*

104. **(A)** Infrasound (subsonic).   *(10:1)*

105. **(B)** Ultrasound.   *(10:1)*

106. **(B)** Audible sound.   *(10:1)*

107. **(B)** The electromagnetic spectrum is a large family of electromagnetic waves. Light, x-rays, and infrared and ultraviolet rays are among its spectrum; ultrasound is not.   *(1:1–3)*

108. **(D)** Cycle per second (cps).   *(10:1)*

109. **(B)** Electrical energy into mechanical energy and vice versa.   *(2:48)*

110. **(E)** All of the answers given are correct.   *(2:48)*

111. **(D)** Increase or decrease depending on the polarity applied.   *(2:49)*

112. **(D)** 1 mega = 1 million. Therefore, 5 MHz = 5 million cycles per second or 5 million Hz.   *(10:1)*

113. **(G)** The damping material reduces pulse duration and spatial pulse length, and as a result it improves axial resolution.   *(2:51)*

114. **(A)** Velocity of ultrasound transmitted through a medium depends on the properties of the medium: (1) temperature, (2) elasticity, and (3) density. The speed of ultrasound varies with temperature. However, temperature/velocity in human soft tissue can usually be ignored because body temperature is usually constant within a narrow range, for example: 94°F (low) to 106°F (high). The velocity of ultrasound in soft tissue at 37°C or 98.6°F (body temperature) is 1540 meters per second (1540 m/s).   *(11:3; 9:55; 10:5)*

115. **(C)** A single cycle.   *(11:2)*

116. **(A)** Particle motion parallel to (or in the same direction of) the axis of wave propagation.   *(7:4)*

117. **(C)** Particle motion perpendicular to the axis of wave propagation.   *(7:4)*

118. **(B)** Condensations.   *(7:4)*

119. **(C)** Rarefactions.   *(7:4)*

120. **(D)** Pressure.   *(11:9)*

121. **(F)**   *(2:64)*

122. **(F)**   *(2:64)*

123–131. See Fig. 1–8 in the Study Guide.   *(1:367; 2:98)*

132–140. See Fig. 1–23 in the Study Guide.   *(12:2; 1:373)*

141. **(A)** If frequency increases, the wavelength decreases.   *(2:140–141)*

142. **(B)** If frequency decreases, the wavelength increases.   *(2:140–141)*

143. **(A)** As frequency increases, the penetration decreases.   *(2:140–141)*

144. **(B)** As frequency increases, the resolution increases.   *(2:140–141)*

145. **(A)** Higher frequency transmits shorter pulse and narrower beam width.   *(9:31)*

146. **(F)** Air, bone, and barium sulfate ($BaSO_4$). The contrast material used for intravenous pyelogram (IVP) does not prevent the propagation of ultrasound.   *(12:2; 13:413)*

147. **(C)** Barium sulfate ($BaSO_4$). A coupling medium is a liquid medium placed between the transducer and the skin to eliminate air gap. Air has a reflection coefficient approaching 100%, which results in almost zero transmission. Water or saline can also be used but they dry out faster than gel.   *(13:10–11; 11:52)*

148. **(A)** The progressive weakening of the sound beam as it travels. Attenuation occurs because of (1) absorption, (2) reflection, and (3) scatter. Barium sulfate and air impair ultrasound transmissions.   *(11:4)*

149. **(C)** When crystals are subjected to pressure resulting in electrical charge on their surfaces, it is called a piezoelectric effect.   *(10:12)*

150. **(B)** When crystals are subjected to electrical impulse and generate ultrasound as a result, it is called reverse piezoelectric effect.   *(10:12)*

151. **(B)** Attenuation is the amount of energy lost per unit of depth into the tissue. The parameter used to express the energy loss is the decibel (dB).

$$dB = 10 \log_{10} \frac{I_2}{I_1}$$

   (12:5)

152. **(C)** Waves carry energy from one place to another through a medium.   *(14:1)*

153. **(A)** A mechanical wave causes particles to oscillate around its equilibrium point.   *(14:2)*

154. **(C)** Wavelength is the distance between two identical points on the waveform.   *(14:4)*

155. **(A)** Ultrasonic waves are mechanical. A medium is required for propagation of sounds.   *(14:1)*

156. **(B)** Acoustic impedance is defined as the density of tissue × the speed of sound in tissue ($Z = pc$). *(15:30)*

157. **(D)** Amplitude is defined as the height of the wave. For amplitude, dB = 20 log (amplitude ratio).   *(15:3)*

158. **(B)** Ultrasound is above 20,000 cycles per second (Hz) and is above the audible range of sound.   *(15:2)*

159. **(D)** The equation for period is:

$$period = \frac{1}{frequency}$$

   (14:2)

160. **(D)** The direction of the returning echo is related to the beam angle. The more perpendicular the beam gets to an organ interface, the greater the specular reflection.   *(15:5)*

161. **(A)** A decibel is the ratio of two sound intensities, highest to lowest (or vice versa).   *(14:1)*

162. **(C)** Azimuthal is another name for *lateral* resolution.   *(14:6)*

163. **(B)** Bone has the highest sound velocity due to its stiffness.   *(14:8)*

164. **(B)** No significant biologic effects have been proven in mammals exposed below 100 mW/cm² spatial peak, temporal average (SPTA).   *(2:175)*

165. **(A)** Temporal peak intensity is measured at the time the pulse is present.   *(14:5)*

166. **(D)** SATA has the lowest intensity since the intensity is averaged over the whole beam profile (SA), and over the whole duration of exposure (TA).   *(2:21)*

167. **(B)** The beam uniformity ratio is defined as the spatial peak intensity (measured at the beam center) divided by the spatial average intensity (the average intensity across the beam).   *(2:19)*

168. **(C)** The duty factor is the fraction of time the transducer is emitting sound. In a pulsed echo system it is normally less than 1%.   *(14:5)*

169. **(D)** Axial resolution is defined as one-half the spatial pulse length. Therefore, the shorter the spatial pulse length the better the axial resolution.   *(14:6)*

170. **(B)** V = velocity of sound (cm/sec); f = frequency (cycle/sec); and λ = wavelength (cm).   *(1:364)*

171. **(D)** Attenuation of an ultrasound beam can occur by divergence of a beam, scattering, and reflection. It can also occur by absorption.   *(14:8)*

172. **(A)** Attenuation coefficient of sound is defined by dB/cm/MHz.   *(14:12)*

173. **(C)** Transducer Q factor (quality factor) is equal to the operating frequency divided by the bandwidth. Therefore, if the transducer Q factor is low, the bandwidth is wide.   *(14:6)*

174. **(A)** Axial resolution can be improved by shortening pulse length, increasing damping, and a higher-frequency transducer.   *(14:6)*

175. **(B)** Axial resolution is primarily affected by spatial pulse length. Because the spatial pulse length is the product of wavelength, reducing the wavelength or increasing the frequency will affect axial resolution.   *(2:64)*

176. **(D)** Increasing transducer frequency will improve both lateral and axial resolution but decrease depth of penetration.   *(2:69)*

177. **(C)** Range resolution is another name for *axial* resolution.   *(2:65)*

178. **(B)** The duty factor is the fraction of time that sound is being emitted from the transducer. In continuous wave the sound is being emitted 100% of the time.   *(2:20)*

179. **(A)** Acoustic impedance (Z) is defined as density (p) × propagation speed (c). $Z = pc$.   *(2:10)*

180. **(D)** Acoustic impedance is defined by the unit rayl. Density is defined by kg/m³, and propagation speed by meters per second.   *(2:10)*

181. **(A)** Acoustic impedance is dependent on density and stiffness. It does not depend on frequency.   *(2:10)*

182. **(A)** The height of the vertical spike corresponds to the strength of the echo received by the transducer.   *(6:60)*

183. **(B)** B-mode is an acronym for brightness modulation. Both real-time and static scanning are B-mode display.   *(6:60)*

184. **(A)** The correct equation for calculating reflection percentage is:

$$R = \left(\frac{Z_2 - Z_1}{Z_2 + Z_1} \right)^2 \times 100$$

(31:14–15)

185. **(D)** The reflection coefficient between water and air interface is nearly 100%. Air prevents the sound from entering the body. It is for this reason that a coupling gel is necessary.   *(13:8)*

186. **(B)** Beyond the critical angle, 100% of the sound beam is reflected and 0% is transmitted.   *(13:9)*

187. **(A)** Rayleigh scattering occurs when the particle size is smaller than a wavelength (for ultrasound typically in the 1-mm range).   *(13:9)*

188. **(B)** Particle displacement is an acoustic parameter which is related to the intensity of an ultrasound wave. Other intensity-related factors include sound velocity, pressure, amplitude, and density of the medium.   *(13:4)*

189. **(C)** Power is defined as the rate at which work is done or energy is transferred (energy per unit time). *(2:269)*

190. **(A)** Lateral resolution is the minimum separation between two reflectors perpendicular to the sound path. *(2:65)*

191. **(D)** In most soft tissues the attenuation coefficient increases directly with frequency. As frequency is increased the attenuation coefficient increases, thereby limiting depth of perception. *(13:9)*

192. **(A)** Absorption is the conversion of sound into heat. Absorption, scattering, and reflection are all factors of attenuation. *(2:23)*

193. **(D)** The rule of thumb for attenuation in soft tissue is 0.5 dB per centimeter per megahertz. Therefore an ultrasound beam of 1-MHz frequency will lose 0.5 dB of amplitude for every centimeter traveled. *(11:4)*

194. **(C)** Reverberations produce false echoes. *(2:142)*

195. **(D)** The acoustic mismatch between fat and muscle is small; therefore, approximately 99% of the sound beam is transmitted. *(14:10)*

196. **(A)** Huygens' principle states that all points on a wavefront can be considered as a source for secondary spherical wavelets. *(14:3)*

197. **(B)** Enhancement is the "burst of sound" visualized posterior to weak attenuations. *(2:151)*

198. **(A)** Half-value layer (HVL—sometimes called half-intensity depth) is defined as the thickness of tissue that reduces the beam intensity by half. *(13:10)*

199. **(D)** Propagation speed error. The ultrasound machine assumes a speed of 1540 meters per second (1540 m/s). If the sound passes through a medium of a different velocity, the result is an error in the range equation. *(2:146)*

200. **(B)** Range equation explains the distance to the reflector, which is equal to one-half of the propagation speed × the pulse round-trip time. *(2:44)*

201. **(A)** For a specular reflector, the angle of incidence is equal to the angle of reflection. *(14:9)*

202. **(C)** Propagation speed is determined by the medium. Amplitude, period, and intensity are determined by the transducer. *(2:5)*

203. **(D)** Acoustic variables include density, pressure, temperature, and particle motion. *(2:5)*

204. **(B)** Time gain compensation. *(15:19)*

205. **(B)** The propagation speed for fat is 1440 meters per second (1440 m/s), which is lower than that of average soft tissue. *(2:10)*

206. **(D)** Muscle has a propagation speed of 1585 meters per second (1585 m/s), which is very close to average soft tissue at 1540 m/s. *(14:8)*

207. **(A)** A is correct, with the propagation velocity in this order respectively: 331 m/s, 1450 m/s, 1585 m/s, and 4080 m/s. *(2:9, 180)*

208. **(C)** Backscatter is increased by increasing frequency and increasing heterogeneous media. *(2:32)*

209. **(A)** Critical angle is the angle at which sound is totally reflected and none is transmitted. *(13:9)*

210. **(D)** The pulse repetition frequency (PRF) is the number of pulses occurring per second. The PRF is inversely proportional to the pulse repetition period. *(2:16)*

211. **(D)** The duty factor is the fraction of time that the transducer is emitting a pulse. It is unitless. *(2:15)*

212. **(A)** The attenuation coefficient is the attenuation per unit length of sound travel. Its typical value is 3 dB/cm, for 6 MHz sound in soft tissue (0.5 dB/cm/MHz × 6 MHz = 3 dB/cm). *(2:28)*

213. **(B)** Normal incidence is also known as perpendicular incidence. At normal incidence sound may be reflected or transmitted in various degrees. *(2:32)*

214. **(A)** The difference (mismatch) of acoustic impedance between two media is what determines how much energy will be transmitted and/or reflected. *(14:10)*

215. **(A)** Acoustic impedance is equal to the product of the density of a substance and the velocity of sound. The propagation speed in solids is higher than in liquids, and the propagation speed in gas is low. The increase in propagation speed is caused by increasing stiffness of the media, not by the density. *(2:180)*

216. **(A)** According to Snell's law,

$$\frac{\sin i}{\sin r} = \frac{V_1}{V_2}$$

the transmission angle is proportional to the incidence angle times the medium 2 propagation speed divided by the medium 1 propagation speed. *(2:30)*

217. **(C)** The propagation speed of the medium must be known in order to calculate the distance to the reflector. In addition, the round-trip must be measured. The distance to the reflector is equal to the product of the propagation speed and the pulse round-trip time divided by 2. *(2:45)*

218. **(D)** The mirror image artifact occurs around strong reflectors, for example the diaphragm. *(2:144–146)*

219. **(C)** The comet tail artifact is a type of reverberation artifact. The greater the acoustic impedance mismatch, the greater the possibility of this artifact to occur. *(16:7)*

220. **(C)** The acoustic impedance mismatch between tissue and gas is very great; therefore, it may produce the comet tail artifact. *(16:7)*

221. **(B)** Fat has a slower velocity than the liver. Therefore, the returning time of the echo to the transducer is delayed. Since the ultrasound machine assumes that everything in its path has a velocity of 1540 meters per second (1540 m/s), the diaphragm posterior to the fat is registered as farther than it actually is. *(19:58)*

222. **(D)** By increasing damping one also increases the bandwidth. Bandwidth is the range of frequency involved in a pulse. *(2:54)*

223. **(A)** Output affects the amount of energy leaving the transducer. It does not affect the amplification of echoes that are received. *(14:12)*

224. **(B)** The compression controls on some sonographic equipment, when adjusted, will reduce the dynamic range. Compression is the process of decreasing the difference between small and large amplitude echoes. *(14:13)*

225. **(A)** Ultrasound transducers generally can resolve reflectors along the sound path better than it can those perpendicular to it. *(2:69)*

226. **(D)** The number of electrical pulses produced per second is typically 1000 Hz. *(2:77)*

227. **(D)** Brightness modulation mode. This display is used in two-dimensional ultrasound images, real-time and static. *(6:60)*

228. **(B)** With a typical PRF of 1000 Hz, each pulse-receive interval is 1 millisecond (1000 microseconds) long. Since an average pulse is 1 microsecond long, this leaves 999 microseconds for receiving. 999/1000 is 99.9%. *(20:190)*

229. **(C)** Frequency equals velocity divided by wavelength. Since velocity is standard at 1540 m/s, doubling the frequency will result in decreasing the wavelength by one-half. *(2:8)*

230. **(A)** Real-time transducers display two formats: sector and rectangular. The linear-sequenced array transducer displays a rectangular format. *(2:120)*

231. **(C)** Z is the acoustic impedance; P is the material density; and V is the propagation velocity. *(12:2)*

232. **(A)** Lead zirconate titanate (PZT) is a ceramic material with piezoelectric properties. It is most commonly used in transducers because of its greater efficiency and sensitivity. *(6:50)*

233. **(B)** Transmit–delay focusing creates a narrow beam, which improves lateral resolution. *(14:19)*

234. **(D)** Pulse repetition frequency is equal to lines per frame and is related to time frame rate. Frequency has no relationship to this equation. *(2:77)*

235. **(A)** Pulse repetition frequency is the number of pulses emitted per second or pulse rate. *(2:140)*

236. **(D)** The pulser produces the electric voltage pulses; this in turn drives the transducer to emit ultrasound pulses. It also tells both the memory and receiver when the ultrasound pulses were produced. *(2:77)*

237. **(A)** Demodulation converts the voltage delivered to the receiver from one form to another by rectification and smoothing. *(2:82)*

238. **(C)** Demodulation and compression are not operator adjustable. Amplification, compensation, and rejection functions are operator adjustable. *(2:85)*

239. **(A)** Lateral resolution is dependent on beam diameter, which varies with distance from the transducer. *(2:65)*

240. **(C)** A period is the time it takes for one full cycle to occur. *(2:7)*

241. **(B)** Half-intensity depth decreases with increasing frequency. *(2:64)*

242. **(C)** Redirection of a portion of the sound beam from a boundary. *(11:5)*

243. **(D)** Computers use a special number system called binary numbers. The system uses two digits, 0 and 1. *(18:8.2)*

244. **(A)** Bit is an acronym for binary digit and represents the basic unit for storing data in the main computer memory. *(18:8.1)*

245. **(A)** Eight bits equal 1 byte. A bit is a unit of data in binary notation and assumes one of two states: "on" representing the number 1, or "off" representing the number 0. *(17:136)*

246. **(B)** A computer and its peripherals are categorized into hardware and software. Hardware is the term used to describe any of the physical embodiments of the computer, for example, the keyboard, disk drive, CRT, and printer. Computer programs are software. The software in turn runs the hardware. *(17:139)*

247. **(B)** Random-access memory. This type of memory is called random because it provides access to any storage location in the memory. *(18:8.13)*

248. **(A)** Read-only memory. This type of program memory provides access to read out only. *(18:8.13)*

249. **(B)** Any set of computer devices that transfers information or data from an external medium into the internal storage of the computer is called an input device. A printer is an output device. *(18:3.2)*

250. **(B)** ROM (read-only memory) is programmed into the computer at the time of manufacture. PROM (programmable read-only memory) can be written to by the programmer. *(18:8.13)*

251. **(D)** Erasable programmable read-only memory (EPROM) can be reprogrammed or erased. *(18:8.13)*

252. **(B)** Central processing unit (CPU). *(18:8.1)*

253. **(B)** Most microprocessors use 8-, 16- or 32-bit word length. The most common is a 16-bit. *(18:8.1–8.17)*

254. **(C)** While the symbol K represents kilo or 1000 in metric, in computer terminology K = 1024. The amount that can be stored in memory is then $128 \times 1024 \times 8$ bits = 1,048,576 bits, referred to as 1 megabit. *(18:8.1–8.17)*

255. **(D)** Contents of EPROM are erased by exposing them to ultraviolet light. *(18:8.13)*

256. **(B)** Modem. *(18:11.5)*

257. **(C)** BASIC. *(18:13.8)*

258. **(D)** Baud rate. The measured speed is expressed in the number of bits per second (bps). *(18:11.9)*

259. **(B)** Hard disks have a larger storage capacity and faster access than do floppy disks. *(18:9.9)*

260. **(C)** Beginner's all-purpose symbolic instruction code (BASIC). *(18:13.8)*

261. **(C)** A modem is an acronym for modulator/demodulator. It is a device that translates digital data to analog signals and vice versa over standard telephone lines. *(18:11.5)*

262. **(B)** Two: off or on. "Off" represents the number 0. "On" represents the number 1. *(19:33; 17:137)*

263. **(C)** Two (0 or 1). *(19:31)*

264. **(E)** The number 30 is represented by 011110. To convert from decimal to binary, repeatedly divide by two and note the remainder.

$30 \div 2 = 15$ remainder 0 $3 \div 2 = 1$ remainder 1
$15 \div 2 = 7$ remainder 1 $1 \div 2 = 0$ remainder 1
$7 \div 2 = 3$ remainder 1 $0 \div 2 = 0$ remainder 0

(2:259)

265. **(D)** The binary system, which is used in digital scan converter memory, is based on the powers of two. For four bits, 2^4 ($2 \times 2 \times 2 \times 2$) or 16 different gray levels can be represented. Another way of looking at this is to list all possible states:

0000	0100	1000	1100
0001	0101	1001	1101
0010	0110	1010	1110
0011	0111	1011	1111

There are 16 possible unique states. *(19:32)*

266. **(B)** Digital memory, where the electronic components are either on (1) or off (0), is based on the binary number system. We can say that the number of discrete levels possible, N, is equal to 2 raised to the power of that number of bits. $N = 2^n$. Therefore, to make 64 shades of gray would require 2^6 bit memory.

$(2 \times 2 \quad 4 \times 2 \quad 8 \times 2 \quad 16 \times 2 \quad 32 \times 2 = 64)$
$1 \qquad 2 \qquad 3 \qquad 4 \qquad 5 \qquad 6$

(19:32)

267. **(B)** At high ultrasound intensities, tissue damage has been observed to be caused by heat and cavitation. *(7:185)*

268. **(C)** The receiver processes echoes detected by the transducer. These echoes may be amplified (gain), compensated for depth (TGC), compressed (to fit into the dynamic range of the system), and rejected (eliminating low-level signals). *(19:27)*

269. **(D)** The greater the pulse amplitude (electronic voltage applied to the transducer), the greater the amplitude of the ultrasound pulse provided by the transducer. *(2:77)*

270. **(B)** The pulser produces electric voltage pulses which drive the transducer and at the same time tell the receiver that the transducer has been driven. *(2:77)*

271. **(D)** Components of a pulse–echo system include the *pulser* that produces the electrical pulse which drives the *transducer*. For each reflection received from the tissue by the transducer, an electrical voltage is produced that goes to the *receiver,* where it is processed for display. Information on transducer position and orientation is delivered to the *image memory*. Electric information from the memory drives the *display* (oscilloscope). *(2:75)*

272. **(B)** Transducers may be focused by using a curved piezoelectric transducer element (internal focusing) or by using an acoustic lens. *(19:20)*

273. **(E)** Quality factor (Q factor) is equal to the operating frequency divided by the bandwidth, and is unitless. *(2:54)*

274. **(E)** Reduction in echoes from a region distal to an attenuating structure. *(2:216)*

275. **(G)** An increase in echoes from a region distal to a weakly attenuating structure or tissue. *(2:212)*

276. **(A or F)** A structure that is echo-free. Not necessarily cystic unless there is good through transmission. A solid mass can be anechoic but will not have good through transmission. *(15:27)*

277. **(D)** An echo that does not correspond to the real target. *(21)*

278. **(I)** A structure that possesses echoes. *(15:27)*

279. **(H)** Echoes of higher amplitude than the normal surrounding tissues. *(21)*

280. **(B)** Echoes of lower amplitude than the normal surrounding tissues. *(21)*

281. **(C)** The surface forming the boundary between two media having different acoustic impedances. *(15:28)*

282. **(A or F)** A structure without echoes and with low absorption. Not necessarily cystic unless there is good through transmission. *Sonolucent* is a misnomer for *anechoic*. *(15:29; 21)*

283. **(C)** Air. There are numerable backing materials used for damping. Pulse–echo transducer backing materials are: (1) epoxy resin, (2) tungsten, (3) cork, and (4) rubber. Continuous-wave Doppler transducers have little or no backing materials. They are usually air backed. *(9:263; 22:33)*

284. **(D)** Surgical, therapeutic, and Doppler. Diagnostic application uses a pulse–echo transducer. *(9:311; 19:23; 22:33)*

285. **(A)** Not all waves are visible. Waves that appear on the surface of water (water waves) are visible. X-rays, radio waves, and sound waves are invisible waves. *(17:3)*

286. **(C)** In order for ultrasound to propagate a medium, the medium must be composed of particles of matter. A vacuum is a space empty of matter; therefore, ultrasound cannot travel in a vacuum. *(10:1; 25:19)*

287. **(B)** Wavelength. *(17:5)*

288. **(A)** Period. *(17:5)*

289. **(B)** Hertz (Hz) represents cycle per second (cps). Therefore, 20 cps = 20 Hz. *(17:5)*

290. **(C)** One MHz. *(17:5)*

291. **(C)** Ultrasound is produced by piezoelectric crystal. The crystal, damping material, and matching layer are enclosed in a device called a transducer. *(17:31)*

292. **(A)** A-mode is an acronym for amplitude mode. This mode is presented graphically with vertical spikes arising from a horizontal baseline. The height of the vertical spikes represents the amplitude of the deflected echo. *(22:2)*

293. **(B)** B-mode is an acronym for brightness modulation. This mode presents a two-dimensional image of internal body structures displayed as dots. The brightness of the dots is proportional to the amplitude of the echo. B-mode display is employed in all two-dimensional images, static or real-time. *(6:60; 22:2)*

294. **(C)** M-mode is an acronym for time–motion modulation. This mode is a graphical display of movement of reflecting structures related to time. M-mode is used almost exclusively in echocardiography. *(6:60; 22:2)*

295. **(C)** The cathode-ray tube (CRT) is formed by three essential elements: (1) the electron gun, (2) the fluorescent screen, and (3) the deflection system (vertical and horizontal plates). Silicon is a nonmetallic element found in the earth and used in computer semiconductors.   *(24:234)*

296. **(B)** The cathode-ray tube (CRT) is enclosed by a glass tube containing a high vacuum. The manufacturer normally "degases" the tube (removes trapped air or gas) in order to provide a free passage for electrons.   *(17:88; 9:13–15)*

297. **(A)** The anode is the counterpart of the cathode and is positively (+) charged.   *(17:88)*

298. **(B)** The cathode consists of the electron gun and filament and is negatively (−) charged.   *(17:88)*

299. **(C)** The intensity of the ultrasound beam depends on the beam diameter. Intensity is defined as the beam power divided by the beam cross-sectional area.   *(2:18)*

300. **(C)** Huygens' principle   *(1:362)*

301. **(A)** The fraction of time that a pulsed ultrasound is actually producing ultrasound is called the duty factor.

$$\text{duty factor (DF)} = \frac{\text{pulse duration (PD)}}{\text{pulse repetition period (PRP)}}$$

(2:55)

302. **(C)** Real-time ultrasound instrumentation is classified as

1. Sector — Linear-phased array (pie shaped) / Wobbler or rotating wheel (pie shaped)

2. Linear-sequenced array——rectangular image

3. Annular——employs both mechanical and electronic (combination systems)

(3:15–30; 22:6–9)

303. **(B)** The speed at which ultrasound propagates within a medium depends primarily on the compressibility of the medium.   *(34:1)*

304. **(C)** The reverberation artifact occurs when two or more reflections are present along the path of the beam. This gives rise to multiple reflections, which will appear behind one another at intervals equal to the separation of the real reflectors.   *(11:40; 19:50)*

305. **(C)** Gain is the ratio of electric power. Gain governs the electric compensation for tissue attenuation and is expressed in decibels (dB).   *(2:80; 9:89)*

306. **(C)** Multipath reverberation artifacts result from sound reflected from a highly curved specular surface when the echo takes an indirect path back to the transducer.   *(6:28–29)*

307. **(B)** Both analog and digital scan converters are memory devices. An analog converter stores image information gathered during the scanning process and then retrieves and reads out the information to a vacuum tube similar to a CRT oscilloscope without the phosphor screen. A digital scan converter takes the incoming analog signals from the detector and converts them to binary numbers that are used to represent signal levels. These numbers are then stored in memory.   *(19:31–32)*

308. **(B)** Echo signals that are in analog format as they emerge from the receiver are transferred to a digital format by an analog-to-digital (A–D) converter. Preprocessing then produces the best possible digital representation of the analog signal.   *(19:32)*

309. **(D)** By increasing frequency (f) and/or transducer diameter, the near zone length is increased, as shown in the equation:

$$\text{near zone length} = \frac{(\text{transducer diameter})^2 f}{6}$$

(2:59)

310. **(B)** Mass divided by volume.   *(2:209–217)*

311. **(H)** Progression or travel.   *(2:209–217)*

312. **(D)** Number of cycles per unit time.   *(2:209–217)*

313. **(A)** Rate at which work is done.   *(2:209–217)*

314. **(G)** The product of pulse duration and pulse repetition rate.   *(2:209–217)*

315. **(F)** Range of frequencies contained in the ultrasound pulse.   *(2:209–217)*

316. **(E)** Density multiplied by sound propagation speed.   *(2:209–217)*

317. **(C)** Conversion of sound to heat.   *(2:209–217)*

318. **(I)** Operating frequency divided by bandwidth.   *(2:209–217)*

319. (J) Power divided by area.   (2:209–217)

320. (B) The damping material reduces spatial pulse length, efficiency, and sensitivity.   (2:15)

321. (C) Gain is electric compensation for tissue attenuation.   (15:19)

322. (A) Spectral analysis allows the determination of the frequency spectrum of a signal.   (17:16)

323. (C) Analog scan converters store any increment of signal amplitude, whereas digital scan converters store the signal amplitude in discrete steps.   (17:30)

324. (C) Gray-scale resolution is the ability of a gray-scale display to distinguish between echoes of slightly different amplitudes or intensities. The first step in this problem is to figure out how many shades of gray are contained in a 5-bit digital system. The total number of shades of gray is 32 (2^5 = 32). The next step is to divide the dynamic range (42 dB) by the number of levels. This will give the number of dB per level. 42 dB ÷ 32 gray levels = 1.3 dB/gray level.   (2:93)

325. (B)

$$Distance = velocity \times time$$
$$= 1540 \text{ m/s} \times 0.01 \text{ s}$$
$$= 15.4 \text{ m}$$

However, 0.1 seconds is only the time to reach the echo source. The time of the round trip must be calculated by multiplying by 2. Round-trip distance = 15.4 m × 2 = 30.8 m.   (14:2)

326. (B) An edge artifact. Edge shadowing results from refraction and reflection of the ultrasound beam on a rounded surface, for example, the fetal skull.   (28:42)

327. (A) A split image artifact (ghost artifact) may produce duplication or triplication of an image, resulting in ultrasound beam refraction at a muscle–fat interface.   (26:29–34; 27:49–52)

328. (A) Multipath, mirror image, and side lobe artifacts are most likely to produce a pseudomass. A comet tail artifact is least likely.   (28:27–43)

329. (A) Split image artifact is more noticeable in athletic and mesomorphic habitus patients.   (27:49–52)

330. (C) Split image artifact (ghost artifact) is *not* caused by a gas bubble. The most likely cause is refraction of the sound beam at a muscle–fat interface. The artifact is more evident at an interface between subcutaneous fat and abdominal muscle or between rectus muscle and fat in the pelvis. The artifact can also be produced by an abdominal scar.   (26:29–34; 27:49–52)

331. (C) The most likely cause of beam thickness artifact is partial volume effect. This type of artifact occurs most often when the ultrasound beam interacts with a cyst or other fluid-filled structures.   (28:27–45)

332. (C) Beam thickness artifacts depend on beam angulation, not gravity. Therefore, if an image of the gallbladder has what appears to be sludge, a change in the patient's position relative to the beam could differentiate pseudosludge caused by artifact from layering of biliary sludge.   (28:27–45)

333. (D) Side lobe artifact is apparent in both static and real-time images.   (28:27–45)

334. (B) Shotgun pellets and metallic surgical clips produce a trail of dense continuous echoes. Bone, gas, and gallstones produce distal acoustic shadow.   (28:27–45)

335. (A) The most common type of artifact observed in patients with shotgun pellets or metallic surgical clips is the comet tail artifact. This type of reverberation artifact is characterized by a trail of dense continuous echoes distal to a strongly reflecting structure.   (16:1–17; 29:225–230)

336. (D) A ring-down artifact is characterized sonographically as high-amplitude parallel lines occurring at regular intervals distal to a reflecting interface. This type of artifact is commonly associated with bowel gas.   (30:21–28)

337. (A) It is possible to calculate the displacement in split images by using Snell's law.   (26:29–34)

338. (C) The first vertical deflection at the start of the A-mode is called "main bang," or transducer artifact.   (11:26–27)

339. (C) Annular-array real-time uses a combination of mechanical and electronic devices. The annular-array is used for dynamic focusing, the mechanical part for beam steering.   (22:9)

340. (A) A decrease in the amplitude of the returning echo results in a fade-away picture.   (11:52; 22:21)

341. (D) Hard copy is a term applied to any form of picture storage. A videotape recorder is hardware, whereas videotape is a hard copy (storage medium).   (11:35; 22:23)

342. (C) M-mode stands for time-motion modulation. This mode displays a graphic representation of motion of reflecting surfaces. It is used primarily in echocardiography. *(10:44)*

343. (A) B-mode stands for brightness modulation. This mode displays a two-dimensional view of internal body structures in cross-section or sagittal section. The images, displayed as dots on the monitor, result from interaction between ultrasound and tissues. The brightness of the dots is proportional to the amplitude of the echo. Both static and real-time equipment use B-mode. *(10:44; 22:2)*

344. (B) A-mode stands for amplitude modulation. This mode displays a graphic representation of vertically deflected echoes arising from a horizontal baseline. The height of the vertical deflection is proportional to the amplitude of the echo, and the distance from one vertical deflection to the next represents the distance from one interface to another. A-mode is one-dimensional. *(10:44; 11:26; 22:2)*

345. (B) The effects of ultrasound on human soft tissue are called bioeffects or biologic effects. *(2:2)*

346. (A) 1.54 millimeters per microsecond (1.54 mm/µs) or 1540 meters per second (1540 m/s).

347. (C) Slope.

348. (B) Delay.

349. (D) Far gain.

350. (A) Near gain.

DIAGRAM OF TGC CURVE

(17:299–318; 19:26–27)

351. (C) Progressive weakening of the sound beam as it travels through a medium. *(2:209–217)*

352. (F) Having two stages (on or off), black-and-white image, no range of gray. *(2:209–217)*

353. (G) Binary digit. *(2:209–217)*

354. (B) The production and behavior of bubbles in sound at high intensities. *(2:209–217)*

355. (D) A liquid placed between the transducer and the skin. *(2:209–217)*

356. (H) A method of reducing pulse duration by mechanical or electrical means. *(2:209–217)*

357. (E) The number of intensity levels between black and white. *(2:209–217)*

358. (J) Plastic material placed in front of the transducer face to reduce the reflection at the transducer surface. *(2:209–217)*

359. (A) Picture element. *(2:209–217)*

360. (I) Single-frame imaging. *(2:209–217)*

361. (D) W/cm^2. *(17:242)*

362. (A) 100 mW/cm^2 SPTA. *(2:168)*

363. (C) Spatial peak temporal average. *(17:242)*

364. (B) kg/m^3. *(2:261)*

365. (D) m/s. *(2:261)*

366. (F) Hz. *(2:261)*

367. (E) J. *(2:261)*

368. (A) W/cm^2. *(2:261)*

369. (C) m. *(2:261)*

370. (G) dB. *(2:261)*

371. (B) 0.002 W/cm^2–0.5 W/cm^2 SPTA. *(17:250)*

372. (A) 0.5 W/cm^2–2.0 W/cm^2 SPTA. *(17:250)*

373. (C) Under normal intensity ranges, diagnostic ultrasound is atraumatic, nontoxic, noninvasive, and nonionizing. It is nonionizing because the intensity in diagnostic ultrasound range is not sufficient to eject an electron from an atom. *(10:26)*

374. (D) Heat. However, at the diagnostic intensity range, the heat produced has no known effect. *(10:26)*

375. (A) The production and behavior of gas bubbles (microbubbles) is called cavitation. Cavitation occurs when dissolved gases grow into microbubbles during the negative pressure phase of ultrasound wave propagation. There are two types of cavitation, stable and transient. Stable cavitation is a phenomenon in which microbubbles are formed and persist in a diameter with the passing pressure variations of the ultrasound wave. In transient cavitation, the microbubbles continue to grow in size until they collapse, producing shock waves. *(10:26–27; 35:156)*

376. (D) There are two types of cavitation, stable and transient. Stable cavitation is a phenomenon in which bubbles are formed and persist. In transient cavitation the bubbles continue to grow in size until they collapse. *(10:26–27)*

377. **(A)** Doppler. *(10:61)*

378. **(A)** When an interface is smooth or "mirror-like," or larger than the wavelength, it is called a specular reflector. When the ultrasound beam strikes a specular reflector, the angle of reflection is equal to the angle of incidence. Therefore, reflection can be a critical factor when performing sonograms. The maximum amount of reflected echo occurs when the transducer is perpendicular to the interface. *(11:6; 12)*

379. **(B)** When an interface is smaller than the wavelength, usually less than 3 mm, it is called a nonspecular reflector. Nonspecular reflectors are not beam-angle dependent. *(11:6; 12)*

380. **(B)** Spatial average temporal average. *(17:242)*

381. **(C)** Spatial peak pulse average. *(17:242)*

382. **(A)** Since Doppler instruments are used for moving structures, static imaging does not apply. The Doppler instrument employs pulsed or continuous waves. The signal is amplified by a loudspeaker; thus the resulting sound is audible. *(22:10)*

383. **(A)** 5-MHz, short-focus. The choice of focal zone depends on what structure is to be imaged. The choice of transducer frequency depends on the amount of penetration and/or resolution needed. High-frequency transducers display good axial resolution but reduced tissue penetration. For superficial structures, a high-frequency transducer is most useful; for deep structures, low frequency is most useful. *(4:26–29)*

384. **(B)** 3-MHz, long-focus. See explanation for Question 383. *(4:26–29)*

385. **(A)** Pixel is short for picture element. *(11:32)*

386. **(A)** Under normal circumstances, the human eye can distinguish as many as 16 shades of gray. *(4:38)*

387. **(A)** $512 \times 512 \times 6$-bit deep. *(11:32)*

388. **(C)** "Aliasing" results when the velocity exceeds the pulse repetition frequency (PRF). Aliasing is an artifact seen in Doppler ultrasound. *(34:1)*

389. **(D)** All of the above. *(4:43)*

390. **(A)** As ultrasound propagates through body tissue it undergoes attenuation, which is the progressive weakening of the sound wave as it travels. The causes of attenuation are:

1. absorption
2. reflection
3. scattering

When the sound wave is absorbed, it is then converted to heat. The heat generated from absorption is mostly removed by conduction. *(10:28; 11:5, 19:74)*

391. **(D)** Most commercial and standard CRT monitors use 525 horizontal lines. *(11:34)*

392. **(B)** CRT monitors display 30 frames per second. *(11:34)*

393. **(B)** Every one-sixtieth of a second reduces the flicker. *(11:34)*

394. **(B)** 20–25 dB. *(11:34)*

395. **(A)** Digital memory stores information divided into squares. The number of rows and columns of squares is called a matrix. *(11:32)*

396. **(A)** Digital memory is similar to squares on a checkerboard in which echoes are stored in a square corresponding to the location of the scanning plane. *(11:32)*

397. **(A)** Echo-free. *(21)*

398. **(B)** Echogenic. *(21)*

399. **(C)** Impedance cannot be measured by a hydrophone. *(2:163)*

400. **(B)** The hydrophone is made up of transducer elements. *(2:163)*

401. **(C)** When a beam is applied for 2–3 minutes on laboratory animals, the results are growth retardation and hemorrhage. These effects were observed in laboratory animals, not humans, and with continuous wave ultrasound. *(17:251)*

402. **(C)** Refraction and diffraction are least likely associated with attenuation. Refraction is the bending of the sound beam as it crosses an acoustic impedance mismatch. The spreading-out of an ultrasound beam is referred to as diffraction. *(9:48, 11:5)*

403. **(B)** Conversion of sound to heat. *(11:5)*

404. **(A)** The spreading-out of an ultrasound beam is referred to as diffraction. *(9:48, 11:5)*

405. **(D)** Redirection of the sound beam in several directions. *(2:215; 11:5; 9:60)*

406. **(C)** The transducer's piezoelectric ceramic is heat sensitive and should not be subjected to excessive heat sterilization, because the crystal in the transducer housing could become depolarized and lose its piezoelectric properties. Transducers are made up of a variety of materials, including plastic, crystals, bonding seals, steel or metal casing, but they are not all constructed alike. A disinfectant that is safe for some transducers may be destructive to others. The recommended method for sterilizing transducers is available from the manufacturer's user manual or from the manufacturer's technical support department. Any product used on transducers against the manufacturer instructions or precautionary measures could result in damage to the transducer and loss of the transducer warranty.

(33:130–131)

407. **(A)** An acoustic window is a pathway through which the sound beam travels without interference. Examples are the liver and the urinary bladder.

(31:77)

408. **(A)** The decimal number 10 may also be represented by the binary number 1010. *(2:96)*

409. **(B)** Real-time imaging is similar to x-ray fluoroscopy in that each displays motion of internal body parts. *(31:167)*

410. **(C)** The frame rate for real-time systems vary from 15 frames per second to 60 frames per second. A slow frame rate causes flickering. A frame rate higher than 15 frames per second is required to produce a flicker-free image. For fast-moving structures, a high frame rate is needed. *(4:34; 31:167)*

411. **(A)** All images of transverse scans should be viewed from the patient's feet, supine or prone.

(31:86)

412. **(B)** In longitudinal (sagittal) scans the images are presented with the patient's head to the left of the image and feet to the right of the image in both supine and prone positions. *(31:86)*

413. **(C)** Within the receiver, a number of signal-processing functions take place: amplification, compensation, demodulation, compression, and rejection. *(2:84)*

414. **(B)** Because the particles in ultrasound waves oscillate in the same direction of wave propagation, no plane is defined. Therefore, ultrasound waves cannot be polarized. *(9:359; 10:1)*

415. **(D)** Quartz is the transducer crystal most likely to be employed. *(9:310)*

416. **(D)** All of the above. *(9:310)*

417. **(C)** PZT-5. *(9:310)*

418. **(D)** Two hundred fifty-six (256), or the number 2 raised to the power of 8 (the number of bits per memory element): $256 = 2^8$. *(34:32)*

419. **(B)** A real-time mechanical sector transducer allows greater maneuverability for small intercostal space scanning. *(3:173–174)*

420. **(G)** Both ultrasound and fluoroscopy evaluate moving structures in movie-like appearance. However, ultrasound is nonionizing because its intensity is insufficient to eject an electron from the atom. Fluoroscopy is ionizing and results in potential biologic effects. *(10:26)*

421. **(F)** The contrast media used for roentgenographic oral cholecystogram (x-ray of the GB) and intravenous pyelogram (x-rays of the kidneys) do not obscure the propagation of ultrasound. *(10:329)*

422. **(I)** A device used to focus sound beams. *(2:209–217)*

423. **(C)** Picture element. *(2:209–217)*

424. **(D)** Pie shaped. *(2:209–217)*

425. **(F)** A device that changes sound waves into visible light patterns. *(2:209–217)*

426. **(B)** The portion of the sound beam outside of the main beam. *(2:209–217)*

427. **(H)** Imaginary surface passing through particles of the same vibration as an ultrasound wave.

(2:209–217)

428. **(A)** Unit of impedance. *(2:209–217)*

429. **(G)** The ratio between the angle of incidence and the refraction. *(2:209–217)*

430. **(E)** A change in frequency as a result of reflector motion between the transducer and the reflector.

(22:233–238)

431. **(B)** The lateral resolution is defined as being equal to the beam diameter. *(32:32)*

432. **(F)** Perspex, aluminum, and polystyrene. Ethylene oxide is a gas, not a material used for lenses. *(9:317)*

433. **(C)** Both ultrasound and light can be focused and defocused by mirrors and lenses. *(9:317)*

434. **(A)** 0.1–1.5 mm. *(10:7)*

435. (C) Individual cells cannot be identified because they are smaller than the wavelength used in the medium. *(10:10)*

436. (D) Mass per unit volume. *(10:5)*

437. (D) The longer the distance traveled, the greater the absorption. Absorption increases with increased frequency, and the amount of frictional force encountered by the propagating sound wave (viscosity) determines the amount of absorption. *(10:18)*

438. (D) There are no confirmed biologic effects on human tissue exposed to intensities used in the diagnostic range below 100 m/Wcm². However, laboratory experiments on pregnant mice with intensities far greater than that used in the diagnostic range resulted in growth retardation in the offspring of the mice. *(17:251; 2:168)*

439. (C) Pregnant mice exposed to continuous wave ultrasound, applied for 2 to 3 minutes, experienced neurocranial damage, hemorrhage, and growth retardation. *(2:168)*

440. (B) A combination of low frequency and high intensity is most likely to cause cavitation resulting in tissue damage. *(17:250)*

441. (H) Living human tissue. *(21:1–12; 32:1–3)*

442. (E) Tissue cultures in a test tube. *(21:1–12; 32:1–3)*

443. (F) A method of analyzing a waveform. *(21:1–12; 32:1–3)*

444. (G) The property of a medium characterized by energy distortion in the medium and irreversibly converted to heat. *(21:1–12; 32:1–3)*

445. (B) Elimination of small amplitude echo. *(21:1–12; 32:1–3)*

446. (C) A process of acoustic energy absorption. *(21:1–12; 32:1–3)*

447. (A) An in vivo phenomenon, characterized by erythrocytes within small vessels stopping the flow and collecting in the low pressure regions of the standing wave field. *(21:1–12; 32:1–3)*

448. (D) Energy transported per unit time. *(21:1–12; 32:1–3)*

449. (G) All of the statements are false or unconfirmed at the present time. Experimental studies were conducted on pregnant mice, not pregnant women. The intensity, frequency, and exposure time were far greater than those used in a diagnostic setting.

Continuous ultrasound was used in many of the experiments. *(17:251; 2:173–174)*

450. (D) At present, there are no known exposure injuries in humans in the clinical setting. Injuries have been reported only in laboratory animals. *(17:251; 2:173–174)*

451. (A) No distinction. All real-time scans are B-scans, and both static and real-time instruments employ B-mode. *(28:44–45)*

452. (D) The word transonic implies a region uninhibited to the propagation of ultrasound. An echo-free (anechoic) region does not guarantee the region to be transonic. For example, a homogenous solid mass can be echo-free but not transonic. Conversely, a region can exhibit echoes and be transonic. *(2:179)*

453. (B) Real-time is also referred to as dynamic imaging. A-mode and M-mode are also real-time modes. *(2:179)*

454. (A) The TGC is comprised of near gain, delay, slope, knee, and far gain. *(31:58–61)*

455. (A) The range of pulse repetition frequencies used in diagnostic ultrasound is 0.5 to 4 kHz. *(2:192)*

456. (C) Cycles, wavelength. The spatial pulse length (SPL) is defined as the product of the wavelength multiplied by the number of cycles in a pulse. *(35:61)*

457. (B) A-mode and M-mode. *(2:105–107)*

458. (C) Used in some Doppler instruments. Doppler instruments use both continuous or pulse waves. *(2:128)*

459. (C) Doppler. Doppler instruments employ an audio mode. *(10:62)*

460. (C) Continuous wave mode. Continuous wave mode requires two crystals, one for transmitting and the other for receiving. *(10:14)*

461. (B) Acoustic mirror. See Fig. 1–10B, p. 10, in the Study Guide.

462. (D) Piezoelectric crystal.

463. (C) Scanner head.

464. (A) Motor.

465. (B) 0.2–400 mW/cm². *(2:123)*

466. **(A)** Higher frequency than the incident frequency.
(2:123)

467. **(B)** Lower frequency than the incident frequency.
(2:123)

468. **(C)** Bidirectional. *(2:128)*

469. **(A)** Color Doppler is not beneficial. Color Doppler is very helpful in improving the ability to depict abnormal blood flow. *(2:129)*

470. **(B)** Control used to suppress or increase echoes in the near field. *(15:19–22)*

471. **(A)** Control used to suppress or increase echoes in the far field. *(15:19–22)*

472. **(D)** Control the upward incline of the TGC. Used to display an even texture throughout an organ.
(15:19–22)

473. **(C)** Control used to delay the start of the slope.
(15:19–22)

474. **(E)** Controls the point where the slope ends.
(15:19–22)

475. **(B)** Bandwidth. Bandwidth is the range of frequencies contained in an ultrasound pulse. *(2:210)*

476. **(A)** Q factor. The Q factor is unitless. *(2:54)*

477. **(B)** A fluid-filled mass. Fluid-filled masses are characterized by sharp posterior walls and distal acoustic enhancement. The enhancement is associated with low attenuation. Solid and calcified masses demonstrate a different phenomenon, distal attenuation, the degree of which is determined by the attenuating properties of the mass. *(13:32)*

478. **(C)** A calcified mass. Calcified masses, gallstones or any high reflective or attenuating structure can produce an acoustic shadow. This results from failure of the sound beam to pass through the object. The urinary bladder, gallbladder, and any fluid-filled structure will demonstrate acoustic enhancement. In some circumstances both acoustic enhancement and acoustic shadowing can be seen, for example, a gallbladder with stones. *(2:216; 15:29)*

479. **(B)** 2. Continuous-wave Doppler uses two piezo-electric crystals, one for transmitting and the other for receiving the returning echoes. *(1:391)*

480. **(C)** When the beam strikes a vessel at a 30° angle. Doppler angle is the angle between the direction of propagation of the ultrasound beam and the direction of flow. Unlike real-time imaging of the abdom-

inal organs in which the best images are obtained when the ultrasound beam has a perpendicular incidence, Doppler has a minimum shift at 90° (perpendicular) incidence, and a maximum shift when the transducer is oriented parallel to the direction of flow, even though parallel transducer orientation is not possible in most cases. Doppler application employs a Doppler angle of 30° to 60° with respect to the vessel. *(1:391)*

481. **(B)**

20 dB.
$$dB = 10 \log \left(\frac{\text{power out}}{\text{power in}} \right)$$
$$= 10 \log (100) = 20 \text{ dB}$$

(34:3)

482. **(D)** Depth-gain compensation. *(1:376)*

483. **(D)** Refraction, propagation speed. Refraction occurs only if there is a change in propagation speed.
(1:367)

484. **(A)** Better axial resolution. Axial resolution is related to the length of the pulse. The shorter the pulse, the better the axial resolution. *(1:378)*

485. **(A)** 0.25 mW/cm². The reflection fraction R:

$$R = \left(\frac{Z_2 - Z_1}{Z_2 + Z_1} \right)^2 = \left(\frac{75 - 25}{75 + 25} \right)^2 = 0.25$$

(1:366)

486. **(B)** Frequency and diameter. Near zone length (NZL) is the same as the Fresnel zone:

$$NZL = \frac{D^2}{4\lambda}$$

where D is diameter transducer (cm) and λ is wavelength (cm). *(1:362)*

487. **(D)** The element thickness.

$$\text{thickness} = \frac{1}{2} \text{ wavelength} \qquad (2:50)$$

488. **(B)** Refraction. Refraction is described by Snell's Law which relates the incident angle (ϕ_i) and the transmitted angle (ϕ_t) to the relative velocities of the two media.

$$\frac{\sin \phi_i}{\sin \phi_t} = \frac{V_1}{V_2}$$

When there is normal incidence, $\phi_i = 0$, and the

sound will only change velocity and will not be bent. *(1:367)*

489. **(C)** 1.54 mm/μs or 1540 m/s. *(1:353)*

490. **(C)** 1.0%

$$DF = \frac{PD}{PRP} = \frac{5}{500} = \frac{1}{100} = 1\%$$

(2:155)

491. **(B)** 20 kHz (or 20,000 Hz). This is the upper limit of the audible range for human beings. *(34:1)*

492. **(C)** Tissue attenuation. Tissue attenuation increases with increased frequency. *(1:369)*

493. **(C)** 3.5 dB.

total attenuation = attenuation coefficient
× path length

dB = 1.75 dB/cm × 2 cm
= 3.5 dB

The attenuation coefficient in dB/cm is by a rule-of-thumb equal to one half the frequency in MHz, ie, at 3.5 MHz, the attenuation coefficient is 1.75 dB/cm. *(2:23)*

494. **(D)** Propagation speed.

$$Z = \rho C,$$

where ρ is density and C is propagation speed. *(34:7)*

495. **(B)** False. Intensity depends upon beam diameter which is not constant.

$$intensity = \frac{power}{beam\ area}$$

(34:2)

496. **(C)** 70%.

100% = percent reflected + percent transmitted
(1:366)

497. **(A)** Frequencies. *(1:360)*

498. **(C)** Distance, velocity, and time

distance = velocity × time

(34:1)

499. **(A)** Spatial pulse length. (See answer for question 456.) *(2:64)*

500. **(C)** 90°

$$Doppler\ shift\ frequency = \frac{2fV}{C}\ \cos\ \theta$$

where V = velocity of blood flow; f, transducer frequency; c, velocity of sound. Since, cos 90 is 0, then the Doppler shift frequency is 0. *(1:386)*

501. **(B)** False. Frame rate depends upon the velocity of sound, the image depth, and the number of lines in an image. *(34:14)*

502. **(A)** The ratio of the maximum to the minimum intensity. *(2:6)*

503. **(B)** Smaller. The scan converter dynamic range is determined by its bit depth. *(34:30)*

504. **(A)** Compensates for attenuation effects. *(1:376)*

505. **(D)** Computer memory. *(34:32)*

506. **(B)** False. Frame rate is determined by the velocity of sound, the depth of the image, and the lines per frame and does not necessarily get reduced by the mechanical scanner. *(34:14)*

507. **(B)** Weakly attenuating structures. *(2:146)*

508. **(B)** False. Preprocessing alters the echo amplitudes before storage; thus, changes will cause the memory content to change. *(34:32)*

509. **(A)** Is equal to the beam diameter. *(2:65)*

510. **(B)** Increased frame rate. If the line density is kept constant, then the number of lines per image will decrease, making the time required per image smaller. *(34:14)*

511. **(D)** Reject control. *(1:376)*

512. **(A)** Too close to. The arrival time will be sooner than expected, causing the system to position the echoes too close. *(1:353)*

513. **(D)** Some Doppler systems. *(34:34)*

514. **(C)** 15 dB. For every change of 3 dB, the intensity will change by a factor of 2. *(2:255)*

515. **(C)** Decreases the maximum depth imaged. The pulse repetition period is the length of time allowed to collect echoes for each image line; a shorter PRP means less image depth. *(34:14)*

516. **(D)** Measures spatial resolution—using different rod-sets in the phantom, estimates of both axial and lateral resolution may be made. *(2:155)*

517. **(B)** False. Real-time scanning is achieved using a number of different designs of mechanically steered single-element transducers. *(34:26)*

518. **(A)** Increase with increased steering angle. In electronic array systems, minimum grating lobe artifacts are generated when the beam is projected normal to the plane of the array. Beams steered away from the normal will experience greater grating lobe artifacts. *(34:29)*

519. **(C)** dB/cm. Total attenuation is expressed in terms of dB, intensity in units of mW/cm² and power in units of mW. *(34:6)*

520. **(C)** Wavelength, velocity and frequency

$$C = \lambda f,$$

where C = velocity; λ, wavelength, f, frequency. *(34:1)*

521. **(B)** Sensitivity. *(2:155)*

522. **(A)** Thermal and cavitation. Thermal or heating effects are normally unmeasurable with diagnostic instruments. Further cavitation is also unlikely at current diagnostic levels. Cavitation refers to the growth and behavior of gas bubbles produced in tissue by ultrasound. *(34:17)*

523. **(B)** Frequency and transducer diameter. High frequencies and/or large diameter transducers produce long near-zones (Fresnel) lengths. *(1:362)*

524. **(B)** No confirmed. *(2:168)*

525. **(C)** Highest at the focal zone. This is true since the intensity is equal to the power/beam area, and the beam area is smallest at the focal zone. *(2:18)*

526. **(B)** 0.3 mm.

$$\lambda = \frac{V}{f} = \frac{1.54 \text{ mm/}\mu\text{s}}{5 \text{ MHz}}$$

$$\lambda = 0.3 \text{ mm}$$

(2:8)

527. **(C)** Two times smaller. A 3-dB attenuation change would correspond to a factor-of-two reduction, ie, one-half. For each decrease in intensity of 3 dB, the intensity is decreased by one-half. Thus, for 6 dB

attenuation, the intensity is decreased by one-fourth. *(1:356)*

528. **(B)** False. A low Q factor implies a short spatial pulse length which means higher spatial resolution. *(1:359)*

529. **(A)** A wide band of frequencies centered at 5 MHz. *(1:360)*

530. **(D)** Thickness, resonance frequency. Specifically, thickness equals one-half wavelength, where wavelength is velocity divided by frequency. *(1:358)*

531. **(A)** Increased damping, sensitivity. Increased damping does improve axial resolution by making the spatial pulse length shorter; however, the result is to make the transducer less sensitive to small echoes. *(1:360)*

532. **(A)** Piezoelectric. *(34:4)*

533. **(C)** Matching. Usually a matching layer is added to the front surface of the transducer acoustic impedance intermediate between the impedance of the transducer and that of soft tissue. *(1:370)*

534. **(D)** Constructive interference. *(1:361)*

535. **(A)** Highly attenuating structures. *(2:139)*

536. **(B)** Occur with multiple strong reflectors. Reverberation artifacts are present when two or more strong reflectors are located in the beam. One of these may be the transducer itself. The sound in essence gets trapped between these reflectors. *(2:142)*

537. **(A)** Good axial resolution. A large bandwidth is equivalent to a short spatial pulse length. *(1:360)*

538. **(B)** Fresnel zone. The far zone is also known as the Fraunhofer zone. *(1:363)*

539. **(D)** With normal incidence of the ultrasound beam. At oblique incidence, a sound beam will be bent if there is a change in propagation speed across the boundary. With normal incidence, however, the beam will either slow down or speed up but not bend. *(34:7)*

540. **(C)** The pulser voltage spike. The larger the applied voltage, the greater the deformation of the crystal and consequently, the amplitude of the pressure wave produced. However, a larger crystal (same thickness) experiencing the same voltage will produce more acoustic energy. *(34:8)*

541. **(B)** The reflecting surface is large and smooth with respect to the wavelength. Reflectors whose boundaries are smooth relative to the wavelength behave as mirrors and reflect all frequencies equally. Small reflectors (diffuse or nonspecular) scatter the sound in all directions and show a frequency dependence.   *(2:42)*

542. **(C)** Snell's law.   *(34:6)*

543. **(B)** Is mechanically steered. An annular array is capable of focusing the beam electronically in both *x* and *y* directions, but is unable to electronically steer. It must be steered, therefore, by physically moving the transducer or alternatively an acoustic mirror.   *(34:31)*

544. **(A)** 90–100%. Since the acoustic impedance of gas is so much smaller than that of soft tissue, there is almost 100% of the energy reflected.   *(1:366)*

545. **(C)** 1–10%

$$Z_{fat} = 1.38$$

$$Z_{muscle} = 1.70$$

$$R = \left(\frac{1.70 - 1.38}{1.70 + 1.38} \right)^2 = 0.011 \ (1.1\%)$$

where *R* is the percent of beam reflected.   *(1:366)*

546. **(B)** Focal zone moved to skin surface. Often a detachable water path is used to allow the focal zone of a fixed focus transducer to be placed at a superficial location.   *(34:28)*

547. **(D)** Longitudinal compression waves. Longitudinal implies that the variation in the pressure occurs in the direction of propagation. This is opposed to a transverse wave where variations occur perpendicular to the propagation. Transverse waves can occur in bone.   *(34:1)*

548. **(A)** Short wavelength and less penetration. The wavelength is inversely related to the frequency and the attenuation is directly related to frequency.

$$\text{the half-intensity depth (cm)} = \frac{3dB}{f}$$

where *f* is the frequency in MHz.   *(34:6)*

549. **(A)** Ring-down time. A long ring-down time is undesirable. It increases the spatial pulse length and thus decreases axial resolution.   *(1:360)*

550. **(B)** Electronically focus in two dimensions rather than one. An annular phased array can be focused dynamically in two dimensions. A linear array can

be focused dynamically only in the plane of the array. In the slice-thickness direction, perpendicular to the array plane, focusing is achieved by shaping the transducer elements or by acoustic lens. This is often referred to as double focusing.   *(34:30)*

551. **(C)** Gas, muscle, bone. This ordering proceeds along increasing stiffness or lack of compressibility.   *(34:2)*

552. **(A)** Resolution, penetration—At low frequencies, the axial resolution becomes unacceptable (< 1 MHz), while at high frequencies the depth of penetration in the body becomes prohibitively small (10 MHz).   *(34:6)*

553. **(B)** False. Color Doppler is basically a pulsed Doppler system with color encoding. As such, it suffers from aliasing at high flow velocities, ie, shift frequencies greater than one-half the pulse repetition frequency.   *(34:37)*

554. **(B)** SPTP is always equal to or greater than SPTA. SPTP refers to spatial peak-temporal peak and SPTA refers to spatial peak-temporal average. In all cases, peak values will be at least as great as the average values by definition. For continuous wave ultrasound, there is no variation of the intensity in time, and peak values will be equal.   *(2:21)*

555. **(C)** A hydrophone. A hydrophone is a small piezoelectric crystal that is moved in front of a transducer in a manner so that the beam pattern is mapped. A radiation force balance is used to quantify the total beam power. Other phantoms can be used to give qualitative estimates of beam profiles.   *(2:163)*

556. **(A)** Electronic or mechanical. Electronic generally also refers to a transducer array, either linear or annular. Mechanical generally refers to a single element or physically moved annular arrays.   *(34:26)*

557. **(B)** Schlieren method. Schlieren photography gives a two-dimensional photograph of the beam pressure profile.   *(1:362)*

558. **(D)** Time. Pulse duration is equal to the period of a wave times the number of waves in a pulse, usually microseconds in length.   *(2:14)*

559. **(C)** The frequency. The propagation speed does not significantly depend upon frequency, and thus the frame rate is not dependent.   *(34:14)*

560. **(B)** W/cm². SPTA refers to intensity, which is power (watts) per unit beam area (cm²).   *(2:21)*

561. **(C)** Curie point. Crystals heated above the Curie point lose their piezoelectric property. The Curie point for quartz is 573°C and for PET-4 is 328°C.

(1:358)

562. **(C)** Increased ninefold. $I = A^2 = (3)^2 = 9$, where I is intensity and A is amplitude. *(1:388)*

563. **(B)** False. In many cases, electronic and mechanical scanners demonstrate a frame rate lower than 30 frames/s. *(34:32)*

564. **(D)** Velocity, unchanged. The velocity is essentially independent of frequency and is rather dependent upon the physical properties of the medium. *(34:1)*

565. **(B)** Electronic time-delay pulsing. The delay pulsing of the array elements can be used to form a wavefront which is directed at different angles. Pulsing can also be used to focus the beam at different depths. *(34:30)*

566. **(A)** Is made possible by array-based systems. Dynamic focusing is possible only with array-based systems since it is necessary to individually monitor echoes received from each location. *(34:30)*

567. **(B)** False. Quality assurance is essential for all systems in order to operate in a reproducible manner.
(34:37)

568. **(C)** 1.54 mm. The velocity of ultrasound in tissues is 1.54 mm/μs. *(34:2)*

569. **(A)** Ring-down artifact. The arrow points to a ring-down artifact produced most probably by gas bubbles resulting in a tail of reverberation echoes.
(30:21–28)

570. **(A)** Rods for measuring ring-down. The small open arrows point to a rod group used in measurement of the transducer dead-zone or ring-down distance.
(17:261–276)

571. **(B)** A simulated solid lesion. *(17:261–276)*

572. **(C)** A simulated cyst. *(17:261–276)*

REFERENCES

1. Christensen EE, Curry T, Dowdey J. *Introduction to the Physics of Diagnostic Radiology,* 3rd ed. Philadelphia: Lea & Febiger, 1984

2. Kremkau FW. *Diagnostic Ultrasound: Principles, Instrumentation and Exercises,* 2nd ed. New York: Grune & Stratton, 1984.

3. Fleischer AC, James E. *Real-Time Sonography.* Norwalk, CT: Appleton-Century-Crofts, 1984.

4. Sanders R, James E. *The Principles and Practice of Ultrasonography in Obstetrics and Gynecology,* 3rd ed. Norwalk, CT: Appleton-Century-Crofts, 1984.

5. Wells PNT. *Biomedical Ultrasonics.* London: Academic Press, 1977.

6. Raymond H, Zwiebel W, et al. *Seminars in Ultrasound: Physics* 4(1), New York: Grune & Stratton, 1983.

7. Rose J, Goldberg B. *Basic Physics in Diagnostic Ultrasound.* New York: Wiley, 1979.

8. Wells PNT. *Physical Principles of Ultrasonic Diagnosis.* New York: Academic Press, 1969.

9. McDicken W. *Diagnostic Ultrasonics: Principles and Use of Instruments,* 2nd ed. New York: Wiley, 1981.

10. Goldberg B, Kotler M, Ziskin M, et al. *Diagnostic Uses of Ultrasound.* New York: Grune & Stratton, 1975.

11. Bartrum R, Crow H. *Real-Time Ultrasound: A Manual for Physicians and Technical Personnel.* Philadelphia: WB Saunders, 1983.

12. Powis R. *Ultrasound Physics: For the Fun of It.* Denver: Unirad, 1978.

13. Sarti D, Sample W. *Diagnostic Ultrasound Text and Cases.* Boston: GK Hall, 1980.

14. Pinkney N. *A Review of the Concept of Ultrasound Physics and Instrumentation.* Philadelphia: Sonior, 1983.

15. Saunders R. *Clinical Sonography: A Practical Guide.* Boston: Little, Brown, 1984.

16. Ziskin MC, Thickman DI, Goldberg NJ. The comet tail artifact. *J Ultrasound Med* **1:**1–7, 1982.

17. Powis R, Powis W. *A Thinker's Guide to Ultrasonic Imaging.* Baltimore: Urban & Schwarzenberg, 1984.

18. Shelly G, Cashman T. *Computer Fundamentals for an Information Age.* Brea, CA: Anaheim Publishing, 1984.

19. Hagen-Ansert S. *Textbook of Diagnostic Ultrasonography,* 2nd ed. St. Louis: CV Mosby, 1983.

20. Skelly A: Beyond 100 mW/cm². *A Bioeffects Primer: Part 1—Fundamentals,* vol 1, no 5. Philadelphia: JB Lippincott, Sept–Oct 1985.

21. Eggleton R. *American Institute of Ultrasound in Medicine: Recommended Nomenclature: Physics and Engineering.* Oklahoma City: AIUM, Aug 1979.

22. Wells P, Ziskin M. New Techniques and Instrumentation in Ultrasonography. In *Clinics in Diagnostic Ultrasound,* vol 5. New York: Churchill Livingstone, 1980.

23. Beiser A. *Modern Technical Physics,* 2nd ed. Menlo Park, CA: Cummings, 1973.

24. Rose J, Goldberg B. *Basic Physics in Diagnostic Ultrasound.* New York: Wiley, 1979.

25. Hussey M. *Diagnostic Ultrasound: An Introduction to the Interactions Between Ultrasound and Biological Tissues.* Glasgow: Blackie & Son, 1975.

26. Sauerbrei E. The split image artifact in pelvic ultrasonography: The anatomy and physics. *J Ultrasound Med* 4:29–34, 1985.

27. Buttery B, Davison G. The ghost artifact. *J Ultrasound Med* 3:49–52, 1984.

28. Laing F. Commonly encountered artifacts in clinical ultrasound. In Raymond H, Zwiebel W (eds). *Seminars in Ultrasound: Physics* 4(1), New York: Grune & Stratton, 1983.

29. Thickman D, Ziskin M, Goldenberg J, et al. Clinical manifestations of the comet tail artifact. *J Ultrasound Med* 2:225–230, 1983.

30. Avruch L, Cooperberg P. The ring-down artifact. *J Ultrasound Med* 4:21–28, 1985.

31. Wicks J, Howe K. *Fundamentals of Ultrasonographic Technique*. Chicago: Yearbook, 1983.

32. Edmonds P. *American Institute of Ultrasound in Medicine: Appendix relating to ultrasound tissue signatures*. Oklahoma City: AIUM-11375, April 1976.

33. Odwin C, Fleischer AC, Kepple D, et al. Probe covers and disinfectants for transvaginal transducers. *J Diagnostics Med Sonogr* 6(3):130–134.

34. Fleischer AC, Romero R, Manning FA, et al. *The Principles and Practice of Ultrasonography in Obstetrics and Gynecology*, 4th ed. Norwalk, CT: Appleton & Lange, 1991.

35. Bushong SC, Archer BR. Diagnostic Ultrasound: Physics, Biology, and Instrumentation. St. Louis: Mosby-Year Book, 1991.

CHAPTER 2

DOPPLER COLOR FLOW IMAGING INSTRUMENTATION

Raymond L. Powis

Study Guide

Color flow imaging arrived on the medical scene in answer to a basic medical need: to look at blood flow noninvasively. The technology emerged from the development of multigate Doppler systems, which first appeared in 1975.[1] Although these systems used color Doppler only inside an M-mode display, they established both the multigate approach and the use of color to encode motion. In 1983 the first real-time echocardiography color flow system became available commercially.[2] The first commercially available color flow vascular imaging device followed in 1986. Since then, nearly all ultrasound manufacturers have added color flow imaging capabilities to their product line.

The current applications of color flow imaging are extensive and increasing vigorously. Basic and clinical research is extending the usefulness of this imaging modality. And within the research engineering departments of many ultrasound companies, new technologies are shaping the speed and capabilities of color flow imaging. As in other parts of ultrasound, understanding the instrumentation can go a long way toward understanding how to conduct clinical examinations and read the images. This chapter briefly reviews color flow imaging instrumentation and how it fits into the major applications of imaging.

THE ESSENTIAL COLOR FLOW IMAGE

The primary feature of the color flow image is the coincident depiction of stationary soft tissues in gray scale and moving soft tissues in color. For the most part, the moving soft tissue is blood within the cardiovascular system. This relationship opens the use of color flow imaging to two major applications: cardiac imaging and vascular imaging. But, as you will discover, any moving echo source within and sometimes outside the scanning field can produce color in the image. Setting up the system correctly,

however, will limit the color flow information to moving blood.

Color flow imaging is a direct extension of duplex imaging and Doppler multigate analysis. Duplex imaging is older than multigate analysis and has several different forms. It includes the combination of either a continuous-wave or a single-point (pulsed-Doppler) spectrum with an image.[4] The image can be an M-mode trace, a real-time B-mode image, or, almost paradoxically, a color flow image. (The paradox is not real, however. Color flow imaging and a single-point spectrum look at the same events, but they do so from different points of view. As a result, they can be profitably combined into a common presentation.)

Multigate analysis is a method of collecting Doppler data from several adjacent spatial locations. The system analyzes each sampling site for flow events using Doppler signal processing. The limitation of this form of signal treatment is time. Multigate systems look at each site serially; thus, as the number of sites increases, the time required to make an image also increases.[3] Conversely, as the image frame time increases, the image frame rate decreases.

Current machines use a number of modern signal-handling techniques to keep the image frame rates as high as possible. The essential color flow presentation provides the following pieces of information directly from the image: (1) the existence of flow, (2) its location in the image, (3) its location in the anatomy, (4) its direction relative to the transducer, (5) its direction relative to the anatomy, and (6) its pattern over space and time.

Because the color image shows flow over space and time, we can use the image to locate specific characteristics of the flow pattern. For example, the higher-velocity flow segments (major streamlines and poststenotic jets) are visible within the heart and larger vessels. In addition, the image clearly shows the difference between complex flow patterns resulting from anatomy and poststenotic flow patterns (turbulence) associated with disease.[5]

The ability to clearly show the patterns of flow depends on advanced technologies focused on asking the right technologic questions. Everything comes together at the image, where we begin the discussion.

COLOR FLOW IMAGING TECHNOLOGY

Production of the Image

Color flow imaging begins by making a multigate image for both the gray-scale and the Doppler segments of the image. The system divides each beam location in the scanning plane into a series of small sampling sites, each of which translates into a specific location in the digital scan converter image.[6] Fig. 2–1 shows an example of this division using a linear array. The digital scan converter in the ultrasound machine determines the size and spacing of these sampling sites.

The sampling sizes depend on the type of image. For example, a gray-scale image requires sampling intervals no greater than one wavelength.[7] In this form of imaging, the system detects the echo signal amplitudes and converts them into gray-scale intensities. Sampling intervals that are greater than one wavelength simply do not display tissue texturing well enough to support good gray-scale imaging. To show the differences among tissues, a gray-scale image must be able to show the differences between the various tissue textures.

Sampling for Doppler information has a different set of requirements. Doppler signal processing requires more time than does amplitude detection. For example, a single pulse–listen cycle can provide the information for a single gray-scale image line of sight. Doppler, however, requires anywhere from 4 to 100 pulse–listen cycles to build a single Doppler image line of sight.[3] Practicalities will limit the dwelling time on each line of sight to a range of 4 to 32 cycles. As a result, the sampling intervals are usually larger and fewer than in gray-scale imaging. The smallest Doppler sampling sites are at one-wavelength in-

Figure 2–2. Flow image resolution and sampling intervals. W is the vessel wall, NV is the normal velocity profile, LS is the profile with large-interval sampling, and SS is the profile with small-interval sampling. The smaller the sampling, the better the depiction of flow.

tervals. Often, to shorten the time to form one frame of a real-time image, the Doppler sampling sites may be several wavelengths long. For vascular imaging, sampling sites larger than 1 mm provide a poor depiction of vascular flow patterns. Fig. 2–2 shows how the sampling intervals affect the depiction of flow patterns in a vessel.

The heart poses a different set of requirements. Because we do not need to see the same detailed flow patterns required in vascular imaging, color flow imaging in the heart can use larger sampling intervals.[2] By reducing the time required to make the colored portion of an image, frame rates can be speeded up enough to depict events in both adult and pediatric hearts. Even these techniques, however, may not be adequate. Higher frame rates may still require reducing the number of Doppler lines of sight in an image. Limiting Doppler signal processing to a specific region or window can help restore the frame rates to usable levels. Usually, the window can be moved to permit interrogating the entire image for flow. At each Doppler sampling site, the color flow imaging system looks at the returning echo signals for changes in phase and the Doppler shift frequencies.

Changes in Phase. The changes in echo signal phase or timing show that an echo source is moving and reveal the direction of its motion.[8] The reference for this motion is the transducer. As in duplex imaging, movement toward the transducer is called *forward* motion; movement away from the transducer is called *reverse*. The color flow system encodes this directional information into color, typically red and blue. Fig. 2–3 shows this color assignment geometry for a linear array. These same rules apply to every ultrasound beam in both sector and linear scanning fields. Because no universally accepted standard exists for assigning color to direction, most systems have a flow-reverse button that switches the color assignment. This often permits setting arterial flow in red and venous flow in blue.

Doppler Shift Frequencies. Each Doppler image sampling site is a range gate that represents the position of the Doppler sample volume. If the sample volume is within a pattern of flowing blood, a spectrum of Doppler

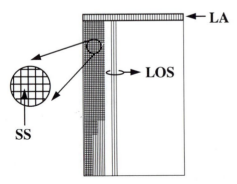

Figure 2–1. Sampling the scanning beams. LA is the linear array, SS is a sample site, and LOS represents the scanning lines of sight. Each sampling site represents a position in the digital scan converter.

Figure 2–3. Color assignment to the direction of flow. LA is the linear array, B is the ultrasound beam, SG is the scanning field geometry, F is forward motion, R is reverse motion, and H is a horizontal line. Flow vectors pointing on the F arc are all one color. Flow vectors pointing on the R arc are the opposite color. Anatomy further restricts blood flow to the anatomy of the vessel.

shift frequencies appears. The system, however, cannot display a spectrum within each colored pixel that makes a color flow image. Instead, most color flow systems determine a representative frequency and encode this frequency into a color quality.[9]

All current color flow systems use some form of average frequency to represent the Doppler shift frequency within a sample site. The average frequency is a good choice because it is less sensitive to noise than are most alternatives. In some systems, the average frequency comes from an on-line spectral analysis.[9] In others, autocorrelation and signal-averaging techniques produce the average value.[2] Regardless of the type of system, the signal processing encodes the average frequency into one of several color qualities.

Color has three inherent qualities we can use to encode information: hue, brightness, and saturation. The hue of a color represents its basic frequency or wavelength. For example, red and blue are different hues; so are yellow and green. Some systems encode the Doppler shift frequency information into hue, presenting a variety of different colors, each representing a different Doppler shift frequency.[2]

The brightness of a color represents its energy content. For example, increasing or decreasing the illumination on a color patch changes the brightness of the color without changing its hue. In general, current designs avoid using color brightness to encode the average frequency, but may employ it to smooth the edges of the color boundaries.

Saturation is a measure of a color's purity. A color with 100% saturation is pure. For example, a pure or 100%-saturated red would appear on the screen as a deep red. Changing the saturation means adding some white light to the color; thus, a less saturated red appears whiter. Several systems use color saturation to encode the average frequency information.[10] In these images, jets and major streamlines appear whiter than the surrounding color.

Beam Contributions to Sampling

Forming the ultrasound beam and its subsequent motion have a strong role to play in making a color flow image. Most color flow imaging systems use a phased array, linear array, or curved linear array transducer. Only a few systems use a mechanical scan. This preference for electronic scanning is not merely a matter of chance.

The Doppler effect does not distinguish between a moving ultrasound beam and stationary echo sources or between a stable ultrasound beam with moving echo sources. A mechanical scanner has a steadily moving beam (Fig. 2–4). This continuous motion means that the Doppler signal processing always sees some movement between the tissue echo sources and the ultrasound beam. Common to the few color flow systems that use mechanical scanning is an inability to look at extremely slow blood velocities. This form of insensitivity appears as the system filters out the Doppler shift frequencies produced by the moving ultrasound beam. Along with the moving beam frequencies goes all the low-velocity information.

One clear advantage of the electronic systems is the formation of a stationary ultrasound beam (Fig. 2–4). In this scanning pattern, each beam appears at a fixed line-of-sight position in the scanning plane.[11] However, electronic beam forming and steering have a price as well. Every transducer, regardless of size, acts as if it were a hole or aperture in space.[12] In this model (Fig. 2–5), the ultrasound comes from a point source behind the aperture. As the waves travel through, the interaction of the aperture and the waves produces a diffraction pattern. Most of the energy comes through to form a large central lobe of energy. The remaining energy diffracts into a set of side lobes that broaden and smear the beam.

An array of transducers (linear and curved) produces a similar set of side lobes. Because these lobes come from the summation of side lobes from each transducer element, they are called grating lobes. When the electronic

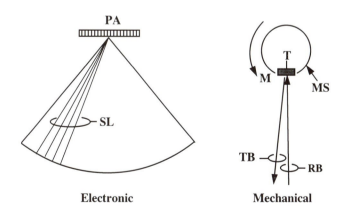

Electronic　　　　　**Mechanical**

Figure 2–4. Electronic and mechanically steered beams. PA is a phased array, SL represents the scanning lines, MS is the mechanical scanning head, T is a transducer, M is the direction of motion, TB is the position of the transmit beam, and RB is the position of the receive beam. Electronic steering permits fixed positions for each scan line.

Because the two scanning fields have different orientations, the color imaging and the gray-scale images do not entirely correspond to one another (Fig. 2–11). Portions of the steered Doppler image are outside the gray-scale field, whereas portions of the gray-scale field are outside the Doppler field. To keep the overall image frame rate high, a system often confines the color to a small mobile window. This is a common practice for all color flow systems—both vascular and cardiac.

PRACTICAL ISSUES

Cardiac Imaging Requirements

In general, viewing the heart with ultrasound requires intercostal and subcostal imaging with low-frequency ultrasound.[2] For parasternal color flow imaging, the beam is placed at angles approximately 90° to the flow. As a result, apical and subcostal views of the heart are needed to place flow patterns parallel to the ultrasound beams. The phased array and the short-radius, curved linear arrays are the transducers of choice for viewing through these thoracic and abdominal windows. The sector angles range from 30° to 90°.

Because blood is a low attenuator (0.15 dB/cm per MHz), viewing the heart with ultrasound does not require the front-end design (delay lines and receivers) that vascular imaging requires. In addition, the high frame rates, combined with large fields of view, impose large sampling intervals on the cardiac image. And the scanning is on a sector format. All these factors combine to make the cardiac color flow device right for the heart and wrong for the vascular system.

Because the Doppler sampling intervals can be relatively large in echocardiography, detecting a regional turbulence is not always easy. To help find any disorganization of flow (spectral broadening) in a given location, most cardiac systems determine not only the mean frequency at a sample site but the signal variance as well.[2] In many cardiac devices, color coding for an increasing variance introduces green to the primary color.

Vascular Imaging Requirements

Vascular color flow imaging involves all available vessels, including the large, upper thoracic vessels and the deeper vessels in the abdomen. The linear array is used to view the peripheral vessels. This linear scanning field sets the stage for using changes in color to show changes in the direction of flow. In contrast, a sector scan of a linear vessel has a continuously changing Doppler angle (Fig. 2–12) and, thus, continuously changing color.

Sector scanning transducers such as the phased array and the curved linear array are used to view abdominal vessels. These transducers permit both subcostal and intercostal scanning to visualize the deeper abdominal vessels.

The sector fields, however, make reading the images more difficult. Identifying arteries and veins requires knowing both the direction of flow and the pulsatility of the flow. Large fields of view and longer processing times

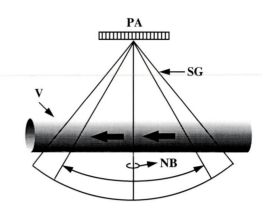

Figure 2–12. Vascular imaging with a sector scanning field. PA is a phased array, SG is the scanning field geometry, V is the vessel, and NB is the beam perpendicular to flow in the vessel (arrows). Because each beam position has a different Doppler angle, the colors in the image change rapidly.

for the color flow image often make the frame rates too low to permit easy determination of pulsatility. The single-point spectrum and color flow image as well as reduced color regions can yield information about pulsatility.

Displays of Frequency and Velocity

All current color flow images using Doppler are two-dimensional maps of the Doppler shift frequencies. After all, color flow is Doppler, too.

Many systems show the color values in velocity (cm/s) rather than frequency. Such a color image display suggests a direct measurement of velocity. As in all color-flow Doppler determinations of velocity, the values represent a solution to the Doppler equation (Fig. 2–13). However, the velocity is not the absolute velocity of the red cells. Instead, it represents the closing velocity along the ultrasound beam. Absolute velocities would require continuous correction of angles for all flow patterns throughout the image. Fig. 2–14 shows the closing velocity relationship.

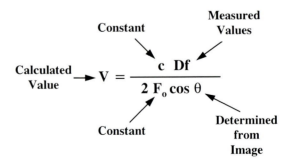

$$V = \frac{c \; Df}{2 \; F_o \cos \theta}$$

Calculated Value · Constant · Measured Values · Constant · Determined from Image

Figure 2–13. Calculation of velocity with the Doppler equation. V is the velocity, c is the ultrasound propagation velocity, Df is the Doppler shift frequency, F_o is the carrier frequency, and θ is the Doppler angle. Doppler machines measure frequency and calculate velocity.

Because the two scanning fields have different orientations, the color imaging and the gray-scale images do not entirely correspond to one another (Fig. 2–11). Portions of the steered Doppler image are outside the gray-scale field, whereas portions of the gray-scale field are outside the Doppler field. To keep the overall image frame rate high, a system often confines the color to a small mobile window. This is a common practice for all color flow systems—both vascular and cardiac.

PRACTICAL ISSUES

Cardiac Imaging Requirements

In general, viewing the heart with ultrasound requires intercostal and subcostal imaging with low-frequency ultrasound.[2] For parasternal color flow imaging, the beam is placed at angles approximately 90° to the flow. As a result, apical and subcostal views of the heart are needed to place flow patterns parallel to the ultrasound beams. The phased array and the short-radius, curved linear arrays are the transducers of choice for viewing through these thoracic and abdominal windows. The sector angles range from 30° to 90°.

Because blood is a low attenuator (0.15 dB/cm per MHz), viewing the heart with ultrasound does not require the front-end design (delay lines and receivers) that vascular imaging requires. In addition, the high frame rates, combined with large fields of view, impose large sampling intervals on the cardiac image. And the scanning is on a sector format. All these factors combine to make the cardiac color flow device right for the heart and wrong for the vascular system.

Because the Doppler sampling intervals can be relatively large in echocardiography, detecting a regional turbulence is not always easy. To help find any disorganization of flow (spectral broadening) in a given location, most cardiac systems determine not only the mean frequency at a sample site but the signal variance as well.[2] In many cardiac devices, color coding for an increasing variance introduces green to the primary color.

Vascular Imaging Requirements

Vascular color flow imaging involves all available vessels, including the large, upper thoracic vessels and the deeper vessels in the abdomen. The linear array is used to view the peripheral vessels. This linear scanning field sets the stage for using changes in color to show changes in the direction of flow. In contrast, a sector scan of a linear vessel has a continuously changing Doppler angle (Fig. 2–12) and, thus, continuously changing color.

Sector scanning transducers such as the phased array and the curved linear array are used to view abdominal vessels. These transducers permit both subcostal and intercostal scanning to visualize the deeper abdominal vessels.

The sector fields, however, make reading the images more difficult. Identifying arteries and veins requires knowing both the direction of flow and the pulsatility of the flow. Large fields of view and longer processing times

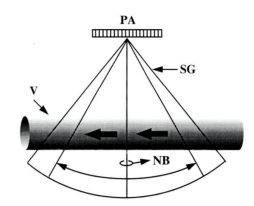

Figure 2–12. Vascular imaging with a sector scanning field. PA is a phased array, SG is the scanning field geometry, V is the vessel, and NB is the beam perpendicular to flow in the vessel (arrows). Because each beam position has a different Doppler angle, the colors in the image change rapidly.

for the color flow image often make the frame rates too low to permit easy determination of pulsatility. The single-point spectrum and color flow image as well as reduced color regions can yield information about pulsatility.

Displays of Frequency and Velocity

All current color flow images using Doppler are two-dimensional maps of the Doppler shift frequencies. After all, color flow is Doppler, too.

Many systems show the color values in velocity (cm/s) rather than frequency. Such a color image display suggests a direct measurement of velocity. As in all color-flow Doppler determinations of velocity, the values represent a solution to the Doppler equation (Fig. 2–13). However, the velocity is not the absolute velocity of the red cells. Instead, it represents the closing velocity along the ultrasound beam. Absolute velocities would require continuous correction of angles for all flow patterns throughout the image. Fig. 2–14 shows the closing velocity relationship.

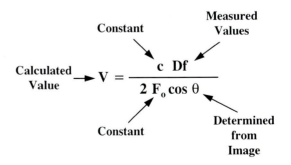

Figure 2–13. Calculation of velocity with the Doppler equation. V is the velocity, c is the ultrasound propagation velocity, Df is the Doppler shift frequency, F_o is the carrier frequency, and θ is the Doppler angle. Doppler machines measure frequency and calculate velocity.

Figure 2–3. Color assignment to the direction of flow. LA is the linear array, B is the ultrasound beam, SG is the scanning field geometry, F is forward motion, R is reverse motion, and H is a horizontal line. Flow vectors pointing on the F arc are all one color. Flow vectors pointing on the R arc are the opposite color. Anatomy further restricts blood flow to the anatomy of the vessel.

shift frequencies appears. The system, however, cannot display a spectrum within each colored pixel that makes a color flow image. Instead, most color flow systems determine a representative frequency and encode this frequency into a color quality.[9]

All current color flow systems use some form of average frequency to represent the Doppler shift frequency within a sample site. The average frequency is a good choice because it is less sensitive to noise than are most alternatives. In some systems, the average frequency comes from an on-line spectral analysis.[9] In others, autocorrelation and signal-averaging techniques produce the average value.[2] Regardless of the type of system, the signal processing encodes the average frequency into one of several color qualities.

Color has three inherent qualities we can use to encode information: hue, brightness, and saturation. The hue of a color represents its basic frequency or wavelength. For example, red and blue are different hues; so are yellow and green. Some systems encode the Doppler shift frequency information into hue, presenting a variety of different colors, each representing a different Doppler shift frequency.[2]

The brightness of a color represents its energy content. For example, increasing or decreasing the illumination on a color patch changes the brightness of the color without changing its hue. In general, current designs avoid using color brightness to encode the average frequency, but may employ it to smooth the edges of the color boundaries.

Saturation is a measure of a color's purity. A color with 100% saturation is pure. For example, a pure or 100%-saturated red would appear on the screen as a deep red. Changing the saturation means adding some white light to the color; thus, a less saturated red appears whiter. Several systems use color saturation to encode the average frequency information.[10] In these images, jets and major streamlines appear whiter than the surrounding color.

Beam Contributions to Sampling

Forming the ultrasound beam and its subsequent motion have a strong role to play in making a color flow image. Most color flow imaging systems use a phased array, linear array, or curved linear array transducer. Only a few systems use a mechanical scan. This preference for electronic scanning is not merely a matter of chance.

The Doppler effect does not distinguish between a moving ultrasound beam and stationary echo sources or between a stable ultrasound beam with moving echo sources. A mechanical scanner has a steadily moving beam (Fig. 2–4). This continuous motion means that the Doppler signal processing always sees some movement between the tissue echo sources and the ultrasound beam. Common to the few color flow systems that use mechanical scanning is an inability to look at extremely slow blood velocities. This form of insensitivity appears as the system filters out the Doppler shift frequencies produced by the moving ultrasound beam. Along with the moving beam frequencies goes all the low-velocity information.

One clear advantage of the electronic systems is the formation of a stationary ultrasound beam (Fig. 2–4). In this scanning pattern, each beam appears at a fixed line-of-sight position in the scanning plane.[11] However, electronic beam forming and steering have a price as well. Every transducer, regardless of size, acts as if it were a hole or aperture in space.[12] In this model (Fig. 2–5), the ultrasound comes from a point source behind the aperture. As the waves travel through, the interaction of the aperture and the waves produces a diffraction pattern. Most of the energy comes through to form a large central lobe of energy. The remaining energy diffracts into a set of side lobes that broaden and smear the beam.

An array of transducers (linear and curved) produces a similar set of side lobes. Because these lobes come from the summation of side lobes from each transducer element, they are called grating lobes. When the electronic

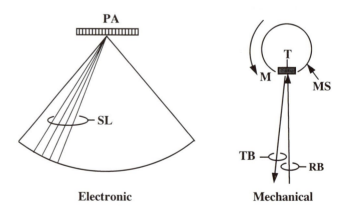

Electronic   **Mechanical**

Figure 2–4. Electronic and mechanically steered beams. PA is a phased array, SL represents the scanning lines, MS is the mechanical scanning head, T is a transducer, M is the direction of motion, TB is the position of the transmit beam, and RB is the position of the receive beam. Electronic steering permits fixed positions for each scan line.

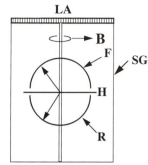

Figure 2–3. Color assignment to the direction of flow. LA is the linear array, B is the ultrasound beam, SG is the scanning field geometry, F is forward motion, R is reverse motion, and H is a horizontal line. Flow vectors pointing on the F arc are all one color. Flow vectors pointing on the R arc are the opposite color. Anatomy further restricts blood flow to the anatomy of the vessel.

shift frequencies appears. The system, however, cannot display a spectrum within each colored pixel that makes a color flow image. Instead, most color flow systems determine a representative frequency and encode this frequency into a color quality.[9]

All current color flow systems use some form of average frequency to represent the Doppler shift frequency within a sample site. The average frequency is a good choice because it is less sensitive to noise than are most alternatives. In some systems, the average frequency comes from an on-line spectral analysis.[9] In others, autocorrelation and signal-averaging techniques produce the average value.[2] Regardless of the type of system, the signal processing encodes the average frequency into one of several color qualities.

Color has three inherent qualities we can use to encode information: hue, brightness, and saturation. The hue of a color represents its basic frequency or wavelength. For example, red and blue are different hues; so are yellow and green. Some systems encode the Doppler shift frequency information into hue, presenting a variety of different colors, each representing a different Doppler shift frequency.[2]

The brightness of a color represents its energy content. For example, increasing or decreasing the illumination on a color patch changes the brightness of the color without changing its hue. In general, current designs avoid using color brightness to encode the average frequency, but may employ it to smooth the edges of the color boundaries.

Saturation is a measure of a color's purity. A color with 100% saturation is pure. For example, a pure or 100%-saturated red would appear on the screen as a deep red. Changing the saturation means adding some white light to the color; thus, a less saturated red appears whiter. Several systems use color saturation to encode the average frequency information.[10] In these images, jets and major streamlines appear whiter than the surrounding color.

Beam Contributions to Sampling

Forming the ultrasound beam and its subsequent motion have a strong role to play in making a color flow image. Most color flow imaging systems use a phased array, linear array, or curved linear array transducer. Only a few systems use a mechanical scan. This preference for electronic scanning is not merely a matter of chance.

The Doppler effect does not distinguish between a moving ultrasound beam and stationary echo sources or between a stable ultrasound beam with moving echo sources. A mechanical scanner has a steadily moving beam (Fig. 2–4). This continuous motion means that the Doppler signal processing always sees some movement between the tissue echo sources and the ultrasound beam. Common to the few color flow systems that use mechanical scanning is an inability to look at extremely slow blood velocities. This form of insensitivity appears as the system filters out the Doppler shift frequencies produced by the moving ultrasound beam. Along with the moving beam frequencies goes all the low-velocity information.

One clear advantage of the electronic systems is the formation of a stationary ultrasound beam (Fig. 2–4). In this scanning pattern, each beam appears at a fixed line-of-sight position in the scanning plane.[11] However, electronic beam forming and steering have a price as well. Every transducer, regardless of size, acts as if it were a hole or aperture in space.[12] In this model (Fig. 2–5), the ultrasound comes from a point source behind the aperture. As the waves travel through, the interaction of the aperture and the waves produces a diffraction pattern. Most of the energy comes through to form a large central lobe of energy. The remaining energy diffracts into a set of side lobes that broaden and smear the beam.

An array of transducers (linear and curved) produces a similar set of side lobes. Because these lobes come from the summation of side lobes from each transducer element, they are called grating lobes. When the electronic

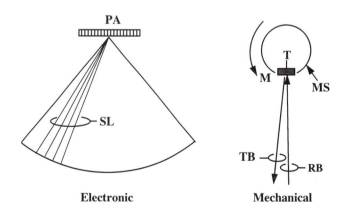

Electronic   **Mechanical**

Figure 2–4. Electronic and mechanically steered beams. PA is a phased array, SL represents the scanning lines, MS is the mechanical scanning head, T is a transducer, M is the direction of motion, TB is the position of the transmit beam, and RB is the position of the receive beam. Electronic steering permits fixed positions for each scan line.

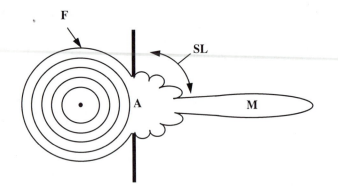

Figure 2–5. The transducer is a diffracting aperture. F is the virtual ultrasound field behind the aperture, A is the aperture, SL represents the diffraction side lobes, and M is the main beam. Each transducer acts like a diffracting hole in space.

control steers the beam perpendicular to the array, the grating lobes can be relatively small. By using several different cancellation techniques, engineers can suppress the grating lobes −60 dB (1/1000th) or more below the main lobe of energy. When the steered beam points off to the side, however, the number and size of the grating lobes increase (Fig. 2–6).[2] Again, the result is a smearing of the ultrasound beam and a loss of lateral resolution—a loss that can affect the accurate placement of color within an image.

Signal Processing

Once the echo signals are inside the machine, they face a diverse set of analyses. When and how these analyses occur will determine the character of the final color flow image.

Within the various machines, signal processing takes on two different forms. First, a system can use the same signal to make both the gray-scale and Doppler images. This is synchronous signal processing.[3] Second, the sys-

tem can use different signals to form the gray-scale and Doppler images. This is asynchronous signal processing.[3] These two forms of signal processing are sufficiently different that they even have different names. High-resolution synchronous processing is currently called angiodynography,[6] whereas low-resolution synchronous imaging and both high- and low-resolution asynchronous imaging are termed color flow imaging. Angiodynography is, of course, a special form of color flow imaging.

Synchronous Signal Processing. Fig. 2–7 shows the basic organization of a synchronous signal-processing system. Replacing the linear array with a single transducer and replacing the B-mode image with an M-mode trace produced the earliest synchronous system: the M/Q system.[12] This system used the same signals to produce both an M-mode display and a point spectrum. All synchronous systems use the same transducer, coherent transmitter, and receiver because they extract different information from a common signal. After reception, the signals divide into two pathways: one for the gray-scale image, the other for the Doppler image.

Most cardiac color flow systems are synchronous.[2] Because they do not separate the signal processing events for gray scale and color, they permit higher frame rates. These systems focus on the phased array to form and steer the ultrasound beams (Fig. 2–8). At the same time, beam steering spreads the beam with grating lobes; the effects of these lobes appear in both the gray-scale and color images.

In synchronous vascular imaging, or angiodynography, the system shapes and focuses an ultrasound beam along a line of sight perpendicular to the linear array. Fig. 2–9 shows the organization of this system. The beam scans down the array to form a rectangular scanning field. Zone focusing on "transmit" and dynamic focusing on "receive" provide a narrow beam over the field of view.[13]

The system tests each sample site along each beam for flow. If flow exists, the corresponding image pixel becomes colored; if not, the pixel becomes gray scale. In this man-

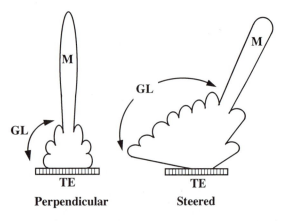

Figure 2–6. Grating lobe formation with beam steering. TE represents transducer elements, GL represents grating lobes, and M is the main lobe. Steering increases the formation of side lobes, smearing the ultrasound beam.

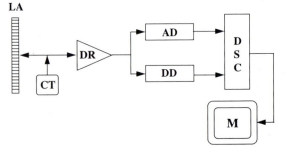

Figure 2–7. Synchronous signal processing. LA is the linear array, CT is a coherent transmitter, R is a receiver, AD represents amplitude detection, DD represents Doppler detection, DSC is the digital scan converter, and M is the color monitor. Synchronous signal processing uses the same signal to make the gray-scale and Doppler images.

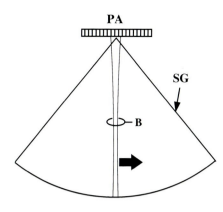

Figure 2–8. Formation of a phased array beam and steering. PA represents the phased array elements, B is the beam, SG is the scanning field geometry, and the arrow shows beam movement. The phased array has a limited aperture size that limits the focal spot size and focal range. Thus, focusing is poorest at the edges of the sector.

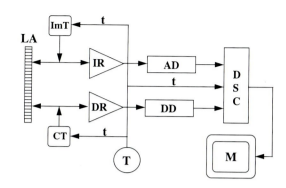

Figure 2–10. Asynchronous signal processing. LA is the linear array, ImT is the imaging transmitter, CT is the coherent transmitter, R is a receiver, AD represents amplitude detection, DD represents Doppler detection, DSC is the digital scan converter, M is the color monitor, T is a common timer with control signals (t), IR is the gray scale imaging receiver, and DR is the Doppler receiver. Asynchronous signal processing uses different signals for the gray-scale and color portions of the image.

ner, the processing builds the image on a sample-site by sample-site basis.

Gray-scale imaging depends on a mix of specular and scattering reflections. Doppler imaging, however, needs an angle of less than 90° between the beam and the flow streamlines. Synchronous vascular imaging systems use a mechanical wedge to establish the Doppler angle.[6] The wedge displaces one edge of the array about 18°, which in turn sets the ultrasound beams about 72° in relation to the vessels that are parallel or nearly parallel to the skin. In general, the wedge is a water-filled plastic device that slips on and off the array as needed. The choice of plastics and the internal architecture of the wedge reduces its attenuating effect on the echo signals to about 0.3 dB. The wedge does not affect focusing of the ultrasound beam, yet it suppresses reverberations within the wedge.

Asynchronous Signal Processing. Asynchronous signal-processing systems use different ultrasound beams and signals to create the gray-scale and Doppler images.

Typically, they use separate transmitters for gray-scale and Doppler signals. Only the transducer array and a central coordinating timer are common throughout most of the signal pathway to the scan converter. In Fig. 2–10 the organization of this imaging system is illustrated.

Most asynchronous systems use beam steering to obtain the Doppler image, and they keep the beams perpendicular to form the gray-scale image. Fig. 2–11 shows how the two scanning fields interact. Because the system uses two different transmitters, the Doppler carrier frequency can be different from the imaging frequency. For example, imaging might be at 5.0 MHz and Doppler might be at 3.0 MHz.

The operating cycle interweaves the Doppler and gray-scale beams to produce two separate images. This interweaving reduces the potential frame rates for the system. Because the sample sites for the two fields of view do not coincide, they cannot accumulate into a common memory. Instead, they pass to separate memories and finally overlay one another in the digital scan converter.

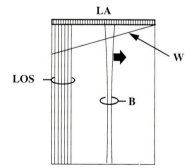

Figure 2–9. Scanning organization in angiodynography. LA is the linear array, LOS represents the scanning lines of sight, W is the wedge, B is the beam, and the arrow shows beam motion. The wedge provides a Doppler angle between the moving blood and the ultrasound beam.

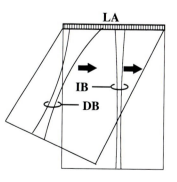

Figure 2–11. Scanning organization for asynchronous signal processing. LA is the linear array, DB is the Doppler beam, IB is the gray-scale beam, and the arrows show beam motion. Beam steering provides a Doppler angle for making the Doppler image. The Doppler and gray-scale frequencies can differ.

Because the two scanning fields have different orientations, the color imaging and the gray-scale images do not entirely correspond to one another (Fig. 2–11). Portions of the steered Doppler image are outside the gray-scale field, whereas portions of the gray-scale field are outside the Doppler field. To keep the overall image frame rate high, a system often confines the color to a small mobile window. This is a common practice for all color flow systems—both vascular and cardiac.

PRACTICAL ISSUES

Cardiac Imaging Requirements
In general, viewing the heart with ultrasound requires intercostal and subcostal imaging with low-frequency ultrasound.[2] For parasternal color flow imaging, the beam is placed at angles approximately 90° to the flow. As a result, apical and subcostal views of the heart are needed to place flow patterns parallel to the ultrasound beams. The phased array and the short-radius, curved linear arrays are the transducers of choice for viewing through these thoracic and abdominal windows. The sector angles range from 30° to 90°.

Because blood is a low attenuator (0.15 dB/cm per MHz), viewing the heart with ultrasound does not require the front-end design (delay lines and receivers) that vascular imaging requires. In addition, the high frame rates, combined with large fields of view, impose large sampling intervals on the cardiac image. And the scanning is on a sector format. All these factors combine to make the cardiac color flow device right for the heart and wrong for the vascular system.

Because the Doppler sampling intervals can be relatively large in echocardiography, detecting a regional turbulence is not always easy. To help find any disorganization of flow (spectral broadening) in a given location, most cardiac systems determine not only the mean frequency at a sample site but the signal variance as well.[2] In many cardiac devices, color coding for an increasing variance introduces green to the primary color.

Vascular Imaging Requirements
Vascular color flow imaging involves all available vessels, including the large, upper thoracic vessels and the deeper vessels in the abdomen. The linear array is used to view the peripheral vessels. This linear scanning field sets the stage for using changes in color to show changes in the direction of flow. In contrast, a sector scan of a linear vessel has a continuously changing Doppler angle (Fig. 2–12) and, thus, continuously changing color.

Sector scanning transducers such as the phased array and the curved linear array are used to view abdominal vessels. These transducers permit both subcostal and intercostal scanning to visualize the deeper abdominal vessels.

The sector fields, however, make reading the images more difficult. Identifying arteries and veins requires knowing both the direction of flow and the pulsatility of the flow. Large fields of view and longer processing times

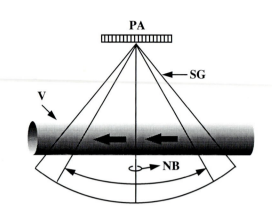

Figure 2–12. Vascular imaging with a sector scanning field. PA is a phased array, SG is the scanning field geometry, V is the vessel, and NB is the beam perpendicular to flow in the vessel (arrows). Because each beam position has a different Doppler angle, the colors in the image change rapidly.

for the color flow image often make the frame rates too low to permit easy determination of pulsatility. The single-point spectrum and color flow image as well as reduced color regions can yield information about pulsatility.

Displays of Frequency and Velocity
All current color flow images using Doppler are two-dimensional maps of the Doppler shift frequencies. After all, color flow is Doppler, too.

Many systems show the color values in velocity (cm/s) rather than frequency. Such a color image display suggests a direct measurement of velocity. As in all color-flow Doppler determinations of velocity, the values represent a solution to the Doppler equation (Fig. 2–13). However, the velocity is not the absolute velocity of the red cells. Instead, it represents the closing velocity along the ultrasound beam. Absolute velocities would require continuous correction of angles for all flow patterns throughout the image. Fig. 2–14 shows the closing velocity relationship.

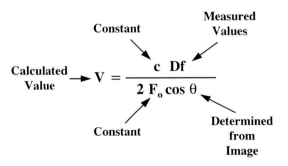

Figure 2–13. Calculation of velocity with the Doppler equation. *V* is the velocity, *c* is the ultrasound propagation velocity, *Df* is the Doppler shift frequency, F_o is the carrier frequency, and θ is the Doppler angle. Doppler machines measure frequency and calculate velocity.

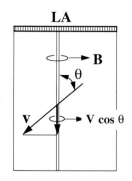

Figure 2–14. The closing velocity geometry. LA is the linear array, B is the ultrasound beam, SG is the scanning field geometry, *V* is the target velocity, and *V* cos θ is the closing velocity. Closing velocity is the component of motion along the ultrasound beam.

Color Flow Imaging Artifacts

Because color flow imaging incorporates both B-mode imaging and Doppler signal processing, it is subject to the same artifacts that affect ultrasound in general. Three primary sources of confusion in color flow imaging are (1) range ambiguity artifacts, (2) Doppler high-frequency aliasing, and (3) soft-tissue vibrations.

Fig. 2–15 shows the organization required to obtain a range ambiguity artifact. The high power and fast frame rates typical of color flow imaging offer ample opportunities for this artifact.[14] In color flow imaging, the artifact appears as diffuse nonpulsatile colors, suggesting flow that may not actually exist.

High-frequency aliasing occurs when the Doppler shift frequency exceeds the pulse repetition frequency (PRF) of the system.[8] As a result, the colors and spectra wrap around the display format and confuse the appearance of flow. To remove aliasing, a sonographer must ei-

ther increase the PRF (shorten the field of view) or decrease the Doppler shift frequency.[12] The Doppler shift frequency can be decreased by either decreasing the Doppler carrier frequency or moving the Doppler angle closer to 90°.

A not uncommon problem is the mechanical vibration of soft tissues. For example, vibrations can occur if a patient talks. Such vibrations can fill an image of a carotid artery with diffuse colors. The low-frequency pulse from the heart also can fill an abdominal image with a burst of color. More often, the vibration comes from turbulent flow patterns within vessels that vibrate the surrounding soft tissues.[15]

Applying the Technology to Real Images

With some idea of how the various color flow systems work, we are now in a position to examine some examples of color flow imaging. They range from the depiction of flow within an M-mode recording to high-resolution imaging of the vascular system.

Fig. 2–16 shows the combination of an M-mode recording with color flow imaging. All motion in this image is referenced to the transducer as a closing velocity; that is, only as motion toward or away from the transducer. In this example, the Doppler frequencies have been calculated into closing velocities, which do not necessarily represent the true velocities of the cardiac blood flow. This system shows the increased Doppler shift frequencies (spectral broadening) by adding green to the primary di-

Figure 2–15. The range ambiguity artifact. LA is the linear array, PL1 is the initial pulse–listen cycle, IU1 is the incident ultrasound from PL1, S1 is an echo source inside the field boundary (FB), S2 is an echo source outside the scanning field, DR1 is the deeper returning echo, and SA represents the simultaneous arrival of the two echo signals. Range ambiguity occurs when echo sources outside the scanning field appear in the image.

Figure 2–16. Color flow imaging of a mitral valve. This M-mode tracing views the mitral valve from the upper portion of the cardiac window, which is aimed down toward the mitral valve. Red is flow toward the transducer; blue is flow away. Closing velocity values (aliasing limits) appear on the color bar. The red flow between the interventricular septum and the closed mitral valve is ejection through the left ventricular outflow tract. During ventricular filling, the blue-green flow along the anterior mitral valve leaflet is reversed turbulent flow produced by an aortic regurgitation. Depth markers are at the right of the image, and an EKG trace provides timing at the bottom of the image. *(Reproduced with permission from Advanced Technology Labs, Bothell, WA.)*

rectional colors. As a result, the aortic regurgitation is quite evident in the color flow pattern.

Determining the true flow pattern is easier with a two-dimensional image of the heart. Fig. 2–17 provides a clear view of the heart in long axis, with the blood flow confined to the heart's chambers. Again, the Doppler frequency map is calculated into closing velocity values. True velocities would require a continuous angle correction throughout the image, which is not possible with current imaging technologies. This image shows a nonaxial regurgitating jet extending from the aortic root into the left ventricle. In this case, the color flow images show not only the existence of the jet but its nonaxial geometry.

Fig. 2–19 depicts a carotid artery with higher resolution, synchronous color flow imaging (angiodynography). The sampling rate in this image is at one-wavelength intervals (0.2 mm at 7.5 MHz) for both the gray scale image and the color portion of the image. The internal flow pattern of the vessel shows a normal flow separation and reversal in the carotid bulb. The flow direction is from image right to left, away from the transducer, causing the vessel to appear red. The higher Doppler shift frequencies are whiter, which clearly depicts the higher-velocity portions of the flow.

The beam steering that is typical of asynchronous signal processing changes the appearance of a similar carotid artery. This system also depicts different average Doppler shift frequencies with different color hues. As in Fig. 2–19, the image clearly shows the flow separation and reversal that is typical of a normal carotid bulb. This image also shows one of the hallmarks of normal blood flow, the nonaxial location of the higher-flow velocities.

Figure 2–18. Color flow imaging of a carotid artery. This long-axis view of a normal carotid artery bifurcation shows the common carotid artery branching into internal (upper branch) and external (lower branch) carotid arteries. Flow is right to left, away from the transducer (red bar at the top of the image). The vessel above the carotid (blue) is the jugular vein. Within the carotid bulb is a normal flow separation and reversal (blue). Because higher Doppler shift frequencies are whiter, the major streamlines appear white in the image. The required Doppler angle comes from the wedge standoff (black triangular space at the top of the image). The peripheral dots are 1-cm markers, and the aliasing frequencies appear at the top and bottom of the color bar. (*Reproduced with permission from Quantum Medical Systems, Issaquah, WA.*)

Figure 2–17. Cardiac color flow imaging. This parasternal long-axis view of the heart shows (from the top down) the right ventricle, the interventricular septum, and the left ventricle containing the mitral valve leaflets. Red is flow toward the transducer; blue is away. Closing velocity values (aliasing limits) appear on the color bar. The color-imaging window (blue boundary) shows a nonaxial blue-green turbulent jet (regurgitation) originating at the aortic root. Without color, the nonaxial quality of the jet could not be easily determined. (*Reproduced with permission from Advanced Technology Labs, Bothell, WA.*)

Figure 2–19. Color flow imaging of a carotid artery. The image shows the internal carotid artery and bulb. Flow in the artery (red) is from right to left, with a flow separation and reversal in blue. The major, nonaxial streamline (yellow) in the bulb is along the anterior wall. A small segment of aliasing (green) appears in the streamline. The more anterior blue vessel is the jugular vein. The Doppler angle for this image comes from beam steering. The white parallelogram shows the steering angle and the boundary for color signal processing in the image. The aliasing frequency limits appear on the color bar, with depth markers and a transmit focal point position on the right side of the image. (*Reproduced with permission from Advanced Technology Labs, Bothell, WA.*)

The beam steering in this image will not show flow throughout the image, but moving the color flow processing window and changing the scanning position permits a full interrogation of most vessels.

Any highly vascular tissue or structure is a good candidate for color flow imaging when trying to separate out ambiguous anatomy. Flow within major fetal vessels appears in Fig. 2–20. This image is formed with a convex linear array, producing a sector image pattern. Because of the complexity of the vascular anatomy and the changing angle between the vessels and the beams, color does not always indicate arteries and veins. Instead, the vessel pulsatility and its position relative to internal anatomical landmarks tell the story. If the system frame rate is too slow, then the single point, pulsed Doppler will be the most reliable means of determining the pulsatile flow patterns of arteries and the steady flow patterns of veins.

When wall disease in a vessel disturbs the flow pattern, a single point spectrum does not show the source or character of the disturbances. However, high-resolution color flow imaging, as in Fig. 2–21, clearly shows not only the irregularities of the vessel walls but the flow disturbances that result from these changes.

In the presence of stenosis, the flow within the narrowing increases velocity. The narrowing also often appears in the image as a physical narrowing of the color distribution, following the vessel. Fig. 2–22 shows these two results, the narrowing of the color distribution and the acceleration (whiter segments of the color) due to a carotid artery stenosis.

When frame rates are high enough and the Doppler sampling is fine enough, we begin to see some of the subtler flow physiology. Each pulse in the vascular system is a wave that travels down the vessels, only to reflect a por-

Figure 2–21. Color flow imaging of a carotid artery. This artery has irregular walls that cause flow disturbances (blue) at the walls. Flow is from right to left toward the transducer. The blue bar at the top represents flow away from the transducer. The color saturation shows a white major streamline that is crossing the vessel from the posterior to the anterior wall. The deviation of flow is more than 15° steeper than the vessel walls. The peripheral dots are 1-cm markers, and the aliasing frequencies appear at the top and bottom of the color bar. The black space at the top is a wedge standoff. (*Reproduced with permission from Quantum Medical Systems, Issaquah, WA.*)

Figure 2–20. Color flow imaging of a fetal abdomen. This image shows the fetal aorta with renal and iliac branches. Flow away from the transducer is blue; flow toward the transducer is red. The peripheral dots are 1-cm markers, and the aliasing frequencies appear at the top and bottom of the color bar. A convex curved array forms the sector scanning field. (*Reproduced with permission from Quantum Medical Systems, Issaquah, WA.*)

Figure 2–22. Color flow imaging of a carotid artery. This artery has a significant stenosis that is narrowing the flow channel (narrow color) and causing poststenotic turbulence (mixed colors). Flow is right to left, away from the transducer and is therefore colored red (red bar at the top represents flow away from the transducer). The peripheral dots are 1-cm markers, and the aliasing frequencies appear at the top and bottom of the color bar. The black space at the top of the image is a wedge standoff. (*Reproduced with permission from Quantum Medical Systems, Issaquah, WA.*)

Figure 2–23. Color flow imaging of a superficial femoral artery and vein. These normal vessels show typical flow patterns during the cardiac and respiratory cycle. Arterial flow is from left to right, with a distally reflected pulse wave (blue) arriving to cross the incident pulse wave (red). The superficial femoral vein (blue posterior vessel) is flowing right to left as flow and color fill the vein's residual lumen. This color flow image clearly shows that the reversal of flow in a tri- or biphasic flow pattern comes from a traveling pulse wave. The peripheral dots are 1-cm markers, and the aliasing frequencies appear at the top and bottom of the color bar. The black space at the top of the image is a wedge standoff. *(Reproduced with permission from Quantum Medical Systems, Issaquah, WA.)*

tion of the energy at changes in hydraulic impedance. Fig. 2–23 shows the intersection of two traveling pulse waves: The red portion is the incident wave and the blue portion is the reflected wave. The color flow image and the Doppler spectrum show the connection between the triphasic flow pattern of this high-resistance vessel and the passing of forward and reversed pulse waves with the artery.

SUMMARY

Color flow imaging is a combination of gray-scale anatomical information and a colored depiction of flow events. It is an integrated image of form and function—anatomy and physiology. The color portion of the image is not an image of blood however; it is an image of motion.

Within each color flow system, the amplitudes of echo signals become gray-scale intensities, whereas the frequency content of the signals becomes color. The echo signals for both may be the same or be different even in carrier frequency. This imaging modality depends on the sophistication and speed of the signal processing. It also is an imaging modality that is changing, and will continue to change, the fields of ultrasound and medicine.

REFERENCES

See page 97.

Questions

1. Duplex imaging combines gray scale with Doppler and can appear as

   (A) M-mode and spectrum
   (B) B-mode and spectrum
   (C) color flow imaging and spectrum
   (D) all of the above

2. Color flow imaging produces an image composed of

   (A) tissue echoes in gray scale and blood echoes in color
   (B) soft-tissue echoes in gray scale and blood motion in color
   (C) stationary tissues in gray scale and moving tissues in color
   (D) stationary tissues in gray scale and stationary blood in color

3. Angiodynography is a term used to describe

   (A) a form of high-resolution color flow imaging
   (B) a form of high-resolution magnetic resonance imaging
   (C) a new form of imaging relying on high-speed propagation velocities in soft tissues
   (D) the coloring of conventional angiograms

4. The Doppler effect occurs

   (A) only to waves traveling more than 1000 m/s
   (B) only to ultrasound waves with intensities greater than 500 mW/cm², SPTA
   (C) to all waves coming from a moving wave source
   (D) in ultrasound, but only when the targets are moving faster than 1.0 m/s

5. The Doppler effect depends on

   (A) the carrier frequency, the angle between echo source velocity and beam axis, and the reflectivity of blood
   (B) the closing velocity between transducer and tissue, carrier frequency, and ultrasound propagation velocity
   (C) the lowest Doppler-shift frequency detectable and the highest frequency without aliasing
   (D) the largest change in acoustical impedance within the moving blood

6. To calculate blood velocity using color flow imaging, a sonographer must

   (A) place a sample volume in the major streamline or jet within the vessel and set an angle correction parallel to the vessel wall
   (B) assume that all flow is parallel to the vessel wall
   (C) locate the major streamline and place the sampling angle at 60° to the vessel wall
   (D) place a sample volume in the major streamline or jet and set the angle correction parallel to the streamline

7. To preserve gray-scale texture, digital sampling for gray-scale images must be at intervals of

   (A) 0.6 mm
   (B) one wavelength or less
   (C) 1.0 mm
   (D) 3 dB

8. To preserve flow detail, digital Doppler sampling intervals for a vascular color flow image must be at intervals of

   (A) 1–2 mm
   (B) 1–2 cm
   (C) one wavelength or more but less than 1 mm
   (D) −6 dB

9. Gray-scale tissue texture in a color flow imaging system depends on

   (A) transmit focusing only
   (B) receive focusing only
   (C) the product of transmit and receive focusing
   (D) the speed at which the ultrasound beam is moved by the scanhead

10. The shape of the sample volume in pulsed Doppler has a major effect on the content of the Doppler signal

    (A) true
    (B) false

11. To form the color patterns in a color flow image, a color flow system samples down each Doppler image line of sight for

    (A) the amplitude of the Doppler signal
    (B) the velocities of red blood cells
    (C) the average Doppler shift frequency
    (D) the velocity spread within the sample site

12. The Doppler portion of a color flow image is a map of red-cell velocities

    (A) true
    (B) false

13. Separating moving soft tissue from moving blood in a color flow image tests for

    (A) Doppler signal amplitudes only
    (B) tissue signal amplitudes only
    (C) Doppler signal frequencies only
    (D) the relationship between the amplitudes and frequencies of the Doppler signals

14. A curving vessel within a color flow image shows color in the vessel when the beam and vessel are parallel and shows no color as the vessel turns. The loss of color means that

    (A) the vessel is occluded
    (B) the vessel is open, but the blood velocity is too low to complete the image
    (C) the dark region is diseased
    (D) the Doppler effect works only when the vessel is parallel to the ultrasound beam

15. The smallest vessels that appear in a color flow image are about 1 mm in diameter. The smaller vessels are absent because

    (A) arterial blood velocities are too low in vessels that are less than 1 mm in diameter
    (B) the smaller vessels are shadowed by the surrounding soft tissue
    (C) soft tissue does not have many vessels that are less than 1 mm in diameter
    (D) the smaller vessels do not reflect ultrasound as well as the larger vessels do

16. The color flow image provides information on (1) the existence of flow, (2) the location of flow in the image, (3) flow direction relative to transducer, (4) the maximum flow velocity.

    (A) all of the above
    (B) 1, 3, and 4

(C) 3 and 4
(D) 1, 2, and 3

17. Detecting flow in a color flow imaging system depends on the detection of

    (A) changes in Doppler signal amplitude
    (B) changes in Doppler signal frequency content
    (C) changes in echo signal phase and frequency content
    (D) changes in echo signal phase

18. One begins reading a color flow image by

    (A) determining the maximum systolic frequency
    (B) knowing the position of the scan plane on the patient's body
    (C) knowing the direction of flow relative to the transducer
    (D) determining the Doppler carrier frequency

19. Changes in the Doppler shift frequencies within a color flow image sample site appear in the image as

    (A) nothing; the image only shows changes in phase
    (B) different colors (hues)
    (C) different levels of color saturation (purity)
    (D) different colors (hues) or different levels of saturation (purity)

20. An angiodynogram shows changes in the frequency content of a Doppler sample site by

    (A) changes in color
    (B) changes in saturation
    (C) changes in color texture
    (D) the introduction of green markers

21. Cardiac color flow imaging shows changes in the frequency content of the Doppler sample site by

    (A) changes in color
    (B) changes in saturation
    (C) changes in color texture
    (D) the introduction of red markers

22. Color flow imaging systems determine the maximum Doppler shift frequency at each sample site.

    (A) true
    (B) false

23. A measurement of the peak systolic frequency in a carotid artery with a single point spectrum will be lower than a measurement of the color-encoded frequency at the same point.

    (A) true
    (B) false

24. The synchronous signal processing in angiodynography uses a Doppler carrier frequency that is the same as the imaging center operating frequency.

(A) true
(B) false

25. Asynchronous signal processing in color flow imaging requires the same frequency for both Doppler and gray-scale imaging.
(A) true
(B) false

26. Beam steering in asynchronous color flow imaging is used to provide
(A) a Doppler angle to typical blood flow
(B) a way of looking at the same soft-tissue targets at an angle different from the perpendicular beams
(C) an enlarged Doppler beam to improve Doppler sensitivity
(D) improved Doppler sensitivity to smaller vessels

27. The mechanical wedge in angiodynography is used to provide
(A) improved penetration through impedance matching
(B) improved beam focusing for the gray-scale image
(C) an attenuation system to remove side lobes
(D) a Doppler angle between the typical flow patterns in vessels

28. The ability to see flow in deep vessels is limited by the fact that
(A) blood has scattering units that are about the same size as soft tissue
(B) blood is moving faster than the surrounding tissues
(C) blood has an extremely low attenuation rate
(D) blood reflectivity is about 40 dB to 60 dB below that of soft tissue

29. Levels of output power and intensity for color flow imaging are generally higher than those for conventional gray-scale imaging.
(A) true
(B) false

30. Because Doppler signal processing requires more energy, synchronous signal processing always produces Doppler power levels that are higher than those for gray-scale imaging.
(A) true
(B) false

31. In general, tissue ultrasonic intensity levels are higher for single-point spectra than for color flow imaging with the same system.
(A) true
(B) false

32. Moving from gray scale only to full-screen color flow imaging in a system means that the image frame rate will probably
(A) decrease
(B) increase
(C) stay the same

33. Color flow imaging in the heart uses larger Doppler sampling intervals to increase the image frame rate than does vascular imaging.
(A) true
(B) false

34. Cardiac color flow imaging also works well in the vascular system because the design can handle the high attenuation rates in cardiac imaging.
(A) true
(B) false

35. Sampling intervals for cardiac color flow imaging and vascular color flow imaging are similar.
(A) true
(B) false

36. Cardiac color flow imaging is limited with a mechanical sector scanner because
(A) the cardiac attenuation rate is too high
(B) the ultrasound beams are always moving
(C) the beam has a fixed focal point
(D) the beam has too many side lobes

37. The phased array sector scanner and the linear array share common beam forming properties of (1) a stationary beam at each line of sight, (2) increased grating lobes with beam steering, (3) three dimensional dynamic focusing on receive, (4) the same aperture sizes for dynamic focusing.
(A) 1 and 2
(B) 1, 2, and 4
(C) 2, 3, and 4
(D) all of the above

38. Color flow imaging and angiodynography in the peripheral vascular system typically use
(A) the phased sector scan
(B) the linear array scan
(C) the curved linear scan
(D) a combination of A and B

39. Color flow imaging in the heart typically uses
(A) the phased sector scan
(B) the linear array scan
(C) the curved linear scan
(D) a combination of A and C

40. You are imaging a small vessel using 7.5 MHz color flow imaging with the lowest portrayable velocity of 6.0 cm/s. Changing only the carrier frequency to 5.0 MHz will change the lowest portrayable velocity to

(A) 1.5 cm/s
(B) 9 cm/s
(C) 6.0 cm/s; the vessel does not change
(D) 15 cm/s

41. Color flow imaging is unique because it does not have a major problem with high-frequency aliasing.

(A) true
(B) false

42. Both the color and a point spectrum in a stenosis show high-frequency aliasing. One strategy for removing the aliasing involves

(A) doing nothing. Aliasing cannot be removed from the system
(B) decreasing the system PRF
(C) decreasing the carrier frequency
(D) decreasing the Doppler angle toward zero

43. Increasing output power levels and PRFs to increase penetration and frame rates opens the system to the following artifact:

(A) high-frequency aliasing
(B) loss of low velocities
(C) tissue mirroring
(D) range ambiguity

44. The color coding of red arteries and blue veins and the slow high-resolution frame rates make the identity of arteries and veins in the abdomen direct and easy.

(A) true
(B) false

45. Turbulence in a vascular color flow image appears as

(A) a mottled pattern of colors
(B) a mottled pattern of red and blue with changing saturations
(C) a mottled green region
(D) A or B

46. Turbulence in a cardiac color flow image appears as

(A) a mottled pattern of colors
(B) a mottled pattern of red and blue with changing saturations
(C) a bright red region
(D) a mottled green region

Answers and Explanations

1. **(D)** All of the above. Color flow images can be used to locate a pulsed Doppler sample volume, as is the case with more conventional duplex imaging. *(5:1241)*

2. **(C)** Stationary tissue in gray scale and moving tissues in color. All moving tissues in a color flow imaging can produce color. Thus, stationary tissues are in gray scale, whereas moving tissues, including blood, are in color. *(3:236)*

3. **(A)** A form of high-resolution color flow imaging. Angiodynography is a form of high-resolution color flow imaging. It uses one-wavelength sampling intervals along each image line of sight. *(3:236, 5:1241, 9:27)*

4. **(C)** To all waves coming from a moving wave source. The Doppler effect happens to all waves coming from a moving source regardless of propagating velocity or power levels. *(12:172)*

5. **(B)** The closing velocity between transducer and tissue, carrier frequency, and ultrasound propagation velocity. The Doppler equation looks like the following,

$$Df = 2\,(f_o/c)\,V\cos\theta,$$

where f_o is the carrier frequency, c is the propagation velocity, and θ is the Doppler angle. $V\cos\theta$ is the closing velocity between the transducer and moving tissue. *(12:173)*

6. **(D)** Place a sample volume in the major streamline or jet and set the angle correction parallel to the streamline. Because the color pattern shows the location of the major streamline or jet, calculating velocity requires correction relative to the flow geometry, not the vessel. *(12:195)*

7. **(B)** One wavelength or less. This is necessary for textural information to reach the display in a digital scan converter. *(7:654)*

8. **(C)** One wavelength or more but less 1 mm. Digital sampling for vascular flow information requires such an interval because larger intervals cannot show the flow patterns within the vessel. *(3:236)*

9. **(C)** The product of transmit and receive focusing. The effective beam width results from the mathematical product of both functions. *(13:155, 11:620)*

10. **(A)** True. The sample volume and flow interact in a manner that depends on the geometry of the sample volume. *(8:9)*

11. **(C)** The average Doppler shift frequency. At each sample site, the color flow system determines the average Doppler shift frequency. *(3:236)*

12. **(B)** False. At each sample site, the system determines the average Doppler shift frequency. The display is then either these average frequencies or, in some cases, the calculated closing velocity. This velocity is the rate at which the flow is approaching or moving away from the transducer along the line of sight. *(3:236)*

13. **(D)** The relationship between the amplitudes and frequencies of the Doppler signals. The system will then avoid coloring strong slow-moving echo sources (tissue) but still color moderately fast weak echo sources (blood). *(15:647)*

14. **(B)** The vessel is open, but the blood velocity is too low to complete the image. As the vessel curves away from the beam, the Doppler frequencies become too low to be portrayed. The completeness of the image depends on the velocity of the blood flow, which is too slow for complete portrayal. *(2:19, 44)*

15. **(D)** The smaller vessels do not reflect ultrasound as well as the larger vessels do. Every living cell in the body is no more than two cell layers away from a red blood cell. The smaller vessels, however, are not sufficiently echogenic and vanish from the color display first because of their small echo signals. *(8:7)*

16. **(D)** 1, 2, and 3. Color provides information about the existence of flow, its location in the image, its location in the anatomy, the direction of the flow relative to the transducer, the direction of flow within the vessel, the flow pattern within the vessel, and the pulsatility of the flow. It does not indicate the velocity of the flow. *(5:1245)*

17. **(D)** Changes in echo signal phase. Like all directional Doppler systems, color flow systems detect the existence of motion with a change in echo signal phase. By measuring the direction of the phase change, the system shows whether the direction of motion is toward or away from the transducer. *(8:34)*

18. **(B)** Knowing the position of the scan plane on the patient's body. The expected flow pattern in any vessel comes from knowing how the scan plane is positioned on the patient. For example, the patient's head is always placed on the image left in long axis scans, and the patient's right side is on the image left in cross sectional scans. *(12:407)*

19. **(D)** Different colors (hues) *or* different levels of saturation (purity). The average frequency within each Doppler sample site is portrayed as a change in either color saturation (purity or whiteness) or hue (color). The object is to use the color to show flow patterns within the vessel lumen or heart chambers. *(2:44)*

20. **(B)** Changes in saturation. The angiodynogram uses only color saturation to show the average changes in Doppler shift frequency in each sampling site. *(3:236, 9:27)*

21. **(A)** Changes in color. Cardiac systems change color hues (frequencies) along red and blue lines to show changes in Doppler shift frequencies. Broadening frequencies in a sample site become shades of green. *(2:44)*

22. **(B)** False. Because only one frequency can come to the screen for each Doppler image pixel, all current systems use some estimate of the mean frequency. *(3:236)*

23. **(B)** False. Because color uses the average frequency at each location, the maximum systolic frequency will always be greater than the mean value. *(3:236, 9:27, 10:591)*

24. **(A)** True. Because synchronous signal processing uses the same echo signal for both Doppler and gray-scale signal processing, the frequency must be the same. *(3:236)*

25. **(B)** False. Asynchronous signal processing can, and often does, use different frequencies for the gray-

scale image and the Doppler image. For example, it could image at 5.0 MHz and have a Doppler carrier of 3.0 MHz. *(3:236)*

26. **(A)** A Doppler angle to typical blood flow. All Doppler imaging requires a Doppler angle. In asynchronous systems that do not use a wedge, the angle comes from beam steering. *(12:173)*

27. **(D)** A Doppler angle between the typical flow patterns in vessels. Synchronous systems that keep the beams perpendicular to the transducer array (angiodynography) use a mechanical wedge to obtain the Doppler angle to the flow pattern of the vessel. *(9:27, 3:236)*

28. **(D)** Blood reflectivity is about 40 dB to 60 dB below that of soft tissue. The fact that blood reflectivity is about 1/100th to 1/1000th that of soft tissues translates into reflectivities that are much lower than those of soft tissues. *(8:18)*

29. **(A)** True. Because the reflectivity of blood is low, many color flow systems improve color penetration by greatly increasing the power of the transmitted Doppler output. *(3:236)*

30. **(B)** False. Synchronous signal processing systems are limited by the power levels of the common transmitter used for both gray-scale imaging and Doppler imaging. As a result, imaging with and without Doppler produces similar power levels. *(3:236, 9:27)*

31. **(A)** True. The single-point spectrum requires the ultrasound beam to linger over its position longer than is the case in either real-time gray-scale imaging or color flow imaging. *(3:236, 9:27)*

32. **(A)** Decrease. Color flow imaging requires dwelling on each line of sight for as few as 4 pulse–listen cycles to as many as 32 pulse–listen cycles. Various systems have different dwell times. The end result is a reduction in image frame rate for color flow imaging. *(3:236)*

33. **(A)** True. Real-time color flow imaging of the heart requires relatively high frame rates. In general, Doppler requires dwelling on each line of sight for some period of time. In addition, each Doppler sample site requires processing time to extract the average Doppler shift frequency. Restoring suitable cardiac frame rates requires decreasing the number of color flow lines of sight and the number of samples along each line. *(12:17, 9:27)*

34. **(B)** False. Cardiac color flow imaging does not work well for vascular imaging because the Doppler sampling intervals are too large. Imaging the heart also

involves a problem with reflectivities, not with tissue attenuation. *(3:236)*

35. (B) False. Doppler sampling for vascular imaging may be well below intervals of 1 mm. In contrast, sampling for echocardiography may be at 7 mm to 10 mm intervals or more. *(2:17)*

36. (B) The ultrasound beams are always moving. This is the case because mechanical systems lack a special motor that could move the beam in small steps. Because Doppler signal processing is keyed to relative movement and the beam is always moving, color does not work well in mechanical systems. *(2:17)*

37. (A) 1 and 2. The linear phased array and the phased linear array have stationary ultrasound beams at each line of sight in the scanning plane. Both arrays also have increased grating lobes with beam steering. They do not have three-dimensional dynamic focusing or apertures of the same size. *(9:27, 2:21)*

38. (B) The linear array scan. The linear array with a rectangular scanning field is the geometry used for vascular imaging. The sector-scanning geometry makes reading color ambiguous in the straighter segments of a vessel. *(2:44)*

39. (D) A combination of A and C. Color flow imaging of the heart uses the phased-array sector scan and the curved linear-array sector scan. These scanheads permit cardiac imaging from intercostal and subcostal windows. *(2:41)*

40. (B) Nine cm/s. Lowering the Doppler carrier frequency means that the same Doppler shift frequency requires a higher velocity. *(13:280)*

41. (B) False. Like all pulsed Doppler systems, color systems will alias when the Doppler frequencies exceed the PRF sampling limit. *(8:37)*

42. (C) Decreasing the carrier frequency. This moves all Doppler frequencies downward and may bring the high aliasing frequencies below the aliasing limit. *(12:192)*

43. (D) Range ambiguity. High frame rates (high PRFs) and high output power permit structures from outside the field of view to enter the image as a range ambiguity artifact. *(14:83)*

44. (B) False. The large fields of view for abdominal imaging slow the frame rate. In addition, vessel anatomy goes in all directions. Sorting out arteries and veins requires the spectrum to determine pulsatility. *(10:591)*

45. (D) A or B. In vascular color flow imaging, turbulence appears as broken streamlines. The image then takes on a mottled appearance either in color or in color saturation. *(10:591)*

46. (D) A mottled green region. In color flow echocardiography, the sampling intervals are too large to show turbulence. As a result, the system determines the spectral variance at each sampling site and expresses increased turbulence (increased variance) in green. *(2:12)*

REFERENCES

1. Fish PJ. Multichannel, direction resolving Doppler angiography. *Abstracts of 2nd European Congress of Ultrasonics in Medicine,* **72,** 1975.
2. Omoto R, ed. *Color Atlas of Real-Time Two-Dimensional Doppler Echocardiography.* Tokyo: Shindan-To-Chiryo, 1984.
3. Powis RL. Color flow imaging: understanding its science and technology. *JDMS* **4:**236–245, 1988.
4. Burns PN. *Instrumentation and clinical interpretation of the Doppler spectrum: carotid and deep Doppler.* In *Conventional & Color-Flow Duplex Ultrasound Course.* AIUM Spring Education Meeting, 29–38, 1989.
5. Persson AV, Powis RL. Recent advances in imaging and evaluation of blood flow using ultrasound. *Med Clin North Am* **70:**1241–1252, 1986.
6. Powis RL. Angiodynography: a new real-time look at the vascular system. *Applied Radiol* **January/February,** 1986.
7. Ophir J, Maklad NF. Digital scan converters in diagnostic ultrasound imaging. *Proc IEEE* **67:**654–664, 1979.
8. Atkinson P, Woodcock JP. *Doppler Ultrasound and Its Use in Clinical Measurement.* New York: Academic Press, 1982.
9. Powis RL. Color flow imaging technology. In *Basic Science of Flow Measurement.* Syllabus AIUM 1989 Spring Education Meeting, 27–33, 1989.
10. Merritt RBC. Doppler color flow imaging. *J Color Ultrasonography* **15:**591–597, 1987.
11. Havlice JF, Taenzer JC. Medical ultrasonic imaging: an overview of principles and instrumentation. *Proc IEEE* **67:**620–641, 1979.
12. Powis RL, Powis WJ. *A Thinker's Guide to Ultrasonic Imaging.* Baltimore: Urban & Schwarzenberg, 1984.
13. McDicken WN. *Diagnostic Ultrasonics: Principles and Use of Instruments,* 2nd ed. New York: John Wiley & Sons, 1981.
14. Goldstein A. Range Ambiguities in Real-Time Ultrasound. 9:83–90, 1981.
15. Middleton WD, Erickson S, Melson GL. Perivascular color artifact: pathologic significance and appearance on color Doppler US images. *Radiology* **171:**647–652, 1989.

CHAPTER 3

ADULT ECHOCARDIOGRAPHY

Henny Wasser Rudansky and Mark N. Allen

Study Guide

Echocardiography has evolved into a highly specialized field of ultrasound. It serves as an ideal noninvasive method to examine cardiac anatomy in the normal as well as the disease state. In addition, echocardiography provides valuable hemodynamic information regarding cardiac physiology. The combination of anatomical and functional information provided by echocardiography makes it the diagnostic technique of choice in a variety of clinical situations.

The heart is an extremely complex organ. Echocardiography provides a variety of techniques that can be applied to obtain moderately comprehensive information about a very dynamic organ. When performing an echocardiographic examination, it is important to consider not only the two-dimensional imaging information but also the Doppler findings. Both techniques should be performed as an integral part of an echocardiographic examination and should be used to complement one another.

Throughout this chapter M-mode, two-dimensional, and Doppler findings are discussed in each of the normal as well as abnormal conditions. The chapter begins by providing a description of Doppler echocardiography and its physical properties. The rest of the chapter combines these various techniques in a manner similar to that which should be done during an actual examination.

DOPPLER ECHOCARDIOGRAPHY

The Doppler effect was first described in 1842 by Christian Johann Doppler. Its basic principle states that as the source of sound moves toward one's ear, the frequency of that sound increases and the wavelength decreases. This is why a sound source moving toward you increases in loudness and decreases in loudness as it moves away from you. Doppler echocardiography allows quantification of blood flow velocities and direction of blood flow. It is the study of sound-wave reflections from blood cells as they course through the heart. To record these reflections, the sound beam must be parallel to blood flow. This is the opposite of imaging techniques in which the ideal position is perpendicular to the target. Three basic Doppler modalities are available: pulsed-wave, of which color flow mapping is one variation; continuous-wave; and high-pulsed repetition-frequency Doppler.

In pulsed-wave Doppler, a burst of sound waves is produced by electronically stimulating the piezoelectric crystal in the head of the transducer. Because short periods of time elapse between bursts of sound, reflected signals are allowed to return to the transducer. Thus, the time required to send the original signal and to receive can be determined. Given that the speed of sound in soft tissue also is known (1540 m/s), the depth of the target can then be calculated. The area under examination is called the sample volume. Therefore, the principal advantage of pulsed-wave Doppler is the ability to examine flow in one particular area at a given point in time while ignoring flow in other areas. Its major disadvantage is the inability to measure high velocities. Once flow reaches a particular velocity or frequency known as the Nyquist limit, a phenomenon called aliasing occurs. In this case, the Doppler signal appears to be ambiguous and the peak of the signal is not seen. The pulses are sent at a particular frequency, which is a physical characteristic of the machine known as the pulse repetition frequency or PRF. Sound frequencies received are measured if they fall within the PRF of the machine. Received sound frequencies outside the PRF are not well recorded and appear ambiguous.

When color encoding is used, blood flow is assigned colors according to the direction in which the blood is moving. Red indicates blood flowing toward the transducer, whereas blue indicates blood flowing away from the transducer.

Continuous-wave Doppler uses two separate crystals. One crystal transmits the signal; the other receives the incoming signals. The major advantage of continuous-wave Doppler is that peak velocities can be measured.

Aliasing is not a problem because a high pulse-repetition frequency is used. The major disadvantage is the inability to localize specific origins of the signals. Because they are continuously being sent and received, signals all along the path of the beam path are present.

The Doppler equation demonstrates the mathematical relationship between the velocity of the target (blood cells in the case of cardiac examinations) and the Doppler frequency.

$$f_d = f_r - f_t$$

$$f_d = \frac{2f_t \, V \cdot \cos \theta}{c}$$

where f_d = the Doppler frequency, f_t = the transmitted frequency, f_r = the received frequency, V = the velocity of blood cells, c = the speed of sound waves in a medium, and $\cos \theta$ = cosine of the angle between the direction of the moving target and the path of the ultrasound beam.

The ideal angle is 0°. However, an angle of less than 20° will give a frequency shift. Angles greater than 20° will not yield good results.

Two basic types of blood-flow patterns exist within the heart. Laminar flow is the normal condition in which the blood cells are moving in a uniform direction and at a relatively uniform velocity. Cells traveling in the center of the vessel typically move slightly faster, whereas blood cells near the walls move slightly more slowly because of friction. The resulting Doppler signal is a well-defined spectral display.

The second type of flow pattern seen in the heart is turbulent flow. This is observed in narrowed or obstructed valves (stenosis), regurgitation, ventricular septal defect, and several other pathological conditions that are discussed in this chapter. In these conditions, blood cells no longer travel in a uniform direction; instead, they may travel in the opposite direction as they encounter an obstruction. The blood swirls much like water does when it encounters a dam. The modified or simplified Bernoulli equation can be used to calculate the pressure drop across the obstruction:

$$\Delta P = 4V^2,$$

where V is the velocity of blood flow distal to the obstruction and ΔP is the pressure drop across the obstruction.

The pressure half-time formula is useful for quantifying the degree of stenosis of the mitral valve. The theory behind this formula is that the time required for the peak velocity to be reduced by half is related to the degree of mitral stenosis. The formula is relatively simple and yields accurate results. The peak velocity is either divided by the square root of 1.4 or multiplied by 0.7. The time taken from the peak velocity to that value is the pressure half-time. The pressure half-time is then divided into the empirically derived number of 220. The resulting value is the area of the mitral valve.

ANATOMY AND PHYSIOLOGY OF THE HEART

In order to become proficient in the techniques of echocardiography, a thorough understanding of cardiac anatomy is essential. One must know the normal structures and be able to recognize normal variants from pathological states. There are numerous pathologies that affect the heart in the adult. These disease states can cause a variety of primary as well as secondary anatomical changes in the heart. Knowing what these changes are greatly enhances the echocardiographic examination. Once the student has an understanding of heart anatomy, the echocardiographic images are better understood. The basic two-dimensional echocardiographic views are illustrated in Figs. 3–1 through 3–8. These figures are from the American Society of Echocardiography and are the accepted nomenclature for two-dimensional imaging.

Left Ventricle

Anatomy. The left ventricle is the largest cardiac chamber, accounting for 75% of heart mass. It consists of two papillary muscles, has trabeculations in the apex, and a smooth-walled basal area. Its end-diastolic diameter is 3.6–5.2 cm, and its end-systolic diameter is 2.3–3.9 cm. The thickness of its wall in diastole measures 6–12 mm.

Hemodynamics. The ventricle receives oxygenated blood from the left atrium and pumps it through the aortic valve to the body by way of arteries, arterioles, and capillaries. Its systolic pressure is 100–120 mm Hg.

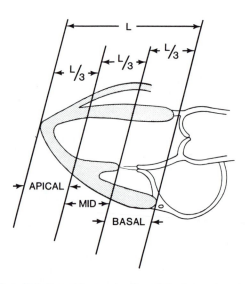

Figure 3–1. Parasternal long-axis view of the heart demonstrating the method of subdividing the myocardial walls along the long axis (L) into three regions of equal length using the left ventricular papillary muscles as landmarks. (*Reprinted with permission from the American Society of Echocardiography. Report of the ASE Committee on Nomenclature and Standards: Identification of Myocardial Wall Segments, November 1982.*)

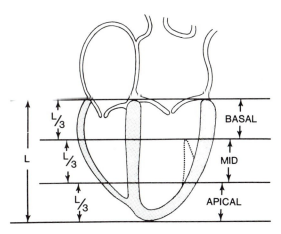

Figure 3–2. Apical four-chamber view of the heart demonstrating the method of subdividing the myocardial walls into three regions using the left ventricular papillary muscles as landmarks. (*Reprinted with permission from the American Society of Echocardiography. Report of the ASE Committee on Nomenclature and Standards: Identification of Myocardial Wall Segments, November 1982.*)

Echocardiographic Views. Almost all the standard views of the left ventricle allow visualization of at least part of the left ventricle. The apical views allow examination of the apex, which can be difficult to see in other views. The maximum internal dimensions are seen at end-diastole and should be measured at the onset of the QRS complex. The minimum internal dimensions are seen at end-systole and should be taken at the peak posterior motion of the interventricular septum.

Left Atrium

Anatomy. The left atrium is a smooth-walled sac, the walls of which are thicker than those of the right atrium.

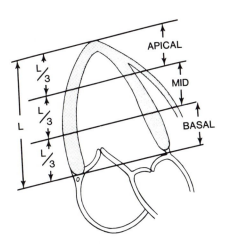

Figure 3–3. Apical long-axis view of the heart demonstrating the method of subdividing the myocardial walls into three regions of equal length. (*Reprinted with permission from the American Society of Echocardiography. Report of the ASE Committee on Nomenclature and Standards: Identification of Myocardial Wall Segments, November 1982.*)

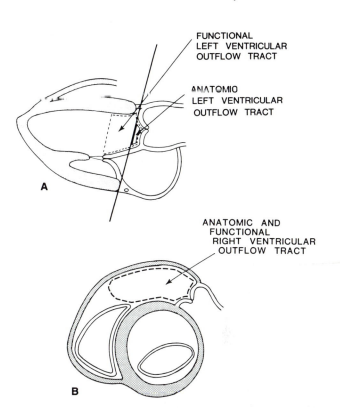

Figure 3–4. The functional and anatomic left ventricular outflow tracts of the heart are diagrammed in the upper panel (**A**), whereas the functional and anatomic right ventricular outflow tract is illustrated in the bottom panel (**B**). (*Reprinted with permission from the American Society of Echocardiography. Report of the ASE Committee on Nomenclature and Standards: Identification of Myocardial Wall Segments, November 1982.*)

The chamber receives four pulmonary veins: two (sometimes three) on the right and two (sometimes one) on the left. The interatrial septum is thin. The left auricle, or left atrial appendage, arises from the upper anterior part of the left atrium and contains small pectinate muscles. The average dimension of the chamber in the adult is 28–38 mm.

Hemodynamics. The mean pressure in the left atrium ranges from 1 mm Hg to 10 mm Hg. Oxygenated blood flows from the lungs and enters the atrium through the pulmonary veins. As left atrial pressure increases over that of the left ventricle, the mitral valve opens and blood then passes through the mitral valve and enters the left ventricle.

Echocardiographic Views. Maximal dimensions should be measured at end-systole. Measurements should be made from the leading edge of the posterior wall of the aorta to the leading edge of the posterior wall of the left atrium. This chamber is best seen from the parasternal long- and short-axis views; however, it also can be seen from the apical and subcostal views. In the left parasternal long-axis view, the descending aorta can be seen running posteriorly to the left atrium. Care must be given when

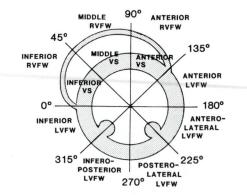

Figure 3–7. Short-axis view of the midventricular region of the heart demonstrating the method of subdividing the myocardial walls into segments using a coordinate system consisting of eight lines that are 45° apart. With this system, the left ventricular free wall (LVFW) is divided into five segments, whereas the ventricular septum (VS) and right ventricular free walls (RVFW) are subdivided into three segments each. (*Reprinted with permission from the American Society of Echocardiography. Report of the ASE Committee on Nomenclature and Standards: Identification of Myocardial Wall Segments, November 1982.*)

Figure 3–5. Diagram of the heart (**A**) and the short-axis views of the basal region (**B**), midventricular region (**C**), and apical region (**D**). (*Reprinted with permission from the American Society of Echocardiography. Report of the ASE Committee on Nomenclature and Standards: Identification of Myocardial Wall Segments, November 1982.*)

measuring the diameter of the left atrium so that the descending aorta is not included in the measurement because this will give an erroneous left atrial diameter.

Right Atrium

Anatomy. The right atrium has two parts: an anterior portion and a posterior portion. The two portions are separated by a ridge of muscle called the crista terminalis.

The smooth-walled posterior portion of the atrium is derived from the embryonic sinus venosus and receives the inferior and superior vena cavae. Guarding the opening (ostium) of the inferior vena cava is a thin fold of tissue called the eustachian valve, which is sometimes

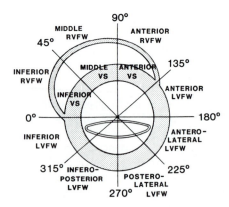

Figure 3–6. Short-axis view of the basal region of the heart demonstrating the method of subdividing the myocardial walls into segments using a coordinate system consisting of eight lines that are 45° apart. With this system, the left ventricular free wall (LVFW) is divided into five segments, whereas the ventricular septum (VS) and right ventricular free walls (RVFW) are subdivided into three segments each. (*Reprinted with permission from the American Society of Echocardiography. Report of the ASE Committee on Nomenclature and Standards: Identification of Myocardial Wall Segments, November 1982.*)

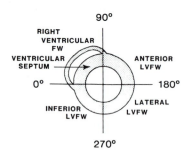

Figure 3–8. Short-axis view of the apical region of the heart demonstrating the method of subdividing the myocardial walls into segments using a coordinate system consisting of four lines that are 90° apart. With this system, the left ventricular free wall (LVFW) is subdivided into three segments, whereas the ventricular septum and right ventricular free wall (FW) are subdivided into one segment each. (*Reprinted with permission from the American Society of Echocardiography. Report of the ASE Committee on Nomenclature and Standards: Identification of Myocardial Wall Segments, November 1982.*)

large and complex and forms a network of tissues known as the network of Chiari. The coronary sinus also enters the right atrium anterior to the inferior vena cava. The coronary sinus also can be guarded by a thin fold of tissue called the thebesian valve.

The anterior portion, which represents the embryonic right atrium, is extremely thin and is trabeculated. The right atrial appendage, or right auricle, arises from the superior portion of the right atrium and contains pectinate muscle. The dimensions of the right atrium in adults range from 26–34 mm.

Hemodynamics. Deoxygenated blood from the body, head, and heart flows into the right atrium through the inferior vena cava, the superior vena cava, and the coronary sinus, respectively. When pressures in the right atrium increase above the pressures in the right ventricle, the tricuspid valve opens, allowing the blood to flow forward into the right ventricle. Mean pressures in this chamber range from 0–8 mm Hg.

Echocardiographic Views. Apical views are best for assessing the right atrium. Others include the subcostal and, to a lesser extent, the parasternal short-axis views.

Right Ventricle

Anatomy. The right ventricle is divided into a posterior inferior inflow portion and an anterior superior outflow portion. The inflow portion contains the tricuspid valve and is heavily trabeculated. The outflow portion, also called the infundibulum, gives rise to the pulmonary trunk. The subpulmonic area is smooth walled.

The right ventricle contains numerous papillary muscles that anchor the tricuspid valve. The ventricle contains numerous bands of muscle. One band, the moderator band, is readily seen in the apex of the ventricle by two-dimensional imaging. Internal diameters range from 7–26 mm.

Hemodynamics. Systolic pressures range from 15–30 mm Hg, and diastolic pressures range from 0–8 mm Hg.

Echocardiographic Views. The right ventricle is seen best from the apical and subcostal views. It also can be seen from the parasternal views.

Aorta

Anatomy. The aorta arises from the base of the heart and enters the superior mediastinum, where it almost reaches the sternum, then courses obliquely backward and to the left over the left bronchus. It then becomes the descending aorta and courses downward anterior to and slightly left of the vertebral column. The aorta is highly elastic and has three layers: (1) a thin inner layer called the tunica intima, (2) a thick middle layer called the tunica media, and (3) a thin outer layer called the tunica adventia. The diameter of the aortic root measures 2.5–3.3 cm.

Hemodynamics. Maximal velocities of blood flow in adults are 1.0–1.7 m/s.

Echocardiographic Views. The aortic root is seen from parasternal views. The ascending aorta, aortic arch, and descending aorta can be seen from the suprasternal view. As was mentioned earlier, part of the descending aorta also can be seen behind the left atrium in the long-axis view. The subcostal views allows visualization of the aortic root and valve.

Main Pulmonary Artery

Anatomy. The main pulmonary artery is located superior to and originates from the right ventricle. Immediately after leaving the pericardium, it bifurcates into a right pulmonary artery and a left pulmonary artery that enter the right and left lung, respectively.

Hemodynamics. This artery delivers deoxygenated blood from the right ventricle to the lungs. Flow velocities range from 0.6–0.9 m/s.

Echocardiographic Views. The artery is seen best from the parasternal short-axis view.

Mitral Valve

Anatomy. The mitral valve is an atrioventricular valve. It is located between the left atrium and left ventricle, is a thin yellowish-white membrane that originates at the annulus fibrous, a fibrous ring that surrounds the orifice of the valve. The valve has an anterior leaflet and a posterior leaflet, both of which have sawtoothlike edges. Both leaflets are attached to papillary muscles by cordae tendinae. The surface on the atrial side of the valve is smooth whereas the surface on the ventricular side is irregular.

Hemodynamics. Flow velocities across the valve range from 0.6–1.3 m/s. The valve's function is to prevent backflow of blood from the left ventricle into the left atrium.

Echocardiographic Views. The mitral valve is seen best from the long- and short-axis parasternal views and the apical view. Doppler measurements are obtained best from the apical four- and two-chamber views.

Aortic Valve

Anatomy. The aortic valve consists of three pocket-shaped thin smooth cusps named according to their location in relation to the coronary arteries. The cusp near the left coronary artery is the left coronary cusp, the cusp near the right coronary artery is the right coronary cusp, and the cusp that is not near a coronary artery is the noncoronary cusp. Because of its lunar or half-moon shape, the aortic valve is referred to as semilunar.

Hemodynamics. The function of the aortic valve is to prevent backflow of blood from the aorta into the left ventricle. The velocity of flow ranges from 1.0–1.7 m/s.

Echocardiographic Views. The valve is seen best from the parasternal views. It also can be seen from the apical four-chamber view with anterior angulation. The best Doppler measurements are obtained from the apical four-chamber view with anterior angulation, from the right parasternal window, and from the suprasternal view.

Tricuspid Valve

Anatomy. The tricuspid valve is an atrioventricular valve. It is located between the right atrium and ventricle. The atrial side is smooth; the ventricular side is irregular. Like the mitral valve, it is a thin yellowish-white membrane that originates at the annulus fibrous, a fibrous ring that surrounds the orifice of the valve. The valve has three leaflets—anterior, posterior, and medial—all of which are sawtoothlike in appearance. Each leaflet is attached to papillary muscles by cordae tendinae.

Hemodynamics. The function of this valve is to prevent backflow of blood from the right ventricle to the right atrium. The velocity of flow ranges from 0.3–0.7 m/s.

Echocardiographic Views. The valve is seen best from the parasternal short-axis and apical four-chamber views. The subcostal view also affords a good look. The best Doppler measurements are taken from the parasternal short-axis and apical four-chamber views.

Pulmonic Valve

Anatomy. The pulmonic valve consists of three thin smooth pocket-shaped cusps. Because of its shape, this valve, like the aortic valve, is called semilunar.

Hemodynamics. The function of this valve is to prevent backflow of blood from the main pulmonary artery to the right ventricle. The velocity of flow ranges from 0.6–0.9 m/s.

Echocardiographic Views. The pulmonic valve is seen best from the parasternal short-axis view. The best Doppler recordings are taken from the left parasternal short axis.

DISEASES AFFECTING THE VALVES

Mitral Valve Disease

Stenosis. Mitral valve stenosis results primarily from rheumatic disease. The valves may not become involved for many decades following rheumatic fever. Congenital mitral stenosis can occur but is extremely rare.

M-mode findings include (1) a flattened E-F slope (reduced diastolic filling), (2) anterior motion of the posterior leaflet, (3) thickened leaflets, and (4) an absent A wave in the absence of atrial fibrillation. Two-dimensional imaging also indicates thickening and shows doming of the leaflets in diastole.

Doppler measurements reveal a reduced rate of decrease in diastolic flow (reduced diastolic slope), a higher-than-normal peak velocity of flow, and spectral broadening on Doppler display. Secondary findings and complications include left atrial dilatation, pulmonary hypertension, a left atrial clot, and an exaggerated diastolic dip of the interventricular septum.

Regurgitation. Mitral regurgitation can occur as a result of mitral annular calcification, rheumatic mitral disease, flail mitral valve leaflet, conditions that may stretch the mitral annulus such as cardiomyopathies, myocardial infarction, mitral valve vegetations or other masses on the mitral valve or within the left atrium, papillary dysfunction, and mitral valve prolapse.

M-mode findings include (1) increased size of the left atrium, (2) exaggerated motion of the interventricular septum, (3) pulsations of the left atrial wall, and (4) preclosure of the aortic valve during systole. The first three findings are the result of volume overload.

Two-dimensional imaging reveals an increase in the size of the left atrium and exaggerated motion of the interventricular septum—all of which are the result of volume overload. In addition, pulsations of the left atrial wall and preclosure of the aortic valve during systole are observed.

Prolapse. The classic clinical findings in mitral valve prolapse are a systolic click (a sound that corresponds with the posterior displacement of the mitral valve leaflet into the left atrium) and a late systolic murmur (a sound that corresponds with the resulting mitral regurgitation that often occurs because of the prolapsing leaflets).

M-mode findings include late systolic posterior displacement of the anterior and posterior leaflets and anterior motion of the mitral valve in early systole. To achieve the best views for making the diagnosis, the ultrasound beam should be perpendicular to the valve from the parasternal windows. The two-dimensional findings reveal that the valve is bowing into the left atrium and, in many cases, thickened.

Flail Leaflet. The most common cause of flail leaflet is rupture of the chordae tendineae, which often occurs secondary to myocardial infarction. Rupture of papillary muscle is a less common etiology.

M-mode findings indicate coarse diastolic fluttering and systolic fluttering of the leaflet and visualization of part of the leaflet in the left atrium. Two-dimensional imaging indicates protrusion of the flail leaflet into the left atrium, noncoaptation of the two leaflets, and systolic and coarse diastolic motion of the flail leaflet. Doppler measurements indicate harsh, turbulent mitral regurgitation.

Annular Calcification. Mitral annular calcification results from the deposition of calcium in the annulus of the mitral valve. This is normally associated with aging. This condition can be caused by mitral regurgitation, conduction abnormalities, aging, or obstruction of the left ventricular outflow tract (LVOF).

M-mode findings reveal high-density echoes between the valve and the posterior wall of the left ventricle. Two-dimensional imaging reveals high-density bright echoes between the valve and the posterior wall of the left ventricle.

Aortic Valve Disease

Stenosis (versus Sclerosis). The cause of stenosis of the aortic valve can be congenital, the result of rheumatic heart disease, or degeneration. The effect is hypertrophy of the left ventricular walls.

M-mode findings indicate thickened cusps and restricted excursion of the cusps to less than 1.5 cm. Two-dimensional imaging not only reveals these M-mode findings but systolic doming of the cusps (the most important sign) as well. Doppler measurements reveal high-velocity jets greater than 1.7 m/s.

Regurgitation. The effects of regurgitation on atria, ventricles, and cardiac vessels result in dilation of the left ventricle. The condition can be caused by any one of the following: congenital (bicuspid cusp), rheumatic heart disease (the most common cause in adults), degeneration of the leaflet caused by infection, or aortic dilatation (Marfan syndrome).

M-mode findings reveal fluttering of the interventricular septum and diastolic fluttering of the mitral valve. Two-dimensional imaging indicates fine diastolic fluttering of the aortic valve, diastolic fluttering of the mitral valve, and fluttering of the interventricular septum. Spectral Doppler studies reveal diastolic flow, which appears above the baseline when in an apical position.

Tricuspid Valve Diseases

Stenosis. In stenotic disease of the tricuspid valve, the effects on atria, ventricles, and vessels cause dilatation of the right atrium.

M-mode findings indicate a reduced diastolic slope and thickening and decreased separation of the leaflets. Two-dimensional imaging reveals the most specific finding, systolic doming, as well as thickening of the leaflets. In Doppler measurements, the sample is placed in the right ventricle; the results indicate turbulent diastolic flow and slowed reduction in the velocity of flow during diastole.

Regurgitation. The primary cause of regurgitation is secondary to pulmonary hypertension. In rare cases, the condition can be caused by rheumatic heart disease, prolapse of the valve, or carcinoid heart disease. A secondary effect is dilatation of the right atrium and ventricle.

M-mode findings indicate a dilated right ventricle and anterior motion of the interventricular septum during isovolumetric contraction. Two-dimensional imaging reveals incomplete closure and diastolic fluttering of the leaflets, ruptured chordae, dilation of the right ventricle, and flattening of the interventricular septum. With Doppler measurements, turbulent flow can be detected in the right atrium during systole.

Pulmonic Valve Diseases

Stenosis. The causes of pulmonic valve disease are atherosclerosis, infectious endocarditis, and papillary fibroma. This disease is extremely rare in adults.

Regurgitation. M-mode findings reveal fluttering of the tricuspid leaflets, and Doppler measurements reveal early diastolic high-velocity, turbulent flow. The cause can be pulmonary hypertension or bacterial endocarditis or be secondary to pulmonary valvotomy.

Endocarditis

Types. Endocarditis can be caused by either bacteria or vegetation (funguslike growth) and, depending on the infecting organism, is classified as acute or subacute. Although the disease can occur in the endocardium of the heart, the infection usually affects the endocardium in specific valves and is more likely to affect the left heart than the right. Infection of the tricuspid and pulmonic valves is usually the result of intravenous (IV) drug abuse.

Bacterial Endocarditis. Predisposing factors for bacterial endocarditis include dental procedures, tonsilloadenoidectomy, cirrhosis, drug addiction, surgery, and burns.

Nonbacterial Endocarditis. Among the nonbacterial forms of the disease are systemic lupus erythematosus (SLE) and fungal (mycotic), nonbacterial thrombotic, Löffler's, marantic, and Libman-Sacks endocarditis. The most common manifestation of SLE is vegetation. Although this nonbacterial form of endocarditis primarily involves the mitral valve, it also can affect the mural endocardium. The mycotic form of the disease is usually subacute and can be caused by a variety of fungi—most commonly, *Candida*, *Aspergillus*, and *Histoplasma*. In the thrombotic form of nonbacterial endocarditis, the vegetation consists of fibrin and other blood elements.

Löffler's endocarditis is characterized by a marked increase of eosinophils. It primarily affects men in their forties who live in temperate climates. The disease affects both ventricles equally. Thickening of the inflow portions of the ventricles and the apices can be observed, as can formation of mural thrombi. Hemodynamically, diastolic filling is impaired because of increased stiffness of the heart. Atrioventricular valve regurgitation is a typical finding.

In the marantic form of the disease, the vegetation is nondestructive and sterile. It occurs in patients with malignant tumors and primarily affects the valves on the left side of the heart. Embolus is the most serious complication.

Libman-Sacks endocarditis is characterized by vegetations or verrucae on the endocardium.

Hemodynamic Mechanisms. One common cause of subacute infectious endocarditis occurs when a high-velocity jet consistently hits a surface. Damage results when blood from a high-pressure area flows to a low-pressure area; this is called the Venturi effect. The site where vegetation has formed will usually be in the low-pressure area. When the mitral valve is involved and mitral regurgitation is present, the atrial side of the leaflets is the susceptible area. In this case, the high-pressure area is the ventricle and, because the mitral leaflets fail to coapt, the low-pressure area is the atrial side of the leaflets. The atrial wall that bears the brunt of the regurgitation also may become infected.

When the aortic valve is involved and aortic insufficiency is present, the aorta is the high-pressure area and the ventricle is the low-pressure area. Vegetations tend to form on the ventricular side of the aortic cusps because the cusps do not close completely in aortic regurgitation. The section of the ventricular wall hit by the regurgitant jet also may be damaged.

In ventricular septal defects (VSDs), the high-pressure area is the left ventricle in left-to-right shunting and the low-pressure area is the right ventricular side of the defect. The right ventricular wall directly across from the defect also can suffer damage and be prone to vegetation.

Echocardiographic Appearance. The presence of a mass on any valve leads to a diagnosis of infection caused by vegetation. However, echocardiography cannot differentiate between a new and old infection. M-mode patterns indicate shaggy echoes on the infected valve and detect 52% of vegetations. The technique of choice is two-dimensional imaging, which detects more than 80% of vegetations, reveals dense echoes on the valve, and often detects mobility of the mass.

Aortic Valve. Vegetation is seen best in diastole and is attached to the ventricular side of the cusps. This condition can cause reduced cardiac output and acute aortic regurgitation. The best views for two-dimensional imaging are the left parasternal long and short axes.

Mitral Valve. Predisposing factors to vegetational infection of the mitral valve include mitral valve prolapse, rheumatic valvulitis, and dysfunction of the papillary muscles with secondary mitral regurgitation and mitral annular calcification. Infection occurs most commonly on the atrial side of the leaflet.

The best views include the left parasternal short and long axes; the apical two- and four-chamber views also can be used. Vegetations as small as 2 mm in diameter are detectable or can be as large as 40 mm in diameter. Whereas M-mode imaging detects 14–65% of the vegeta-

tion, two-dimensional imaging detects 43–100%. Differential diagnoses include myomas, lipomas, and fibromas.

Tricuspid or Pulmonic Valve. Infections of the tricuspid or pulmonic valves are usually caused by IV drug abuse. Such infections are less common than left-sided infections; however, when they occur on the tricuspid valve, the infections can become larger than is typical of left-sided infections. They rarely occur on the pulmonic valve.

Prosthetic Valves

Types. Two types of prosthetic valves are available: mechanical and bioprosthetic. The mechanical types are ball-in-cage, disc-in-cage, and tilting-disc valves. The Starr-Edwards valve is the most common ball-in-cage type. The best view for observing excursion of the ball is the apical view when in the mitral and aortic positions. The disc-in-cage valve has less excursion than does the ball-in-cage type. The most common type of tilting-disc valve is the Bjork-Shiley, which consists of one disc that tilts. The less common St. Jude valve contains two tilting discs.

The most common bioprosthetic valve is the xenograft. A porcine heterograft is the most commonly used tissue; porcine pericardial tissue also can be used. Human homografts and facia lata tissue are sometimes used as valves.

Malfunctions. The following factors cause both types of prosthetic valves to malfunction: thrombi, regurgitation, stenosis, dehiscence, and vegetation.

Thrombi. Blood clots, the most common cause of valve malfunction, reduce the effective orifice and impair motion of the ball, disc, or leaflet tissue. Their major complication is the potential for an embolus. Two-dimensional imaging is the echocardiographic technique of choice for detecting the presence of a clot. The limitation of the technique is the masking effect produced by the highly reflective nature of the prosthetic material. Transesophageal echocardiography has proved to be useful for evaluating the formation of clots on prosthetic valves. In the Bjork-Shiley mitral prosthesis, there is a rounding to the E point on M-mode.

Regurgitation. Regurgitation can occur through the valve or around the sewing ring. Doppler echocardiography is the procedure of choice for detecting the problem. When masking is a problem from apical views, color Doppler is especially useful. Color flow Doppler not only allows spatial orientation but also demonstrates the direction of blood jets. Secondary echocardiographic findings for aortic prosthetic regurgitation include (1) fluttering of the mitral valve, (2) fluttering of the interventricular septum, and (3) evidence of volume overload in the left ventricle. Doppler echocardiography also is a procedure of choice for detecting paravalvular leaks with a high degree of sensitivity and specificity. In the Bjork-Shiley mitral valve, an early diastolic bump is noted by M-mode and two-dimensional imaging.

Stenosis. All prosthetic valves have some degree of obstruction. Doppler echocardiography can detect a valve with moderate to severe stenosis.

Dehiscence. In dehiscence, the valve becomes detached from its sewing bed. Disruption of suture lines securing the prosthesis to the sewing ring is usually the cause. The result is severe regurgitation, heart failure, or both, which can be detected by a Doppler examination. Two-dimensional imaging demonstrates an unusual rocking motion away from its normal excursion. Cinefluoroscopy can be helpful in assessing abnormal rocking motion.

Vegetation. As was mentioned earlier, vegetation is difficult to assess with echocardiographic techniques because it is often masked by the highly reflective properties of the prosthesis. These infections are usually found on bioprosthetic valves, are extremely mobile, and are more common in the aortic than the mitral position.

Degeneration. Degeneration is most common in bioprosthetic valves and usually occurs as a result of calcification of the area where the valve is joined to the surrounding tissue.

DISEASES AFFECTING THE PERICARDIUIM

The pericardium is composed of two layers. The inner layer is a serous membrane called the visceral pericardium, which is attached to the surface of the heart. This layer folds back upon itself to form an outer fibrous layer called the parietal pericardium. Between the two layers is the pericardial space, which is filled with a thin layer of fluid throughout. The functions of the pericardium are to (1) fix the heart anatomically, (2) prevent excessive motion during changes in body position, (3) reduce friction between the heart and other organs, (4) provide a barrier against infection, and (5) help maintain hydrostatic forces on the heart. Pericardial disease can be caused by any one of the following: malignant disease that spreads to the pericardium, pericarditis, acute infarction, cardiac perforation during diagnostic procedures, radiation therapy, SLE, or postcardiac surgery.

Effusion
In the normal pericardium, the pressure within the pericardial space is similar to the intrapleural pressure and lower than the right and left ventricular diastolic pressures. Increased intrapericardial pressure depends on three factors: the volume of the effusion, the rate at which fluid accumulates, and the characteristics of the pericardium. The normal intrapericardial space contains 15–50 mL of fluid, and it can tolerate the slow addition of as much as 1 to 2 L of fluid without increasing the intrapericardial pressure. However, if the fluid is added rapidly, the intrapericardial pressure increases dramatically.

Pericardial effusion can be diagnosed using M-mode and two-dimensional techniques. Three diagnostic criteria can be used: (1) posterior echo-free space, (2) obliteration of echo-free space at the left atrioventricular groove, and (3) decreased motion of the posterior pericardial motion.

Cardiac tamponade results when intrapericardial pressures increase. This problem is characterized by increased intracardiac pressures, impaired diastolic filling of the ventricles, and reduced stroke volume. The following echocardiographic findings are associated with cardiac tamponade:

- increased dimensions of the right ventricle during inspiration,
- decreased mitral diastolic slope (E-F),
- decreased end diastolic dimension of the right atrium or ventricle,
- posterior motion of the anterior wall of the right ventricle,
- collapse of the right ventricular free wall,
- diastolic collapse of the right atrial wall, and
- increased flow velocities across the tricuspid and pulmonic valve during inspiration.

Several findings can create a false positive diagnosis of pericardial effusion:

- Epicardial fat located on the anterior wall.
- Misinterpretation of normal cardiac structures such as the descending aorta or coronary sinus.
- Other abnormal cardiac or noncardiac structures.
- Confusion of pleural effusions with pericardial effusions.

Pericardial effusion can be differentiated from pleural effusion in several ways. First, in pericardial effusion, a large amount of fluid can collect posterior to the heart without any anterior collection. Second, a pericardial effusion tapers as it approaches the left atrium; a pleural effusion does not. Third, if both types of effusion occur simultaneously, a thin echogenic line should be noted between the two collections of fluid. And fourth, the descending aorta lies posterior to a pericardial effusion, whereas it lies anterior to a pleural effusion.

Pericarditis
Pericarditis comes in two forms: acute and constrictive. In acute pericarditis, the pericardium is inflamed. This form of the disease has a variety of etiologies: idiopathic causes, viruses, uremia, bacterial infections, acute myocardial infarction, tuberculosis, malignancies, and trauma. Echocardiography reveals thickening of the pericardium, with or without pericardial effusion.

In constrictive disease, the pericardium thickens and restricts diastolic filling of the heart chambers. Like the acute form, it has a variety of causes: tuberculosis, hemodialysis used to treat chronic renal failure, connective tissue disorders (eg, SLE, rheumatoid arthritis), metastatic infiltration, radiation therapy to the mediastinum, fungal or parasitic infections, and complications of surgery. Echocardiographic findings may include

- thickened pericardium,
- flattening of the left ventricular wall in mid and late systole,
- a rapid mitral valve E-F slope,
- exaggerated anterior motion of the interventricular septum,
- mid-diastolic premature opening of the pulmonic valve,
- inspiratory dilatation of hepatic veins and the inferior vena cava, and
- inspiratory leftward motion of the interatrial and interventricular septa.

DISEASES AFFECTING THE MYOCARDIUM

The term cardiomyopathy is used to describe a variety of cardiac diseases that affect the myocardium. Cardiomyopathies have been classified into three categories: (1) hypertrophic, which may or may not obstruct the left ventricular outflow tract, (2) dilated, and (3) restrictive. The classification depends on the anatomical characteristics of the left ventricular cavity as well as systolic-ejection and diastolic-filling properties of the left ventricle.

Hypertrophic Cardiomyopathy

Hypertrophic cardiomyopathy is characterized by concentric or asymmetric left ventricular hypertrophy, which results in an increase in left ventricular mass, with normal or reduced dimensions of the left ventricular cavity. Normal systolic function usually is preserved. Although asymmetric hypertrophy can occur anywhere within the left ventricle, the most common site is the proximal portion of the ventricular septum near the outflow tract. Asymmetric septal hypertrophy can be diagnosed when the ratio of septal thickness to posterior wall thickness is 1.3 to 1. When asymmetric hypertrophy is present obstruction most frequently occurs. Concentric hypertrophy may or may not lead to obstruction. A number of names are used to describe the obstructive forms of cardiomyopathy, including idiopathic hypertrophic subaortic stenosis, muscular subaortic stenosis, asymmetric septal hypertrophy, and hypertrophic obstructive cardiomyopathy.

Several echocardiographic findings, when found in conjunction, are highly specific for the diagnosis of obstructive cardiomyopathy. M-mode and two-dimensional findings include systolic anterior motion of the mitral valve, asymmetric septal hypertrophy, premature midsystolic closure of the aortic valve, septal hypokinesis, and anterior displacement of the mitral valve. The size of the left ventricle is small to normal. Doppler examination reveals a decreased E wave in mitral flow with an exaggerated A wave. These findings suggest a decrease in diastolic compliance and an increase in left ventricular end diastolic pressures. In aortic flow, there is a midsystolic reduction of velocity. Fifty percent of patients demonstrate regurgitation in the mitral valve. Pulsed-wave Doppler is used to determine the obstructed area.

At rest, systolic anterior motion of the mitral valve may not be demonstrated. Because this motion is a diagnostic indication for this disease, provocative maneuvers are used to bring it out. Such techniques include the Valsalva's maneuver, amyl nitrate, and IV isoproterenol.

Dilated Cardiomyopathy

Dilated cardiomyopathy is characterized by globally reduced systolic function, with an ejection fraction of less than 40%, increased end-systolic and end-diastolic volumes, and, eventually, congestive heart failure. M-mode findings include increased end-diastolic and end-systolic dimensions of the left ventricle, reduced septal and posterior wall excursion, increased E point-to-septal separation, decreased aortic root movement, and a structurally normal aortic valve that opens slowly and drifts closed during systole because of reduced cardiac output. The principal two-dimensional echocardiographic findings include left ventricular dilatation and dysfunction, abnormal closure of the mitral valve, and dilatation of the left atrium. The abnormal closure of the aortic valve also is noted. Mitral regurgitation is a frequent Doppler finding in dilated cardiomyopathy. Hemodynamically, the left ventricle demonstrates signs of increased diastolic pressure in the left ventricle and decreased compliance. The walls of the left ventricle are normal in size. The right heart also may become enlarged as a result of the increased diastolic pressures in the left heart. The most common complication of dilated cardiomyopathy is the formation of thrombi and a potential cardiac source of emboli.

Dilated cardiomyopathies can be the result of a familial or x-linked cardiomyopathy, pregnancy, systemic hypertension, ingestion of toxic agents such as alcohol or other drugs, and a variety of viral infections. They also can be of unknown cause or idiopathic. This form of cardiomyopathy also can be found in severe coronary artery disease.

Restrictive Cardiomyopathy

Restrictive cardiomyopathy falls into two categories: endomyocardial fibrosis and infiltrative myocardial disease, which includes amyloidosis, sarcoidosis, hematochromatosis, Pompe's disease, and Fabry's disease. The characteristic feature of restrictive cardiomyopathy is increased resistance to left ventricular filling. The associated cardiac findings include elevated diastolic pressure in the left ventricle, hypertension and enlargement of the left atrium, and secondary pulmonary hypertension. The echocardiographic features include an increase in the thickness and mass of the left ventricular wall, a small-to-normal sized left ventricular cavity, normal systolic function, and a pericardial effusion. Restrictive cardiomyopathies are most common in East Africa; they account for only 5% of noncoronary cardiomyopathies in the western world.

Endomyocardial fibrosis involves formation of fibrotic sheets of tissue in the subendocardium. These sheets vary in thickness and result in increased stiffness of the ventricles. The bright reflective characteristic of this tissue is easily seen with two-dimensional echocardiography. Other characteristic echocardiographic findings include a normal-sized left ventricle, increased thickness of the left ventricular wall, thrombus, and left atrial enlargement, which usually occurs because of elevated diastolic pressure of the left ventricle. The right heart is normal in size, with mildly reduced systolic function and increased wall dimensions. Tricuspid regurgitation is present because of the pulmonary hypertension that occurs because of elevated pressures in the left heart.

There are two basic varieties of endomyocardial fibrosis. One form, found primarily in temperate regions, results from hypereosinophilia and is therefore termed hypereosinophilic syndrome. This syndrome, also referred to as Löffler's endocarditis parietalis fibroplastica or Löffler's endocarditis, mainly affects men in their forties and is characterized by increased eosinophils of more than 1500/mm^3. The second form, obliterative endomyocardial fibrosis,[1] occurs primarily in subtropical climates and is especially common in Uganda and Nigeria. It accounts for 10–20% of all cardiac deaths in those countries. Large pericardial effusions are typical in this cardiomyopathy.

CARDIAC MASSES

Benign Tumors

Myxomas. Myxoma is the most common type of benign tumor, accounting for 30–50% of all benign tumors. Three times as many females as males are affected, and 90% of the tumors are found in the atria: 75–86% are found in the left atrium; 8–20% in the right atrium; and 5–11%, in the right atrium or left ventricle but rarely in both atria. Ninety percent of myxomas are pedunculated; the most common site of attachment is the interatrial septum near the fossa avalis. This tumor may be hereditary (autosomal dominant).

M-mode findings reveal echos behind the anterior leaflet of the mitral valve. Two-dimensional imaging reveals an echogenic mass in the affected chamber. The echo may be brightly echogenic to sonolucent because of hemorrhage or necrosis.

The clinical findings include the following: symptoms similar to those of mitral valve disease, embolic phenomena, no symptoms, symptoms similar to those of tricuspid valve disease, sudden death, pericarditis, myocardial infarction, symptoms similar to pulmonic valve disease, and a fever of unknown origin.

Rhabdomyomas. Rhabdomyoma, also called myocardial hamartoma, is the most common cardiac tumor found in infants and children and is associated with tuberous sclerosis. In 90% of the cases, multiple rhabdomyomas are involved. The tumor is yellow gray in appearance, ranges from 1 mm to several centimeters in diameter, and most commonly involves the ventricles. Large tumors may lead to intracavitary obstruction resulting in death.

Lipomas. Lipoma, the second most common benign tumor, affects people of all ages and is found equally often in males and females. Most of these tumors are sessile. Fifty percent are located in the subendocardium, 25% are found in the subepicardium, and 25% are intramuscular. The most common sites are the left ventricle, right atrium, and interatrial septum.

Fibromas. Fibromas occur in the connective tissue and are the second most common benign tumors found predominantly in children (most of whom are younger than 10 years). Almost all of these tumors occur in the ventricular myocardium.

Angiomas. Angiomas are extremely rare. They may occur in any part of the heart.[2]

Teratomas. Teratomas are extremely rare and occur more often in children. They are found most frequently in the right heart, but also can occur in the interatrial or interventricular septum.[2]

Cystic Tumors. Cystic tumors are usually small lesions found in the region of the A-V node.[2]

Malignant Tumors

Primary Cardiac Tumors. Angiosarcomas usually occur in adults and are twice as common in men as in women. They are usually found in the right atrium; the most common site is the interatrial septum. Other primary cardiac tumors are rhabdomyosarcomas, fibrosarcomas, lymphosarcomas, and sarcomas of the pulmonary artery.

Secondary Metastatic Tumors. Metastatic tumors usually invade the right heart. Usually they are clinically silent. However, they can cause superior vena cava syndrome because of obstruction, supraventricular arrhythmias, myocardial infarction, cardiomegaly, congestive heart failure, or nonbacterial endocarditis. Bronchogenic carcinomas, breast carcinomas, malignant melanomas, and leukemia's account for the vast majority of metastases to the heart. Bronchogenic carcinomas are the most common, followed by breast carcinomas, malignant melanomas, and leukemias. Spread of these tumors varies. Bronchogenic carcinomas spread via direct extension; breast carcinomas spread via the lymphatic channels; and metastases of malignant melanomas spread through the blood. Usually metastases involve the pericardium or the myocardium.[2]

Cardiac Thrombi

Left Ventricular Thrombi. Thrombi of the left ventricle occur in myocardial infarctions, left ventricular aneurysms, and cardiomyopathies. They usually form in the apex of the ventricle. Two-dimensional imaging can diagnose the clot with 90% sensitivity and specificity. Echocardiography reveals that the clot has distinct margins, is usually located near an akinetic or dyskinetic area, and may protrude within the ventricle or move with the adjacent wall. Protruding thrombi tend to be more echodense than mural thrombi, whereas mural thrombi have a layered appearance and are often echolucent along the endocardial border.

Thrombi form within the first 4 days after an infarction and occur in 30% of all anterior wall infarctions; they rarely occur in inferior wall infarctions. If they do not dissolve spontaneously, they may disappear with the use of anticoagulants.

Left Atrial Thrombi. Thrombi usually form in the left atrium in the presence of mitral valve disease (stenosis), an enlarged left atrium, and atrial fibrillation—conditions that predispose to blood stasis. The most common site is the atrial appendage. The echocardiographic appearance of these thrombi varies. In many cases, they are attached to the atrial wall and can be round or ovoid in shape. Their borders are often well defined, they demonstrate mobility, and their texture is uniform. Occasionally, they appear as a flat immobile mass or as a free-floating ball.

Thrombi of the Right Heart. Most thrombi form in the right heart in the presence of right ventricular infarction, cardiomyopathies, or cor pulmonale. They usually are immobile, heterogeneous sessile masses. In addition, secondary thrombi may occur. Their source is embolization from deep-vein thrombosis. Echocardiography typically reveals a long, serpentine, apparently free-floating mass with no obvious site of attachment. Patients are at a much higher risk for an embolus when the thrombus in any area of the heart is protruding or free floating.

Other Cardiac Masses. Because a number of foreign objects can mimic a thrombus, one must be aware of their presence and location. For example, right-heart catheters are often seen in both the right atrium and the right ventricle. These appear as highly reflective linear echoes.

Normal cardiac structures also can mimic intracardiac masses. The moderator band seen in the apex of the right ventricle appears as a thick muscular band extending from the free wall of the right ventricle to the interventricular septum. Occasionally, a prominent eustachian valve can be seen in the right atrium at the junction of the inferior vena cava. It appears as a thin, long, mobile structure in the right atrium, which also may contain thin filamentous structures known as the Chiari network that is a remnant of embryonic structures. The left ventricle also may contain long thin fibers known as false tendons or ectopic chordae tendineae. These filamentous structures traverse the left ventricle and typically are brightly reflective structures of no clinical significance.

DISEASES OF THE AORTA

Aortic Dilatation

The aorta is considered dilated when its diameter is greater than 37 mm. The average diameter of the adult aorta is 33–37 mm. M-mode measurements of the aorta should be taken at the level of the aortic annulus and the

sinus of Valsalva. Aortic dilatation is seen most frequently in patients with annuloaortic ectasia or Marfan syndrome. In these patients, the medial layer of the aorta weakens and the aorta dilates. The dilatation occurs not only in the wall of the aorta but in the aortic annulus as well. This often leads to aortic insufficiency because the cusps of the aorta are unable to coapt during closure. Two-dimensional echocardiography can easily detect a dilated aorta.

Aortic Aneurysm

An aortic aneurysm can occur anywhere along the thoracic aorta. The most common sites are the arch and descending aorta, with most occurring just beyond the left subclavian artery. Aneurysms of the thoracic aorta often extend into the abdominal aorta.

A dissecting aortic aneurysm results from intimal tears of the aortic wall. The driving force of the blood destroys the media further and strips the intimal layer from the adventitial layer. Aortic dissections are classified according to the area and extent of the intimal tear. Type I tears extend from the ascending aorta and continue beyond the arch. Type II tears also begin a few centimeters from the aortic valve but are confined to the ascending aorta. Type III tears begin in the descending aorta, usually just distal to the origin of the left subclavian artery. More than 90% of patients with dissecting aneurysms experience severe pain. Dissections occur twice as often in men as in women and usually in the sixth and seventh decade of life. M-mode findings reveal extra linear echos within the aorta. Two-dimensional imaging is the echocardiographic tool of choice. Two-dimensional imaging allows visualization of the intimal flap, which divides the true lumen of the aorta from the false lumen. Color flow Doppler can be invaluable in localizing the site of intraluminal communication. Other echocardiographic evidence for dissection includes aortic regurgitation—the most commonly noted complication. Doppler is useful for detecting disturbed flow patterns in the left ventricular outflow tract. The left ventricle may become enlarged because of volume overload from the aortic regurgitation; pericardial effusion can be noted, and left pleural effusion also may be noted. The diagnosis of dissection should be made when an intima flap is seen in more than one view.

Aneurysms that occur in the sinus of Valsalva are seen best using two-dimensional imaging. They are observed most easily in the short-axis view during diastole. Rupture usually occurs into the right side of the heart, but it also can occur in the left heart and interventricular septum. Sinus of Valsalva aneurysms can be acquired or congenital in nature.

CONGENITAL HEART DISEASE

Aortic Stenosis

Abnormalities of the left ventricular outflow tract are the most common congenital heart disease found in the adult population. Obstruction can occur at the subvalvular, supravalvular, or valvular level. Congenital abnormalities of the aortic valve occur in 1% of the population, with a higher prevalence among males. The most common malformation of the aortic valve is a bicuspid valve. Aortic coarctation, VSD, and isolated pulmonic stenosis are associated with the condition, As the valve ages, it becomes fibrotic and may calcify. By the fourth decade, 50% of all bicuspid aortic valves become stenotic.

Subvalvular stenosis also can occur. There are two types of subvalvular stenosis: discrete and subaortic. In discrete stenosis, a thin membrane obstructs the outflow tract or a more fibromuscular ridge obstructs the flow of blood. Subaortic stenosis, too, is more common in males. Aortic regurgitation is a frequent finding in subaortic stenosis. Discrete subvalvular stenosis is primarily an acquired rather than a congenital problem when it is present in adults.

Supravalvular stenosis also can be classified into two categories. The most frequent supravalvular narrowing is found in the ascending aorta just above the valve. Less frequently, the obstruction involves the ascending aorta, the aortic arch, and the descending aorta. Supravalvular obstruction can be a familial finding, but it also can be sporadic or as a result of rubella infection. When found in association with mental retardation, a diagnosis of Williams syndrome can be made.

Patients with congenital outflow obstruction usually present with left ventricular systolic hypertension and develop concentric left ventricular hypertrophy. The physical examination reveals a harsh systolic ejection murmur over the right parasternal border. Echocardiography has become the diagnostic tool of choice in making this diagnosis. M-mode echocardiography reveals a thickened valve with an eccentric closure line. Normally, the closure line of the aortic valve is centrally located. In a bicuspid aortic valve, however, the closure line is displaced toward either the anterior or the posterior wall of the aorta. Two-dimensional echocardiography reveals systolic doming of the cusps, which is seen in the left parasternal long-axis view. The left parasternal short-axis view reveals the presence of only two cusps. Pulsed-wave Doppler echocardiography can localize the area of obstruction and determine what type of obstruction is present. Continuous-wave Doppler examination allows quantification of peak and mean pressure gradients across the obstruction. Color flow Doppler examination allows assessment of blood flow direction.

Atrial Septal Defects

Atrial septal defects (ASD) is the second most common congenital abnormality found in adults. There are three classifications of ASDs, depending on their location: ostium secundum defects, ostium primum defects, and sinus venosus defects. Ostium secundum defects make up 70% of all ASDs found in adults. These are located near the fossa ovalis. Women are three times more likely than men to have this defect. Twenty percent of patients with this type of ASD have associated mitral valve prolapse. Other associated findings include mitral or pulmonic stenosis and atrial septal aneurysm. When an ASD and mitral

stenosis exist simultaneously, the condition is called Lutembacher's syndrome. In isolated mitral stenosis, the left atrium is dilated because the valve area is reduced. In ASD the blood can escape across the atrial defect, thereby preserving the size of the left atrium.

Fifteen percent of all ASDs are the ostium primum type. These defects occur in the region of the ostium primum or the lower portion of the atrial septum. A common associated finding is a clefted anterior mitral valve leaflet.

Sinus venosus ASDs account for the other 15%. These defects occur in the upper portion of the atrial septum near the orifice of the inferior vena cava. The most common finding associated with this defect is partial anomalous pulmonary venous drainage.

Two-dimensional and M-mode echocardiography reveal a volume overload in the right heart. Findings indicative of right-sided volume overload include a dilated right ventricle and a flattening of the septum in diastole Two-dimensional imaging of the atrial septum allows direct visualization and localization of the defect. The views most commonly used to assess the atrial septum include the parasternal short-axis, the apical four-chamber, and the subcostal views. The latter view is the best one for visualizing the atrial septum. In addition to the secondary findings already described, two-dimensional imaging allows direct visualization of the defect. In septal defects, a dropout of echos is noted in the area of the defect. On echocardiography, the dropout of echos is characterized by a bright echo perpendicular to the atrial septum. This finding has been described as the "T" sign.

Doppler echocardiography also can help detect ASDs. In the absence of elevated pressures in the right heart, blood flows from the higher-pressure left ventricle to the lower-pressure right heart. In the subcostal view, a pulsed Doppler sample gate can be placed in the right heart near the atrial septum. The spectral display will reveal turbulent flow toward the transducer in late systole and throughout diastole. Color flow Doppler allows visualization of the interatrial shunt by superimposing a color coding on a two-dimensional image.

Contrast echocardiography can be used when imaging and when Doppler are unable to clearly identify the atrial defect. When used in conjunction with two-dimensional imaging, 92–100% of ASDs can be detected. Contrast agents injected into a vein enter the right heart, which is often highly opacified. In the presence of an ASD, small amounts of contrast material can be seen crossing the atrial septum into the left atrium and to the left ventricle. When the shunt is left to right, which is normally the case, a negative contrast effect can be noted. Contrast enhancement can be increased by having the patient perform the Valsalva maneuver or cough.

Patent Foramen Ovale

Patent (open) foramen ovale can be found in 27% of older patients. Left-to-right shunting does not normally occur when pressures are normal. A potential complication of the condition is paradoxical embolus.

Ventricular Septal Defects

VSDs are the most common defects found in infants and children. In the adult, ASDs are much more common. VSDs fall into two major classifications: muscular septal defects and membranous defects. Like ASDs, VSDs are classified according to the region involved.

Muscular Septal Defects. Muscular septal defects are entirely surrounded by muscle. Outlet defects occur in the most superior portion of the septum and make up part of the outflow region of the left ventricle. They are also referred to as outflow defects, subpulmonic or infundibular defects, or bulbar defects. These defects are bordered by the trabecula septomarginalis (right ventricular septal band) and the pulmonary valve annulus. Thus, they are the most difficult VSDs to image and are seen best from the subcostal and high parasternal positions.

A special form of outlet defect occurs above the crista supraventricularis. This defect is known as the supracristal ventricular defect; it also is referred to as the doubly committed subarterial defect because of its proximity to both semilunar valves. This defect also is seen best from the subcostal and high parasternal positions. Associated findings in this defect include (1) aortic valve prolapse because of lack of support, usually involving the right coronary cusp, (2) dilatation of the right coronary sinus of Valsalva, and (3) aortic insufficiency. The defect is usually small.

Inlet ventricular defects are bordered superiorly by the tricuspid valve annulus, apically by the tips of the papillary muscles, and anteriorly by the trabecula septomarginalis. They are also referred to as endocardial cushion defects, retrocristal defects, sinus defects, and inflow defects, which can be seen in several planes, including the parasternal, apical, and subcostal views. Because these defects are usually large, they can be confused with a double-inlet ventricle.

Trabecular defects are bordered by the chordal attachments of the papillary muscle to the apex. They extend from the smooth outlet septum to the inlet septum, are heavily trabeculated, and are usually large. They also can be multiple. These defects typically lead to hypertension of the right ventricle and may produce a right-to-left shunt if the pressures in the right heart exceed those in the left. A special type of muscular septal defect that occurs in the muscular septum is characterized by numerous small defects resembling Swiss cheese. This "Swiss cheese" defect occurs primarily in the apex.

Membranous Defects. Membranous septal defects occur in the region bordered by the inlet and outlet septums and the junctions between the right and noncoronary cusps of the aortic valve. This part of the septum is located at the base of the heart. Defects in this area are often referred to as perimembranous because they usually involve part of a surrounding muscular septum. Almost all planes can be used to image these defects, which occur more frequently than the muscular varieties.

Using two-dimensional imaging allows visualization of the septum. When the defect is large, a dropout of echoes is appreciated. In addition, a "T" artifact is observed. When imaging does not allow localization of the defect, color flow Doppler can be used. High-velocity turbulent flow usually can be seen as a mosaic color pattern in the area of the jet. Contrast echocardiography also can be used to localize the defect. Agitated solution can be injected into the right heart through a peripheral vein. Even a few bubbles seen entering the left ventricle are indicative of a right-to-left shunt when right-sided pressures are slightly elevated.

Tetralogy of Fallot

In adults, tetralogy of Fallot is the primary congenital disease producing cyanosis. In this condition, four specific findings are noted. The aorta overrides the perimembranous VSD. Infundibular or valvular pulmonic stenosis is present, resulting in right ventricular hypertrophy. M-mode criteria for diagnosing tetralogy of Fallot includes a break in the continuity of the anterior wall of the aorta from that of the interventricular septum as well as a narrowing of the right ventricular outflow tract. Two-dimensional imaging, however, allows direct visualization of the cardiac anatomy and is therefore the echocardiographic procedure of choice. Imaging often allows visualization of the VSD and gives valuable information about the amount of aortic override. Doppler echocardiography allows quantification of gradients across the obstruction of right ventricular outflow.

Pulmonic Stenosis

Eighty percent of all congenital obstructions of right ventricular outflow occur at the level of the pulmonic valve. The valve is often thickened with fusion of the cusps and can be seen doming in systole. Right ventricular hypertrophy occurs as a result of the increased resistance to flow. Two-dimensional imaging allows visualization of the valve, which usually appears thickened and with reduced excursion.

Persistent Ductus Arteriosis

Persistent ductus arteriosus (PDA) occurs when the ductus fails to close after birth. In utero, communication exists between the pulmonary circulation and the systemic circulation, the purpose of which in fetal circulation is to direct the flow of desaturated blood away from the coronary and cerebral circulation and toward the placenta. The ductus is located near the isthmus of the aorta near the origin of the left subclavian artery; it extends to the left pulmonary artery just beyond the bifurcation. In the absence of elevated pulmonary pressures, blood flows from the aorta to the pulmonary artery. In adults, the most common symptom of a PDA is dyspnea on exertion. In persistent ductus, the increased blood flow to the lungs results in dilatation of the pulmonary arteries, the left atrium and ventricle, and the aorta. If pulmonary pressure increases, the blood flow may reverse and travel from the pulmonary circulation toward the aorta. This condition is known as Eisenmenger's complex and is characterized by right-to-left shunting.

Coarctation of the Aorta

Twice as many men as women are likely to have coarctation of the aorta. Most patients with this condition are asymptomatic. The coarctation is manifested as left ventricular hypertension. On physical examination, a systolic murmur can be heard. The most common site of narrowing occurs in the thoracic aorta just distal to the left subclavian artery. This condition is often found in association with other congenital abnormalities such as VSD, PDA, a bicuspid aortic valve, and mitral valve abnormalities. It is the most common cardiac malformation found in Turner's syndrome.

The suprasternal notch offers the best view of the ascending aorta, the arch, and the descending aorta. Direct visualization of the coarctation is possible using two-dimensional imaging. Doppler echocardiography typically reveals increased velocities across the site of coarctation.

Ebstein's Anomaly

Ebstein's anomaly is characterized by downward displacement of the anterior or septal leaflet of the tricuspid valve into the right ventricle. As a result, the ventricle becomes "atrialized" and loses some of its pumping capacity. Associated findings include secundum-type ASDs, pulmonic stenosis or atresia, VSD, and mitral valve prolapse. Symptoms may not be evident until the patient is between 30 and 40 years old. The most common complication of this abnormality is failure of the right ventricle.

The M-mode criterion for this anomaly includes visualization of a large tricuspid valve leaflet, simultaneously seen with the anterior leaflet of the mitral leaflet. A delay time in closure of the tricuspid valve of 80 m/s or more to that of closure of the mitral valve is the second M-mode finding. Two-dimensional imaging allows direct visualization of the anatomy. Specific findings in imaging include an apically located tricuspid leaflet and a functionally small right ventricle. Ebstein's anomaly can be diagnosed if the leaflet is displaced 20 mm or more.

HYPERTENSIVE DISEASE

Systemic Hypertension

There are two basic types of systemic hypertension: essential or idiopathic and secondary hypertension. Both affect the diastolic and systolic pressure. The classification of blood pressure is shown in Table 3–1.

The cause of essential hypertension is unknown. Although several mechanisms may come into play, no specific cause has been well described. Secondary hypertension results in high blood pressure associated with any of the following: renal disease, endocrine disease, coarctation of the aorta, pregnancy, neurological disorders, acute stress, increased intravascular volume, alcohol and other drug abuse, increased cardiac output, and rigidity of the aorta.

The hemodynamic properties of systemic hyperten-

TABLE 3–1. CLASSIFICATION OF BLOOD PRESSURE

Range (mm Hg)	Category
Diastolic	
<85	Normal blood pressure
85–89	High normal blood pressure
90–104	Mild hypertension
105–114	Moderate hypertension
≥115	Severe hypertension
Systolic, when diastolic blood pressure is <90 mm Hg	
<140	Normal blood pressure
140–159	Borderline isolated systolic hypertension
≥160	Isolated systolic hypertension

Reprinted with permission from "The 1984 Report of the Joint National Committee on Detection, Evaluation, and Treatment of High Blood Pressure." Arch Intern Med 144, May 1984.

sion, whatever the cause, are similar. Initially, cardiac output increases, as does fluid volume. This increased fluid volume is transferred to the various organs and tissues. Once tissues receive more blood than they need, the blood vessels that deliver the blood constrict. This is known as vasoconstriction, which is an intrinsic property of systemic vessels such as arterioles and arteries. If this state continues, the vessels continue to exert resistance on the incoming blood (peripheral resistance). As a result, the heart beats against greater resistance and the vessels themselves become thicker.

As is the case with any muscle, hypertrophy occurs when stress is exerted. Just as the bicep increases in size when one does curls, so does the heart increase in size as it is forced to pump blood against increased peripheral resistance. Therefore, the main echocardiographic findings are increased muscle mass of the heart, especially the left ventricle. By M-mode criteria, the walls of the left ventricle are thick. The principal Doppler findings include (1) decreased transmitral E wave, (2) increased A wave, and (3) increased A-to-E-wave ratios.

Pulmonary Hypertension

In normal physiology, the pulmonary blood flow allows passage of blood to the lungs for three basic functions: oxygenation, filtration, and pH balance by excreting carbon dioxide. Blood coming in from the various tissues and organs of the body is directed to the right heart through the superior and inferior vena cavae. Once this deoxygenated blood enters the right atrium, it passes through the tricuspid valve into the right ventricle across the pulmonic valve and into the main pulmonary artery, which bifurcates into a left and right branch and directs blood to the left and right lobes of the lungs. Normally, the pulmonary circulation offers little resistance to blood flow: The normal peak systolic pressure ranges from 18–25 mm Hg, and the normal diastolic pressure ranges from 6–10 mm Hg. Pulmonary artery pressure in excess of 30 mm Hg systolic pressure and 20 mm Hg diastolic pressure represents elevated pulmonary pressures, or pulmonary hypertension.

Pulmonary Hypertension

Like systemic hypertension, pulmonary hypertension has two basic forms: primary and secondary. Primary pulmonary hypertension—also known as idiopathic, essential, or unexplained pulmonary hypertension—has no known discernible cause. Secondary pulmonary hypertension can be the result of any one of the following factors:

- increased resistance to pulmonary venous drainage,
- elevated left ventricular diastolic pressure,
- left atrial hypertension (mitral stenosis),
- pulmonary parenchymal disease, or
- pulmonary venous obstruction (cor triatriatum or pulmonary veno-occlusive disease).

Cor triatriatum is a congenital abnormality in which the common embryonic pulmonary vein is not incorporated into the left atrium. Instead, the pulmonary veins empty into an accessory chamber and communicate with the left atrium through a small opening. The result is obstruction of pulmonary venous flow that simulates mitral stenosis. In pulmonary veno-occlusive disease, the veins and venules of the lung become fibrotic.

M-mode findings reveal an absent or decreased A wave in the absence of right ventricular failure: a lack of respiratory variation in the A wave; an extended preejection period; midsystolic closure of the pulmonic valve, also known as midsystolic notch; and reduced ejection time of the right ventricle. Two-dimensional imaging indicates a dilated pulmonary artery and abnormalities in interventricular septal motion.

Doppler measurements reveal the following: a decreased acceleration time, a longer preejection period, a shorter ejection time, and tricuspid regurgitation. The acceleration time is the time interval between the onset of flow and the peak systolic flow. In pulmonary hypertension, the velocity of blood flow increases rapidly and peaks early in systole. This measurement is made by identifying the beginning of the Doppler signal and the peak velocity of the same signal. The time between the two is the acceleration time.

The preejection period is the time interval between the onset of the QRS complex to onset of flow in the pulmonary artery. In pulmonary hypertension, this time period increases.

Ejection time is the time from the onset of flow to the cessation of flow. In pulmonary hypertension, this time period becomes shorter. This measurement is made by taking the time between the beginning and end of the Doppler signal.

Tricuspid regurgitation occurs in the majority of patients with elevated pressures in the pulmonary artery. Continuous-wave Doppler can be used to localize the regurgitant jet and obtain the peak transtricuspid gradient using the modified Bernoulli equation. The peak gradient is the difference in systolic pressure between the right atrium and right ventricle. Estimation of the pulmonary pressures is accomplished by adding the right atrial pressures, which are determined by visual inspection of the jugular venous pulse. A more common way is to add the constant "10" to the peak systolic transtricuspid gradient. When stenosis of the pulmonic valve is present, however, one cannot determine pulmonary artery pressures using the peak transtricuspid regurgitant gradient.

CORONARY ARTERY DISEASE

The normal right and left coronary arteries supply the heart muscle with oxygenated blood (Table 3–2). The left coronary artery originates from the left coronary sinus of Valsalva, which bifurcates into two branches: the anterior interventricular or descending branch, also known as the left anterior descending branch, and the circumflex branch. The right coronary artery originates from the right coronary sinus of Valsalva.

The coronary anatomy can vary considerably in humans. In 67% of cases, the right coronary artery is the dominant artery. In these cases, this artery supplies the parts of the left ventricle and septum. In 15% of cases, the left coronary artery is the dominant one and supplies blood to all of the left ventricle and septum. In 18% of cases, the two arteries are equal; this situation is called the balanced coronary arterial pattern.

Abnormal Wall Motion

When the blood supply to the heart muscle is interrupted, the muscle is damaged and immediate changes in motion can be observed. The affected area can be identified using the various echocardiographic views. The wall segment

TABLE 3–2. NORMAL BRANCHES OF THE CORONARY ARTERIES

Coronary Artery	Major Branches	Area Supplied
Left coronary	Left anterior descending	Anterior left ventricular wall
		Anterior two-thirds of apical septum
		Anteroapical portions of left ventricle
		Anterior-lateral papillary muscle
		Midseptum
		Bundle of His
		Anterior right ventricular papillary muscle
	Circumflex*	Lateral left ventricular wall
		Left atrium
Right coronary	Numerous branches	Anterior right ventricular wall
		Posterior third (or more) of the interventricular septum
		Diaphragmatic wall of right ventricle
		Atrioventricular node

*If the circumflex terminates at the crux of the heart, it supplies the entire left ventricle and interventricular septum.

should be identified using the American Society of Echocardiography's recommendations (see the section of wall segment in the "Normal Anatomy" section).[3]

Complications of Ischemic Heart Disease

Ventricular Aneurysm. One complication of ischemic heart disease is ventricular aneurysm. Although aneurysms can form in any part of the left ventricle, more than 80% form in the apex and are the result of an anterior infarction. Of the 5–10% that form in the posterior wall, nearly half are false aneurysms.

The echocardiographic appearance of aneurysms includes thin walls that do not thicken in systole, a bulging wall, and dyskinetic motion to the affected area.

There are three types of ventricular aneurysms: anatomically true, functionally true, and anatomically false aneurysms. An anatomically true aneurysm is composed of fibrous tissue, may or may not contain a clot, and protrudes during both diastole and systole. Its mouth is wider or as wide as its maximum diameter, and its wall is the former left ventricular wall. An anatomically true aneurysm almost never ruptures once healed. A functionally true aneurysm also consists of fibrous tissue but protrudes only during ventricular systole.

An anatomically false aneurysm always contains a clot. Its mouth is considerably smaller than its maximum diameter, and it protrudes during both systole and diastole and may even expand. Its wall is composed of parietal pericardium. Because a false aneurysm often ruptures, immediate surgery is usually required.

Ventricular Septal Defect. A VSD occurs when a rupture occurs in the septum. Several echocardiographic techniques can be used to make the diagnosis. Two-dimensional imaging allows direct visualization of the defect. With contrast echocardiography with imaging, contrasting material can be seen filling the right ventricle and entering the left ventricle as blood moves back and forth through the defect. Negative contrast effect also can be noted. Doppler measurements can detect turbulent high-velocity signals on the right side of the ventricular septum. The best views include the left parasternal long- and short-axis views and the apical four-chamber view. Color Doppler can demonstrate communication between the left and right ventricles. The color jet appears as a mosaic pattern of high-velocity flow.

Thrombus. Thrombus, the most common complication of infarction, usually occurs in the apex in areas of dyskinesis. It can be laminar, lay close to the wall of the ventricle, or protrude into the cavity and be highly mobile. The diagnosis should be made when the thrombus is seen in several views.

Valve Dysfunction. An infarction is most likely to affect the mitral valve. Mitral regurgitation results if the papillary muscle is ruptured; if it becomes fibrosed; or if the mitral annulus is affected, resulting in incomplete closure of the leaflets.

Right Ventricular Involvement. Involvement of the right ventricle occurs primarily when the infarction is in the inferior wall or when the proximal right coronary artery is obstructed. Echocardiography reveals that the ventricle is dilated and its free wall moves abnormally.

REFERENCES

1. Feigenbaum H. *Endocardiopathy,* 4th ed. Philadelphia: Lea & Febiger, 1986.
2. Braunwald, E. *Heart Disease: A Textbook of Cardiac Medicine,* 3rd ed. Philadelphia: WB Saunders, 1988.
3. Report of the American Society of Echocardiography Committee on Nomenclature and Standards: Identification of Myocardial Wall Segments. 1982.

Questions

GENERAL INSTRUCTIONS: For each question, select the best answer. Select only one answer for each question, unless otherwise specified.

1. Which of the following views would best demonstrate all four cardiac chambers simultaneously?

   (A) left parasternal
   (B) right parasternal
   (C) subcostal
   (D) suprasternal

2. The three orthogonal planes for two-dimensional echocardiographic imaging are termed

   (A) long axis, short axis, and four chamber
   (B) apical, subcostal, and parasternal
   (C) suprasternal, right sternal border, and left sternal border
   (D) anterior, posterior, and coronal

3. Which of the following abnormalities are usually best demonstrated with the subcostal four-chamber view?

   (A) atrial septal defects and ventricular septal defects
   (B) mitral regurgitation and tricuspid regurgitation
   (C) mitral stenosis and tricuspid stenosis
   (D) aortic insufficiency and pulmonic insufficiency

4. The control that suppresses near-field echoes and enhances the intensity of the far-field echoes is called

   (A) attenuation
   (B) time-gain compensation
   (C) reject
   (D) compression

5. The tricuspid valve opens when
   (A) the right ventricular pressure drops below the right atrial pressure
   (B) the papillary muscle contracts
   (C) the velocity of blood flow in the right ventri-

cle exceeds the velocity of flow in the right atrium
   (D) the pulmonic valve opens

6. Which of the following is *not* a remnant of the fetal circulation?

   (A) the eustachian valve
   (B) the coronary ligament
   (C) the foramen ovale
   (D) the ligamentum arteriosus

7. Blood normally flows from the right ventricle to the

   (A) pulmonary artery
   (B) aorta
   (C) right atrium
   (D) pulmonary vein

8. A pulmonary vein is normally attached to the

   (A) right ventricle
   (B) left ventricle
   (C) left atrium
   (D) right atrium

9. Which of the following statements regarding cardiac anatomy is false?

   (A) The heart tends to assume a more vertical position in tall thin people and a more horizontal position in short heavy people
   (B) The ligamentum arteriosum runs from the left pulmonary artery to the descending aorta
   (C) The coronary arteries arise from the sinuses within the pockets of the left and right coronary cusps of the aortic valve
   (D) The left ventricle constitutes most of the ventral surface of the heart

10. Left ventricular ejection time can be assessed from an M-mode echocardiogram by measuring the distance between the

   (A) aortic valve opening and closing points
   (B) mitral D and C points

(C) R wave and T wave

(D) mitral valve closure and aortic valve opening

11. Often, the best two-dimensional view for examining patients with chronic obstructive pulmonary disease is

(A) parasternal
(B) apical
(C) suprasternal
(D) subcostal

12. The two best transducer positions for Doppler investigation of systolic blood flow across the aortic valve are

(A) parasternal and suprasternal
(B) apical and right sternal border
(C) suprasternal and subcostal
(D) subcostal and apical

13. The size of the left atrium is measured on the M-mode

(A) at end-systole
(B) at the peak of the R wave
(C) with the onset of aortic valve opening
(D) at the beginning of the P wave

14. Doming of any cardiac valve on two-dimensional echocardiography is consistent with

(A) regurgitation
(B) decreased cardiac output
(C) stenosis
(D) congenital malformation

15. Two-dimensional images are best obtained when the ultrasound beam is directed _____ to the structure of interest. Doppler signals are best obtained when the ultrasound beam is directed _____ to the flow of blood.

(A) oblique, perpendicular
(B) parallel, perpendicular
(C) perpendicular, parallel
(D) perpendicular, oblique

16. Right ventricular systolic pressure overload can be caused by

(A) pulmonary insufficiency
(B) an atrial septal defect
(C) aortic stenosis
(D) pulmonary hypertension

17. Left ventricular measurements should be obtained from the parasternal long-axis view at the level of the

(A) mitral valve annulus
(B) tips of the mitral leaflets
(C) chordae tendineae
(D) papillary muscle

18. All of the following can cause paradoxical interventricular septal motion except

(A) left bundle branch block
(B) postpericardiotomy
(C) left ventricular volume overload
(D) severe tricuspid regurgitation

19. In a patient with volume overload of the right ventricle, the onset of ventricular systole is likely to show the interventricular septum moving

(A) toward the right ventricular free wall
(B) toward the left ventricular wall
(C) laterally
(D) not at all

20. A murmur that is associated with a thrill is likely to be

(A) organic in origin
(B) insignificant
(C) functional
(D) the result of an atrial septal defect

21. The Valsalva maneuver and the inhalation of amyl nitrite are techniques that are sometimes used during an echocardiographic examination when checking for

(A) mitral valve prolapse or systolic anterior motion of the mitral valve
(B) aortic stenosis or mitral stenosis
(C) aortic stenosis or aortic regurgitation
(D) a ventricular septal defect or pulmonic stenosis

22. Clubbing of the fingers and nail beds is a sign of

(A) cyanotic heart disease
(B) Marfan syndrome
(C) Barlow syndrome
(D) increased cardiac output

23. Even though two-dimensional echocardiography has largely replaced M-mode echocardiography for cardiac diagnosis, M-mode still has the advantage of

(A) defining spatial relationships of cardiac structures
(B) providing enhanced temporal resolution
(C) providing dynamic assessment of the velocity of blood flow
(D) providing superior lateral resolution

24. When attempting a parasternal short-axis view, if the left ventricle appears oval rather than circular, the echocardiographer should move the transducer

(A) medially
(B) laterally
(C) to a higher intercostal space
(D) to a lower intercostal space

25. A Doppler tracing of the mitral valve in which the A point is higher than the E point indicates

   (A) high cardiac output
   (B) low cardiac output
   (C) decreased left ventricular compliance
   (D) high left ventricular end-diastolic pressures

26. Which of the following is usually not a secondary finding in patients with mitral stenosis?

   (A) a dilated left atrium
   (B) a dilated right atrium
   (C) a left ventricular thrombus
   (D) a left atrial thrombus

27. The Doppler signal obtained from the apex in a patient with mitral stenosis is most likely to demonstrate all of the following except

   (A) an increased diastolic peak velocity
   (B) spectral broadening
   (C) a decreased E-F slope
   (D) a peak gradient occurring in late diastole

28. Torn chordae tendineae will cause

   (A) aortic insufficiency
   (B) myocardial infarction
   (C) mitral insufficiency
   (D) mitral stenosis

29. All of the following can produce false positive signs of mitral valve prolapse on an M-mode except

   (A) pericardial effusion
   (B) premature ventricular contractions
   (C) improper placement of the transducer
   (D) hypertrophic obstructive cardiomyopathy

30. Which of the following is a secondary echocardiographic finding in mitral regurgitation?

   (A) a dilated left atrium
   (B) left ventricular hypertrophy
   (C) a hypokinetic left ventricle
   (D) a dilated aortic root

31. The degree of mitral regurgitation is best estimated by measuring the

   (A) width and length of the systolic jet by color Doppler
   (B) peak velocity of the continuous-wave Doppler systolic mitral signal
   (C) pressure half-time of the continuous-wave Doppler diastolic signal
   (D) integral of the continuous-wave systolic curve

32. Which of the following is least likely to occur as a sequela of rheumatic fever?

   (A) mitral stenosis
   (B) mitral insufficiency
   (C) aortic stenosis
   (D) pulmonic stenosis

33. The two-dimensional echocardiogram of a patient with combined mitral and aortic stenosis is most likely to demonstrate

   (A) a dilated left atrium and left ventricular hypertrophy
   (B) a dilated left atrium and a dilated left ventricle
   (C) a small left atrium and a small left ventricle
   (D) systolic anterior motion of the mitral valve and left ventricular hypertrophy

34. The M-mode of the mitral valve in mitral stenosis is often missing an A wave. The reason is

   (A) high initial diastolic pressures in the left ventricle
   (B) concurrent atrial fibrillation
   (C) decreased compliance of the left ventricle
   (D) a dilated left atrium

35. A Doppler tracing that demonstrates a late diastolic mitral inflow velocity (A point) that is higher than the initial diastolic velocity (E point) can be seen with which of the following pathologies?

   (A) aortic insufficiency
   (B) hypertrophic cardiomyopathy
   (C) mitral regurgitation
   (D) a ventricular septal defect

36. If the two-dimensional examination demonstrates a markedly dilated and hyperkinetic left ventricle and a left atrium of normal size, one should suspect the presence of

   (A) mitral regurgitation
   (B) aortic regurgitation
   (C) a ventricular septal defect
   (D) aortic stenosis

37. Which group of echocardiographic findings would give a definitive diagnosis of mitral stenosis?

   (A) a decreased E-F slope, a dilated left atrium, and a small left ventricle
   (B) a thickened mitral valve, a dilated left atrium, and a small left ventricle
   (C) a decreased E-F slope, a thickened mitral valve, and diastolic doming of the mitral valve
   (D) a thickened mitral valve and a mitral diastolic velocity >1.5 m/s

38. A patient with mitral stenosis will usually have all of the following except

(A) a diastolic rumble on auscultation
(B) an increased E-F slope on M-mode
(C) a history of rheumatic fever
(D) a dilated left atrium

39. To obtain the true circumference of the mitral valve, one should obtain a short-axis view at the level of the

    (A) papillary muscle
    (B) chordae tendineae
    (C) tips of the mitral leaflets
    (D) mitral annulus

40. Secondary echocardiographic findings of mitral stenosis include all of the following except

    (A) a dilated left atrium
    (B) a dilated right atrium
    (C) a dilated left ventricle
    (D) a left atrial thrombus

41. A successful mitral valve commissurotomy would be *least* likely to demonstrate

    (A) doming of the mitral valve
    (B) mitral valve thickening
    (C) an increase in pressure half-time
    (D) a dilated left atrium

42. Left ventricular dilatation in a patient with mitral stenosis suggests

    (A) severe mitral stenosis
    (B) concomitant mitral regurgitation
    (C) aortic stenosis
    (D) hypertrophic cardiomyopathy

43. Early diastolic closure of the mitral valve is usually a sign of

    (A) severe acute aortic regurgitation
    (B) a left bundle branch block
    (C) poor function of the left ventricle
    (D) first-degree A-V block

44. Degenerative calcification of the mitral annulus can be accelerated by all of the following conditions except

    (A) systemic hypertension
    (B) aortic stenosis
    (C) hypertrophic obstructive cardiomyopathy
    (D) a ventricular septal defect

45. A mitral valve pressure half-time of 220 msec is consistent with a mitral valve area of

    (A) 0.6 cm^2
    (B) 1 cm^2
    (C) 2.2 cm^2
    (D) 5 cm^2

46. Echocardiographic findings of significant aortic stenosis include all of the following except

    (A) reduced separation of the aortic valve cusp
    (B) diastolic fluttering of the anterior mitral leaflet
    (C) Doppler systolic velocities greater than 4 m/s
    (D) thickened left ventricular walls

47. Which of the following causes the left ventricular walls to appear thick on an echocardiogram?

    (A) mitral stenosis
    (B) aortic insufficiency
    (C) mitral regurgitation
    (D) systemic hypertension

48. The presence of a systolic ejection murmur should alert one to look for

    (A) a ventricular septal defect
    (B) mitral regurgitation
    (C) aortic stenosis
    (D) patent ductus arteriosis

49. All of the following statements regarding a bicuspid aortic valve are true except

    (A) the problem is a congenital one
    (B) it may be associated with aortic stenosis
    (C) it is often seen in conjunction with mitral stenosis
    (D) it may be associated with coarctation of the aorta

50. The continuity equation is used to calculate the _____. It is most helpful in patients with _____.

    (A) mitral valve area, mitral stenosis
    (B) aortic valve area, poor left ventricular function
    (C) aortic valve velocity, systemic hypertension
    (D) degree of shunting, a ventricular septal defect

51. In patients with combined aortic stenosis and aortic insufficiency, which of the following parameters is best for assessing the severity of aortic stenosis?

    (A) the maximum pressure gradient
    (B) the mean pressure gradient
    (C) the high pulse-repetition frequency
    (D) the analog waveform

52. Which of the following two-dimensional views will best illustrate a color Doppler jet of aortic insufficiency?

    (A) the apical long-axis view
    (B) the suprasternal view
    (C) the subcostal fine-chamber view
    (D) the short axis view of the base

53. Which of the following is a secondary echocardiographic sign of aortic stenosis?

    (A) a thickened aortic valve
    (B) left ventricular hypertrophy
    (C) a hyperdynamic left ventricle
    (D) a dilated left ventricle

54. An M-mode finding of fine diastolic fluttering of the anterior mitral leaflet is consistent with

    (A) aortic insufficiency
    (B) mitral stenosis
    (C) atrial fibrillation
    (D) a prolonged heart rate

55. Diastolic velocity signals were detected in a patient's left ventricular outflow tract using pulsed Doppler. They could be detected between the tip of the anterior mitral leaflet and the aortic valve from the parasternal position. This is

    (A) normal
    (B) consistent with severe mitral regurgitation
    (C) consistent with severe aortic regurgitation
    (D) consistent with moderate aortic regurgitation
    (E) consistent with moderate mitral regurgitation

56. The referring physician hears an Austin-Flint murmur. The M-mode echocardiogram of this patient is most likely to demonstrate

    (A) a thickened mitral valve with a decreased E-F slope
    (B) fine diastolic fluttering and possible flattening of the anterior mitral leaflet
    (C) a thickened aortic valve with a decreased opening
    (D) systolic posterior motion of the tricuspid valve

57. The best approach for obtaining the maximum aortic velocity in patients with aortic stenosis is from the

    (A) left sternal border
    (B) left supraclavicular region
    (C) subcostal region
    (D) right sternal border view

58. The best way to rule out an aortic dissection is with

    (A) M-mode echocardiography
    (B) transthoracic two-dimensional imaging
    (C) color Doppler
    (D) transesophageal echocardiography

59. Which echocardiographic finding is not associated with tricuspid insufficiency?

    (A) a dilated right atrium
    (B) tricuspid prolapse

    (C) a dilated right ventricle
    (D) a thickened anterior right ventricle wall

60. A tricuspid regurgitant velocity of 4 m/s indicates the presence of

    (A) tricuspid stenosis
    (B) severe tricuspid regurgitation
    (C) a flail tricuspid leaflet
    (D) pulmonary hypertension

61. Which of the following regarding tricuspid stenosis is *not* true?

    (A) it occurs as a sequela to rheumatic fever
    (B) Doppler echocardiography demonstrates a decreased pressure half-time
    (C) two-dimensional echocardiography shows diastolic doming, and M-mode reveals a decreased E-F slope
    (D) it is usually seen as part of the aging process

62. A peripheral contrast injection into the arm of a patient with severe tricuspid regurgitation is likely to demonstrate

    (A) contrast in the pulmonary veins during diastole
    (B) right-to-left shunting
    (C) contrast in the inferior vena cava during ventricular systole
    (D) left-to-right shunting

63. If the physician suspects carcinoid heart disease, the echocardiographer should pay special attention to the

    (A) mitral valve
    (B) tricuspid valve
    (C) inferior vena cava
    (D) interatrial septum

64. The velocity of a tricuspid regurgitant jet can be used to calculate

    (A) the severity of tricuspid regurgitation
    (B) right ventricular systolic pressure
    (C) the severity of pulmonic regurgitation
    (D) left atrial pressure

65. Coarse systolic fluttering of the pulmonic valve with an extremely high systolic velocity in the right ventricular outflow tract is most likely to be found in a patient with

    (A) pulmonic regurgitation
    (B) paradoxical interventricular septal motion
    (C) infundibular pulmonic stenosis
    (D) pulmonary hypertension

66. The most common window used to record peak pulmonic systolic velocity is

(A) suprasternal
(B) apical
(C) right parasternal
(D) left parasternal

67. The pulmonic valve is located where in relation to the aortic valve?

(A) cranial and lateral
(B) caudal and lateral
(C) cranial and medial
(D) caudal and medial

68. All of the following echocardiographic findings are associated with pulmonic stenosis except

(A) right ventricular hypertrophy
(B) M-mode demonstration of a steep pulmonic A wave
(C) midsystolic notching noted on M-mode
(D) systolic pulmonic Doppler velocities greater than 3 m/s

69. Valvular vegetations are best detected with

(A) M-mode echocardiography
(B) two-dimensional echocardiography
(C) Doppler echocardiography
(D) contrast injection

70. A 30-year-old intravenous drug abuser presents with an embolus to the right leg. The most likely cause of the embolic event is the presence of

(A) a left atrial myxoma
(B) mitral valve vegetation
(C) a right ventricular thrombus
(D) a myocardial abscess

71. Color Doppler assessment of prosthetic heart valves is especially helpful when checking for the

(A) presence of valve stenosis
(B) presence of paravalvular regurgitation
(C) presence of a clot
(D) valve area

72. A normally functioning Starr-Edwards valve

(A) may exhibit high Doppler velocities
(B) will echocardiographically resemble a bioprosthetic valve
(C) has a major and a minor orifice
(D) may exhibit mild-to-moderate regurgitation

73. A Bjork-Shiley is

(A) an example of a mechanical heart valve
(B) an example of a bioprosthetic heart valve
(C) not noticeable on the two-dimensional image
(D) a surgical procedure used to correct for transposition of the great vessels

74. Which of the following echocardiographic examinations is best used for evaluating the function of a prosthetic valve

(A) M-mode echocardiography
(B) high-pulse repetition-frequency Doppler echocardiography
(C) transesophageal echocardiography
(D) contrast echocardiography

75. All of the following are examples of mechanical prosthetic valves except

(A) St. Jude
(B) Bjork-Shiley
(C) Starr-Edwards
(D) Hancock

76. To check for prosthetic valve dehiscence, the echocardiographer should look for

(A) decreased valve excursion
(B) an abnormal mass of echoes on the valve
(C) abnormal rocking motion of the valve
(D) Doppler evidence of stenosis

77. A 26-year-old woman with significant mitral insufficiency is about to receive a mitral valve replacement. The surgeons are most likely to use a porcine valve because

(A) it tends to last longer
(B) it preserves myocardium better
(C) it often makes anticoagulation unnecessary
(D) it obstructs flow less

78. Prophylactic antibiotics are often recommended for individuals with mitral valve prolapse who are undergoing dental or surgical procedures

(A) because these patients are at a higher risk for endocarditis
(B) to prevent possible mitral regurgitation
(C) to prevent pneumonia
(D) because incisions on patients with mitral valve prolapse usually take longer to heal

79. One can be reasonably certain that a large amount of pericardial effusion is present by noting

(A) echocardiographic signs of cardiac tamponade
(B) a crescent-shaped pattern on the short-axis view
(C) a "swinging heart" on the two-dimensional examination
(D) a posterior echo-free space

80. Constrictive pericarditis

    (A) impairs diastolic filling
    (B) is sometimes referred to as "Dressler's syndrome"
    (C) is detected by noting increased echogenicity of the pericardium
    (D) is usually associated with a large pericardial effusion

81. Cardiac tamponade is most likely to occur when

    (A) pressure in the pericardial cavity rises to equal or exceed the diastolic pressure in the heart
    (B) there is a small pericardial effusion
    (C) there is a large chronic pericardial effusion
    (D) the pericardium becomes a sheath of fibrous tissue that interferes with diastolic filling

82. Which one of the following statements about pericardial effusion is false?

    (A) pericardial effusion may be confused with epicardial fat
    (B) an effusion may accumulate anteriorly without accumulating posteriorly
    (C) a pericardial effusion can consist of blood or clear fluid
    (D) In Dressler's syndrome, a pericardial effusion develops as a result of renal disease

83. A 38-year-old woman with a history of breast cancer is referred for an echocardiogram because she is experiencing shortness of breath. The echocardiogram is most likely to reveal

    (A) metastasis to the left atrium
    (B) metastasis to the right atrium
    (C) a left atrial myxoma
    (D) a pericardial effusion

84. All of the following can lead to a false-positive diagnosis of pericardial effusion on M-mode except

    (A) the descending aorta
    (B) a calcified mitral annulus
    (C) ascites
    (D) mitral valve prolapse

85. A false-negative sign of tamponade may occur in patients with

    (A) pulmonic stenosis
    (B) a pleural effusion
    (C) mitral regurgitation
    (D) loculated effusions

86. The pericardium appears as an extremely bright linear structure on the echocardiogram because

    (A) it is a thick structure
    (B) it is a fibrous band

    (C) there is a large acoustic mismatch between lung tissue and pericardial tissue
    (D) it contains calcium

87. Two echocardiographic techniques that are useful when evaluating for the presence of pericardial effusion are

    (A) increasing reject and decreasing frame-rate
    (B) decreasing time-gain control and increasing overall gain
    (C) decreasing overall gain and increasing depth setting
    (D) increasing reject and decreasing depth setting

88. The structure that often aids in differentiating a pericardial effusion from a pleural effusion on two-dimensional examination is the

    (A) liver
    (B) inferior vena cava
    (C) pleural sac
    (D) descending aorta

89. Flat mid-diastolic motion of the posterior wall on an M-mode echocardiogram suggests

    (A) constrictive pericarditis
    (B) left ventricular volume overload
    (C) myocardial infarction
    (D) dilated cardiomyopathy

90. The most striking echocardiographic feature of patients with an absent pericardium is

    (A) excessive cardiac motion
    (B) absence of bright linear pericardial echoes
    (C) hypokinesis of the heart
    (D) dyskinetic motion of the heart

91. The effect of systemic hypertension on the heart is

    (A) thickening of the right ventricular free wall
    (B) decreased systolic function of the left ventricle
    (C) reduced compliance of the left ventricle
    (D) right ventricular dilatation

92. Echocardiographic signs of outflow tract obstruction in hypertrophic cardiomyopathy include all of the following *except*

    (A) midsystolic notching of the aortic valve
    (B) left ventricular hypertrophy
    (C) systolic anterior motion of the mitral valve
    (D) high systolic velocity in the left ventricular outflow tract

93. A definitive diagnosis of amyloid heart disease is best made with

(A) M-mode echocardiography
(B) transthoracic echocardiography
(C) transesophageal echocardiography
(D) endomyocardial biopsy

94. All of the following can cause dilated (congestive) cardiomyopathy *except*

(A) coronary artery disease
(B) sarcoidosis
(C) viral myocarditis
(D) long-term alcohol abuse

95. All of the following are echocardiographic findings seen in dilated cardiomyopathy *except*

(A) increased systolic velocity in the left ventricular outflow tract
(B) dilated chambers
(C) global hypokinesis
(D) an increased E point-to-septal separation

96. Cardiac contusion

(A) is more likely to affect the right ventricle than the left ventricle
(B) is the same as a myocardial infarction
(C) occurs when there is underlying coronary artery disease
(D) leads to hypercontractility of the left ventricle

97. A 64-year-old man presents with an acute myocardial infarction of the anterior wall and an embolus to the right leg. Before beginning the examination, the echocardiographer should suspect the possibility of (choose the most likely diagnosis)

(A) an apical aneurysm with a mural thrombus
(B) mitral stenosis and a left atrial clot
(C) a right ventricular infarct with a clot
(D) vegetation on the mitral or aortic valve

98. All of the following echocardiographic findings are consistent with diastolic dysfunction of the left ventricle except

(A) M-mode demonstration of a mitral valve B notch
(B) M-mode demonstration of a high mitral A wave
(C) two-dimensional demonstration of an ejection fraction lower than 50%
(D) Doppler demonstration of a mitral valve E-to-A ratio >1.0

99. Akinesis of the anterior left ventricular wall is most likely to indicate obstruction of the

(A) right coronary artery
(B) left circumflex artery

(C) left anterior descending artery
(D) posterior descending artery

100. Pseudoaneurysms

(A) are usually hyperkinetic
(B) have a low risk of rupture
(C) have walls comprised of endocardium, myocardium, epicardium, and pericardium
(D) have a narrow neck

101. An increased E point-to-septal separation is usually a good indicator of

(A) high end-diastolic pressures in the left ventricle
(B) a reduced ejection fraction
(C) high initial diastolic pressures
(D) poor compliance of the left ventricle

102. A segment of the left ventricle that lacks systolic wall thickening and motion is best described as

(A) hypokinetic
(B) akinetic
(C) dyskinetic
(D) aneurysmal

103. Aneurysms in the inferior wall of the left ventricle may be associated with all of the following except

(A) an increased E point-to-septal separation
(B) thrombus formation
(C) mitral regurgitation
(D) occlusion of the left anterior descending coronary artery

104. The echocardiogram of a patient with a ruptured papillary muscle will exhibit

(A) mitral valve prolapse
(B) severe mitral regurgitation
(C) some degree of aortic insufficiency
(D) dyskinesis of the posterior left ventricular wall

105. Stress echocardiography

(A) is used instead of standard stress testing
(B) studies the acoustic properties of the myocardium
(C) allows for visualization of myocardial perfusion
(D) is used in diagnosing ischemic heart disease

106. Which of the following statements regarding left atrial myxomas is not true?

(A) they usually attach to the interatrial septum
(B) they may be pedunculated
(C) they do not recur once they are surgically removed
(D) clinically, they can mimic mitral stenosis

107. The QP/QS ratio is used to evaluate the severity of

    (A) pulmonic stenosis
    (B) ventricular septal defects
    (C) aortic stenosis
    (D) systemic hypertension

108. Which of the following would best describe the pulsed Doppler pattern of a patent ductus arteriosis if the sample volume were placed in the pulmonary artery from a short-axis view of the base of the heart?

    (A) systolic flow below baseline
    (B) continuous flow (systolic and diastolic) above baseline
    (C) diastolic flow above baseline
    (D) a biphasic systolic flow pattern below baseline

109. The best way to detect a small atrial septal defect is with

    (A) two-dimensional echocardiography
    (B) contrast injection echocardiography
    (C) M-mode echocardiography
    (D) pulsed-wave Doppler echocardiography

110. The most common type of atrial septal defect is

    (A) primum
    (B) secundum
    (C) fenestrated
    (D) sinus venosus

111. A ventricular septal defect with right-to-left shunting is consistent with

    (A) Ebstein's anomaly
    (B) tetralogy of Fallot
    (C) Eisenmenger's syndrome
    (D) a double-outlet right ventricle

112. Which of the following is not associated with Ebstein's anomaly?

    (A) an abnormally large tricuspid valve
    (B) infundibular pulmonic stenosis
    (C) "atrialization" of the right ventricle
    (D) an atrial septal defect

113. The echocardiogram of a patient with an endocardial cushion defect might exhibit

    (A) a muscular ventricular septal defect and tricuspid valve vegetation
    (B) a hypokinetic left ventricle and mitral valve vegetation
    (C) overriding of the aorta and subpulmonic stenosis
    (D) ostium primum atrial septal defect and an inlet ventricular septal defect

114. An echocardiographic diagnosis of coarctation of the aorta can be made by detecting a high-velocity Doppler jet in the

    (A) left branch of the pulmonary artery
    (B) aortic arch, proximal to the subclavian artery
    (C) descending thoracic aorta
    (D) abdominal aorta

115. The four principal components of tetralogy of Fallot include all of the following except

    (A) a ventricular septal defect
    (B) an override of the aorta
    (C) an obstruction of pulmonary blood flow
    (D) an atrial septal defect

116. Cor triatriatum

    (A) is a fairly common congenital abnormality
    (B) is a congenital malformation in which a fibrous membrane divides the left atrium into an upper and lower chamber
    (C) results in mitral stenosis
    (D) is a condition in which the pulmonary veins drain into the right atrium

117. The echocardiographic finding most commonly associated with left bundle branch block is

    (A) left ventricular hypertrophy
    (B) a hypercontractile interventricular septum
    (C) paradoxical septal motion
    (D) a dilated left ventricle

118. The echocardiographic pattern of the mitral valve in Fig. 3–9 is consistent with

    (A) mitral stenosis
    (B) mitral valve vegetation
    (C) a mechanical prosthetic valve
    (D) a calcified mitral valve annulus

Figure 3–9. Apical four-chamber view.

Figure 3–10. M-mode echocardiogram at the level of the mitral valve.

Figure 3–11. Continuous-wave Doppler tracing obtained from the apical position.

119. The M-mode pattern in Fig. 3–10 suggests that the ejection fraction of the left ventricle is

(A) normal
(B) mildly increased
(C) significantly increased
(D) significantly decreased

120. What other hemodynamic information could be derived from the M-mode (Fig. 3–10)?

(A) cardiac output is increased
(B) left ventricular end-diastolic pressure is increased
(C) the systolic ejection period is prolonged
(D) atrial flutter is present

121. The Doppler tracing in Fig. 3–11 demonstrates

(A) aortic stenosis and aortic insufficiency
(B) mitral stenosis and mitral regurgitation
(C) tricuspid stenosis and tricuspid regurgitation
(D) mitral stenosis and aortic stenosis

122. The echocardiographic findings in Fig. 3–12 indicate that the patient probably has a history of

(A) hypertension
(B) diabetes mellitus
(C) rheumatic fever
(D) coronary artery disease

123. The arrow in Fig. 3–12 is pointing to

(A) a side-lobe artifact
(B) papillary muscle
(C) chordae tendineae
(D) the anterior mitral leaflet

124. Fig. 3–13 demonstrates echoes within the left ventricular cavity. These echoes are

(A) artifactual
(B) caused by a mural thrombus
(C) caused by stagnant blood
(D) caused by a high near-gain setting

Questions 125 through 131: Match the numbered structures in Fig. 3–14 with the correct term given in Column B.

COLUMN A	COLUMN B
125. _____	(A) left ventricle
126. _____	(B) coronary sinus
127. _____	(C) left atrium
128. _____	(D) right ventricle
129. _____	(E) pericardial effusion
130. _____	(F) descending aorta
131. _____	(G) pleural effusion
	(H) aortic root
	(I) right atrium

132. Fig. 3–15 demonstrates

(A) a large pleural effusion
(B) pneumomediastinum
(C) ascites
(D) a large pericardial effusion

133. The echocardiographic examination of this patient should include analysis of the motion of the

(A) interventricular septum
(B) right ventricular wall
(C) left ventricular wall
(D) tricuspid valve

Figure 3–12. Split-screen display of a two-dimensional long-axis (left) and a correlating M-mode pattern (right). Note M-mode scan plane indicated by cursor (arrow).

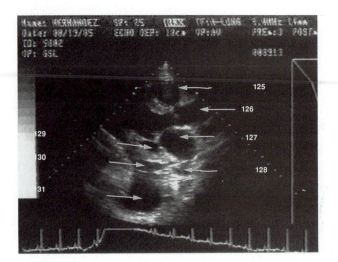

Figure 3–14. Parasternal long-axis view with an increased depth setting.

134. Color Doppler interrogation of the aortic valve shown in Fig. 3–16 is most likely to demonstrate

    (A) a narrow diastolic jet directed at the anterior mitral leaflet
    (B) a diastolic jet filling the left ventricular outflow tract and extending deep into the left ventricle
    (C) a normal pattern of blood flow
    (D) a narrow systolic jet directed at the anterior mitral leaflet

135. The arrow in Fig. 3–17 is pointing to

    (A) a fistula between the aorta and right ventricle
    (B) the coronary sinus
    (C) the left main coronary artery
    (D) the origin of the right coronary artery

136. The right ventricular outflow tract is located medial to the arrow in Fig. 3–17.

    (A) true
    (B) false

137. The contrast study in Fig. 3–18 shows

    (A) left-to-right shunting at the atrial level
    (B) no shunting of blood
    (C) right-to-left shunting at the atrial level
    (D) right-to-left shunting at the ventricular level

138. A secondary finding noted on Fig. 3–18 is a moderate-sized pericardial effusion.

    (A) true
    (B) false

Figure 3–13. Apical four-chamber view showing a dilated left ventricle.

Figure 3–15. Apical four-chamber view.

Figure 3–16. Narrow sector parasternal long-axis view.

Figure 3–18. Subcostal four-chamber view with contrast injection.

139. The arrow in Fig. 3–18 is pointing to

(A) lung tissue
(B) liver parenchyma
(C) a mediastinal tumor
(D) the spleen

140. The absence of an A wave and midsystolic notching of the pulmonic valve on the M-Mode in Fig. 3–19 is consistent with

(A) pulmonic stenosis
(B) tricuspid stenosis
(C) mitral stenosis
(D) pulmonary hypertension

141. What other abnormality should be ruled out in the presence of the abnormality noted on the M-mode of the tricuspid valve in Fig. 3–20?

(A) tricuspid stenosis
(B) pulmonary hypertension
(C) mitral valve prolapse
(D) atrial septal defect

142. An 85-year-old woman with a long history of chest pain is sent for an echocardiogram. The M-mode of the mitral valve is shown in Fig. 3–21. The M-mode of the aortic valve would be likely to demonstrate

(A) diastolic fluttering
(B) delayed opening
(C) midsystolic notching
(D) systolic fluttering

Figure 3–17. Short-axis view of the base of the heart.

Figure 3–19. M-mode of the pulmonic valve.

Figure 3–20. M-mode of the tricuspid valve.

Figure 3–22. Parasternal long-axis view.

143. An extremely tall slender young man was referred for an echocardiogram because he has a murmur. Echocardiographic findings in Fig. 3–22 include

    (A) a biscupid aortic valve
    (B) a cleft mitral valve
    (C) a dilated aortic root
    (D) left ventricular hypertrophy

144. Which echocardiographic view would be best for further evaluation of this abnormality?

    (A) the long-axis suprasternal view
    (B) the short-axis view of the base of the heart
    (C) the apical four-chamber view
    (D) the subcostal four-chamber view

145. The left ventricle in Fig. 3–23 demonstrates

    (A) hypertrophic cardiomyopathy
    (B) an infiltrative tumor
    (C) a large apical thrombus
    (D) a myxoma

146. The mitral valve in Fig. 3–24 is

    (A) normal
    (B) flail
    (C) stenotic
    (D) prolapsing

147. The arrow in Fig. 3–25 is pointing to the

    (A) left subclavian artery
    (B) right pulmonary artery
    (C) superior vena cava
    (D) left pulmonary vein

Figure 3–21. M-mode echocardiogram at the level of the mitral valve.

Figure 3–23. Apical four-chamber view.

Figure 3–24. Parasternal long-axis view.

Figure 3–26. Apical four-chamber view.

148. Posterior to this structure is an echo-free space. This represents

    (A) the left atrium
    (B) a pleural effusion
    (C) pericardial effusion
    (D) the superior vena cava

149. The curved arrow in Fig. 3–26 is directed at

    (A) a pacemaker wire
    (B) the Chiari network
    (C) false chordae tendineae
    (D) the moderator band

150. The arrow in Fig. 3–26 is pointing to a structure that most likely represents

    (A) a right atrial myxoma
    (B) a left atrial thrombus

    (C) the left pulmonary vein
    (D) the eustachian valve

151. The echocardiographic findings in the long-axis view presented in Fig. 3–27 include

    (A) a dilated left atrium, mitral stenosis, and a pericardial effusion
    (B) aortic stenosis, a calcified mitral annulus, and basal septal hypertrophy
    (C) a dilated coronary sinus, left ventricular hypertrophy, and mitral valve vegetation
    (D) a dilated aortic root, a dilated left ventricle, and a thickened mitral valve

Figure 3–25. Suprasternal notch long-axis view of the aorta and transverse arch.

Figure 3–27. Parasternal long-axis view with slightly increased depth setting.

152. These findings are most consistent with

    (A) rheumatic heart disease
    (B) congenital heart disease
    (C) subacute bacterial endocarditis
    (D) an aged heart

153. The mitral valve diastolic waveforms in Fig. 3–28C are not uniform. This is caused by

    (A) high end-diastolic pressure of the left ventricle
    (B) faulty technique
    (C) inspiration
    (D) atrial fibrillation

The following study is of a 58-year-old woman who vaguely remembers a childhood illness that included pain in her joints. She was presented with a trans-ischemic attack and atrial fibrillation. For questions 154 through 156, refer to Fig. 3–28A, B, and C.

154. The mitral valve demonstrates

    (A) systolic prolapse
    (B) diastolic doming
    (C) myxomatous degeneration
    (D) hyperkinesis

155. Which chamber is significantly dilated?

    (A) the left atrium
    (B) the left ventricle
    (C) the right atrium
    (D) the right ventricle

156. Auscultation of this patient is most likely to reveal

    (A) a midsystolic click
    (B) a systolic ejection murmur
    (C) a systolic rumble
    (D) an opening snap

157. The arrow in Fig. 3–28B is pointing to the

    (A) coronary sinus
    (B) inferior vena cava

A

B

C

Figure 3–28. (A) Parasternal long-axis view; **(B)** apical four-chamber view; **(C)** continuous-wave Doppler tracing of mitral inflow from the apical position.

(C) descending aorta

(D) left pulmonary vein

158. The pressure half-time derived from the Doppler tracing of the mitral valve in Fig. 3–28C can be used to estimate

(A) the mitral valve area

(B) the mitral valve gradient

(C) the severity of aortic insufficiency

(D) the ejection fraction

A 52-year-old woman presents with chronic dyspnea. Chest x-ray reveals cardiomegaly. For questions 159 through 162, refer to Fig. 3–29A and B.

159. The most striking feature of this echocardiogram is

(A) left atrial compression

(B) mitral valve doming

(C) left ventricular hypertrophy

(D) right ventricular dilatation

160. Additional findings on this echocardiogram include

(A) a dilated aortic root, mitral valve prolapse, and a dilated coronary sinus

(B) a thickened mitral valve, a prominent interatrial septum, a small left ventricle, and a pericardial effusion

(C) a calcified mitral annulus, an extracardiac mass, and pleural effusion

(D) left atrial dilatation, systolic anterior motion of the mitral valve, and a thickened aortic valve

161. Given all the above information, the most likely diagnosis is

(A) hypertrophic obstructive cardiomyopathy

(B) Marfan syndrome

(C) endomyocardial fibrosis

(D) amyloid cardiomyopathy

162. The best way to substantiate this diagnosis is by obtaining

(A) a CT scan

(B) an endomyocardial biopsy

(C) a cardiac catheterization

(D) an electrocardiogram

A 64-year-old male sustained a myocardial infarction one week before this echocardiogram. He developed congestive heart failure and became hypotensive. A new murmur was detected on auscultation. For questions 163 through 167, refer to Fig. 3–30A and B.

163. The echocardiogram reveals a

(A) dilated cardiomyopathy

(B) ventricular septal defect

(C) cleft mitral valve

(D) pseudoaneurysm

164. Which of the following would be the most helpful in confirming the diagnosis

(A) color flow Doppler imaging

(B) M-mode echocardiography

(C) continuous-wave Doppler imaging

(D) pulsed-wave Doppler imaging

165. The arrow in Fig. 3–30B is pointing to a linear structure called the

(A) coronary sinus

(B) left anterior descending coronary artery

(C) left pulmonary vein

(D) left circumflex coronary artery

A

B

Figure 3–29. (**A**) Parasternal long-axis view; (**B**) apical four-chamber view.

A   B

Figure 3–30. (A) Parasternal short-axis view at the level of the papillary muscles; **(B)** modified apical four-chamber view: The transducer is angled posteriorly and the depth setting is decreased.

166. This linear structure contains

(A) serous fluid
(B) deoxygenated blood
(C) oxygenated blood
(D) air

167. In Fig. 3–30B, in what direction would the transducer need to be directed to visualize the left ventricular outflow tract?

(A) anteriorly
(B) medially
(C) laterally
(D) inferiorly

A 34-year-old woman is extremely nervous at the time of the examination. She states that she often experiences chest pain and palpitations. Ausculta-

tion reveals a systolic murmur. For questions 168 through 171 refer to Fig. 3–31A and B.

168. The mitral valve demonstrates

(A) diastolic doming
(B) prolapse of the anterior leaflet
(C) prolapse of the posterior leaflet
(D) systolic anterior motion

169. Continuous-wave Doppler evaluation of the mitral valve from the apical position would most likely demonstrate a

(A) systolic curve below baseline greater than 3 m/s
(B) diastolic signal above baseline with a decreased pressure half-time
(C) systolic curve above baseline less than 3 m/s

A   B

Figure 3–31. (A) Narrow sector parasternal long-axis view; **(B)** apical four-chamber view.

A

B

Figure 3–32. (A) M-mode tracing at the aortic valve level; (B) Continuous-wave Doppler tracing of aortic flow from the right sternal border (calibration marks are 1 m/s).

(D) diastolic curve below baseline greater than 3 m/s

170. The arrow in Fig. 3–31B is pointing to the posterior wall of the left ventricle.

(A) true
(B) false

171. The dropout of echoes in the interatrial septum in Fig. 3–31B is most likely

(A) a primum atrial septal defect
(B) a secundum atrial septal defect
(C) artifactual
(D) the result of interatrial septal prolapse

A 23-year-old male was referred for an echocardiogram because a systolic ejection murmur was heard on auscultation. For questions 172 through 175, refer to Fig. 3–32A and B.

172. The M-mode of the aortic valve in Fig. 3–32A demonstrates

(A) slight thickening of the valve with a normal opening
(B) the absence of aortic valve echoes
(C) systolic fluttering of the aortic valve
(D) a thickened aortic valve with a markedly decreased opening

173. According to the Doppler tracing in Fig. 3–32B, the peak aortic gradient using the simplified Bernoulli formula is approximately

(A) 4 mm Hg
(B) 16 mm Hg

(C) 36 mm Hg
(D) 100 mm Hg

174. The most likely diagnosis for this patient is

(A) aortic valve vegetation
(B) congenital aortic stenosis
(C) moderate aortic insufficiency
(D) rheumatic heart disease

175. Two-dimensional examination of the aortic valve is most likely to demonstrate

(A) systolic doming
(B) a mass of echoes in the left ventricular outflow tract
(C) diastolic doming
(D) four aortic cusps

A 38-year-old woman, who recently had extensive dental work performed, presented with fever, chills, and a transischemic attack. Auscultation revealed a grade 2/6 systolic murmur. For questions 176 through 181, refer to Fig. 3–33A, B, and C.

176. The mitral valve is

(A) normal
(B) doming
(C) exhibiting shaggy irregular echoes
(D) flail

177. The most likely diagnosis for this patient is

(A) rheumatic heart disease
(B) subacute bacterial endocarditis
(C) ruptured papillary muscle
(D) mitral valve prolapse

simultaneously and may have to relinquish quality in one to obtain excellent-quality images in the others. *(1:104)*

16. **(D)** Pulmonary hypertension. The constant pressure overload of pulmonary hypertension causes right ventricular hypertrophy until the ventricle fails, at which point the right ventricle wall dilates. *(3:217)*

17. **(C)** Chordae tendineae. Left ventricular dimensions have been standardized to be obtained at the level of the chordae tendineae. *(7:1072)*

18. **(C)** Left ventricular volume overload. Right ventricular volume overload may cause paradoxical interventricular septal motion (anterior motion of the interventricular septum at the onset of systole). *(1:164)*

19. **(A)** Toward the right ventricular free wall. Right ventricular volume overload causes paradoxical septal motion, whereby the septum moves toward the right side of the heart in systole rather than toward the left side of the heart. *(1:164)*

20. **(A)** Organic in origin. A thrill is a murmur that produces a vibratory sensation when palpated. It is almost always organic in origin. *(8:51)*

21. **(A)** Mitral valve prolapse or systolic anterior motion of the mitral valve. The Valsalva maneuver and the inhalation of amyl nitrite decrease left ventricular volume and reduce the diameter of the left ventricular outflow tract, thereby stimulating mitral valve prolapse or systolic anterior motion of the mitral valve. *(3:222)*

22. **(A)** Cyanotic heart disease. Clubbing occurs when there is widening and cyanosis of the distal ends of the fingers and toes. *(9:18)*

23. **(B)** Providing enhanced temporal resolution. M-mode is still used in many laboratories to take measurements and to evaluate events that occur too rapidly for the eye to perceive, such as diastolic fluttering of the anterior mitral leaflet. This is the case because M-mode provides far better temporal (time) resolution than does two-dimensional echocardiography and allows for better analysis of intracardiac events. *(3:78)*

24. **(C)** To a higher intercostal space. If the transducer is placed too low relative to the position of the heart, the sector plane passes obliquely through the left ventricle, producing an ovoid image. *(3:110)*

25. **(C)** Decreased left ventricular compliance. This situation, referred to as reversed E-to-A ratio, in-

dicates decreased left ventricular diastolic compliance. Conditions that cause this include left systemic hypertension, hypertrophic cardiomyopathy, and coronary artery disease. *(3:240)*

26. **(C)** A left ventricular thrombus. Left ventricular function is not impaired in mitral stenosis. Because thrombi tend to form in areas of poor blood flow, the likelihood of finding a left ventricular thrombus is low. *(1:489)*

27. **(D)** A peak gradient occurring in late diastole. The peak gradient in mitral stenosis usually occurs in early diastole. *(10:132)*

28. **(C)** Mitral insufficiency. Ruptured chordae tendineae always result in mitral regurgitation, the onset of which is often abrupt and acute. *(3:189)*

29. **(D)** Hypertrophic obstructive cardiomyopathy. This causes anterior motion of the mitral valve. It is not a source of confusion for mitral valve prolapse, in which the mitral valve moves posteriorly in systole. *(11:211)*

30. **(A)** A dilated left atrium. This is a secondary sign of mitral regurgitation. The left ventricle usually dilates as well and becomes hyperkinetic in response to the volume overload. *(1:266)*

31. **(A)** Width and length of the systolic jet by color Doppler. Color Doppler provides a spatial display of regurgitant flow. Quantification of the severity of mitral regurgitation is based roughly on the size and configuration of the regurgitant jet. *(12:87)*

32. **(D)** Pulmonic stenosis. The pulmonic valve is the valve that is least likely to be deformed by rheumatic fever. When pulmonic stenosis is noted on an echocardiogram, it is usually a congenital abnormality rather than a sequela of rheumatic fever. *(9:1711)*

33. **(A)** A dilated left atrium and left ventricular hypertrophy. Mitral stenosis causes the left atrium to dilate, and aortic stenosis leads to left ventricular hypertrophy. *(3:186,206)*

34. **(B)** Concurrent atrial fibrillation. Mitral stenosis often leads to atrial fibrillation. The A wave of the mitral valve corresponds to the P wave on the electrocardiogram. Because the P wave is absent in atrial fibrillation, the A wave will be absent as well. *(11:333)*

35. **(B)** Hypertrophic cardiomyopathy. Under normal circumstances, the mitral E point, which represents rapid ventricular filling, is higher than the mitral A point, which corresponds to atrial contraction.

simultaneously and may have to relinquish quality in one to obtain excellent-quality images in the others.   *(1:104)*

16. **(D)** Pulmonary hypertension. The constant pressure overload of pulmonary hypertension causes right ventricular hypertrophy until the ventricle fails, at which point the right ventricle wall dilates.   *(3:217)*

17. **(C)** Chordae tendineae. Left ventricular dimensions have been standardized to be obtained at the level of the chordae tendineae.   *(7:1072)*

18. **(C)** Left ventricular volume overload. Right ventricular volume overload may cause paradoxical interventricular septal motion (anterior motion of the interventricular septum at the onset of systole).   *(1:164)*

19. **(A)** Toward the right ventricular free wall. Right ventricular volume overload causes paradoxical septal motion, whereby the septum moves toward the right side of the heart in systole rather than toward the left side of the heart.   *(1:164)*

20. **(A)** Organic in origin. A thrill is a murmur that produces a vibratory sensation when palpated. It is almost always organic in origin.   *(8:51)*

21. **(A)** Mitral valve prolapse or systolic anterior motion of the mitral valve. The Valsalva maneuver and the inhalation of amyl nitrite decrease left ventricular volume and reduce the diameter of the left ventricular outflow tract, thereby stimulating mitral valve prolapse or systolic anterior motion of the mitral valve.   *(3:222)*

22. **(A)** Cyanotic heart disease. Clubbing occurs when there is widening and cyanosis of the distal ends of the fingers and toes.   *(9:18)*

23. **(B)** Providing enhanced temporal resolution. M-mode is still used in many laboratories to take measurements and to evaluate events that occur too rapidly for the eye to perceive, such as diastolic fluttering of the anterior mitral leaflet. This is the case because M-mode provides far better temporal (time) resolution than does two-dimensional echocardiography and allows for better analysis of intracardiac events.   *(3:78)*

24. **(C)** To a higher intercostal space. If the transducer is placed too low relative to the position of the heart, the sector plane passes obliquely through the left ventricle, producing an ovoid image.   *(3:110)*

25. **(C)** Decreased left ventricular compliance. This situation, referred to as reversed E-to-A ratio, in-

dicates decreased left ventricular diastolic compliance. Conditions that cause this include left systemic hypertension, hypertrophic cardiomyopathy, and coronary artery disease.   *(3:240)*

26. **(C)** A left ventricular thrombus. Left ventricular function is not impaired in mitral stenosis. Because thrombi tend to form in areas of poor blood flow, the likelihood of finding a left ventricular thrombus is low.   *(1:489)*

27. **(D)** A peak gradient occurring in late diastole. The peak gradient in mitral stenosis usually occurs in early diastole.   *(10:132)*

28. **(C)** Mitral insufficiency. Ruptured chordae tendineae always result in mitral regurgitation, the onset of which is often abrupt and acute.   *(3:189)*

29. **(D)** Hypertrophic obstructive cardiomyopathy. This causes anterior motion of the mitral valve. It is not a source of confusion for mitral valve prolapse, in which the mitral valve moves posteriorly in systole.   *(11:211)*

30. **(A)** A dilated left atrium. This is a secondary sign of mitral regurgitation. The left ventricle usually dilates as well and becomes hyperkinetic in response to the volume overload.   *(1:266)*

31. **(A)** Width and length of the systolic jet by color Doppler. Color Doppler provides a spatial display of regurgitant flow. Quantification of the severity of mitral regurgitation is based roughly on the size and configuration of the regurgitant jet.   *(12:87)*

32. **(D)** Pulmonic stenosis. The pulmonic valve is the valve that is least likely to be deformed by rheumatic fever. When pulmonic stenosis is noted on an echocardiogram, it is usually a congenital abnormality rather than a sequela of rheumatic fever.   *(9:1711)*

33. **(A)** A dilated left atrium and left ventricular hypertrophy. Mitral stenosis causes the left atrium to dilate, and aortic stenosis leads to left ventricular hypertrophy.   *(3:186, 206)*

34. **(B)** Concurrent atrial fibrillation. Mitral stenosis often leads to atrial fibrillation. The A wave of the mitral valve corresponds to the P wave on the electrocardiogram. Because the P wave is absent in atrial fibrillation, the A wave will be absent as well.   *(11:333)*

35. **(B)** Hypertrophic cardiomyopathy. Under normal circumstances, the mitral E point, which represents rapid ventricular filling, is higher than the mitral A point, which corresponds to atrial contraction.

Answers and Explanations

1. **(C)** Subcostal. Standard parasternal and suprasternal views do not demonstrate all four cardiac chambers. Only the apical and subcostal windows allow visualization of all cardiac chambers. *(1:80)*

2. **(A)** Long axis, short axis, and four chamber. The American Society of Echocardiography has standardized two-dimensional views of the heart into three basic orthogonal planes for which all views can basically be categorized. *(2:212)*

3. **(A)** Atrial septal defect and ventricular septal defect. If the ultrasound beam is not oriented perpendicular to the interatrial and interventricular septum, there may be false dropout of echoes. The subcostal approach allows the ultrasound beam to be perpendicular to the cardiac chambers, thereby allowing a better demonstration of atrial or ventricular septal defects. In addition, any gap noted in the interatrial or interventricular septum when the subcostal four-chamber view is used should be considered real. *(1:92)*

4. **(B)** Time-gain compensation. The time-gain compensation control allows the echocardiographer to selectively increase or decrease the gain at different depths of tissue. The objective is to achieve a uniform echocardiographic image without artifactually adding or eliminating information. *(3:52)*

5. **(A)** The right ventricular pressure drops below the right atrial pressure. The atrioventricular valves open when ventricular pressure drops below atrial pressure. *(3:38)*

6. **(B)** The coronary ligament. This ligament defines the bare area of the liver and is the only choice that does not represent a remnant of fetal circulation. *(4:30)*

7. **(A)** Pulmonary artery. The right side of the heart pumps deoxygenated blood through the pulmonary artery to the lungs for reoxygenation. (The pulmonary artery is the only artery in the body that carries deoxygenated blood.) *(3:9)*

8. **(C)** Left atrium. Four pulmonary veins transport oxygenated blood from the lungs to the left atrium. (The pulmonary veins are the only veins in the body that carry oxygenated blood.) *(3:9)*

9. **(D)** The left ventricle constitutes most of the ventral surface of the heart. The right ventricle, although less muscular than the left ventricle, dominates the ventral surface of the heart. *(3:25)*

10. **(A)** Aortic valve opening and closing points. Left ventricular ejection time—the time it takes for blood to be ejected from the left ventricle—can be obtained from an M-mode tracing of the aortic valve by measuring the time interval between opening and closing of the valve. *(3:156)*

11. **(D)** Subcostal. Lung expansion in patients with chronic obstructive pulmonary disease often obliterates the apical and parasternal position. This lung expansion also tends to shift the heart inferiorly, making the subcostal view the best approach for scanning the heart. *(5:79)*

12. **(B)** Apical and right sternal border. The most common windows used to record systolic blood flow across the aortic valve are the apical, right parasternal, and suprasternal. *(6:128)*

13. **(A)** At end-systole. M-mode measurements of the left atrium, left ventricle, and right ventricle are done at a point when the chambers are at their largest. The left atrium is largest at end-systole. *(3:82)*

14. **(C)** Stenosis. Doming is a main two-dimensional feature of any stenotic valve. The valve domes when it opens because the commissures are fused, causing the body of the valve to separate more widely than the tips. *(1:251)*

15. **(C)** Perpendicular, parallel. Because of the differences in transducer orientation for optimum two-dimensional and Doppler studies, one rarely obtains excellent-quality images and wave forms

A

B

C

Figure 3–33. (A) Parasternal long-axis view; **(B)** parasternal short-axis view at the papillary muscle level; **(C)** apical four-chamber view.

178. The mitral valve excursion is most likely

(A) reduced
(B) increased
(C) normal
(D) absent

179. Apical continuous-wave Doppler examination of the mitral valve is most likely to demonstrate a

(A) systolic waveform below baseline
(B) diastolic waveform below baseline
(C) diastolic waveform above baseline greater than 3 m/s
(D) systolic waveform above baseline

180. By referring to all three echocardiographic views presented in this case, one could suggest that the mass of echoes on the mitral valve

(A) is stationary
(B) prolapses into the left atrium
(C) prolapses into the left ventricle
(D) prolapses into the left atrium and left ventricle

181. The arrow in Fig. 3–33B points to

(A) a mural thrombus
(B) the posteromedial papillary muscle
(C) vegetation
(D) a cleft mitral valve

Figure 3–32. (**A**) M-mode tracing at the aortic valve level; (**B**) Continuous-wave Doppler tracing of aortic flow from the right sternal border (calibration marks are 1 m/s).

(D) diastolic curve below baseline greater than 3 m/s

170. The arrow in Fig. 3–31B is pointing to the posterior wall of the left ventricle.

    (A) true
    (B) false

171. The dropout of echoes in the interatrial septum in Fig. 3–31B is most likely

    (A) a primum atrial septal defect
    (B) a secundum atrial septal defect
    (C) artifactual
    (D) the result of interatrial septal prolapse

A 23-year-old male was referred for an echocardiogram because a systolic ejection murmur was heard on auscultation. For questions 172 through 175, refer to Fig. 3–32A and B.

172. The M-mode of the aortic valve in Fig. 3–32A demonstrates

    (A) slight thickening of the valve with a normal opening
    (B) the absence of aortic valve echoes
    (C) systolic fluttering of the aortic valve
    (D) a thickened aortic valve with a markedly decreased opening

173. According to the Doppler tracing in Fig. 3–32B, the peak aortic gradient using the simplified Bernoulli formula is approximately

    (A) 4 mm Hg
    (B) 16 mm Hg

(C) 36 mm Hg
(D) 100 mm Hg

174. The most likely diagnosis for this patient is

    (A) aortic valve vegetation
    (B) congenital aortic stenosis
    (C) moderate aortic insufficiency
    (D) rheumatic heart disease

175. Two-dimensional examination of the aortic valve is most likely to demonstrate

    (A) systolic doming
    (B) a mass of echoes in the left ventricular outflow tract
    (C) diastolic doming
    (D) four aortic cusps

A 38-year-old woman, who recently had extensive dental work performed, presented with fever, chills, and a transischemic attack. Auscultation revealed a grade 2/6 systolic murmur. For questions 176 through 181, refer to Fig. 3–33A, B, and C.

176. The mitral valve is

    (A) normal
    (B) doming
    (C) exhibiting shaggy irregular echoes
    (D) flail

177. The most likely diagnosis for this patient is

    (A) rheumatic heart disease
    (B) subacute bacterial endocarditis
    (C) ruptured papillary muscle
    (D) mitral valve prolapse

This relationship between the two points is altered when there is decreased left ventricular compliance (as is the case with hypertrophic cardiomyopathy).

(6:155)

36. **(B)** Aortic regurgitation. Aortic regurgitation causes a left ventricular volume overload pattern on the echocardiogram (a dilated and hypercontractile left ventricle). Mitral regurgitation usually causes dilatation of both the left atrium and the left ventricle.

(5:231)

37. **(C)** A decreased E-F slope, a thickened mitral valve, and a mitral distal velocity >1.5 m/s. Both thickening of the mitral valve and a reduced E-F slope must be noted to be sure the pathology is mitral stenosis. Diastolic doming of the mitral valve also is a specific sign of mitral stenosis. *(1:251)*

38. **(B)** An increased E-F slope on M-mode. One M-mode criterion for mitral stenosis is a decreased E-F slope.

(1:249)

39. **(C)** Tips of the mitral leaflets. The mitral valve is funnel shaped, with the true orifice at the narrow end. Measurement of the size of the orifice should therefore be done at the tips of the leaflets at the point where the chordae tendineae merge with the body of the valve. *(3:161)*

40. **(C)** A dilated left ventricle. Unless there is concomitant mitral regurgitation, the size of the left ventricle will be normal or smaller than normal. *(13:64)*

41. **(C)** An increase in pressure half-time. A successful mitral valve commissurotomy should lead to a decrease in the pressure half-time. The other findings will usually remain, although the left atrium may decrease slightly in size. *(13:65)*

42. **(B)** Concomitant mitral regurgitation. Pure mitral stenosis leads to a dilated left atrium and a normal or smaller-than-normal left ventricle. Aortic stenosis and hypertrophic cardiomyopathy cause the left ventricular walls to appear thickened. Only concomitant mitral regurgitation will cause left ventricular dilatation as well. *(1:139)*

43. **(A)** Severe acute aortic regurgitation. Severe acute aortic insufficiency can cause an elevated left ventricular diastolic pressure, which in turn causes the mitral valve to close early. *(1:295)*

44. **(D)** A ventricular septal defect. Conditions such as systemic hypertension that stress the area of the mitral annulus can lead to premature calcification of the mitral annulus. *(9:1035)*

45. **(B)** 1 cm². Studies done by Hatle and co-workers found that a mitral valve with an area of 1 cm² exhibits a Doppler pressure half-time of 220 m/s.

(14:1096)

46. **(B)** Diastolic fluttering of the anterior mitral leaflet. This is a finding of aortic insufficiency. *(3:210)*

47. **(D)** Systemic hypertension. This produces pressure overload of the left ventricle that, in turn, leads to left ventricular hypertrophy. Choices B and C cause a left ventricular volume overload pattern on the echocardiogram (dilated and hyperkinetic left ventricle). *(15:104)*

48. **(C)** Aortic stenosis. A systolic ejection murmur can be heard with this disorder. *(3:204)*

49. **(C)** It is often seen in conjunction with mitral stenosis. A bicuspid aortic valve is a congenital abnormality in which one of the aortic commissures is fused, leading to the formation of two aortic cusps instead of the usual three. Bicuspid valves tend to become stenotic in adulthood. Although they are sometimes seen in conjunction with coarctation of the aorta, a bicuspid valve and mitral stenosis have no direct association. *(3:202)*

50. **(B)** The aortic valve area, poor left ventricular function. When aortic stenosis is found in conjunction with a poorly moving left ventricle, standard estimations of the degree of aortic stenosis will be inaccurate. The continuity equation compensates for ventricular hypocontractility, allowing for a more accurate estimate of the aortic valve area.

(3:207, 16:105)

51. **(B)** The mean pressure gradient. Aortic insufficiency may cause a high initial instantaneous gradient. When there is combined aortic stenosis and insufficiency, the mean pressure gradient is more specific for estimating the severity of aortic stenosis. *(6:137)*

52. **(A)** The apical long-axis view. All Doppler procedures are best performed with the ultrasound beam directed parallel to the flow of blood. Of the choices presented, the apical long-axis view provides the optimum angle to image acquisition. *(1:104)*

53. **(B)** Left ventricular hypertrophy. Aortic stenosis causes pressure overload of the left ventricle. This overload leads to left ventricular hypertrophy.

(11:203)

54. **(A)** Aortic insufficiency. The anterior mitral leaflet flutters rapidly when hit by an aortic insufficiency

jet. These oscillations are best detected by M-mode. Atrial fibrillation causes coarse diastolic fluttering of the anterior mitral leaflet.   *(1:294)*

55. **(D)** Consistent with moderate aortic regurgitation. The grading of aortic insufficiency with Doppler echocardiography is similar to the grading method used in cardiac catheterization laboratories. An aortic insufficiency jet that extends from the aortic valve to the tips of the anterior mitral leaflet is consistent with moderate aortic regurgitation.

    (17:339)

56. **(B)** Fine diastolic fluttering and possible flattening of the anterior mitral leaflet. An Austin-Flint murmur represents functional mitral stenosis caused by inhibition of anterior leaflet motion resulting from compression by a strong aortic insufficiency jet. This would appear on M-mode as fine diastolic fluttering of the anterior mitral leaflet with inhibition of opening.   *(9:77)*

57. **(D)** The right sternal border. When obtainable, the right sternal border approach is usually best for acquiring maximum aortic valve velocities. The patient is turned onto his or her right side, and the Doppler probe is directed into the aortic root.   *(18:89)*

58. **(D)** Transesophageal echocardiography. Because of the high-resolution images it provides of the thoracic aorta, transesophageal echocardiography has been highly successful in evaluating patients with suspected aortic dissection.   *(19:216)*

59. **(D)** A thickened anterior right ventricle wall. Thickening of the right ventricular walls is usually caused by right ventricular pressure overload. Tricuspid insufficiency causes right ventricular volume overload.   *(1:162)*

60. **(D)** Pulmonary hypertension. The right ventricular systolic pressure in this ventricle is approximately 74 mm Hg (using the formula $4 V^2 + 10$). Because right ventricular pressures are basically equal to pulmonary artery pressures, the pulmonary artery pressure in this instance is roughly 74 mm Hg, thus indicating the presence of pulmonary hypertension.   *(3:161)*

61. **(D)** It is usually seen as part of the aging process. Tricuspid stenosis is a rare condition that usually occurs as a sequela to rheumatic fever. Its echocardiographic findings are similar to those of mitral stenosis.   *(3:198)*

62. **(C)** Contrast in the inferior vena cava during ventricular systole. With severe tricuspid regurgitation, the regurgitant volume extends all the way back into the right atrium and sometimes into the inferior vena cava as well. By injecting contrast, this regurgitant volume can be "seen" with M-mode or two-dimensional echocardiography.   *(1:305)*

63. **(B)** Tricuspid valve. The echocardiographer should pay special attention to this valve because carcinoid heart disease presents as thickening and rigidity of the tricuspid valve leaflets. Severe tricuspid regurgitation is usually detected with Doppler.   *(1:305)*

64. **(B)** Right ventricular systolic pressure. By using the modified Bernoulli equation and an estimate of jugular venous pressure, systolic pressure in the right ventricle can be determined.   *(3:112)*

65. **(C)** Infundibular pulmonic stenosis. This is caused by hypertrophied muscle bands in the right ventricular outflow tract. Echocardiographically, it can be distinguished from valvular pulmonic stenosis by noting a step-up in Doppler velocities proximal to the pulmonic valve. In addition, the muscular ridge produces turbulence of blood, which hits the pulmonic valve and causes it to flutter.   *(1:393)*

66. **(D)** Left parasternal. Pulmonary artery flow velocities are usually obtained from the left parasternal short-axis view at the level of the aortic root.   *(10:80)*

67. **(A)** Cranial and lateral. This relationship is best appreciated from the short-axis view of the base of the heart.   *(3:27)*

68. **(C)** Midsystolic notching noted on M-mode. Midsystolic notching is a sign of pulmonary hypertension.   *(3:388)*

69. **(B)** Two-dimensional echocardiography. The spatial orientation of two-dimensional echocardiography provides for a better assessment of the size, location, and motion of valvular vegetations.   *(3:277)*

70. **(B)** Mitral valve vegetation. Intravenous drug abusers have an increased incidence of endocarditis because of microorganisms that enter the bloodstream via unsterile needles. Vegetations usually form on the valves of the right side of the heart, but they may settle on left-sided valves as well. One complication of valvular vegetation is an embolic event.   *(3:276)*

71. **(B)** Presence of paravalvular regurgitation. The spatial orientation of color Doppler allows for a quick assessment of blood flow in the region surrounding the prosthetic valve.   *(12:141)*

72. **(A)** May exhibit high Doppler velocities. The normal Doppler velocities across any prosthetic valve will be slightly higher than those of a native valve.

A Starr-Edwards, or ball-in-cage valve, tends to exhibit the highest velocities.   *(3:349)*

73. **(A)** An example of a mechanical heart valve. The Bjork-Shiley is a tilting-disc mechanical heart valve.   *(3:314)*

74. **(C)** Transesophageal echocardiography. This is a major application in the evaluation of prosthetic heart valves, particularly in the mitral position.   *(3:358)*

75. **(D)** Hancock. This valve is an example of a heterograft (bioprosthetic) valve.   *(3:334)*

76. **(C)** Abnormal rocking motion of the valve. Valve dehiscence refers to a condition in which the prosthetic valve loosens or separates from the sewing ring and causes an abnormal rocking motion and a paravalvular leak.   *(3:346)*

77. **(C)** It often makes anticoagulation unnecessary. Mechanical valves require constant anticoagulation. Women during childbearing years would therefore be more likely to receive a bioprosthetic valve, which would not require anticoagulation.   *(20:1392)*

78. **(A)** Because these patients are at a higher risk for endocarditis. Because bacteremias occur during dental or surgical procedures, prophylactic antibiotics are often administered to susceptible patients (such as mitral valve prolapse patients) in an attempt to prevent bacterial endocarditis.   *(20:1151)*

79. **(C)** A "swinging heart" on the two-dimensional examination. Excessive motion of the heart can sometimes be noted with massive pericardial effusion.   *(1:558)*

80. **(A)** Impairs diastolic filling. The rigid and fibrotic pericardial sac impairs diastolic filling of the cardiac chambers.   *(3:268)*

81. **(A)** Pressure in the pericardial cavity rises to equal or exceed the diastolic pressure in the heart. Tamponade occurs when intrapericardial pressures rise and impair cardiac filling. Although cardiac tamponade is usually seen in association with a large pericardial effusion, a small effusion may cause tamponade if the rate of accumulation of pericardial fluid exceeds the ability of the pericardium to accommodate the increased volume.   *(15:213)*

82. **(D)** In Dressler's syndrome, a pericardial effusion develops as a result of renal disease. Dressler's syndrome, also known as postmyocardial infarction syndrome, is the development of pericardial effusion 2-to-10 weeks after infarction.   *(9:1287)*

83. **(D)** A pericardial effusion. Neoplasms from the thoracic region often lead to pericardial effusion.   *(20:1254)*

84. **(D)** Mitral valve prolapse. The descending aorta, a calcified mitral annulus, and ascites can cause echo-free spaces that may be misleading on an echocardiogram. Although a large effusion in which the heart exhibits excessive motion may lead to false mitral valve prolapse, prolapse will not lead to a false-positive diagnosis of pericardial effusion.   *(1:552)*

85. **(A)** Pulmonic stenosis. Diastolic collapse of the right ventricular walls is a good indicator of tamponade. Pulmonic stenosis, or any other form of right ventricular pressure overload, leads to thickening of the right ventricular walls. A thickened wall is unlikely to collapse in diastole.   *(1:565)*

86. **(C)** There is a large acoustic mismatch between lung tissue and pericardial tissue. A greater mismatch between two structures results in brighter reflected echoes from the interface between them. Because there is an extremely large acoustic mismatch between lung (air) and pericardium (tissue), the interface created by the two will cause a bright echo to appear on the echocardiogram.   *(1:2)*

87. **(C)** Decreasing overall gain and increasing depth setting. Decreasing the gain allows for differentiation between the pericardium and epicardium, and increasing the depth setting helps define the borders of the effusion.   *(11:249)*

88. **(D)** Descending aorta. Because the descending aorta lies posterior to the pericardial effusion and anterior to the pleural effusion, it often aids in differentiating between the two.   *(1:554)*

89. **(A)** Constrictive pericarditis. The pericardium limits cardiac motion. When the pericardium is surgically removed (eg in constrictive pericarditis), the heart expands and exhibits excessive motion.   *(1:575)*

90. **(A)** Excessive cardiac motion. Again, because the pericardium limits cardiac motion, the heart exhibits excessive motion when the pericardium is surgically removed.   *(1:575)*

91. **(C)** Reduced compliance of the left ventricle. Systemic hypertension causes pressure overload of the left ventricle. As in all pressure-overload situations (eg aortic stenosis), the left ventricle hypertrophies and may become noncompliant, leading to diastolic dysfunction.   *(11:273)*

92. (B) Left ventricular hypertrophy. This condition can be present in the absence of an obstruction.
(1:522)

93. (D) Endomyocardial biopsy. Several echocardiographic signs are suggestive of amyloid heart disease, but a definitive diagnosis can be made only with an endomyocardial biopsy performed in the catheterization laboratory.   *(20:1215)*

94. (B) Sarcoidosis. This is an infiltrative process that can lead to restrictive cardiomyopathy.   *(11:317)*

95. (A) Increased systolic velocity of the left ventricular outflow tract. Velocities are low because of decreased cardiac output.   *(3:230)*

96. (A) Is more likely to affect the right ventricle than the left ventricle. Cardiac contusion may be seen following a blunt trauma to the chest (such as a steering-wheel injury). Because the right ventricle is the most anterior structure of the heart, it is the one most susceptible to injury.   *(3:301)*

97. (A) An apical aneurysm with a mural thrombus. Apical aneurysms sometimes develop following an anterior wall myocardial infarction. Because aneurysms are a likely site for thrombus, choice A is the most likely answer.   *(1:489)*

98. (C) Two-dimensional demonstration of an ejection fraction lower than 50%. The ejection fraction is a measure of systolic left ventricular function. *(20:51)*

99. (C) Left anterior descending artery. This artery supplies the anterior wall of the left ventricle and the anterior portion of the interventricular septum.
(3:237)

100. (D) Have a narrow neck. The best way to differentiate a true aneurysm from a pseudoaneurysm is to look at the width of its neck. Pseudoaneurysms tend to have a narrow neck because they result from a tear in the myocardium.   *(1:486)*

101. (B) A reduced ejection fraction. An E point-to-septal separation of more than 10 mm correlates with a reduced ejection fraction.   *(11:205)*

102. (B) Akinetic. Lack of systolic thickening and motion is referred to as akinesis.   *(11:287)*

103. (D) Occlusion of the left anterior descending coronary artery. Blood to the inferior wall of the left ventricle is usually supplied by the right coronary artery.   *(1:467, 21:93)*

104. (B) Severe mitral regurgitation. Doppler interrogation of a patient with ruptured papillary muscle will usually demonstrate this condition.   *(3:249)*

105. (D) Is used in diagnosing ischemic heart disease. Stress echocardiography is used as an adjunct to standard stress testing in diagnosing patients with suspected coronary artery disease. Resting wall motion is compared to wall motion during and after stress.   *(3:250)*

106. (C) They do not recur once they are surgically removed. Although characterized as a benign tumor, a myxoma may recur if some cells remain after excision of the tumor.   *(20:1285)*

107. (B) Ventricular septal defects. The QP/QS ratio refers to the ratio of pulmonary-to-systemic blood flow. It can be calculated echocardiographically to determine the magnitude of left-to-right shunting of blood.   *(6:161)*

108. (B) Continuous flow (systolic and diastolic) above baseline. Shunting of blood from the aorta to the pulmonary artery occurs in both systole and diastole.   *(18:220)*

109. (B) Contrast injection echocardiography. Even a small atrial septal defect can be detected by noting the presence or absence of microbubbles.   *(1:406)*

110. (B) Secundum. Atrial septal defects occur most commonly in the area of the foramen ovale, where they are termed ostium secundum defects.   *(3:381)*

111. (C) Eisenmenger's syndrome. In this syndrome, the pulmonary vascular resistance is equal to or greater than the systemic vascular resistance, leading to right-to-left shunting.   *(20:589)*

112. (B) Infundibular pulmonic stenosis. In Ebstein's anomaly, the tricuspid valve is large and partially adherent to the walls of the right ventricle so that the valve orifice is displaced apically. Therefore, most of the right ventricle functions as part of the right atrium. It is frequently associated with an atrial septal defect. Infundibular pulmonic stenosis is not part of the spectrum of this disorder.   *(3:406)*

113. (D) Ostium primum atrial septal defect and an inlet ventricular septal defect. Endocardial cushion defects occur when the atrial and ventricular components of the cardiac septum fail to develop properly.   *(3:381)*

114. (C) Descending thoracic aorta. Coarctation of the aorta is a constrictive malformation of the aortic arch, usually located just distal to the origin of the left subclavian artery. The obstruction increases the velocity of blood flow beyond the point of constriction.   *(3:396)*

115. **(D)** An atrial septal defect. The fourth component is right ventricular hypertrophy.   *(3:421)*

116. **(B)** Is a congenital malformation in which a fibrous membrane divides the left atrium into an upper and lower chamber. Cor triatriatum is a rare abnormality in which an embryonic membrane in the left atrium fails to regress. It can be detected echocardiographically by noting a linear echo traversing the left atrium. Doppler echocardiography will detect high-velocity flow across a hole in the membrane.   *(3:402)*

117. **(C)** Paradoxical septal motion. Left bundle branch block often causes this motion.   *(1:231)*

118. **(C)** A mechanical prosthetic valve. This high echogenicity of the mitral valve is characteristic of a mechanical prosthetic valve.   *(3:347)*

119. **(D)** Significantly decreased. The M-mode demonstrates a dilated and hypokinetic left ventricle. The markedly increased E point-to-septal separation is consistent with a decreased left ventricular ejection fraction.   *(23:140)*

120. **(B)** Left ventricular end-diastolic pressure is increased. There is a mitral valve B notch, which is consistent with high end-diastolic pressure in the left ventricle.   *(24:69)*

121. **(A)** Aortic stenosis and aortic insufficiency. The systolic waveform below baseline is consistent with moderate aortic stenosis. A mitral regurgitation waveform would be wider and is usually of higher velocity. The diastolic waveform above baseline is too high a velocity to be caused by mitral or tricuspid stenosis and is consistent with aortic insufficiency.   *(6:78)*

122. **(D)** Coronary artery disease. The interventricular septum is hypokinetic and more echogenic than the posterior left ventricular wall. These findings are consistent with an old myocardial infarction. *(1:478)*

123. **(C)** Chordae tendineae. The M-mode cursor in this long-axis view is directed beyond the tips of the mitral leaflets at the level of the chordae tendineae—the level at which left ventricular measurements are obtained.   *(11:12)*

124. **(C)** Caused by stagnant blood. The cloud of fuzzy smokelike echoes in the left ventricle is the result of blood stasis. It is usually seen when there is a severe decrease in left ventricular contractibility.   *(1:492)*

125–131. If you are having a difficult time orienting yourself to an echocardiographic image, find a structure that is easy for you to recognize and work your way from there. For example, if you can identify the aortic root, you can then follow the anterior wall of the root as it continues into the interventricular septum. The posterior wall of the root will follow into the anterior mitral leaflet, and so on. 125. right ventricle, 126. aortic root, 127. left atrium, 128. descending aorta, 129. left ventricle, 130. pericardial effusion, 131. pleural effusion.   *(1:558)*

132. **(D)** A large pericardial effusion. A massive circumferential pericardial effusion is demonstrated in this four-chamber view.   *(11:253)*

133. **(B)** Right ventricular wall. The presence of tamponade should be ruled out in patients with pericardial effusion, especially a massive one. A fairly specific echocardiographic sign of tamponade is diastolic collapse of the right ventricle, the right atrium, or both.   *(25:561)*

134. **(B)** A diastolic jet filling the left ventricular outflow tract and extending deep into the left ventricle. This long-axis view demonstrates a flail right coronary cusp of the aortic valve. The cusp is seen extending into the left ventricular outflow tract in diastole. Color Doppler would be likely to demonstrate severe aortic insufficiency, which choice B describes.   *(12:100)*

135. **(D)** The origin of the right coronary artery. With slight superior angulation from a standard short-axis view of the aortic valve, the ostia and proximal segments of the right coronary artery can be visualized.   *(11:23)*

136. **(B)** False. The right ventricular outflow tract is located lateral to the origin of the right coronary artery.   *(1:102)*

137. **(A)** Left-to-right shunting at the atrial level. There is a washout effect in the right atrium as blood from the left side of the heart enters the contrast-filled right atrium.   *(11:355)*

138. **(B)** False. A pericardial effusion would appear on a subcostal four-chamber view as an echo-free space anterior to the right ventricle.   *(11:251)*

139. **(B)** Liver parenchyma. To obtain a subcostal four-chamber view, the transducer is placed on the abdo-

men and angled in a cephalic direction. Therefore, liver parenchyma will occupy the near field of the image.   *(3:129)*

140.   **(D)** Pulmonary hypertension. An absent A wave and midsystolic notching (flying W sign) are consistent with this condition.   *(3:388)*

141.   **(C)** Mitral valve prolapse. The M-mode in Fig. 3—20 demonstrates late-systolic tricuspid valve prolapse. Tricuspid valve prolapse almost always occurs in patients with concomitant mitral valve prolapse.   *(1:305)*

142.   **(C)** Midsystolic notching. Fig. 3–21 is an example of systolic anterior motion of the mitral valve. This is one classic echocardiographic sign of hypertrophic obstructive cardiomyopathy. The midsystolic obstruction of the left ventricular outflow tract will often be demonstrated on the M-mode of the aortic valve as well as by midsystolic notching.   *(26:6)*

143.   **(C)** A dilated aortic root. This patient exhibits characteristic findings of Marfan syndrome, a connective tissue disorder. There is a linear echo near the aortic valve suggesting aortic root dissection, another complication of Marfan syndrome. This syndrome often causes ascending aortic dilatation as well as myxomatous degeneration of the aortic and mitral valves.   *(11:242)*

144.   **(A)** The long-axis suprasternal view. Because the aortic root is dilated, echocardiographic evaluation should follow the length of the aorta to determine the extent of the aneurysm. The suprasternal long-axis view allows for visualization of the aortic arch and the proximal portion of the descending aorta. Further investigation should include a modified apical two-chamber view for evaluating the thoracic aorta and a subcostal approach for interrogating the abdominal aorta.   *(3:121, 137)*

145.   **(C)** A large apical thrombus. This thrombus is seen filling the apex, with a piece of the medial segment protruding into the left ventricle. Most thrombi are associated with anterior infarctions and are located in the apex in the majority of cases.   *(1:489)*

146.   **(B)** Flail. The tip of the posterior leaflet can be seen protruding into the left atrium, which is consistent with a flail mitral valve.   *(27:1383)*

147.   **(B)** Right pulmonary artery. The artery is seen in its short axis.   *(11:36)*

148.   **(A)** The left atrium. This atrium can sometimes be visualized posterior to the right pulmonary artery on the suprasternal long-axis view.   *(11:36)*

149.   **(D)** The moderator band. This is a muscular strip located in the apical third of the right ventricle. It is sometimes misdiagnosed as a right ventricular apical thrombus.   *(3:117, 294)*

150.   **(B)** A left atrial thrombus. This is seen protruding into the left atrium. (The bright linear echo in the right atrium originates from a pacemaker wire.)   *(1:592)*

151.   **(B)** Aortic stenosis, a calcified mitral annulus, and a pericardial effusion. The aortic valve is markedly calcified; there is a bright echo posterior to the mitral valve, representing a calcified mitral annulus; and the base of the interventricular septum is hypertrophied. The posterior echo-free space represents pleural effusion, as opposed to a pericardial effusion, because it does not taper at the descending aorta.   *(1:345, 283)*

152.   **(D)** An aged heart. When seen together, these findings usually indicate signs of aging.   *(9:1658)*

153.   **(D)** Atrial fibrillation. The electrocardiogram at the top of the Doppler tracing indicates this fibrillation. The variations from beat to beat reflect the altering lengths in diastolic filling periods that occur with atrial fibrillation.   *(11:333)*

154.   **(B)** Diastolic doming. The mitral valve is bulging into the left ventricle in diastole because the valve is stenotic and cannot accommodate all the blood available for delivery into the left ventricle.   *(1:251)*

155.   **(A)** The left atrium. Even without using the centimeter markers as a gauge, one can determine that the left atrium is dilated. On the long axis-view, the aortic root and left aorta should be approximately the same size. The apical four-chamber view is extremely useful for assessing relative chamber size. The right and left atria should be roughly the same size (although the left atrium is usually slightly larger), and they should be smaller than the ventricles.   *(11:368)*

156.   **(D)** An opening snap. The opening snap often affords the first clue to the diagnosis of mitral stenosis.   *(20:185)*

157.   **(C)** Descending aorta. A portion of the aorta can be seen lying behind the left atrium on the apical four-chamber view.   *(1:98)*

158.   **(A)** The mitral valve area. The pressure half-time, or the time it takes for the initial pressure drop of the mitral valve to be halved, can be used to measure mitral valve area. A pressure half-time of 220 msec has been shown to correlate with a valve area of 1.0 cm².   *(18:117)*

159. **(C)** Left ventricular hypertrophy. The left ventricular walls are thickened and exhibit increased echogenicity. *(28:188)*

160. **(B)** A thickened mitral valve, a prominent interatrial septum, a small left ventricle, and pericardial effusion. The mitral valve and interatrial septum are slightly thickened, there is a small-to-moderate-sized pericardial effusion, and the left ventricle is small. *(1:535)*

161. **(D)** Amyloid cardiomyopathy. This patient exhibits classic features of this disease. The infiltrative process of the disease causes thickening of the ventricles, interatrial septum and valves. Pericardial effusion is another finding sometimes associated with this disease. *(3:232)*

162. **(B)** An endomyocardial biopsy. This has been shown to be helpful in identifying amyloid cardiomyopathy. *(3:232)*

163. **(B)** Ventricular septal defect. The short-axis and modified four-chamber views demonstrate a gap in the posterior aspect of the midsection of the interventricular septum. Given the patient's history and the irregular borders on the echocardiogram, one can assume that this defect is acquired rather than congenital. *(29:506)*

164. **(A)** Color-flow Doppler imaging. This is particularly useful for quickly determining the location and quantifying the extent of abnormal blood flow in patients with ventricular septal defects. *(3:243)*

165. **(A)** Coronary sinus. When imaged from the apical two-chamber view, the coronary sinus appears as a circular structure in the atrioventricular groove. By rotating to a four-chamber view and angling posteriorly, one can follow the coronary sinus as it courses along the length of the posterior atrioventricular groove. *(20:29)*

166. **(B)** Deoxygenated blood. The coronary sinus carries venous blood to the right atrium. *(30:211)*

167. **(A)** Anteriorly. By tilting the scan plane anteriorly from this posteriorly directed apical four-chamber view, the aorta and left ventricular outflow tract can be imaged. *(3:131)*

168. **(C)** Prolapse of the posterior leaflet. The posterior mitral leaflet bulges beyond the plane of the mitral annulus, which is consistent with prolapse. *(3:189)*

169. **(A)** A systolic curve below baseline greater than 3 m/s. Mitral valve prolapse, especially to the degree shown in this study, is most likely to be accompanied by some degree of mitral regurgitation, which is detected from the apical window with Doppler echocardiography by noting a systolic curve below baseline usually greater than 3 m/s. *(6:74)*

170. **(B)** False. The arrow is pointing to the lateral wall of the left ventricle. *(11:25)*

171. **(C)** Artifactual. A dropout of echoes in the interatrial septum is not an uncommon finding when visualized from the apical four-chamber view. If this were a true atrial septal defect, a "T sign" would likely be noted. *(1:404)*

172. **(A)** Slight thickening of the valve with a normal opening. This thickening is noted best in diastole. The leaflets appear to open widely in systole. (They open in close proximity to the walls of the aortic root.) *(1:279)*

173. **(C)** 36 mm Hg. Using the simplified Bernoulli equation, the peak aortic gradient can be obtained by squaring the peak velocity (in this case 3 m/s) and then multiplying by four. *(18:23)*

174. **(B)** Congenital aortic stenosis. In this disorder, the valve may be thin or minimally thickened, and M-mode may demonstrate a normal opening if the cursor was directed at the body of the leaflets rather than at the restricted tips. The best way to determine if congenital aortic stenosis is present is by noting Doppler evidence of increased velocities across the valve. *(1:384)*

175. **(A)** Systolic doming. This occurs in congenital aortic stenosis because the body of the leaflets expands to accommodate systolic flow while the tips of the leaflets restrict blood flow. (Normally, the tips of the aortic valve open wide and lie parallel to the aortic root in systole.) *(1:383)*

176. **(C)** Exhibiting shaggy irregular echoes. The mitral valve has a mass of shaggy echoes with irregular borders attached to it. *(3:277)*

177. **(B)** Subacute bacterial endocarditis. Because of the patient's history and the echocardiographic demonstration of an irregular mass attached to the mitral valve, this is the most likely diagnosis. *(20:1141)*

178. **(B)** Increased. Unlike calcium, which tends to inhibit valve opening, vegetations are likely to increase valve excursion. Because calcium and vegetations can look similar echocardiographically this difference can aid in the diagnosis. *(3:277)*

179. **(A)** Systolic waveform below baseline. A mitral valve vegetation will usually cause the mitral valve to be regurgitant. Mitral regurgitation can be de-

tected by continuous-wave Doppler from the apical four-chamber view by noting systolic flow below baseline.   *(6:74)*

180. **(D)** Prolapses into the left atrium and left ventricle. In Fig. 3–33A, the mass is in the left atrium. In Fig. 3–33B and C, the mass appears in the left ventricle. Therefore, one could deduce that the mass is prolapsing into the left atrium in systole and into the left ventricle in diastole.   *(1:312)*

181. **(B)** The posteromedial papillary muscle. On the opposite wall of the left ventricle, one can see the anterolateral papillary muscle. Between the two papillary muscles, the tip of the mitral valve vegetation can be seen protruding into the left ventricle.   *(3:113)*

REFERENCES

1. Feigenbaum H. *Echocardiography,* 4th ed. Philadelphia: Lea & Febiger, 1986.
2. Henry WL, DeMaria A, Gramik R. *Nomenclature and Standardization in Two-Dimensional Echocardiography.* Raleigh, NC: American Society of Echocardiography, 1980.
3. Craig M. *Diagnostic Medical Sonography: A Guide to Clinical Practice. Vol 2. Echocardiography.* Philadelphia: JB Lippincott, 1991.
4. Cosgrove DO, McCready VR. *Ultrasound Imaging: Liver, Spleen, Pancreas.* New York: John Wiley & Sons, 1982.
5. Weyman AE. *Cross-sectional Echocardiography.* Philadelphia: Lea & Febiger, 1982.
6. Kisslo J, Adams D, Mark DB. *Basic Doppler Echocardiography.* New York: Churchill Livingstone, 1986.
7. Sahn DJ, DeMaria A, Kisso J, Weyman A. Recommendations regarding quantitation in M-mode echocardiography: results of a survey of echocardiographic measurements. *Circulation* **58:**1072–1083, 1978.
8. Sokolow M, McIlroy MB, Cheitlin MD. *Clinical Cardiology,* 5th ed. Norwalk, CT: Appleton & Lange, 1990.
9. Braunwald E. *Heart Disease: A Textbook of Cardiovascular Medicine,* 3rd ed. Philadelphia: WB Saunders, 1988.
10. Goldberg SJ, Allen HD, Marx GR, Flinn CJ. *Doppler Echocardiography.* Philadelphia: Lea & Febiger, 1985.
11. Harrigan P, Lee R. *Principles of Interpretation in Echocardiography.* New York: John Wiley & Sons, 1985.
12. Kisso J, Adams DB, Belkin RN. *Doppler Color Flow Imaging.* New York: Churchill Livingstone, 1988.
13. Salcedo E. *Atlas of Echocardiography,* 2nd ed. Philadelphia: WB Saunders, 1985.
14. Hatle L, Angelsen B, Tromsdal A. Noninvasive assessment of atrioventricular pressure half-time by Doppler ultrasound. *Circulation* **60:**1096–1104, 1979.
15. Gravanis MB. *Cardiovascular Pathophysiology.* New York: McGraw-Hill, 1987.
16. Popp RL. Echocardiography, *N Engl J Med* **323:**101–109, 1990.
17. Aobanu J, et al. Pulsed Doppler echocardiography in the diagnosis and estimation of severity of aortic insufficiency. *Am J Cardiol* **49:**339–343, 1982.
18. Hatle L, Angelsen B. *Doppler Ultrasound in Cardiology: Physical Principles and Clinical Applications.* Philadelphia: Lea & Febiger, 1985.
19. Currie PJ. Transesophageal echocardiography: new window to the heart. *Circulation* **80:**215–218, 1989.
20. Hurst JW. *The Heart,* 6th ed. New York: McGraw-Hill, 1986.
21. Wasser HJ, Greengart A, et al. Echocardiographic assessment of posterior left ventricular aneurysms. *J Diagn Med Sonography* **2:**93–95, 1986.
22. Driscoll DJ, Fuster V, McGoon DC. Congenital heart disease in adolescents and adults: atrioventricular canal defect. In Brandenburg RO, Fuster V, Giulani ER, et al. (eds): *Cardiology: Fundamentals and Practice.* Chicago: Year Book Medical Publishers, 1987.
23. D'Cruz IA, Lalmalani GG, et al. The superiority of mitral E point-ventricular septum separation to other echocardiographic indicators of left ventricular performance. *Clin Cardiol* **2:**140, 1979.
24. D'Cruz IA, Kleinman D, Aboulatta H, et al. A reappraisal of the mitral B-bump (B-inflection): its relationship to left ventricular dysfunction. *Echocardiography* **7:**69–75, 1990.
25. Williams GJ, Partidge JB, Right ventricular diastolic collapse: an echocardiographic sign of tamponade. *Br Heart J* **49:**292, 1983.
26. Doi YL, McKenna WJ, et al. M-mode echocardiography in hypertrophic cardiomyopathy: diagnostic criteria and prediction of obstruction. *Am J Cardiol* **45:**6–14, 1980.
27. Child JS, Skorton DJ, Taylor RD, et al. M-mode and cross-sectional echocardiographic features of flail posterior mitral leaflets. *Am J Cardiol* **44:**1383–1390, 1979.
28. Sigueira-Filho AG, Cunha CL, Tajik AJ, et al. M-mode and two-dimensional echocardiographic features in cardiac amyloidosis. *Circulation* **63:**188–196, 1981.
29. Chandraratna PAN, Balachandran PK, Shah PM, Hodges M. Echocardiographic observations on ventricular septal rupture complicating myocardial infarction. *Circulation* **51:**506–510, 1975.
30. Berne RM, Levy MN. *Cardiovascular Physiology,* 4th ed. St. Louis: CV Mosby, 1981.

CHAPTER 4

PEDIATRIC ECHOCARDIOGRAPHY

Diana Kawai Yankowitz

Study Guide

INTRODUCTION

Effective echocardiographic evaluation of congenital heart disease requires an appreciation of malformation severity and cardiovascular hemodynamics. A complete echocardiographic study involves the use of every modality available. Anatomy should be carefully delineated by two-dimensional (2-D) imaging because malformations frequently occur in combination rather than as isolated lesions. Doppler techniques provide information on shunt patterns, flow volumes, gradients through obstructions, and severity of regurgitation. Color flow Doppler facilitates rapid detection of flow abnormalities and qualitative assessment of such flow characteristics as direction, timing, and degree of turbulence. Pulsed-wave (PW) Doppler provides range (spatial) resolution of flow patterns. Quantification of high-velocity flows require the use of continuous-wave (CW) Doppler. M-mode is used primarily to evaluate subtle movements and to measure chamber, vessel, and wall size. Contrast echocardiography is useful in the demonstration of intracardiac and extracardiac shunts, particularly in cases in which 2-D and color flow imaging is suboptimal.

The study outline is intended as a guide for the entry-level pediatric echocardiographer and, as such, includes malformations that occur with relative frequency as well as those that occur rarely but are relatively straightforward. The outline includes a definition of the anatomic malformation, a list of variants, the hemodynamic effect of the lesion, characteristic clinical findings, key echocardiographic concepts, the natural history of the disease, commonly associated cardiac malformations, interventional catheterization techniques, and palliative as well as corrective surgical procedures. Complex malformations such as single ventricle, double-inlet ventricle and double-outlet ventricle are beyond the scope of this chapter. For information regarding these malformations, the reader is referred to more extensive texts.

Sample examination questions are provided following the text to give the reader an appreciation of the scope of knowledge required to perform routine diagnostic pediatric echocardiograms. The questions are *not* intended to be a comprehensive review but to assist the reader in determining what needs to be studied in greater detail.

For discussions of normal anatomy, general scanning technique, echocardiographic physics and instrumentation, and acquired heart disease that is not specific to the pediatric population, the reader is referred to other chapters within this book. Acquired pathologies that occur in the pediatric as well as adult population include mitral valve prolapse, rheumatic heart disease, cardiac masses, cardiomyopathies, pericardial effusions, and bacterial endocarditis. Evaluation of ventricular function in the pediatric population is identical to that of the adult population and, therefore, will not be repeated within this chapter.

SEGMENTAL ANATOMY

When evaluating congenital heart disease, the echocardiographer begins by determining whether the heart is located in the left chest (levocardia), right chest (dextrocardia), or directly posterior to the sternum (mesocardia). The direction in which the apex is pointing is also noted. The echocardiographer should demonstrate segmental anatomy by delineating situs, ventricular looping, and great vessel relationship. This may be done by documenting anatomic landmarks for each chamber and vessel, as follows:

1. Situs[2,49]
   A. Types
      (1) Solitus—normal
         • Descending aorta and left atrium to the left
         • Inferior vena cava to the right
      (2) Inversus—mirror image visceral placement
         • Very rare
      (3) Left atrial isomerism—double left sidedness

- Both atria have left atrial morphology
- 70% have interrupted inferior vena cava with dilated azygos vein located posterior to the aorta on the same side of the spine or direct hepatic vein drainage into atria bilaterally (2-D transverse subcostal views; confirm venous versus arterial structures by Doppler from sagittal views)
- Usually have polysplenia
- Frequently have complex cardiac anomalies

(4) Right atrial isomerism—double right sidedness
- Inferior vena cava located anterior to the aorta on the same side of the spine
- Usually have asplenia
- Frequently have other cardiac lesions

B. Determined by
(1) Positions of descending aorta and inferior venae cavae in the abdomen
(2) Positions of the atria as proven by anatomic landmarks
  a. Right atrium
  - Entrance of superior and inferior venae cavae (contrast echo)[69]
  - Presence of eustachian valve
  - Right atrial appendage (broad connection to atrium)
    —parasternal or subcostal sagittal views
  b. Left atrium
  - Entrance of pulmonary veins (posterior subcostal coronal plane)
  - Left atrial appendage (tubular, with narrow connection)
    —parasternal long or short axis, subcostal, apical four-chamber views

2. Ventricular connection (looping)[12,64,66]
A. Types
(1) Dextro—right ventricle to the right
(2) Levo—right ventricle to the left
B. Determined by positions of the ventricles as proven by anatomical landmarks
(1) Right ventricle
  - Trabeculated endocardial surface
  - Tricuspid valve (three leaflets)
    —annulus inserts more apically than the mitral valve
    —chordal insertion into ventricular septum or free wall
  - Moderator band
(2) Left ventricle
  - Smooth endocardial surface
  - Mitral valve (two leaflets)
  - Two prominent papillary muscles

3. Great vessel relationship[2]
A. Types
(1) Dextro—aortic valve to the right of the pulmonic valve

(2) Levo—aortic valve to the left of the pulmonic valve
B. Determined by positions of the great arteries as proven by anatomical landmarks
(1) Pulmonary artery
  - Bifurcates soon after exiting the heart
  - Posterior course from base of the heart
(2) Aorta
  - Superior course from base of the heart, to form aortic arch
  - Coronary arteries

NORMAL HEMODYNAMICS[1]

chamber/ vessel	mean	diastolic	systolic
Right atrium		<9 mm Hg	<9 mm Hg
Right ventricle		<7 mm Hg	<30 mm Hg
Pulmonary artery	<20 mm Hg		<30 mm Hg
Left atrium	<12 mm Hg		<17 mm Hg
Left ventricle		<12 mm Hg	<140 mm Hg (within 5 mm Hg of arm pressure)
Aorta	determined by blood pressure cuff on arm		

IMPORTANT DOPPLER CALCULATIONS

1. Conversion of frequency shift into velocity by use of the Doppler equation[18]
2. Estimation of pressure gradient by application of the modified Bernoulli equation[18]
3. Determination of flow volume[43]
4. Determination of pulmonary to systemic flow ratio, referred to as Q_p: Q_s[10,58,59]
5. Estimation of valve area by use of the continuity equation[51]

ESTIMATION OF PULMONARY ARTERY PRESSURE

The development and progression of elevated pulmonary artery pressure is of concern in any patient with congenital heart disease. Pulmonary artery pressures rise in response to increased flow volume and/or pressure as pulmonary vascular resistance becomes elevated. Increased flow volume and/or high pressure cause the intimal and medial layers of the pulmonary arterioles to hypertrophy, thereby increasing pulmonary vascular resistance. With prolonged exposure to high-flow volume and/or pressure, the patient develops pulmonary hypertension and eventually pulmonary vascular obstructive disease, which is irreversible. When pulmonary artery pressures exceed systemic pressures, blood flow through intra- and extra-cardiac shunts reverses, such that they become pulmonary to systemic or right to left shunts. Mixing of deoxygenated blood with oxygenated blood leads to cyanosis. The right ventricle eventually fails owing to the increased resistance against which it must work to eject blood. Pulmonary vascular disease that results from prolonged increased volume and pressure to the pulmonary vascular bed from a systemic to pulmonary (left to right) shunt is referred to as Eisenmenger's syndrome.[15]

Echocardiographic Signs of Elevated Pulmonary Artery Pressure (Pulmonary Hypertension)

- Dilated right ventricle with thickened right ventricular free wall
- Disappearance of the "a" wave on the pulmonic valve M-mode[22,27]
- Midsystolic closure of the pulmonic valve on M-mode, also known as the "flying W"[72]
- Tricuspid and/or pulmonic regurgitation in the absence of structural abnormalities of the valves[60]

Estimation of Systolic Pulmonary Artery Pressure

- Peak tricuspid regurgitation gradient plus 7 mm Hg (assumed central venous pressure)[60,73]
- Enhancement of tricuspid regurgitation Doppler tracing by use of echocardiographic contrast[5]

Estimation of Diastolic Pulmonary Artery Pressure

- End-diastolic pulmonary regurgitation gradient plus 7 mm Hg (assumed central venous pressure)[28]

Estimation of Mean Pulmonary Artery Pressure

- Acceleration time (AcT) divided by ejection time (ET) of flow through the right ventricular outflow tract as recorded by PW Doppler[21]

SIMPLE SHUNT LESIONS

Persistent Patent Ductus Arteriosus (PDA)

Anatomy. The ductus arteriosus is a vessel connecting the left pulmonary artery to the descending aorta (immediately distal to the level of the left subclavian artery) that allows blood to bypass the pulmonary circulation during fetal life. Shortly after birth, this vessel should close so blood may enter the pulmonary circulation to be oxygenated. When the vessel remains patent, it is referred to as a persistent patent ductus arteriosus.

Hemodynamics. During fetal life, pulmonary vascular resistance is higher than systemic vascular resistance; therefore, pulmonary pressure is higher than systemic

pressure, so blood flows from the pulmonary artery to the descending aorta. After birth, pulmonary vascular resistance decreases and becomes much lower than systemic vascular resistance. The reversal in pressure differences between the pulmonary and systemic circulations causes a reversal of flow through a persistently patent ductus arteriosus, such that blood from the descending aorta enters the pulmonary circulation. The resulting increase in pulmonary flow continues into the left atrium as a volume overload causing the left atrium and ventricle to dilate. The magnitude of the systemic to pulmonary shunt is determined by the difference between the pulmonary and systemic vascular resistances, the difference in pulmonary artery and descending aortic pressures, and by the luminal diameter of the ductus arteriosus.[1]

Clinical Presentation.[1,11] Patients are usually asymptomatic; in cardiac failure if shunt is large.

- Physical exam: bounding pulses
- Auscultation: systolic murmur in infants, continuous murmer at older age
- ECG (electrocardiogram): variable
- Chest x-ray: enlarged pulmonary artery and aorta, increased vascular markings, ductus "bump" off the descending aorta

Key Echocardiographic Concepts

- 2-D visualization of the ductus entering the pulmonary artery (parasternal short axis or high parasternal view)[42,48]
- 2-D visualization of the ductus entering the descending aorta (suprasternal notch or high parasternal view)[55,56]
- Continuous flow in the pulmonary artery by PW or color flow Doppler[23,39]
- Diastolic flow reversal in the descending aorta distal to the left subclavian artery by PW or color flow Doppler[51,57]
- Demonstration of shunt by contrast echocardiography[3,42]
- Left atrial to aortic root ratio (LA/Ao ratio) greater than 1.2 in the absence of left ventricular failure[3]
- Estimation of pulmonary artery pressure by determining the pressure gradient through the duct by CW Doppler and subtracting this value from the systolic blood pressure[51]

Populations at Increased Risk[1]

- Preterm infant
- Infant born at altitudes greater than 4500 m above sea level
- Rubella syndrome
- Family history
- Complex congenital heart disease[15]

Natural History.[1] A large shunt may cause congestive heart failure, failure to thrive, and recurrent respiratory infections. Pulmonary vascular obstructive disease will develop if left untreated.

Treatment[1]

- Indomethicin: to close ductus medically
- Prostaglandin E_1: to keep ductus patent in the presence of a "duct-dependent" lesion, in which the ductus is necessary to provide pulmonary circulation
- Umbrella closure (interventional catheterization)[36]
- Foam plastic plug closure (interventional catheterization)
- Surgical ligation

Postoperative Echocardiographic Evaluation. Left atrial and ventricular size should regress to normal. Color flow or PW Doppler should be used to check for residual shunting.

Other Systemic to Pulmonary Shunts

Echocardiographic Concepts

- PW Doppler documentation of diastolic descending aortic flow reversal to evaluate patency of the shunt
- Localization of shunt by PW Doppler (determine the level at which the diastolic reversal begins)
- Visualization of shunt on 2-D and color flow Doppler

Types

A. Aorticopulmonary Window: a defect in the walls of the ascending aorta and main pulmonary artery resulting in blood shunting between these structures; Doppler findings similar to persistant patent ductus arteriosus except reversal of flow may be detected in the ascending as well as descending aorta.[51]

B. Surgically Created Systemic to Pulmonary Shunts[1,34]

1. Blalock-Taussig: subclavian artery to pulmonary artery on side opposite the aortic arch; modified versions may be placed on either side; current shunt of choice
2. Central: anastamosis or conduit between the pulmonary artery and aorta
3. Glenn: superior vena cava to right main pulmonary artery; persistent left superior vena cava with innominate vein communication results in a steal phenomenon; occlusion may lead to various complications, including superior vena cava syndrome
4. Potts: descending aorta to pulmonary artery; difficult to control size; older technique
5. Waterston: ascending aorta to right pulmonary artery; difficult to control size; older technique

Atrial Septal Defects (ASDs)

Anatomy. Incomplete septation of the atrial septum results in a "hole" or communication through which blood may flow directly from one atrium into the other. Types of atrial septal defects, as determined by physical location, are listed below.[44,48]

- Secundum: area of the foramen ovale; most common
- Primum: posterior, near the atrioventricular valves; associated with cleft mitral valve and mitral regurgitation
- Sinus venosus: posterior and superior, near the entrance of the superior vena cava; associated with anomalous right pulmonary venous return into the right atrium
- Coronary sinus: area of the entrance of the coronary sinus; rare; associated with persistant left superior vena cava, absent coronary sinus, and complex congenital heart disease[47]

Hemodynamics. Blood is "shunted" from the higher pressure left atrium to the lower pressure right atrium causing a volume overload and, therefore, dilatation of the right atrium, right ventricle, and pulmonary arteries. Doppler interrogation reveals blood flow through the interatrial septum and increased flow velocities through the tricuspid and pulmonic valves.

Clinical Presentation.[1,11] Patients are usually asymptomatic.

- Physical exam: systolic impulse may be felt at the lower left sternal border
- Auscultation: fixed splitting of the second heart sound, systolic crescendo-decrescendo (ejection) murmur that is heard best at the upper left sternal border
- ECG: right ventricular hypertrophy
- Chest x-ray: enlarged heart and increased pulmonary vascular markings

Key Echocardiographic Concepts

- Visualization of defect on 2-D and with color flow Doppler (subcostal long and short, parasternal short axis, and apical four-chamber views)[39,48]
- PW Doppler tracing characteristic of left to right shunt through an atrial septal defect[24]
- Degree of right atrial and ventricular dilatation to estimate severity
- PW Doppler technique to calculate Q_p:Q_s (ie, magnitude of the shunt)
- Use of echocardiographic contrast to confirm the presence of a shunt[13,68]

Associated Disease[3,11]

- Mitral valve prolapse
- Left ventricular inflow obstruction (Lutenbacher's syndrome)
- Subaortic stenosis
- Atrial septal aneurysm

Natural History[1,11]

- May close spontaneously
- Pulmonary vascular obstructive disease may develop, usually in adulthood

Treatment

- Elective surgical suture closure
- Elective surgical patch closure with pericardial or Teflon patch

Postoperative Echocardiographic Evaluation

- Right atrial and ventricular size should regress to normal
- Color flow, PW Doppler, or contrast echo[69] should be used to check for residual shunting around the patch

Ventricular Septal Defects (VSDs)

Anatomy. A communication exits between the ventricles as a result of incomplete septation. Type is determined by location, as listed below.[45,48]

- Perimembranous: including the membranous septum and frequently portions of the muscular septum directly under the aortic valve
- Malalignment: the aorta or pulmonary artery overrides the interventricular septum
- Inflow (atrioventricular canal, endocardial cushion): posterior, at the level of the atrioventricular valves
- Doubly committed subarterial (subpulmonic, supracristal): immediately proximal to the pulmonic valve, in the right ventricular outflow tract
- Muscular: in the body of the ventricular septum
- Apical: in the apical septum
- Left ventricular to right atrial shunt: rare; mimics tricuspid regurgitation[17]

Hemodynamics. Blood from the higher-pressure left ventricle courses through the communication into the lower pressure right ventricle. The greatest volume of blood is shunted during systole when the pressure difference between the ventricles is most pronounced. Because the pulmonic valve is open during systole, the high-velocity jet from the left ventricle proceeds through the right ventricle directly into the pulmonary artery. The pulmonary vasculature, therefore, is affected more by the increased volume and pressure than the right ventricle. The increased blood volume proceeds into the left atrium and ventricle causing dilatation of these chambers.

Clinical Presentation.[11] Patients usually are asymptomatic; may present in cardiac failure if shunt is large

- Physical exam: palpable thrill over the chest
- Auscultation: harsh holosystolic murmur; variably split second heart sound

- ECG: dilated pulmonary artery, pulmonary vessels, left atrium, left ventricle
- Chest x-ray: left ventricular hypertrophy with or without right ventricular hypertrophy

Key Echocardiographic Concepts

- Visualization of defect on 2-D or of the shunt (jet) by color flow Doppler[38,39,48]
- Systolic flow into the right ventricle through the interventricular septum by PW or CW Doppler[58,61]
- Evidence of shunt by contrast echocardiography[45]
- Estimation of right ventricular pressure by determining the pressure gradient through the VSD by CW Doppler and subtracting this value from the systolic blood pressure[32]
- Restrictive versus nonrestrictive VSD[15]
- Estimation of the magnitude of the shunt by calculation of the Q_p:Q_s by Doppler technique

Associated Disease

- Multiple ventricular septal defects may occur
- Aortic insufficiency (particularly with doubly committed subarterial and perimembranous types)[46,48]
- Membranous subaortic stenosis[9]

Natural History[1,15]

- Small defects may close spontaneously
- Risk of developing endocarditis
- Aneurysms of tricuspid valve tissue may partially or completely occlude perimembranous VSDs[45]
- Doubly committed subarterial VSDs may develop aortic valve herniation (prolapse) and subsequent aortic insufficiency of increasing severity[46]
- Development of pulmonary vascular obstructive disease if a significant defect remains open
- Increased risk of progression of pulmonary vascular obstructive disease if closure is delayed beyond 2 years of life

Treatment

- Elective surgical stitch or patch closure
- Repair of aortic valve herniation

Postoperative Echocardiographic Evaluation

- Left atrial and ventricular size should regress to normal[3]
- Assess for peripatch residual shunts by PW Doppler, color flow, or contrast echo[15,23,69]
- Assess for patch dehiscence[3]

Atrioventricular Septal Defects (AVSDs)

Anatomy. A spectrum of malformations that occur at the crux of the heart where the atrioventricular valves, interatrial septum, and interventricular septum intersect. These malformations may also be referred to as endocardial cushion defects or atrioventricular canals. Any combination of the following malformations may exist. When there is atrial, ventricular, and atrioventricular valve involvement, the patient is said to have a complete atrioventricular septal defect[52]:

- Ostium primum atrial septal defect
- Inlet ventricular septal defect
- Atrioventricular valve malformation: including cleft mitral valve, single atrioventricular valve, overriding atrioventricular valve, straddling atrioventricular valve
- Common atrium: interatrial septum is completely absent (associated with atrial isomerism)

Hemodynamics. The defects are generally large; therefore, equalization of pressures may occur between chambers resulting in bidirectional shunting through septal defects. The right heart is dilated due to volume and/or pressure increase. Atrioventricular valve regurgitation may cause atrial dilatation.

Clinical Presentation.[1,11] Patients are usually symptomatic during infancy.

- Physical exam: failure to thrive, fatigue, dyspnea, heart failure, recurrent respiratory infections
- Auscultation: variety of murmurs
- ECG: left axis deviation, biventricular hypertrophy
- Chest x-ray: gross cardiomegaly with increased vascular markings

Key Echocardiographic Concepts

- 2-D evaluation of size and positions of ventricular and atrial septal defects
- Relative right ventricular and left ventricular size by 2-D[52]
- Atrioventricular valve competency by PW or color flow Doppler[58]
- Structure of the atrioventricular valves, particularly chordal attachments[45]
- Assessment of pulmonary artery pressure by Doppler methods

Associated Disease[1,3,52]

- Left heart and aortic obstructive lesions
- Muscular ventricular septal defects
- Atrial isomerisms

Natural History

- Pulmonary vascular obstructive disease develops at an early age[11]

Treatment.[1] Surgery is usually done during the first year of life

- Elective surgical repair of atrioventricular valves and patch closure of septal defects
- Pulmonary artery band: surgical palliation in

which supravalvular pulmonary stenosis is created to limit blood flow to the pulmonary vascular bed to retard progression of pulmonary vascular disease

Postoperative Echocardiographic Evaluation

- After definitive repair, evaluate ventricular function, check for residual shunts and assess competency of atrioventricular valves.
- After pulmonary artery banding, determine the anatomic position of the band and the pressure gradient across it by CW Doppler.

OBSTRUCTIVE LESIONS

Left Ventricular Outflow Obstructions

Anatomy. Various types of obstruction are listed below[1,3,15,48].

- Bicuspid aortic valve: one of the commissures remains fused; the most common type of congenital heart disease; frequently hemodynamically insignificant until adulthood
- Unicuspid aortic valve: in place of a valve, there is a membrane with an orifice
- Discrete subaortic stenosis: membrane or ridge in the left ventricular outflow tract; may also affect the anterior leaflet of the mitral valve
- Dynamic subaortic stenosis (idiopathic hypertrophic subaortic stenosis, hypertrophic obstructive cardiomyopathy): thickened interventricular septum; genetically transmitted
- Tunnel aortic stenosis: diffuse narrowing of the left ventricular outflow tract; rare
- Supravalvular aortic stenosis: localized or diffuse narrowing of the ascending aorta, generally just distal to the sinuses of Valsalva; usually associated with the William syndrome

Hemodynamics. Obstruction increases resistance to flow out of the left ventricle. The left ventricle must therefore generate higher systolic pressures to force the blood past the obstruction. This pressure overload results in thickening of the left ventricular walls.

Clinical Presentation.[1,11] Patients are usually asymptomatic unless obstruction is severe.

- Physical exam: anacrotic notch and prolonged upstroke in peripheral arterial pulse; left ventricular lift and precordial systolic thrill may be palpable
- Auscultation: ejection click and systolic ejection murmur, narrowed splitting of the second heart sound; reversed splitting of the second heart sound if obstruction is severe
- ECG: left ventricular hypertrophy
- Chest x-ray: enlarged left ventricle, dilated ascending aorta

Key Echocardiographic Concepts

General Concepts

- High-velocity, turbulent jet distal to obstruction by PW or color flow Doppler[18,23]
- Increased thickness of left ventricular walls[3]
- Prolonged time to peak velocity (acceleration time to left ventricular ejection time ratio greater than 0.30 suggests pressure greater than 50 mm Hg, greater than 0.55 requires surgery)[18]
- Estimation of pressure gradient through the obstruction by CW Doppler-peak systolic pressure gradient greater than 75 mm Hg with a normal cardiac output is critical aortic stenosis and a surgical emergency[1,18,48]
- Estimation of valve area by continuity equation—area less than 0.5 cm²/m² of body surface area is critical aortic stenosis and a surgical emergency[1]
- Calculation of left ventricular wall stress[3]
- Estimation of left ventricular pressure as posterior left ventricular wall thickness at end systole divided by end-systolic diameter multiplied by 225[6]

Bicuspid Aortic Valve

- Delineation of configuration of cusps by 2-D
- Doming of cusps on 2-D
- Aortic eccentricity index greater than 1.5 determined by M-mode[3]

Discrete Subaortic Stenosis[3,48]

- 2-D visualization of the membrane from the parasternal long axis or apical five-chamber view
- Premature closure or midsystolic notch on the aortic valve M-mode or PW Doppler tracing
- Coarse systolic fluttering of the aortic cusps on M-mode
- Increased velocity of flow proximal to the aortic valve by PW and color flow Doppler

Dynamic Subaortic Stenosis[37]

- 2-D demonstration of distribution of myocardial thickening
- Late systolic peak on CW Doppler tracing

Tunnel Aortic Stenosis

- 2-D visualization of diffusely narrow left ventricular outflow tract, hypoplastic aortic valve with thick cusps, and hypoplastic ascending aorta[48]

Associated Disease[1]

- Bicuspid aortic valve: aortic insufficiency, coarctation of the aorta
- Unicuspid aortic valve: aortic insufficiency
- Discrete subaortic stenosis: aortic insufficiency

Natural History[1]

- Obstruction usually progresses
- Development of aortic regurgitation

Treatment.[1,15] Patients are generally prophylaxed and restricted from participating in competitive sports

- Valvular aortic stenosis: intervention when peak systolic pressure gradient exceeds 75 mm Hg or orifice size decreases to 0.5 cm²/m² of body surface area
  - —Percutaneous balloon valvuloplasty[30]
  - —Commissurotomy
  - —Aortic valve replacement
- Discrete subaortic stenosis: surgical resection of the membrane
- Supravalvular aortic stenosis: surgical resection of obstruction when pressure gradient exceeds 50 mm Hg
- Tunnel aortic stenosis: left ventricular to descending aorta valved conduit,[65] Konno procedure (widening of aortic root and left ventricular outflow tract)

Postoperative Echocardiographic Evaluation. Evaluate for residual or restenosis and aortic insufficiency.

Shone Syndrome

A constellation of left-sided obstructive lesions occur together: supravalvular mitral ring, parachute mitral valve, discrete membranous subaortic stenosis, and coarctation of the aorta.[48]

Coarctation of the Aorta

Anatomy. A discrete or diffuse narrowing of the aorta, most commonly located immediately distal to the left subclavian artery in the area of the ductus arteriosus. Infrequently, the coarctation will occur proximal to the ductus arteriosus or a portion of the aortic arch may be hypoplastic. In either of these cases, patency of the ductus arteriosus may be necessary to perfuse the descending aorta and maintain life.[1]

Hemodynamics. Obstruction to flow at the level of the coarctation results in a build-up of pressure proximal to the obstruction and decreased flow distal to it.[15] Left ventricular walls thicken in response to increased resistance. A high-velocity jet through the obstruction may weaken the aortic wall immediately distal to the obstruction causing poststenotic dilatation.

Clinical Presentation.[1,11] Patients are usually asymptomatic; if severe during infancy, will present in heart failure.

- Physical exam: systemic hypertension, with systolic blood pressure much higher in the upper extremities than in the lower extremities[15]; weak femoral pulses; upper body may be more well developed than the lower body

- Auscultation: systolic murmur along the left sternal border transmitting to back and neck; bruits from collateral vessels in older children
- ECG: right ventricular hypertrophy in symptomatic infants; left ventricular hypertrophy in older children
- Chest x-ray: inverted "3" sign at level of coarctation; prominant descending aorta; rib notching in children older than 8 years

Key Echocardiographic Concepts

- 2-D visualization of obstruction within the aortic lumen[19,35]
- Determination of gradient by CW Doppler tracing through the coarctation[16]
  —Velocity of flow proximal to the obstruction should be taken into consideration[58]
- Decreased pulsatility on the PW Doppler tracing of the descending aorta (blunted acceleration and slow deceleration of flow that does not return to baseline during diastole)[58]

Associated Disease[1,35]

- Bicuspid aortic valve (found in as many as 50% of patients with coarctation of the aorta)
- Additional levels of left heart obstruction
- Ventricular septal defects
- Transposition of the great arteries
- Double-outlet right ventricle

Natural History. If unrelieved, as many as 80% of patients die before reaching the age of 50 years[1]

Treatment.[1,15] Early repair appears to decrease probability of residual systemic hypertension

- Surgical resection of constricted area and primary anastamosis or graft placement
- Subclavian flap procedure: use of proximal portion of left subclavian artery to widen aortic lumen

Postoperative Echocardiographic Evaluation

- Assessment of the lumen size and pressure gradient in the area of the reanastamosis
- PW Doppler spectral tracing of the descending aortic flow may continue to appear somewhat blunted

Hypoplastic Left Heart Syndrome

A spectrum of left-sided hypoplasia in which the left atrium, mitral valve, left ventricle, aortic valve, and aorta may be hypoplastic, stenotic, or atretic. Frequently associated with an atrial septal defect through which pulmonary venous return flows into the right atrium and a patent ductus arteriosus, which in turn supplies the descending aorta.[48]

Treatment[4]

- Cardiac transplantation
- Norwood procedure

Pulmonary Stenosis

Anatomy. Obstruction may occur at various levels along the right ventricular outflow tract and the pulmonary arterial system. Types are listed below.[1,11]

- Valvular stenosis: fusion or dysplasia of cusps
- Infundibular stenosis: hypertrophy of muscle bands in the right ventricular outflow tract; usually associated with a ventricular septal defect or valvular pulmonary stenosis[48]
- Double chamber right ventricle: hypertrophied anomalous muscle bundles in the right ventricle, effectively dividing the right ventricle into two chambers with a communication between them; associated with valvular pulmonary stenosis, perimembranous ventricular septal defects, and subaortic stenosis[9,45]
- Peripheral pulmonary stenosis: may occur as a distinct shelf in the pulmonary artery, discrete narrowing of the pulmonary artery branches, or as diffuse tapered narrowing of the pulmonary artery branches[7]

Hemodynamics. Increased resistance to right ventricular outflow results in a pressure overload to this chamber. The right ventricular walls thicken and the chamber dilates. Blood flow into the pulmonary arterial system is at high velocity and turbulent. Eddy currents produced distal to the obstruction may cause poststenotic dilatation of the pulmonary artery.[48]

Clinical Presentation.[1] Patients are usually asymptomatic.

- Auscultation: systolic ejection murmur
- ECG: right ventricular hypertrophy
- Chest x-ray: prominant pulmonary artery trunk; large right atrium

Key Echocardiographic Concepts

- Thickened right ventricular free wall
- 2-D visualization and measurement of pulmonary valve annulus in candidate for balloon angioplasty of valvular stenosis[54]
- 2-D visualization of anomalous muscle bundle and orifice from parasternal and subcostal views[54]
- Accentuation of the "a wave" on M-mode[1]
- Doppler estimation of pressure gradient from all available positions[14]

Natural History[1]

- Increased risk of endocarditis
- Mild valvular and peripheral stenosis (right ventricular pressure less than 50 mm Hg and a pres-

sure gradient of less than 40 mm Hg) is considered benign and may or may not progress
- Severe stenosis (right ventricular pressure greater than 100 mm Hg and a pressure gradient greater than 80 mm Hg) requires relief
- Infundibular stenosis and anomalous muscle bundles tend to become progressively more obstructive

Treatment. When patient becomes symptomatic or pressure gradient exceeds 50 mm Hg[15]

- Balloon valvuloplasty: to relieve valvular and peripheral stenosis[30]
- Surgical valvotomy[1]
- Surgical resection of infundibular muscle or anomalous muscle bundles

Postoperative Echocardiographic Evaluation

- Assess patency of area of former obstruction
- Assess presence and severity of pulmonary insufficiency

Pulmonary Atresia

Anatomy. Imperforate membrane or thick fibrous band in place of a pulmonary valve or complete absence of the main pulmonary artery.[7]

Hemodynamics. Life is dependent upon a persistent patent ductus arteriosus or collateral vessels. A ventricular septal defect usually coexists and acts as an outlet to systemic venous return.[15]

Clinical Presentation.[1] Severe cyanosis and hypoxemia are seen in the neonate.

- Auscultation: possibly the murmur of a persistent ductus arteriosus
- ECG: right ventricular hypertrophy; right axis deviation
- Chest x-ray: boot-shaped heart; reticular or decreased pulmonary vascular markings

Key Echocardiographic Concepts[1,54]

- 2-D delineation of anatomy
  —right ventricular outflow tract, location and size of main pulmonary artery and branches (subcostal coronal and parasternal short axis)
  —associated malformations
- Contrast echocardiography to delineate anatomy
- Doppler and color flow delineation of flow patterns

Associated Disease[54]

- Persistent ductus arteriosus
- Atrial septal defect or patent foramen ovale
- Malformations of the tricuspid valve
- Coronary arterial sinusoids

Natural History

- Death when the persistent ductus arteriosus closes or systemic to pulmonary collateral flow becomes insufficient to sustain minimal blood oxygenation requirements[1]

Treatment[1,15]

- Prostaglandin E_2: to keep the ductus arteriosus patent
- Palliation with a surgically created systemic to pulmonary shunt
- Surgical reconstruction and/or placement of a prosthetic valve

Postoperative Echocardiographic Evaluation

- Evaluative patency of systemic to pulmonary shunt
- Evaluate patency of reconstructed area

Left Ventricular Inflow Obstruction

Anatomy. Left ventricular inflow is obstructed by a membrane in the left atrium or a decrease in the mitral orifice size. Various forms exist, as listed below.[45,48]

- Valvular mitral stenosis: rare; dysplastic valve leaflets, chordae and papillary muscles
- Parachute mitral valve: all chordae insert onto a single papillary muscle
- Arcade mitral valve: chordae insert onto multiple papillary muscles; may be regurgitant
- Double orifice mitral valve: rare; tissue bridge divides mitral valve into two halves with chordae from each half inserting onto a particular papillary muscle; may be regurgitant; associated with atrioventricular malformation[25]
- Cortriatriatum: rare; left atrial membrane immediately superior to the fossa ovalis and left atrial appendage
- Supravalvular ring: more common than cortriatriatum; left atrial membrane immediately superior to the mitral valve annulus; usually associated with other mitral valve anomalies[44,63]
- Mitral valve hypoplasia: small mitral valve annulus and leaflets
- Mitral atresia: imperforate mitral valve may be associated with a large ventricular septal defect, straddling tricuspid valve, or double-outlet right ventricle

Hemodynamics. Obstruction to left ventricular inflow results in a build-up of pressure in the left atrium causing it to dilate. Pulmonary veins become congested because they cannot empty easily into the left atrium.

Clinical Presentation[1]

- Physical exam: history of recurrent respiratory infections

- Auscultation: diastolic murmur heard best at the apex
- ECG: left atrial enlargement
- Chest x-ray: left atrial enlargement; increased pulmonary vascular markings; right heart enlargement

Key Echocardiographic Concepts

- Delineation of anatomy by 2-D
- Doppler estimation of pressure gradient
- Estimation of orifice size by application of the continuity equation

Associated Disease[1]

- Other levels of left heart obstruction
- Secundum and primum atrial septal defects
- Transposition of the great arteries
- Double-outlet right ventricle

Natural History. Eventually develop pulmonary vascular obstructive disease[1]

Treatment[1]

- Valvular: commissurotomy or valve replacement
- Cortriatriatum and supramitral ring: surgical excision of membrane[54]

Postoperative Echocardiographic Evaluation

- Evaluate residual stenosis and regurgitation

Tricuspid Atresia

Anatomy. A dense band of tissue replaces the tricuspid valve preventing direct communication between the right atrium and ventricle. A large atrial septal defect or patent foramen ovale must coexist to provide an outlet to the right atrium (obligatory shunt).[45] The right ventricle is usually small.[15]

Hemodynamics. Deoxygenated systemic venous blood returns to the right atrium and is shunted into the left atrium where it mixes with oxygenated pulmonary venous return. This mixing of deoxygenated blood with the pulmonary venous return results in desaturation of the oxygenated blood and, therefore, cyanosis. The right atrium and left heart are generally dilated owing to increased flow volume. Because the right ventricle receives blood only indirectly through a ventricular septal defect, it is generally small.[11]

Clinical Presentation.[1,11] Patients are cyanotic with a history of hypoxic spells.

- Physical exam: clubbing of the fingers; delayed growth; hyperactive cardiac impulse at the apex
- Auscultation: single first heart sound; no murmur
- ECG: left ventricular hypertrophy; left axis deviation
- Chest x-ray: decreased vascular markings

Key Echocardiographic Concepts

- 2-D visualization of dense fibrous band across tricuspid annulus and absence of tricuspid valve leaflets
- Dilated right atrium[45]
- Atrial septal defect or single atrium
- Small right ventricle or right ventricular outflow tract

Associated Disease[1,11]

- Atrial septal defect or patent foramen ovale
- Ventricular septal defect and pulmonary stenosis
- Pulmonary atresia
- Transposition of the great vessels

Natural History

- Early death without intervention[1]

Treatment[1]

- Pulmonary artery band (surgical palliation to restrict flow to the pulmonary bed)
- Systemic to pulmonary shunt (surgical palliation to increase flow to the pulmonary bed)
- Balloon atrial septostomy (interventional catheterization to increase interatrial shunting)
- Park blade septostomy (interventional catheterization to increase interatrial shunting)
- Fontan procedure: definitive physiologic correction; the right atrium is connected to the pulmonary artery by placement of a patch or conduit in the hope of increasing pulmonary flow[34]

Postoperative Echocardiographic Evaluation

- Assess for right atrial contractility and adequacy of flow through the pulmonary artery

Tricuspid Hypoplasia/Stenosis

Anatomy. Small tricuspid valve annulus, usually associated with critical pulmonary stenosis, pulmonary atresia with intact interventricular septum, or Ebstein anomaly.[45]

Imperforate Tricuspid Valve

Anatomy. Membrane exists in place of a tricuspid valve, which may be surgically opened.[45]

MALFORMATION OF THE TRICUSPID VALVE

Ebstein Anomaly of the Tricuspid Valve

Anatomy. The septal leaflet is tethered to the interventricular septum and attaches at least 8 mm distal to the tricuspid valve annulus.[3] Other tricuspid leaflets may also adhere to the ventricular wall and be dysplastic.[75]

This malformation results in a large "functional" right atrium and small "functional" right ventricle. The dysplastic nature of the leaflets and chordae prevents effective coaptation resulting in varying degrees of tricuspid insufficiency and stenosis.[45] Contractility of the right ventricle is affected by its size.

Hemodynamics. The right atrium is dilated owing to the volume overload that results from the tricuspid regurgitation. The size of the right ventricle varies with the severity of tricuspid valve leaflet displacement.

Clinical Presentation.[1,11,75] Cyanosis, dyspnea on exertion, and profound weakness or fatigue may be present.

- Physical exam: prominant left chest
- Auscultation: systolic and diastolic murmurs; loud, widely split first heart sound—"sail sound"; triple or quadruple rhythm
- ECG: right atrial hypertrophy; right bundle branch block; Wolff-Parkinson-White syndrome; paroxysmal supraventricular tachycardia
- Chest x-ray: enlarged heart: decreased pulmonary vascular markings; right atrial enlargement

Key Echocardiographic Concepts

- 2-D delineation of the anatomy of the tricuspid valve and degree of displacement and tethering of each leaflet from parasternal short axis, apical four-chamber and subcostal long- and short-axis views[50]
- Determination of the size of the functional right ventricle—if less than 35% of the size of the anatomic right ventricle, prognosis is poor[3]
- Severity of tricuspid regurgitation
- Tricuspid valve closure delayed greater than 90 m/s after mitral valve closure on M-mode[3]

Associated Disease[1,50,75]

- Persistent patent ductus arteriosus
- Atrial septal defect or patent foramen ovale with right to left shunting
- MVP
- Pulmonary stenosis
- Pulmonary atresia with intact ventricular septum
- Congenitally corrected transposition of the great vessels
- Ventricular septal defect

Natural History[1,50,75]

- Increased risk of endocarditis
- Prognosis is better with a larger functional right ventricle
- Prognosis is good if the child survives infancy but generally poor if there are associated lesions

Treatment[1,50,75]

- Annuloplasty: repair of the valve annulus to make it smaller
- Valve replacement
- Valve repair
- Plication of some of the atrialized portion of the right ventricle

Postoperative Echocardiographic Evaluation

- Assess right ventricular function and residual tricuspid insufficiency and/or stenosis

COMPLEX CONGENITAL HEART DISEASE

Tetralogy of Fallot

Anatomy. In this malformation, a large perimembranous ventricular septal defect is associated with a malalignment of the aorta, such that the aortic root overrides the septal defect. The malalignment of the aortic root contributes to the infundibular pulmonary stenosis that occurs as part of this malformation.[54]

Hemodynamics. The large size of the ventricular septal defect allows equalization of left and right ventricular pressures, such that the shunting through the defect is bidirectional. The overriding aorta receives blood from both ventricles, thereby mixing deoxygenated with oxygenated blood.

Clinical Presentation.[1,11] Cyanosis and a history of "tet spells" (transient cerebral ischemia resulting in limpness, paleness, and unconsciousness); history of squatting may present.

- Physical exam: prominant left chest, "clubbing" of fingers; right ventricular heave
- Auscultation: single second heart sound; systolic ejection murmur
- ECG: right ventricular hypertrophy; right axis deviation
- Chest x-ray: boot-shaped heart with decreased vascular markings

Key Echocardiographic Concepts[54]

- 2-D visualization of large perimembranous VSD and assessment of degree of aortic override
- 2-D assessment of degree and levels of right ventricular outflow obstruction
- Size of pulmonary artery and branches from high parasternal short axis and suprasternal notch views (aneurysmally dilated in cases of absent pulmonic valve)[29]
- Thickened RV free wall
- 2-D delineation of coronary artery and aortic arch anatomy to determine surgical approach[8]

Associated Disease[1,3,29,54]

- Valvular pulmonary stenosis or pulmonary atresia
- Congenitally absent pulmonic valve
- Right-sided aortic arch
- Atrial septal defect
- Atrioventricular malformation
- Mitral stenosis
- Coronary artery anomalies
- Persistent left superior vena cava

Natural History.[1]

Severe infundibular stenosis may result in a fatal "tet spell," in which the infundibulum becomes totally occluded. Pulmonary vascular obstructive disease develops.

Treatment[1]

- Palliation by surgical creation of a systemic to pulmonary shunt
- Patch closure of ventricular septal defect and possible myomectomy of the right ventricular outflow tract, or pulmonary valvotomy

Postoperative Echocardiographic Evaluation

- Evaluation of patency of surgically created systemic to pulmonary shunt
- Evaluation of residual right ventricular outflow obstruction and residual shunting around ventricular septal defect

Transposition of the Great Arteries (TGA)

Anatomy.

The aorta arises from the embryologic right ventricle and the pulmonary artery arises from the embryologic left ventricle. Terminology is listed below.

- C-transposition of the great arteries (congenitally corrected, L-transposition): ventricular inversion with the great vessels originating from the incorrect ventricle; blood flow sequence is normal; however, there is a high incidence of associated congenital heart disease
- D-transposition of the great arteries (frequently referred to simply as transposition of the great arteries or complete transposition): the ventricles are concordant with the atria; however the aorta originates from the right ventricle and the pulmonary artery originates from the embryologic left ventricle

Hemodynamics

- C-TGA: Blood flows in the normal sequence—from the systemic veins into the right atrium, through the mitral valve into the left ventricle, and out the pulmonary artery, returns to the left atrium via the pulmonary valves, courses through the tricuspid valve, into the right ventricle and out the aorta.
- D-TGA: Blood flows in two parallel circuits. It flows from the systemic veins into the right atrium, through the tricuspid valve, into the right ventricle and out the aorta, to return again through the systemic veins. Pulmonary venous return flows into the left atrium, through the mitral valve into the left ventricle, and out the pulmonary artery, to return again through the pulmonary veins. In short, deoxygenated blood flows in a continuous loop, and oxygenated blood flows in a separate continuous loop. Unless a communication exists between the systemic and pulmonary circulations (ie, an obligatory shunt), this situation is incompatible with life. In the newborn period, a left to right shunt occurs at the level of the foramen ovale and through a persistent ductus arteriosus, allowing mixing of oxygenated with deoxygenated blood.

Clinical Presentation for D-TGA.[1,11]

Newborns become cyanotic, as the ductus arteriosus closes.

- Physical exam: normal weight, healthy-looking infant
- Auscultation: no murmurs; single second heart sound
- ECG: right ventricular hypertrophy
- Chest x-ray: cardiomegaly; narrow mediastinum; increased vascular markings

Key Echocardiographic Concepts[53]

- Identify situs by delineating anatomic atrial landmarks on 2-D
- Identify ventricular morphology (embryologic origins) by delineating anatomic landmarks on 2-D
- Identify great vessel morphology and relationship (will course in parallel fashion)
- Identity and evaluate magnitude of shunt through the obligatory shunt defect(s)
- Delineate coronary artery anatomy for consideration of surgical approach[8]
- Identify and evaluate associated congenital heart disease

Associated Disease for D-TGA[3,53]

- Patent ductus arteriosus: obligatory shunt; most common associated heart disease
- Aortic arch anomalies: coarctation, hypoplastic segment, interrupted aortic arch
- Atrial septal defect or patent foramen ovale: obligatory shunt
- Ventricular septal defect: obligatory shunt; with or without juxtaposed atrial appendages
- Outflow tract obstruction: fixed or dynamic
- Straddling atrioventricular valve: chordae from one atrioventricular valve attach into both ventricles
- Atrioventricular malformation: rare
- Pulmonary origin of coronary artery

Natural History.

Patients with congenitally corrected transposition may never know they have congenital heart disease unless there is associated congenital heart disease, in which case the natural history is determined by the associated disease.

Patients with D-transposition of the great vessels must be palliated or repaired on an emergent basis because occlusion of the obligatory shunt would result in immediate death. The mortality rate in the absence of intervention is 95% at the end of 2 years of life.[27]

Treatment[1,3,34]

Prostaglandin E₁ Treatment: palliation; to keep ductus arteriosus patent until an atrial shunt or definitive surgical procedure can be performed

Balloon Atrial Septostomy (Rashkind Procedure): palliative interventional catheterization technique in which a distended balloon catheter is torn across a patent foramen ovale or small atrial septal defect creating a large atrial septal defect

Surgical Atrial Septectomy (Blalock-Hanlon Operation): palliation

Mustard Procedure (Atrial Switch): surgical excision of the interatrial septum and placement of a baffle made of pericardium or synthetic material to redirect right atrial flow through the mitral valve into the left ventricle and allow pulmonary venous return to flow around the baffle into the tricuspid valve

Senning Procedure (Atrial Switch): surgical reconstruction of the atrial wall and interatrial septum to create an intra-atrial baffle redirecting venous flow through the atria

Rastelli Procedure (Intraventricular Repair and Extracardiac Conduit): surgical procedure in which a tunnel is constructed through a large ventricular septal defect such that left ventricular outflow is directed to the aortic valve and a valved conduit is placed between the right ventricle and pulmonary artery

Jatene Procedure (Arterial Switch): surgical procedure in which the great arteries are taken off their trunks and moved such that each is reanastomosed to the trunk that will restore a normal blood flow sequence; coronary arteries also are removed and reimplanted into the neoaorta.

Postoperative Echocardiographic Evaluation. Evaluation of left ventricular function

- Balloon atrial septostomy: 2-D visualization of definitive tear in the interatrial septum and calculation of atrial septal defect size to interatrial septal length ratio[27]
- Mustard and Senning procedures: rule out superior vena cava or pulmonary venous obstruction and baffle leaks[1,51] by PW Doppler, color flow Doppler, or contrast echocardiography[69]

- Jatene procedure: evaluate anastomotic sites of great arteries for possible constriction[1]

Truncus Arteriosus

Anatomy.[1,11] A rare malformation in which a single large great artery (common trunk) arises from the heart and receives outflow from both ventricles. In most cases, the common trunk overrides the large ventricular septal defect which must be present. The valve of the common trunk frequently has more than three cusps. Pulmonary circulation occurs in one of the following ways:

- Type I: main pulmonary trunk arises from the common trunk (usually from the posterior aspect) and bifurcates into right and left branches
- Type II: right and left pulmonary arteries arise separately from the left posterolateral aspect of the common trunk
- Type III: right and left pulmonary arteries arise separately from lateral aspects of the common trunk
- Type IV: no pulmonary arteries exist; pulmonary circulation is through bronchiole arteries arising from the descending aorta

Hemodynamics.[1] The large ventricular septal defect causes equalization of pressures between the ventricles. Flow into the pulmonary circulation is at systemic pressures because the pulmonary arteries arise from the aorta and there is no pulmonary valve. There may be decreased flow to the pulmonary circulation if there is stenosis of the pulmonary branches or in type IV.

Clinical Presentation.[1,11] Patients are cyanotic.

- Physical exam: early congestive heart failure or hypoxic spells
- Auscultation: single second heart sound; systolic ejection click and murmur
- ECG: biventricular hypertrophy
- Chest x-ray: cardiomegaly; biventricular enlargement; wide mediastinum

Key Echocardiographic Concepts

- 2-D delineation of anatomy
- Color flow and PW Doppler evaluation of truncal valve (rule out stenosis or insufficiency)
- 2-D and color flow localization of pulmonary arteries (suprasternal notch views may be most helpful)
- Evaluation of size of pulmonary arteries

Associated Disease.[1] Usually, truncus arteriosus is an isolated lesion.

- Right aortic arch
- Truncal valve stenosis and/or insufficiency
- Aortic arch anomalies
- Persistent patent ductus arteriosus
- Coronary ostial anomalies

- Absence of a branch pulmonary artery on the side of the arch
- Atrial septal defect

Natural History.[1] If left untreated, death in infancy from heart failure or later from pulmonary vascular obstructive disease. Without intervention, survival beyond 1 year is unusual.

Treatment[1]

- Removal of the pulmonary arteries from the aorta and placement of a valved conduit between the right ventricle and pulmonary arteries
- Pulmonary artery banding palliation; may make definitive repair difficult or impossible

Postoperative Echocardiographic Evaluation

- Evaluate competency of the conduit valve and evaluate anastomatic areas for stenosis.
- Evaluate placement of pulmonary artery band and gradient across it

ANOMALIES OF THE CORONARY ARTERIES

Kawasaki Syndrome (Mucocutaneous Lymph Node Syndrome)

Anatomy. Acquired coronary artery disease may occur as a sequela to a childhood disease known as Kawasaki disease. Around 15% of patients develop cardiovascular involvement in the form of coronary artery aneurysm formation. The proximal branches appear to be most frequently involved. Distal aneurysms may occur in addition, although rarely without proximal involvement.[31]

Clinical Presentation.[33] Usually seen January to April; patients have fever of over 5 days' duration, lethargy, and irritability.

- Physical exam: bilateral conjunctivitis; dry, fissured lips; strawberry tongue; polymorphous truncal rash; erythema of palms and soles; desquamation of fingertips and toes; cervical lymphadenopathy
- Lab tests: elevated white count, platelet count, erythrocyte sedimentation rate, α_2-globulin, immunoglobulin E, transaminase, and lactic acid dehydrogenase
- ECG: infrequent, minimal changes

Key Echocardiographic Concepts

Acute Phase[8,31]

- Left ventricular dysfunction
- Valvular regurgitation
- Pericardial effusion

Convalescent Phase

- 2-D demonstration of saccular or fusiform coronary

TABLE 4–1. ECHOCARDIOGRAPHIC VIEWS USED TO EVALUATE CORONARY ARTERY ANATOMY

Coronary Artery	Echocardiographic View
Proximal right, left main, proximal left anterior descending, proximal left circumflex	Parasternal short axis High parasternal short axis (caudal angle) Subcostal 4 coronal
Distal right coronary	Subcostal coronal (acute margin of heart) Subcostal short axis (sagittal) Posterior apical 4 chamber (posterior atrioventricular groove)
Posterior descending	Parasternal short axis Subcostal coronal Apical 4 chamber
Left circumflex	Parasternal short Parasternal long Subcostal sagittal
Distal left anterior descending	Parasternal long Parasternal short Subcostal coronal

(Data from references 17 and 66.)

aneurysms (Table 4–1)
- Segmental wall motion abnormalities

Natural History. The majority of aneurysms resolve; however, those with diameters larger than 8 mm are at increased risk for thrombosis, which may result in myocardial infarction.[31]

Treatment. Patients with aneurysms are usually treated with an aspirin per day to decrease the risk of thrombosis. Serial echocardiographic exams are generally performed, with coronary angiography at intervals to determine whether coronary artery bypass surgery is indicated.[1]

Anomalous Origin of the Left Coronary Artery

Anatomy. A rare malformation in which the left coronary artery originates from the main pulmonary artery rather than from the aortic root.[8]

Hemodynamics. The myocardium of the left ventricle is inadequately perfused with oxygen because the blood flowing into the left coronary artery is deoxygenated blood from the pulmonary artery.

Clinical Presentation.[8] Symptomatic in infancy.

- Physical exam: irritable, dyspneic, tachypneic
- Auscultation: mitral insufficiency murmur
- ECG: left ventricular hypertrophy with anterolateral myocardial infarction
- Chest x-ray: enlarged heart

Key Echocardiographic Concepts[8]

- 2-D visualization of left coronary artery originating from the pulmonary artery

- 2-D visualization of a dilated right coronary artery originating from the right sinus of Valsalva
- PW Doppler or color flow demonstration of diastolic flow entering the main pulmonary artery just distal to the pulmonary valve
- Decreased left ventricular contractility
- Mitral insufficiency

Natural History. In the absence of intervention, permanent myocardial damage occurs.

Treatment. Surgery to reimplant the left coronary artery into the aortic root.[8]

Coronary Arteriovenous Fistula

Anatomy. A variably tortuous coronary artery courses along the surface of the heart or within the myocardium to empty into a cardiac chamber or great vessel. Generally, it is the right coronary artery that is involved, and the site of drainage is usually a right heart structure.[8]

Hemodynamics. Rather than perfusing the myocardium, blood from the coronary artery flows into the cardiac chamber or vessel into which it empties.

Clinical Presentation. Generally, patients remain asymptomatic until the fourth decade of life.[26]

- Auscultation: atypical continuous murmur

***Key Echocardiographic Concepts*[71]**

- 2-D demonstration of a dilated coronary artery
  —normal ratios of coronary artery diameter to aortic root diameter
    —left coronary artery = 0.17 ± 0.03
    —right coronary artery = 0.14 ± 0.03
- 2-D demonstration of origin, course, and site of drainage of the fistula
- Color flow Doppler visualization and PW Dopple confirmation of a continuous, turbulent jet entering a cardiac chamber or great vessel in a location in which shunt lesions do not enter
- PW Doppler demonstration of turbulent late systolic, early diastolic flow in a dilated coronary artery supplying the fistula

***Natural History*[71]**

- Spontaneous closure may occur
- Bacterial endocarditis
- Congestive heart failure due to volume overload and myocardial ischemia

Treatment. Elective surgical ligation of the fistula.[71]

Postoperative Echocardiographic Evaluation. Check for residual flow through the fistula.

VENOUS MALFORMATIONS

Persistent Left Superior Vena Cava

Anatomy. In this relatively common malformation (0.5% of the general population and 3–5% of patients with congenital heart disease), a superior vena cava persists in the left chest. The left superior vena cava may empty into coronary sinus (62%), pulmonary venous atrium (21%), common atrium (17%), or rarely into a left-sided pulmonary vein. In most cases, there is also a right superior vena cava, and in 45–60% of cases, a communication exists between the two superior venae cavae.[74]

Hemodynamics. Systemic venous blood returns to the cardiac chamber to which the left superior vena cava connects. Deoxygenated blood mixes with oxygenated blood (right to left shunt) if the left superior vena cava drains into a left heart structure.

***Key Echocardiographic Concepts*[44]**

- Dilated coronary sinus
- Contrast echocardiography[20]
- 2-D and color flow visualization of the left superior vena cava
- Absent or small innominate vein

***Associated Disease*[74]**

- Atrial septal defect
- Complex congenital heart disease

Total Anomalous Pulmonary Venous Return

Anatomy. All of the pulmonary veins drain into something other than the left atrium. The types of anomalous drainage are listed below.[44,70]

- Supracardiac: pulmonary veins drain directly into the superior vena cava or form a vertical vein that empties into the innominate vein, superior vena cava, or persistent left superior vena cava
- Cardiac: pulmonary veins drain into the right atrium or coronary sinus
- Infracardiac: pulmonary veins form a common vein that descends below the diaphragm and empties into the portal vein

Hemodynamics. Increased flow into a systemic vein, right atrium, or coronary sinus[70] and ultimately, the right heart. There is an obligatory right to left shunt at the atrial level.[11]

***Clinical Presentation Without Obstruction.*[11]** Mild cyanosis; asymptomatic.

- Physical exam: poor growth; prominant left chest; right ventricular heave
- Auscultation: fixed, widely split second sound
- ECG: right ventricular hypertrophy

- Chest x-ray: enlarged right heart; increased pulmonary vascular markings; snowman- or figure 8–shaped mediastinum

Clinical Presentation in the Presence of Obstruction.[11] Cyanosis; symptomatic during newborn period.

- Physical exam: tachypnea; dyspnea; right ventricular failure
- Auscultation: no murmurs
- ECG: right ventricular hypertrophy
- Chest x-ray: normal size heart; increased pulmonary vascular markings

Key Echocardiographic Concepts[44,70]

- Absence of normal pulmonary venous return into the left atrium by 2-D and color flow Doppler
- Dilated coronary sinus
- Turbulent flow noted in systemic vein or right atrium by color flow Doppler
- Localization of anomalous venous structures by use of 2-D and color flow Doppler from the subcostal and suprasternal positions
- Color flow Doppler interrogation of anomalous venous structures to rule out obstruction
- Contrast echocardiography

Associated Disease

- Atrial septal defect

Natural History.[11] Obstruction of the common vein or entry into a systemic venous structure will result in pulmonary edema and right heart failure, complete obstruction will cause death. Eventually, pulmonary vascular obstructive disease will develop.

Treatment. Surgical anastamosis of the common vein with the left atrium and closure of the atrial communication.

Postoperative Echocardiographic Evaluation

- Assessment of ventricular function
- Evaluate area of anastamosis to rule out obstruction

INTRAOPERATIVE ECHOCARDIOGRAPHY

Echocardiography is used increasingly in the operating room to enable surgeons to delineate anatomy and evaluate repair effectiveness. The most common method is epicardial echocardiography, in which the transducer and cable are encased in a sterile sheath and left in the sterile field. The surgeon scans "on heart" after the chest is opened and before the patient is put on cardiopulmonary bypass. This technique offers increased resolution when compared with "on chest" scanning because a higher-frequency transducer may be used owing to decreased depth penetration requirements. In some cases, the surgeon may decide to change the surgical approach based on anatomic and hemodynamic information obtained at this time. The role of the echocardiographer is to manipulate the echocardiographic equipment; setting gain and depth, image processing, manipulating Doppler and M-mode functions, and recording the scan. The most useful modalities are 2-D imaging and color flow Doppler. When the repair is completed, the surgeon may choose to image epicardially after the patient is taken off of bypass and before the chest is closed. Should the repair appear to be unsatisfactory, the surgeon may elect to put the patient back on bypass and revise the repair before closing the chest. Comparison of prebypass versus postbypass right and left ventricular function has proven helpful in perioperative medical management. When used routinely, intraoperative echocardiographic imaging and color flow Doppler impacts on as many as 50% of surgical cases.[67]

TRANSESOPHAGEAL ECHOCARDIOGRAPHY

Pediatric transesophageal echocardiography is an invasive technique that has been performed in the operating room, catheterization laboratory, and intensive care unit in patients who are anesthetized or sedated. Currently available transducers image in the transverse plane only and have color flow Doppler and pulsed Doppler capabilities. Uniplane transverse imaging is helpful in the evaluation of the following entities: ventricular function, atrioventricular connection, ventriculoarterial connection, interatrial septum, atrioventricular valve morphology, semilunar valve morphology, normal pulmonary venous connections, and identification of coronary artery origin. Color flow Doppler is useful in evaluating competancy of valves and in searching for residual defects. Owing to limitations in peak velocity resolution and the angle of incidence, pulsed Doppler applications appear to be of limited usefulness.[41] A report of experience with a prototype uniplane longitudinal transesophageal probe confirms improved utility with the addition of this imaging plane. Longitudinal imaging allowed improved imaging of the interatrial septum, interventricular septum, and left ventricular inflow tract. The ventricular outflow tracts and superior vena cava, which were inadequately imaged in the transverse plane were well demonstrated in the longitudinal plane.[40] The utility of this technique will improve with the development of a pediatric-size biplane transducer, improved resolution, and the addition of steerable continuous-wave Doppler. Owing to current limitations, it may best be utilized in the operating room as a complementary technique with epicardial echocardiography.[62]

REFERENCES

1. Adams FH, Emmanouilides GC, Riemenschneider TA (eds): *Moss' Heart Disease in Infants, Children & Adolescents,* 4th ed. Baltimore: Williams & Wilkins, 1989.

2. Anderson R, Ho SY: Echocardiographic diagnosis and description of congenital heart disease: Anatomic principles and philosophy. In St John Sutton M, Oldershaw PJ (eds): *Textbook of Adult and Pediatric Echocardiography and Doppler.* Boston: Blackwell Scientific, 1989, pp 573–606.

3. Armstrong, WF: Congenital heart disease. In Feigenbaum H (ed): *Echocardiography,* 4th ed. Philadelphia: Lea & Febiger, 1986, pp 365–461.

4. Bash SE, Huhta JC, Vick GW, et al: Hypoplastic left heart syndrome: Is echocardiography accurate enough to guide surgical palliation? *J Am Coll Cardiol* 7(3):610–616, 1986.

5. Beard JT, Byrd BF: Saline contrast enhancement of trivial Doppler tricuspid regurgitation signals for estimating pulmonary artery pressure. *Am J Cardiol* 62:486–488, 1988.

6. Brenner JI, Baker KR, Berman MA: Prediction of left ventricular pressure in infants with aortic stenosis. *Br Heart J* 44:406–410, 1980.

7. Burrows PE, Freedom RM, Rabinovitch M, et al: The investigation of abnormal pulmonary arteries in congenital heart disease. *Radiol Clin North Am* 23(4):689–717, 1985.

8. Caldwell RL, Ensing GJ: Coronary artery abnormalities in children. *J Am Soc Echo* 2(4):259–268, 1989.

9. Cassidy SC, Van Hare GF, Silverman NH: The probability of detecting a subaortic ridge in children with ventricular septal defect or coarctation of the aorta. *Am J Cardiol* 66:505–508, 1990.

10. Cloez JL, Schmidt KG, Birk E, Silverman NS: Determination of pulmonary to systemic blood flow ratio in children by a simplified Doppler echocardiographic method. *J Am Coll Cardiol* 11(4):825–830.

11. Fink, BW: Congenital Heart Disease: A Deductive Approach to Its Diagnosis, 2nd ed. Chicago: Year Book Medical, 1985.

12. Foale R, Stefanini L, Rickards A, et al: Left and right ventricular morphology in complex congenital heart disease defined by two-dimensional echocardiography. *Am J Cardiol* 49:93, 1982.

13. Fraker TD, Harris PJ, Behar VS, et al: Detection and exclusion of interatrial shunts by two-dimensional echocardiography and peripheral venous injection. *Circulation* 59(2):379–384, 1979.

14. Frantz, EG, Silverman NH: Doppler ultrasound evaluation of valvar pulmonary stenosis from multiple transducer positions in children requiring pulmonary valvuloplasty. *Am J Cardiol* 61:844–849, 1988.

15. Fuster V, Driscoll DJ, McGoon DC: Congenital heart disease in adolescents and adults. In Brandenburg RO, Fuster V, Giulani ER, McGoon DC (eds): *Cardiology: Fundamentals and Practice.* Chicago: Year Book Medical, 1987, pp 1386–1458.

16. George B, DiSessa TG, Williams R, et al: Coarctation repair without cardiac catheterization in infants. *Am Heart J* 114(6):1421–1425, 1987.

17. Goldfarb BL, Wanderman KL, Rovner M, et al: Ventricular septal defect with left ventricular to right atrial shunt: Documentation by color flow Doppler and avoidance of the pitfall of the diagnosis of tricuspid regurgitation and pulmonary hypertension. *Echocardiography* 6(6):521–525, 1989.

18. Hatle L, Angelsen B: *Doppler Ultrasound in Cardiology: Physical Principles and Clinical Applications,* 2nd ed. Philadelphia: Lea & Febiger, 1985.

19. Huhta JC, Gutgesell HP, Latson LA, et al: Two-dimensional echocardiographic assessment of the aorta in infants and children with congenital heart disease. *Circulation* 70(3):417–424, 1984.

20. Huhta JC, Smallhorn JF, Macartney FJ, et al: Cross-sectional echocardiographic diagnosis of systemic venous return. *Br Heart J* 44:718–723, 1980.

21. Kitabatake A, Inoue M, Asao M, et al: Noninvasive evaluation of pulmonary hypertension by a pulsed Doppler technique. *Circulation* 68:302–309, 1983.

22. Kosturakis D, Goldberg SJ, Allen HD, et al: Doppler echocardiographic prediction of pulmonary arterial hypertension in congenital heart disease. *Am J Cardiol* 53:1110–1114, 1984.

23. Kyo S: Congenital heart disease. In Omoto R. (ed): *Color Atlas of Real-Time Two-Dimensional Doppler Echocardiography.* 2nd ed. Philadelphia: Lea & Febiger, 1987, pp 149–209.

24. Lin F, Fu M, Yeh S, et al: Doppler atrial shunt flow patterns in patients with secundum atrial septal defect: Determinants, limitations and pitfalls. *J Am Soc Echo* 1(2):141–149, 1988.

25. Lipshultz SE, Sanders SP, Mayer JE, et al: Are routine preoperative cardiac catheterization and angiography necessary before repair of ostiuum primum atrial septal defect? *J Am Coll Cardiol* 11(2):373–378, 1988.

26. Lloyd TR, Mahoney LT, Marvin WJ, et al: Identification of coronary artery to right ventricular fistulae by color flow mapping. *Echocardiography* 5(2):115–120, 1988.

27. Marantz P, Capelli H, Ludomirsky A, et al: Echocardiographic assessment of balloon atrial septostomy in patients with transposition of the great arteries: Prediction of the need for early surgery. *Echocardiography* 5(2):99–104, 1988.

28. Masuyama T, Kodama D, Kitabatake A, et al: Continuous wave Doppler echocardiographic detection of pulmonary regurgitation and its application to noninvasive estimation of pulmonary artery pressure. *Circulation* 74:484–492, 1986.

29. McIrvin DM, Murphy DJ, Ludomirsky A: Tetralogy of Fallot with absent pulmonary valve. *Echocardiography* 6(4):363–367, 1989.

30. McKay RG: Balloon valvuloplasty for treating pul-

monic, mitral and aortic valve stenosis. *Am J Cardiol* **61**:102G–108G, 1988.

31. Meyer RA: Echocardiography in Kawasaki disease. *J Am Soc Echo* **2**(4):269–275, 1989.

32. Murphy DJ, Ludomirsky A, Huhta JC: Continuous-wave Doppler in children with ventricular septal defect: noninvasive estimation of interventricular pressure gradient. *Am J Cardiol* **57**:428–432, 1986.

33. Neches WH: Kawasaki syndrome. In Anderson RH, Neches WH, Park SC, Zuberbuhler JR (eds): *Perspectives in Pediatric Cardiology.* Mt Kisco, NY: Futura Publishing, 1988, pp 411–424.

34. NeSmith J, Philips J: The sonographer's beginning guide to surgery for congenital heart disease. *J Am Soc Echo* **1**(5):384–387, 1988.

35. Nihoyannopoulos P, Karas S, Sapsford RN, et al: Accuracy of two-dimensional echocardiography in the diagnosis of aortic arch obstruction. *J Am Coll Cardiol* **10**(5):1072–1077, 1987.

36. Perry SB, Keane JF, Lock JE: Interventional catheterization in pediatric congenital and acquired heart disease. *Am J Cardiol* **61**:109G–117G, 1988.

37. Rakowski H, Sasson Z, Wigle ED. Echocardiographic and Doppler assessment of hypertrophic cardiomyopathy. *J Am Soc Echo* **1**(1):31–47, 1988.

38. Ritter S, Rothe W, Kawai, D, et al: Identification of ventricular septal defects by Doppler color flow mapping. *Clin Res* **36**(3):311A, 1988.

39. Ritter SB: Application of Doppler color flow mapping in the assessment and the evaluation of congenital heart disease. *Echocardiography* **4**(6):543–556, 1987.

40. Ritter SB: Pediatric transesophageal color flow imaging 1990: The long and short of it. *Echocardiography* **7**(6):713–725, 1990.

41. Roberson DA, Muhiudeen IA, Silverman NH: Transesophageal echocardiography in pediatrics: Technique and limitations. *Echocardiography* **7**(6):699–712, 1990.

42. Sahn DJ, Allen HD: Real-time cross-sectional echocardiographic imaging and measurement of the patent ductus arteriosus in infants and children. *Circulation* **58**(2):343–354, 1978.

43. Sahn DJ, Valdes-Cruz LM: Ultrasound Doppler methods for calculating cardiac volume flows, cardiac output, and cardiac shunts. In Kotler MN, Steiner RM (eds): *Cardiac Imaging: New Technologies and Clinical Applications.* Philadelphia: FA Davis, 1986, pp 19–31.

44. Sanders SP: Echocardiography and related techniques in the diagnosis of congenital heart defects Part I: Veins, atria and interatrial septum. *Echocardiography* **1**(2):185–217, 1984.

45. Sanders SP: Echocardiography and related techniques in the diagnosis of congenital heart defects Part II: Atrioventricular valves and ventricles. *Echocardiography* **1**(3):333–391, 1984.

46. Schmidt KG, Cassidy SC, Silverman NH: Doubly committed subarterial ventricular septal defects: Echocardiographic features and surgical implications. *J Am Coll Cardiol* **12**(6):1538–1546, 1988.

47. Schmidt KG, Silverman NH: Cross-sectional and contrast echocardiography in the diagnosis of interatrial communications through the coronary sinus. *Int J Cardiol* **16**:193–199, 1987.

48. Seward JB, Tajik AJ, Edwards WD, Hagler DJ: *Two Dimensional Echocardiographic Atlas.* Vol I: *Congenital Heart Disease.* New York: Springer-Verlag, 1987.

49. Silverman NS, Araujo LML: An echocardiographic method for the diagnosis of cardiac situs and malpositions. *Echocardiography* **4**(1):35–57, 1987.

50. Silverman NS, Birk E: Ebstein's malformation of the tricuspid valve: Cross-sectional echocardiography and Doppler. In Anderson RH, Neches WH, Park SC, Zuberbuhler JR (eds): *Perspectives in Pediatric Cardiology.* Mt Kisco, NY: Futura Publishing, 1988, pp 113–125.

51. Silverman NH, Schmidt KG: The current role of Doppler echocardiography in the diagnosis of heart disease in children. *Cardiol Clin* **7**(2):265–297, 1989.

52. Silverman NH, Zuberbuhler JR, Anderson RH: Atrioventricular septal defects: Cross-sectional echocardiographic and morphologic comparisons. *Int J Cardiol* **13**:309–331, 1986.

53. Smallhorn J: Complete transposition. In St John Sutton M, Oldershaw P (eds): *Textbook of Adult and Pediatric Echocardiography and Doppler.* Boston: Blackwell Scientific, 1989, pp 791–808.

54. Smallhorn J: Right ventricular outflow tract obstruction. In St John Sutton M, Oldershaw P (eds): *Textbook of Adult and Pediatric Echocardiography and Doppler.* Boston: Blackwell Scientific, 1989, pp 761–790.

55. Smallhorn JF: Patent ductus arteriosus—evaluation by echocardiography. *Echocardiography* **4**(2):101–118, 1987.

56. Smallhorn JF, Huhta JC, Anderson RH, et al: Suprasternal cross-sectional echocardiography in assessment of patent ductus arteriosus. *Br Heart J* **48**:321–330, 1982.

57. Snider AR: Doppler echocardiography in congenital heart disease. In Berger M (ed): *Doppler Echocardiography in Heart Disease.* New York: Marcel Dekker, 1987.

58. Stevenson JG: Doppler evaluation of atrial septal defect, ventricular septal defect, and complex malformations. *Acta Paediatr Scand* **329** (suppl):21–43, 1986.

59. Stevenson JG: The use of Doppler echocardiography for detection and estimation of severity of patent ductus arteriosus, ventricular septal defect and atrial septal defect. *Echocardiography* **4**(4):321–346, 1987.

60. Stevenson JG: Comparison of several noninvasive

methods for estimation of pulmonary artery pressure. *J Am Soc Echo* **2**(3):157–171, 1989.

61. Stevenson JG, Kawabori I, Dooley T, et al: Diagnosis of ventricular septal defects by pulsed Doppler echocardiography. *Circulation* **58**(2):322–326, 1978.

62. Stumper O, Kaulitz R, Sreeram N, et al.: Intraoperative transesophageal versus epicardial ultrasound in surgery for congenital heart disease. *J Am Soc Echo* **3**(5):392–401, 1990.

63. Sullivan ID, Robinson PJ, DeLeval M, et al: Membranous supravalvular mitral stenosis: A treatable form of congenital heart disease. *J Am Coll Cardiol* **8**(1):159–164, 1986.

64. Sutherland GR, Smallhorn JF, Anderson RH, et al: Atrioventricular discordance: Cross-sectional echocardiographic morphological correlative study. *Br Heart J* **50**:8, 1983.

65. Sweeney MS, Walker WE, Cooley DA, et al: Apicoaortic conduits for complex left ventricular outflow obstruction: 10-year experience. *Ann Thorac Surg* **42**(6):609–611, 1986.

66. Tani L, Ludomirsky A, Murphy DJ, et al: Ventricular morphology: Echocardiographic evaluation of isolated ventricular inversion. *Echocardiography* **5**(1):39–42, 1988.

67. Ungerleider RM: The use of intraoperative echocardiography with Doppler color flow imaging in the repair of congenital heart defects. *Echocardiography* **7**(3):289–304, 1990.

68. Valdez-Cruz LM, Sahn DJ: Ultrasonic contrast studies for the detection of cardiac shunts. *J Am Coll Cardiol* **3**(4):978–985, 1984.

69. Van Hare GF, Silverman NH: Contrast two-dimensional echocardiography in congenital heart disease: Techniques, indications and clinical utility. *J Am Coll Cardiol* **13**(3):673–686, 1989.

70. Van Hare GF, Schmidt KG, Cassidy SC, et al: Color Doppler flow mapping in the ultrasound diagnosis of total anomalous pulmonary venous connection. *J Am Soc Echo* **1**(5):341–347, 1988.

71. Velvis H, Schmidt KG, Silverman NH, et al: Diagnosis of coronary artery fistula by two-dimensional echocardiography, pulsed Doppler ultrasound and color flow imaging. *J Am Coll Cardiol* **14**(4):968–976, 1989.

72. Weyman AE, Dillon JC, Feigenbaum H, et al: Echocardiographic patterns of pulmonic valve motion with pulmonary hypertension. *Circulation* **50**:905–910, 1974.

73. Yock PG, Popp RL: Noninvasive estimation of right ventricular systolic pressure by Doppler ultrasound in patients with tricuspid regurgitation. *Circulation* **70**(4):657–662, 1984.

74. Zellers TM, Hagler DJ, Julsrud PR: Accuracy of two-dimensional echocardiography in diagnosing left superior vena cava. *J Am Soc Echo* **2**(2):132–138, 1989.

75. Zuberbuhler JR, Anderson RH: Ebstein's malformation of the tricuspid valve: Morphology and natural history. In Anderson RH, Neches WH, Park SC, Zuberbuhler JR (eds): *Perspectives in Pediatric Cardiology*. Mt Kisco, NY: Futura Publishing, 1988, 99–112.

Figure 4–1. Pulsed Doppler spectral tracing of flow in the descending aorta as obtained from the suprasternal notch view.

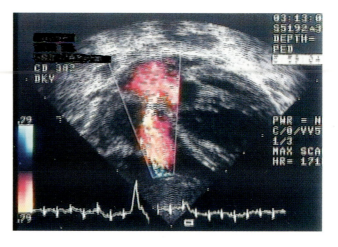

Figure 4–3. Color flow Doppler image of a subcostal four-chamber view presented with the apex down (anatomically correct) presentation. The patient is an 8-month-old female with trisomy 21.

24. An echocardiogram was requested for a premature infant in the neonatal intensive care unit who appeared clinically to be in congestive failure and in whom a murmur was heard. The color flow Doppler image in Fig. 4–2 was taken from the ductus view, which is a parasternal sagittal view. The closed aortic valve may be appreciated in the center of the image. This image demonstrates

(A) a small patent ductus arteriosus
(B) a moderate patent ductus arteriosus
(C) a large patent ductus arteriosus
(D) no ductus arteriosus

25. The image in Fig. 4–3 was taken from an 8-month-old female with trisomy 21. The color flow Doppler

image was taken from the subcostal 4 chamber view. The image demonstrates

(A) a left to right shunt through a primum atrial septal defect
(B) a right to left shunt through a primum atrial septal defect
(C) a left to right shunt through a secundum atrial septal defect
(D) a right to left shunt through a secundum atrial septal defect
(E) a normal heart

26. The images presented in Fig. 4–4 were taken from the cardiac apex of a cyanotic infant. These images demonstrate

(A) a normal heart
(B) an isolated inflow ventricular septal defect
(C) single atrium
(D) tricuspid atresia with ventricular septal defect
(E) tricuspid atresia with intact ventricular septum

27. The color flow Doppler image presented in Fig. 4–5 was taken from an 8-year-old male with a systolic murmur. The image is of the parasternal short axis view during early systole and demonstrates a left to right shunt through a(n)

(A) inflow ventricular septal defect
(B) membranous ventricular septal defect
(C) muscular ventricular septal defect
(D) doubly committed subarterial ventricular septal defect

Figure 4–2. Color flow Doppler image of a modified short-axis parasternal view, known as the "ductus view." The patient is a premature infant in congestive heart failure in whom a murmur is heard.

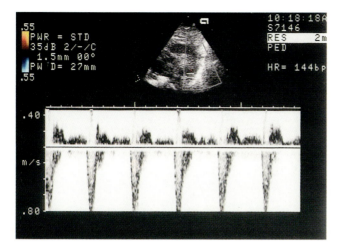

Figure 4–1. Pulsed Doppler spectral tracing of flow in the descending aorta as obtained from the suprasternal notch view.

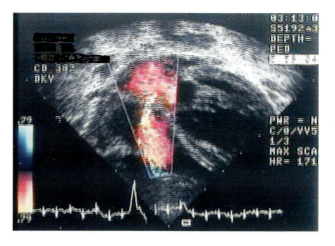

Figure 4–3. Color flow Doppler image of a subcostal four-chamber view presented with the apex down (anatomically correct) presentation. The patient is an 8-month-old female with trisomy 21.

24. An echocardiogram was requested for a premature infant in the neonatal intensive care unit who appeared clinically to be in congestive failure and in whom a murmur was heard. The color flow Doppler image in Fig. 4–2 was taken from the ductus view, which is a parasternal sagittal view. The closed aortic valve may be appreciated in the center of the image. This image demonstrates

(A) a small patent ductus arteriosus
(B) a moderate patent ductus arteriosus
(C) a large patent ductus arteriosus
(D) no ductus arteriosus

25. The image in Fig. 4–3 was taken from an 8-month-old female with trisomy 21. The color flow Doppler

image was taken from the subcostal 4 chamber view. The image demonstrates

(A) a left to right shunt through a primum atrial septal defect
(B) a right to left shunt through a primum atrial septal defect
(C) a left to right shunt through a secundum atrial septal defect
(D) a right to left shunt through a secundum atrial septal defect
(E) a normal heart

26. The images presented in Fig. 4–4 were taken from the cardiac apex of a cyanotic infant. These images demonstrate

(A) a normal heart
(B) an isolated inflow ventricular septal defect
(C) single atrium
(D) tricuspid atresia with ventricular septal defect
(E) tricuspid atresia with intact ventricular septum

27. The color flow Doppler image presented in Fig. 4–5 was taken from an 8-year-old male with a systolic murmur. The image is of the parasternal short axis view during early systole and demonstrates a left to right shunt through a(n)

(A) inflow ventricular septal defect
(B) membranous ventricular septal defect
(C) muscular ventricular septal defect
(D) doubly committed subarterial ventricular septal defect

Figure 4–2. Color flow Doppler image of a modified short-axis parasternal view, known as the "ductus view." The patient is a premature infant in congestive heart failure in whom a murmur is heard.

12. Which of the following is also known as the arterial switch procedure?

   (A) Rashkind procedure
   (B) Mustard procedure
   (C) Jatene procedure
   (D) Senning procedure

13. When the aorta and pulmonary artery are transposed, they course ——— as they exit the heart.

   (A) parallel to each other
   (B) perpendicular to each other
   (C) wound around each other
   (D) in no particular relationship to each other

14. Balloon atrial septostomy is most commonly performed in infants who have

   (A) Ebstein anomaly of the tricuspid valve
   (B) transposition of the great arteries
   (C) truncus arteriosus
   (D) tetralogy of Fallot

15. Of all children who suffer from Kawasaki disease, ——— will develop coronary artery aneurysms.

   (A) 2%
   (B) 15%
   (C) 50%
   (D) 75%
   (E) 100%

16. Which of the following groups is most likely to develop coronary artery aneurysms as a complication of Kawasaki disease?

   (A) toddlers
   (B) infants
   (C) adolescents
   (D) adults

17. Which of the following is not useful in the assessment of pulmonary artery pressure?

   (A) peak Doppler gradient through a patent ductus arteriosus
   (B) peak Doppler gradient of tricuspid regurgitation
   (C) end-diastolic Doppler gradient of pulmonary insufficiency
   (D) acceleration time to ejection time ratio calculated from a right ventricular outflow tract velocity curve
   (E) all of the above are useful in estimating pulmonary artery pressure

18. A child with tetralogy of Fallot is upset and crying during the echocardiogram. The Doppler gradient through the right ventricular outflow tract will be ——— than if the child were sleeping peacefully.

   (A) greater
   (B) less

(C) outflow obstruction in tetralogy of Fallot is not affected by the patient's activity

19. A 3-year-old child with Kawasaki disease is referred to echocardiology. Which of the following views is not really necessary in the 2-D evaluation of the coronary arterial system?

   (A) subcostal transverse
   (B) parasternal short axis
   (C) apical five chamber
   (D) subcostal coronal
   (E) all views are helpful

20. Which of the following Doppler findings is not characteristic of coarctation of the aorta?

   (A) forward flow through the descending aorta extending throughout diastole
   (B) normal or slightly increased velocity of flow in the aorta proximal to the left subclavian artery
   (C) rapid acceleration and deceleration of the Doppler signal taken from the descending aorta
   (D) Doppler signal from the descending aorta does not return to baseline during diastole
   (E) high-velocity flow detected in the descending aorta distal to the left subclavian artery

21. Careful echocardiographic evaluation of a child with complex congenital heart disease reveals absence of the inferior vena cava above the level of the renal arteries. The aorta is to the left of the spine. What is this child's situs most likely to be?

   (A) solitus
   (B) inversus
   (C) left atrial isomerism
   (D) right atrial isomerism

22. The characteristic aortic valve M-mode tracing from a patient with discrete membranous subaortic stenosis demonstrates

   (A) an asymmetric closure line
   (B) early closure and partial reopening
   (C) gradual closure (drifting closed)
   (D) prolonged ejection time

23. Which of the following should not be included in the differential diagnosis when a Doppler tracing such as that in Fig. 4–1 is obtained from the descending aorta?

   (A) patent ductus arteriosus
   (B) severe aortic regurgitation
   (C) arteriovenous malformation
   (D) aortic to pulmonary window
   (E) coarctation of the aorta

Questions

1. The most common type of atrial septal defect is

   (A) primum
   (B) secundum
   (C) sinus venosus
   (D) single atrium

2. Which transducer position is most helpful in the 2-D visualization of atrial septal defects?

   (A) left parasternal
   (B) apical
   (C) subxiphoid
   (D) right parasternal

3. Partial anomalous pulmonary venous return is most commonly associated with which type of atrial septal defect?

   (A) secundum
   (B) priumum
   (C) sinus venosus
   (D) coronary sinus

4. What is the most common congenital heart lesion in the pediatric population?

   (A) mitral stenosis
   (B) atrial septal defect
   (C) ventricular septal defect
   (D) pulmonary stenosis

5. A "T-sign" artifact demonstrated by ———— is useful in the detection of ventricular septal defects.

   (A) M-mode
   (B) 2-D
   (C) pulsed-wave Doppler
   (D) continuous-wave Doppler
   (E) color flow Doppler

6. A small muscular ventricular septal defect may be most easily localized by

   (A) M-mode
   (B) 2-D
   (C) pulsed-wave Doppler
   (D) continuous-wave Doppler
   (E) color flow Doppler

7. Which of the following will *not* cause a reversal of flow in the descending aorta during diastole?

   (A) large patent ductus arteriosus with severe pulmonary hypertension (suprasystemic pulmonary pressures)
   (B) severe aortic insufficiency
   (C) surgically created systemic to pulmonary shunt with normal pulmonary artery pressures
   (D) large patent ductus arteriosus with normal pulmonary artery pressures

8. Which of the following may be associated with valvar aortic stenosis?

   (A) patent ductus arteriosus
   (B) coarctation of the aorta
   (C) ventricular septal defect
   (D) pulmonary stenosis
   (E) all of the above

9. The most commonly associated lesion in patients with coarctation of the aorta is

   (A) ventricular septal defect
   (B) bicuspid aortic valve
   (C) patent ductus arteriosus
   (D) aortic stenosis
   (E) mitral stenosis

10. In the normally related heart, the aortic valve lies

    (A) anterior and to the left of the pulmonary valve
    (B) anterior and to the right of the pulmonary valve
    (C) posterior and to the right of the pulmonary valve
    (D) posterior and to the left of the pulmonary valve

11. Which of the following surgical procedures is *not* frequently used to treat transposition of the great arteries?

    (A) Senning procedure
    (B) Mustard procedure
    (C) Jatene procedure
    (D) Fontan procedure

methods for estimation of pulmonary artery pressure. *J Am Soc Echo* **2**(3):157–171, 1989.

61. Stevenson JG, Kawabori I, Dooley T, et al: Diagnosis of ventricular septal defects by pulsed Doppler echocardiography. *Circulation* **58**(2):322–326, 1978.

62. Stumper O, Kaulitz R, Sreeram N, et al.: Intraoperative transesophageal versus epicardial ultrasound in surgery for congenital heart disease. *J Am Soc Echo* **3**(5):392–401, 1990.

63. Sullivan ID, Robinson PJ, DeLeval M, et al: Membranous supravalvular mitral stenosis: A treatable form of congenital heart disease. *J Am Coll Cardiol* **8**(1):159–164, 1986.

64. Sutherland GR, Smallhorn JF, Anderson RH, et al: Atrioventricular discordance: Cross-sectional echocardiographic morphological correlative study. *Br Heart J* **50**:8, 1983.

65. Sweeney MS, Walker WE, Cooley DA, et al: Apicoaortic conduits for complex left ventricular outflow obstruction: 10-year experience. *Ann Thorac Surg* **42**(6): 609–611, 1986.

66. Tani L, Ludomirsky A, Murphy DJ, et al: Ventricular morphology: Echocardiographic evaluation of isolated ventricular inversion. *Echocardiography* **5**(1):39–42, 1988.

67. Ungerleider RM: The use of intraoperative echocardiography with Doppler color flow imaging in the repair of congenital heart defects. *Echocardiography* **7**(3):289–304, 1990.

68. Valdez-Cruz LM, Sahn DJ: Ultrasonic contrast studies for the detection of cardiac shunts. *J Am Coll Cardiol* **3**(4):978–985, 1984.

69. Van Hare GF, Silverman NH: Contrast two-dimensional echocardiography in congenital heart disease: Techniques, indications and clinical utility. *J Am Coll Cardiol* **13**(3):673–686, 1989.

70. Van Hare GF, Schmidt KG, Cassidy SC, et al: Color Doppler flow mapping in the ultrasound diagnosis of total anomalous pulmonary venous connection. *J Am Soc Echo* **1**(5):341–347, 1988.

71. Velvis H, Schmidt KG, Silverman NH, et al: Diagnosis of coronary artery fistula by two-dimensional echocardiography, pulsed Doppler ultrasound and color flow imaging. *J Am Coll Cardiol* **14**(4):968–976, 1989.

72. Weyman AE, Dillon JC, Feigenbaum H, et al: Echocardiographic patterns of pulmonic valve motion with pulmonary hypertension. *Circulation* **50**:905–910, 1974.

73. Yock PG, Popp RL: Noninvasive estimation of right ventricular systolic pressure by Doppler ultrasound in patients with tricuspid regurgitation. *Circulation* **70**(4):657–662, 1984.

74. Zellers TM, Hagler DJ, Julsrud PR: Accuracy of two-dimensional echocardiography in diagnosing left superior vena cava. *J Am Soc Echo* **2**(2):132–138, 1989.

75. Zuberbuhler JR, Anderson RH: Ebstein's malformation of the tricuspid valve: Morphology and natural history. In Anderson RH, Neches WH, Park SC, Zuberbuhler JR (eds): *Perspectives in Pediatric Cardiology*. Mt Kisco, NY: Futura Publishing, 1988, 99–112.

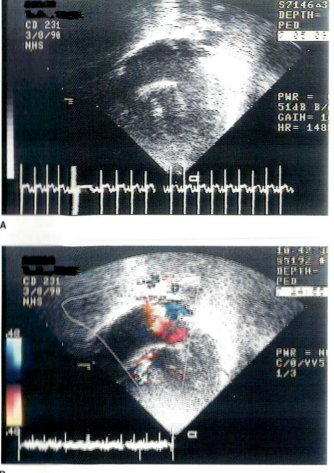

A

B

Figure 4–4. Apical four-chamber view presented with the apex down. (**A**) 2-D image. (**B**) Color flow Doppler image. The patient is a cyanotic infant.

Figure 4–6. 2-D image of the apical four-chamber view presented with the apex down.

28. The 2-D image in Fig. 4–6 was taken from the cardiac apex and demonstrates

(A) a normal apical four-chamber view
(B) tricuspid atresia
(C) Ebstein anomaly of the tricuspid valve
(D) ventricular inversion

29. The 2-D image of the parasternal long-axis view presented in Fig. 4–7 was taken during diastole and demonstrates

(A) a normal heart
(B) valvular aortic stenosis
(C) discrete membranous subaortic stenosis
(D) ideopathic hypertrophic subaortic stenosis

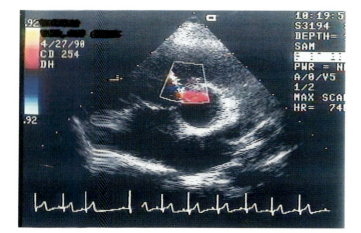

Figure 4–5. Color flow Doppler image of the parasternal short-axis view at the level of the semilunar valves taken in early systole. The patient is an 8-year-old male in whom a systolic murmur may be heard.

Figure 4–7. 2-D image of a parasternal long-axis view taken in diastole.

For each of the following transducer positions, indicate (true or false) whether the position could yield the highest pressure gradient estimate in a patient with valvular pulmonary stenosis.

51. parasternal

52. apical

53. subcostal

54. suprasternal

The 2-D image in Fig. 4–12 was obtained by placing the transducer at the cardiac apex of an infant. The infant was referred to echocardiology because of an enlarged heart on chest x-ray and cardiac failure. A systolic murmur may be heard at the apex. Indicate whether statements 55–60 are true or false for this image.

55. There is a secundum atrial septal defect.

56. There is a primum atrial septal defect.

57. The tricuspid valve appears normal.

58. The left ventricle is significantly smaller in size than the right ventricle.

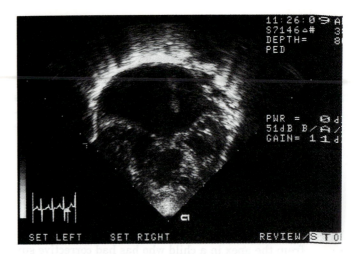

Figure 4–12. 2-D image of an apical four-chamber view presented with the apex down. This infant was in cardiac failure and reportedly had an enlarged heart on chest x-ray. A systolic murmur may be heard at the apex.

59. The diagnosis for this patient is Ebstein anomaly of the tricuspid valve.

60. The systolic murmur is probably due to aortic stenosis.

A

B

Figure 4–4. Apical four-chamber view presented with the apex down. (**A**) 2-D image. (**B**) Color flow Doppler image. The patient is a cyanotic infant.

Figure 4–5. Color flow Doppler image of the parasternal short-axis view at the level of the semilunar valves taken in early systole. The patient is an 8-year-old male in whom a systolic murmur may be heard.

Figure 4–6. 2-D image of the apical four-chamber view presented with the apex down.

28. The 2-D image in Fig. 4–6 was taken from the cardiac apex and demonstrates

   (A) a normal apical four-chamber view
   (B) tricuspid atresia
   (C) Ebstein anomaly of the tricuspid valve
   (D) ventricular inversion

29. The 2-D image of the parasternal long-axis view presented in Fig. 4–7 was taken during diastole and demonstrates

   (A) a normal heart
   (B) valvular aortic stenosis
   (C) discrete membranous subaortic stenosis
   (D) ideopathic hypertrophic subaortic stenosis

Figure 4–7. 2-D image of a parasternal long-axis view taken in diastole.

30. If the left ventricular outflow tract of the patient presented in Fig. 4–7 was interrogated by PW Doppler, what is the most proximal location at which an increase in velocity would be detected?

    (A) just proximal to the aortic valve
    (B) at the aortic valve
    (C) just distal to the aortic valve
    (D) in the aortic root
    (E) distal to the left subclavian artery

31. The 2-D parasternal short-axis view image presented in Fig. 4–8 was taken from a young child who had recently had Kawasaki disease. This view demonstrates

    (A) left coronary artery involvement
    (B) right coronary artery involvement
    (C) both left and right coronary arteries are involved
    (D) normal coronary arteries

32. The 2-D parasternal short-axis view image presented in Fig. 4–9 was taken from an infant who was diagnosed as having tetralogy of Fallot. This image demonstrates

    (A) a normal right ventricular outflow tract
    (B) infundibular pulmonary stenosis only
    (C) infundibular and valvular pulmonary stenosis
    (D) infundibular pulmonary stenosis with hypoplasia of the pulmonary valve and main pulmonary artery

33. Which of the following views would *not* be helpful in delineating the size of left and right pulmonary arteries in the patient imaged for Fig. 4–9?

    (A) suprasternal coronal view
    (B) apical outflow view

Figure 4–8. 2-D image of a parasternal short-axis view at the level of the semilunar valves. The patient is a young child who is in the convalescent phase of Kawasaki's disease.

Figure 4–9. 2-D image of a parasternal short-axis view at the level of the semilunar valves. This infant has been diagnosed as having tetralogy of Fallot.

    (C) subcostal short axis (sagittal) view
    (D) high left parasternal view
    (E) all of the above views would be useful

34. Which of the following methods is most reliable for estimating pulmonary artery pressures?

    (A) thickness of the right ventricular free wall
    (B) determination of the peak regurgitant gradient through the tricuspid valve
    (C) determination of the peak regurgitant gradient through the pulmonic valve
    (D) dividing the acceleration time by the ejection time of flow as obtained from the main pulmonary artery

35. In which of the following surgically created shunts is the subclavian artery used?

    (A) Central
    (B) Glenn
    (C) Waterston
    (D) Blalock-Taussig
    (E) Potts

36. What is needed to estimate $Q_p : Q_s$ in a patient with a ventricular septal defect?

    (A) diameters and peak flow velocities through the pulmonary and aortic valves
    (B) peak pressure gradient through a tricuspid regurgitation jet
    (C) diameters and peak flow velocities through the tricuspid and aortic valves
    (D) diameters and peak flow velocities through the pulmonary and mitral valves

37. The shunt through the atrial septal defect of a patient with tricuspid atresia is

(A) always left to right
(B) always right to left
(C) may be bidirectional
(D) nonexistant

38. The 2-D parasternal view presented in Fig. 4–10 was taken from an adolescent girl with Marfan syndrome. What abnormalities may be seen which are frequently associated with Marfan syndrome?

    (A) dilated aortic root and mitral valve prolapse
    (B) aortic aneurysm dissection
    (C) ideopathic hypertrophic subaortic stenosis
    (D) herniation of the sinus of Valsalva

39. The 2-D image presented in Fig. 4–11 was taken from the apex in a child who has had corrective surgery for transposition of the great arteries. The echogenic line in the left atrium represents

    (A) cortriatriatum
    (B) supramitral ring
    (C) total anomalous pulmonary venous return
    (D) an interatrial baffle

40. If a patient has total anomalous pulmonary venous return, the right atrium should be

    (A) atretic
    (B) small
    (C) normal in size
    (D) dilated

41. The most useful modality in the delineation of anatomy in total anomalous pulmonary venous return is

    (A) 2-D
    (B) M-mode
    (C) PW Doppler
    (D) CW Doppler
    (E) color flow Doppler

Figure 4–11. 2-D image of an apical four-chamber view presented with the apex down. This young child has had a previous repair for transposition of the great vessels.

TRUE OR FALSE: Indicate whether each of the following statements is true or false.

42. Patent ductus arteriosis is more commonly seen in low birth weight premature infants than in term infants.

43. Patency of the ductus arteriosus may be desirable in some cases.

44. In cortriatriatum, the left atrial appendage is continuous with the anatomic left atrium and not with the proximal chamber that receives flow directly from the pulmonary veins.

45. Children with trisomy 21 frequently have partial atrioventricular septal defects.

46. Patients with truncus arteriosus are usually quite cyanotic in infancy.

47. Individuals with Ebstein anomaly of the tricuspid valve are always symptomatic.

48. Distal coronary artery aneurysms are common in the absence of proximal aneurysm formation in patients who have had Kawasaki disease.

49. In patients with coarctation of the aorta, the gradient through the obstruction should approximate the difference in systolic blood pressures taken from the arm and leg of the patient.

50. Persistent left superior vena cava may exist in the absence of a dilated coronary sinus.

Figure 4–10. 2-D image of a parasternal long-axis view. The patient is an adolescent girl thought to have Marfan syndrome.

For each of the following transducer positions, indicate (true or false) whether the position could yield the highest pressure gradient estimate in a patient with valvular pulmonary stenosis.

51. parasternal

52. apical

53. subcostal

54. suprasternal

The 2-D image in Fig. 4–12 was obtained by placing the transducer at the cardiac apex of an infant. The infant was referred to echocardiology because of an enlarged heart on chest x-ray and cardiac failure. A systolic murmur may be heard at the apex. Indicate whether statements 55–60 are true or false for this image.

55. There is a secundum atrial septal defect.

56. There is a primum atrial septal defect.

57. The tricuspid valve appears normal.

58. The left ventricle is significantly smaller in size than the right ventricle.

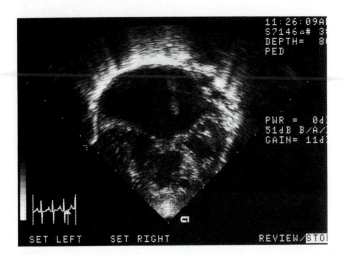

Figure 4–12. 2-D image of an apical four-chamber view presented with the apex down. This infant was in cardiac failure and reportedly had an enlarged heart on chest x-ray. A systolic murmur may be heard at the apex.

59. The diagnosis for this patient is Ebstein anomaly of the tricuspid valve.

60. The systolic murmur is probably due to aortic stenosis.

Answers and Explanations

1. **(B)** Sinus venosus is the rarest form, and single atrium is not considered to be an atrial septal defect because there is complete absence of the atrial septum. *(15:1391)*

2. **(C)** In the subxiphoid position, the sound beam is perpendicular to the interatrial septum, thereby utilizing the axial resolution of the transducer. The atrial septum may also be visualized from the parasternal short axis view but it is more parallel to the sound beam and, therefore, may not be resolved optimally. In the apical position, the sound beam is parallel to the atrial septum, and the atrial septum is a great distance from the transducer, so echocardiographic dropout may be mistaken for an atrial communication. *(48:144–147)*

3. **(C)** Sinus venosus atrial septal defects are bordered posteriorly by the posterior atrial wall and superiorly by the entrance of the superior vena cava. Because of this, the upper right pulmonary vein may empty into the right atrium or superior vena cava. *(1:175)*

4. **(C)** Atrial septal defect and pulmonary stenosis are also common. Mitral stenosis is relatively uncommon in the pediatric population. *(1:190)*

5. **(B)** The "T" artifact is visualized on 2-D echocardiography as a prominence of echoes at the edges of the septal tissue. *(3:415)*

6. **(E)** Muscular VSDs may occur anywhere and be very small. Color flow Doppler allows relatively rapid evaluation of the entire interventricular septum. Visualization of a jet of turbulent flow identifies a VSD. PW or CW Doppler interrogation can be tedious and may miss a small muscular defect in an unusual position. *(39:544–548)*

7. **(A)** When pulmonary pressures exceed systemic pressures, the flow through the patent ductus arteriosus will be right to left; therefore, there would be no reversal in the descending aorta. All of the other choices should cause a reversal of flow in the descending aorta. *(51:285–287)*

8. **(E)** Although patent ductus arteriosus and coarctation of the aorta are more commonly associated with valvar aortic stenosis, ventricular septal defect and pulmonary stenosis may also be associated. *(1:224)*

9. **(B)** Although all of the listed malformations may be associated findings, bicuspid aortic valve has been reported to be an associated finding in as much as 85% of cases. *(1:244)*

10. **(C)** The aortic valve is posterior and to the right of the pulmonic valve in the normally related heart. The aortic valve is located centrally in the base of the heart, whereas the pulmonic valve is anterior and left. *(2:578–581)*

11. **(D)** The Fontan procedure was originally developed to treat patients with tricuspid atresia. Although it is now used in a modified form to treat other forms of complex congenital heart disease, it is not commonly used to treat patients with transposition of the great arteries. *(1:357–359,402–417)*

12. **(C)** The Rashkind procedure is an interventional catheterization technique that also is known as a balloon atrial septostomy. The Mustard and Senning procedures also are known as atrial switches. *(1:402–417)*

13. **(A)** Normally related great vessels course perpendicular to each other. Demonstration of this relationship rules out transposition of the great vessels. *(48:498)*

14. **(B)** The purpose of an atrial septostomy is to mix deoxygenated systemic venous return with oxygenated pulmonary venous return. In truncus arteriosus and tetralogy of Fallot, this mixing occurs through a large ventricular septal defect. In Ebstein

anomaly of the tricuspid valve, blood flow sequence is normal, therefore, mixing is not desirable.

(1:399–400)

15. **(B)** There is about a 15% incidence of coronary artery aneurysm formation in children with Kawasaki disease. *(31:269)*

16. **(B)** Kawasaki disease is a childhood disease. Infants appear to be more likely to develop aneurysms than older children. *(31:273)*

17. **(E)** All of the above that are available should be used. *(18:223; 60:157–171)*

18. **(A)** The right ventricular outflow obstruction of tetralogy of Fallot is a dynamic obstruction; therefore, it may increase when the patient is distressed. *(1:278)*

19. **(E)** Although the proximal portions are the most frequently involved, the coronary system should be evaluated from every available view because aneurysms may occur anywhere. *(31:269–273)*

20. **(C)** In coarctation of the aorta, the descending aortic flow pulsatility is blunted such that the Doppler signal shows a slow acceleration and deceleration.

(18:217–221)

21. **(D)** In situs solitus, the aorta descends anterior and to the left of the spine and the inferior vena cava ascends to the right of the spine. In situs inversus, the opposite is true. In left atrial isomerism, the inferior vena cava is frequently interrupted. *(49:35–56)*

22. **(B)** An asymmetric closure line is suggestive of a bicuspid aortic valve. Gradual closure is suggestive of depressed left ventricular contractility. Ejection time may be prolonged in severe valvular aortic stenosis. *(3:380–386)*

23. **(E)** Reversal of flow during diastole, as shown in Fig. 4–1, may be seen in any of the other conditions. The characteristic PW Doppler pattern in the descending aorta is very different for coarctation of the aorta. *(18:217–228; 51:279–295)*

24. **(B)** From the ECG, we can see that this is an end-diastolic frame. The 2-D image shows closed aortic and pulmonary valves, confirming that this is an end-diastolic frame. Red color representing flow toward the transducer may be appreciated coming into the main pulmonary artery from the patent ductus arteriosus. *(23:161–162,189–190)*

25. **(C)** The red jet seen traversing the interatrial septum represents flow coming toward the transducer, therefore, it is shunting from the left atrium to the

right atrium. Portions of the superior and inferior interatrial septum may be seen on the 2-D image.

(39:548–550)

26. **(D)** The mitral valve is open in Fig. 4–4A. A thick band of tissue appears in place of a normal tricuspid valve. A ventricular septal defect may be appreciated at the top of the ventricular septum in this image. In Fig. 4–4B, flow through the ventricular septal defect into the right ventricle is demonstrated by color flow Doppler during systole. *(3:374–375)*

27. **(B)** Flow through an inflow ventricular septal defect would be visualized at the level of the mitral annulus. Flow through a doubly committed subarterial ventricular septal defect would be visualized just proximal to the pulmonary valve in this view. Flow through a muscular ventricular septal defect would be visualized in the muscular portion of the ventricular septum. This portion of the ventricular septum is visible from the parasternal short axis at the level of the mitral valve and more apically.

(3:155–161, 183–188)

28. **(D)** The mitral valve is always higher on the ventricular septum in the absence of an inflow ventricular septal defect. In this case, the atrioventricular valve of the right-sided ventricle inserts higher on the ventricular septum than the atrioventricular valve of the left-sided ventricle. *(48:324–325)*

29. **(C)** The aortic valve is closed and does not appear thickened. There is an echogenic line that extends posteriorly from the ventricular septum just proximal to the aortic valve. This represents a discrete subaortic membrane. In idiopathic hypertrophic subaortic stenosis, the interventricular septum would be significantly thickened. *(48:424–427)*

30. **(A)** Valvular aortic stenosis would cause the velocity of flow to increase just distal to the valve. Supravalvular aortic stenosis would cause the velocity of flow to increase in the aortic root. Coarctation of the aorta would cause the velocity of flow to increase past the level of the left subclavian artery. *(3:382)*

31. **(C)** The left coronary artery appears mildly dilated, and the large circle noted in the right atrium is the right coronary artery (with aneurysmal dilatation) as it courses within the right atrioventricular groove.

(31:268–273)

32. **(D)** The entire right ventricular outflow tract is small in caliber. *(48:434)*

33. **(E)** The pulmonary artery branches may be imaged from all of these views. *(54:767–782)*

34. **(B)** The thickness of the right ventricular free wall may not be proportionate to the increase in pulmonary artery pressure. The end-diastolic and not peak gradient of pulmonary regurgitation may be used. Acceleration and ejection time should be measured from the right ventricular outflow tract. *(60:157–171)*

35. **(D)** The subclavian artery is used in the construction of the Blalock-Taussig shunt. In a central shunt, the pulmonary artery is connected to the aorta directly or via a conduit. In the Waterston shunt, the ascending aorta is connected to the right pulmonary artery, and in the Potts anastomosis, the descending aorta is connected to the pulmonary artery. *(34:384–385)*

36. **(A)** $Q_p : Q_s$ is a comparison of pulmonary flow to systemic flow used to estimate the amount of blood flow through a systemic to pulmonary shunt. Flow is calculated by multiplying area by velocity of flow. This calculation must be done for the systemic circulation and for the pulmonary circulation. When the shunt is at the level of the ventricles, pulmonary flow may be calculated by using the pulmonary valve or the mitral valve (ie, pulmonary venous return). The systemic flow may be calculated by using the aortic valve or tricuspid valve (ie, systemic venous return). The calculation is done to determine how much more blood is going through the pulmonary vasculature than the systemic vasculature.
(10:825–827; 59:339–344)

37. **(B)** Because the atrial septal defect is the only outlet for the blood in the right atrium, it is an obligatory right to left shunt. *(3:375)*

38. **(A)** Patients with Marfan syndrome are also at risk for aortic dissections, but only a limited amount of the aorta is visualized here. The other two abnormalities are not frequently associated with this syndrome. *(1:792–793)*

39. **(D)** The echogenic line visualized in the left atrium in Fig. 4–11 is an interatrial baffle constructed to redirect blood flow in what is known as an "atrial switch." *(48:552–557)*

40. **(E)** Because pulmonary venous flow returns directly to the right atrium, it will be dilated. *(3:368–371)*

41. **(E)** Color flow aids tremendously in demonstrating the anomalous channels and connections.
(70:341–347)

42. **True.** Constriction of the ductus is physiologically delayed in this group. *(1:209–218)*

43. **True.** Prostaglandin E may be administered to keep the ductus arteriosus patent in infants with severe right ventricular outflow obstruction or atresia or great vessel malformations. *(1:221–222)*

44. **True.** The membrane inserts proximal to the left atrial appendage in cortriatriatum and distal to it in supravalvar mitral ring. *(1:599–602)*

45. **False.** These children more commonly have the complete form of atrioventricular defect. *(1:176)*

46. **False.** Significant cyanosis during infancy occurs only when there is associated pulmonary stenosis.
(1:507)

47. **False.** There is a spectrum of severity in this malformation, and mild forms may remain asymptomatic. *(11:142)*

48. **False.** It is very rare to have distal involvement in the absence of proximal aneurysm formation.
(31:275)

49. **True.** In severe cases, it may be difficult to obtain a reliable Doppler signal because of decreased flow through the area of obstruction. The Doppler derived gradient may be somewhat higher than the systolic pressure differences measured from the arm and thigh because peak systolic pressure occurs at slightly different times in these two areas; therefore the blood pressure method yields a peak to peak pressure difference, whereas the Doppler method yields an instantaneous pressure difference. *(18:217–219)*

50. **True.** Suprasternal coronal evaluation of the extracardiac vessels should be included in patients in whom this may be a concern for planning of surgical procedures. *(74:137)*

51. **True.** This has traditionally been the most common position for evaluation of pulmonary valve stenosis.
(54:765)

52. **True.** The sound beam is angled anteriorly, and the transducer is moved to just below the left nipple.
(14:844–848)

53. **True.** The sound beam is angled anteriorly and slightly to the left. *(54:765)*

54. **True.** In a few cases, this may be the only position from which a diagnostic Doppler signal can be obtained. *(14:844–848)*

55. **False.** The area of the fossa ovalis appears to be intact. *(1:173–174)*

56. **True.** The portion of atrial septum just above the level of the atrioventricular valves is absent.

    (52:309–314)

57. **False.** There is a common atrioventricular valve with chordal insertions onto the ventricular septum.

    (52:315–319)

58. **True.** The left ventricle is about one third the size of the right ventricle. The interventricular septum may be seen bowing into the left ventricle.   *(52:319–330)*

59. **False.** The diagnosis is an unbalanced complete atrioventricular septal defect. In Ebstein anomaly of the tricuspid valve, the tricuspid valve leaflets are adherent to the right ventricular walls.   *(48:293–305)*

60. **False.** The systolic murmur is probably due to atrioventricular valve insufficiency.   *(1:181–187)*

REFERENCES

References appear on page 160.

CHAPTER 5

GENERAL ABDOMINAL SONOGRAPHY

Trudy Dubinsky, Arthur C. Fleischer, and Rena Dubinsky

Study Guide

LIVER

The liver is intraperitoneal. This means that it is surrounded by peritoneum except for a segment known as the bare area posterior to the dome of the liver.

Riedel's lobe is a normal variant of the right lobe of the liver whereby the right lobe projects inferiorly and may be mistaken for a pseudotumor.

Lobes, Ligaments, and Fissures (Figs. 5–1 and 5–2)

Lobes. The liver is divided into three lobes: the *right*—anterior and posterior segments; the *left*—medial (quadrate) and lateral segments; and the *caudate*—lies on the posterosuperior surface of the liver.

Guidelines. Hepatic veins are intersegmental (outlining the segments of the liver). They subdivide the liver as follows: (1) middle hepatic vein—divides the liver into right and left lobes; (2) left hepatic vein—divides the left lobe into medial and lateral segments; and (3) right hepatic vein—divides the right lobe into anterior and posterior segments. Both the right and left hepatic veins drain blood from the caudate lobe.

Since hepatic veins can only be recognized sonographically on superior sections of the liver, additional landmarks such as ligaments and fissures are needed. These landmarks may be used to define segmental anatomy on more caudad sections.

Table 5–1 is a guide to the anatomic structures useful in defining segmental anatomy.

Ligamentum Venosum. The ligamentum venosum is a remnant of the fetal ductus venosus. It divides the caudate lobe from the left lobe. It may be visualized sonographically on transverse and longitudinal scans as an echogenic line extending transversely from the porta hepatis.

Ligamentum Teres. The ligamentum teres is a remnant of the fetal umbilical vein, which lies in the left intersegmental fissure, dividing the left lobe of the liver into medial and lateral segments. Sonographically, it may be visualized on a transverse scan as a round hyperechoic density just to the right of the midline.

Falciform Ligament. The falciform ligament is the portion of the peritoneum reflected around the ligamentum teres, attaching the liver to the diaphragm and abdominal wall.

Main Lobar Fissure. Main lobar fissures separate the right and left lobes and may be visualized sonographically as an echogenic line extending from the porta hepatis to the neck of the gallbladder.

Parenchymal Architecture

The normal liver is homogeneous in texture, and its echogenicity may be compared to renal sinus > pancreas > liver > spleen > renal cortex.

Vasculature of the Liver—Hepatic Vein, Portal Vein, Hepatic Artery

Hepatic Vein. There are three hepatic veins: right, middle, and left. These veins drain into the inferior vena cava.

Portal Vein. The portal vein is formed by the confluence of the splenic vein and the superior mesenteric vein. It courses cephalad and rightward into the porta hepatis, bifurcating into right and left. The main *undivided* portal trunk lies immediately anterior to the inferior vena cava, just cephalad to the head of the pancreas and caudal to the caudate lobe.

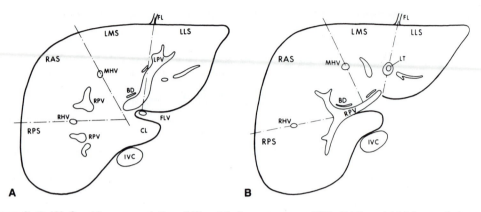

Figure 5–1. (A) Graphic representation. IVC = inferior vena cava; RPS, RAS = right lobe posterior and anterior segments; LMS, LLS = medial and lateral segments of left lobe; FLV = fissure of ligamentum venosum; RPV = right portal vein branch; RHV, MHV = right and middle hepatic veins; BD = bile duct. **(B)** Graphic representation. IVC = inferior vena cava; RPS, RAS = right lobe posterior and anterior segments; LMS, LLS = medial and lateral segments of left lobe; FL = falciform ligament; LT = ligamentum teres. *(Reprinted with permission from Sexton CC, Zeman RK. Correlation of computed tomography, sonography and gross anatomy of the liver. AJR 141:711–718, 1983.)*

Figure 5–2. (A) Lobes, ligaments, and fissures. **(B)** Anterior projection of the liver. **(C)** Posterior projection of the liver.

TABLE 5–1. ANATOMIC STRUCTURES USEFUL FOR DIVIDING AND IDENTIFYING THE HEPATIC SEGMENTS

Structure	Location	Usefulness
RHV	Right intersegmental fissure	Divides cephalic aspect of anterior and posterior segments of right hepatic lobe and courses between anterior and posterior branches of RPV
MHV	Main lobar fissure	Separates right and left lobes
LHV	Left intersegmental fissure	Divides cephalic aspects of medial and lateral segments of left lobe
RPV (anterior)	Intrasegmental in anterior segment of right hepatic lobe	Courses centrally in anterior segment of right hepatic lobe
RPV (posterior)	Intrasegmental in posterior segment of right hepatic lobe	Courses centrally in posterior segment of right hepatic lobe
LPV (initial)	Courses anterior to caudate lobe	Separates caudate lobe posteriorly from medial segment of left lobe anteriorly
LPV (ascending)	Turns anteriorly in left intersegmental fissure	Divides medial and lateral segments of left lobe
IVC fossa	Posterior aspect of main lobar fissure	Separates right and left hepatic lobes
GB fossa	Main lobar fissure	Separates right and left hepatic lobes
Ligamentum teres	Left intersegmental fissure	Divides caudal aspect of left hepatic lobe into medial and lateral segments
Fissure of ligamentum venosum	Left anterior margin of caudate lobe	Separates caudate lobe from medial and lateral segments of left lobe

Reprinted with permission from Callen PW: J Clin Ultrasound 7(2):81, 1979, and John Wiley & Sons, Inc.

The left portal vein is also the umbilical portion of the portal vein, which is of variable size. Organs of the gastrointestinal tract, the gallbladder, the pancreas, and the spleen are drained by the tributaries of the portal vein that enter the liver via the main portal vein to bring nutrients to the liver cells.

How does one differentiate sonographically between portal veins and hepatic veins?

1. Portal veins have brighter walls owing to collagen within the wall
2. The branching angles have different orientation:
   a. Portal veins branch horizontally and are oriented toward the porta hepatis
   b. Hepatic veins branch longitudinally and are oriented toward the inferior vena cava
3. The caliber of a hepatic vein increases as it courses toward the diaphragm and inferior vena cava
4. The caliber of the portal vein increases as it nears the porta hepatis
5. Hepatic veins will vary in size during respiration

How does one differentiate sonographically between portal vein and bile duct? These are not to be confused in the normal liver because one does not see intrahepatic bile ducts unless there is dilatation due to disease or obstruction.

Hepatic Artery. The hepatic artery is visualized normally on transverse scans at the level of the hepatoduodenal ligament (just cephalad to the head of the pancreas and adjacent to the porta hepatis). Both the common bile duct and hepatic artery lie anterior to the portal vein at this level, with the common bile duct being more lateral.

PORTAL TRIAD

Portal vein
Hepatic artery } All travel together in a collagenous sheath (Glisson's capsule) extending throughout the liver.
Bile duct

Common Bile Duct. The common bile duct runs posterior to the head of the pancreas to enter the duodenum. This can be visualized on a sagittal or a right anterior oblique scan.

Several diseases of the liver with clinical findings, supporting laboratory data and sonographic anatomy are detailed in Tables 5–2 to 5–5.

Table 5–6 offers a simplified guide to laboratory tests for specific liver diseases.

GALLBLADDER

The gallbladder is a pear-shaped structure lying in a fossa on the visceral surface of the liver. It is attached to the lateral portion of the porta hepatis at the cystic duct. The cystic duct runs inferiorly and joins the common hepatic duct to form the common bile duct.

The gallbladder has a fundus, body, and neck. Hartmann's pouch is that portion of the neck that is closest to the cystic duct. Stones tend to accumulate at this point and cause obstruction. The cystic duct is markedly tortuous at its junction with the neck of the gallbladder. This is termed the spiral valve of Heister, which is a misnomer because it is not a true valve; bile flows freely in both

TABLE 5–2. FOCAL DISEASE OF THE LIVER

	Clinical Findings	Laboratory Data	Sonographic Anatomy
Cysts			
Congenital			
Simple liver cyst	Asymptomatic, may cause hepatomegaly	Normal liver function	Echo-free Smooth regular walls Posterior enhancement, usually solitary
Polycystic disease	More than 50% associated with renal polycystic disease; produces gross hepatomegaly and usually does not interfere with liver function	Normal liver function	Multiple cysts of various sizes found within the liver parenchyma
Acquired Lesions			
Traumatic (hematoma)	RUQ pain, hepatomegaly, hypotension	Drop in hematocrit Leukocytosis	Mixed echo pattern; may be predominantly cystic (fresh blood) to predominantly echogenic, chronic condition (old blood) Irregular walls Some through transmission—less than a cyst but more than a solid structure
Inflammatory lesions (abscess)	Fever, chills, RUQ pain, hepatomegaly	Leukocytosis	Predominantly fluid filled; with variable amounts of echos and irregular borders An abscess may contain gas or calcification—watch for shadowing
Hydatid cysts	Asymptomatic or RUQ pain and hepatomegaly—the tapeworm *Echinococcus* causes infection, with sheep, pigs, or cows being the intermediate host	Positive Casoni test Eosinophilia	Well-circumscribed cystic mass with smaller cysts surrounding or within it to give a multilocular appearance; the smaller cysts may contain echoes and/or calcification; when only one cyst is present, it cannot be differentiated from a simple cyst
Primary Solid Tumor			
Benign			
Liver cell adenoma	Most common in women who used oral contraceptive pills Patients present with palpable abdominal mass	Normal liver function	Well-defined solid mass of increased echogenicity
Focal nodular hyperplasia (FNH)	Similar to adenoma occurs in both sexes	Normal liver function	Variable sonographic pattern, usually echogenic
Cavernous hemangioma (most common benign tumor)	Generally asymptomatic; most lesions are small but may become quite large		Variable and nonspecific—cannot be distinguished, eg, from hepatomas, adenomas

Malignant
  Primary hepatic tumors
    Hepatomas (hepatocellular carcinoma) associated with longstanding cirrhosis
    Hepatoblastoma—found in children
    Angiocarcinoma
    Bile duct tumor
    Sarcoma
	Primary findings (acute): jaundice, weight loss, hepatomegaly, palpable mass; (chronic): ascites, portal hypertension, splenomegaly	Abnormal hepatocellular function, increased alkaline phosphatase, increased levels of α-fetoprotein in serum	Variable and nonspecific, small or large, diffuse or circumscribed—cannot be distinguished from a benign or metastatic tumor
			Portal vein thrombosis, highly suggestive of hepatoma

(continued)

TABLE 5–2. (*Continued*)

	Clinical Findings	Laboratory Data	Sonographic Anatomy
Metastatic Solid Tumor			

Metastatic spread to the liver is common	Hepatomegaly, weight loss, RUQ pain, ascites, jaundice, splenomegaly	Abnormal hepatocellular function, increased serum bilirubin
		
		Increased alkaline phosphatase
			Variable patterns
			  Well-defined echogenic mass—search the intestines and urogenital tract for the primary
			  Well-defined echo-poor mass—may come from any primary
			  Defined calcific masses—may come from ovary, colon, or rectum
			  Diffuse, miliary—may come from any primary
			  Cystic mass—mucin secreting, especially ovary and pancreas

Lymphoma	Hepatomegaly, splenomegaly retroperitoneal nodes		Decreased echogenicity
Diffuse Liver Disease			
Fatty change—accumulation of fat within the hepatocytes	Causes: alcoholism, by-pass surgery for obesity, corticosteroid administration, malignancy, diabetes mellitus, obesity, protein malnutrition	Abnormal hepatocellular function	Liver enlarges especially the left and/or caudate lobe Regenerating nodules Liver is unduly bright and echogenic As the disease progresses, there is a loss of through transmission; decreased visibility of vessels
Cirrhosis—diffuse fibrotic process that involves the entire liver	Chronic injury to hepatocyte. May develop portal hypertension, ascites, splenomegaly, collateral circulation; jaundice may be seen Alcohol abuse is by far the most common cause	Abnormal hepatocellular function Slight increase in AST (SGOT) and ALT (SGPT) Alkaline phosphatase may or may not be elevated	Liver is shrunken and very echogenic; disproportionate enlargement of caudate lobe Through transmission is very poor Irregular shape; regenerating nodules Ascites Collateral vessels will be seen in the region Patent umbilical vein in severe portal hypertension; cannot trace the course of the major hepatic veins
Hepatitis			
Viral hepatitis is a diffuse inflammatory process of the liver; types: A, B, and non-A, non-B	Malaise, nausea, fever, and pain followed by jaundice. Liver is enlarged and tender	Elevation of SGOT and SGPT over 1000 units Serum bilirubin increased Alkaline phosphatase increased	Acute hepatitis—the echogenicity of the liver is reduced, the renal cortex being more echogenic than the liver Chronic hepatitis—the echogenicity is that of a bright liver as in early cirrhosis with increased echogenicity of portal veins Acute and/or chronic hepatitis—patchy liver, areas of increased and decreased echogenicity; hepatomegaly

(*continued*)

TABLE 5–2. (Continued)

	Clinical Findings	Laboratory Data	Sonographic Anatomy
Chronic Passive Congestion of the Liver			
	History of heart failure Hepatomegaly, dilatation of the inferior vena cava	Normal or slightly abnormal hepatocellular function	Texture changes are similar to those seen in fatty infiltrate of the liver; changes are accompanied by dilatation of the hepatic veins, inferior vena cava, mesenteric, and splenic veins, hepatomegaly
Glycogen Storage Disease			
Groups of hereditary disorders of carbohydrate metabolism resulting in glycogen accumulation in hepatocytes	Hypoglycemia Decreased glucose-6-phosphatase		Hepatomegaly Diffuse increased liver echogenicity Splenomegaly

TABLE 5–3. VASCULAR ABNORMALITIES WITHIN THE LIVER

	Etiology	Clinical Findings	Sonographic Findings
Portal hypertension	Owing to cirrhosis in >90% of cases. May be due to obstruction, tumors, or prolonged congestive heart failure	Ascites—46% Formation of collateral venous channels Splenomegaly GI bleeding as a consequence of abnormal venous channels	Portal vein enlargement, >1.3 cm Lack of distension of the splenic and superior mesenteric veins during respiration Patent umbilical vein >3 mm bull's-eye pattern in the ligamentum teres Splenorenal, gastrorenal, hemorrhoidal, intestinal varices
Portal vein obstruction	Related to thrombosis or direct invasion of the portal vein by tumors	Associated with hepatocellular carcinoma, pancreatic, GI cancer or lymphoma	Nonvisualization of the portal vein Echogenic material within the portal vein Dilatation of the splenic and superior mesenteric veins proximal to the point of obstruction
Budd-Chiari syndrome	Caused by obstruction of the hepatic veins	The liver becomes enlarged and tender with ascites. The most common finding is unexplained partial or complete fibrous obliteration of the major hepatic veins	An enlarged and hypoechoic caudate lobe Reduced or nonvisualization of hepatic veins Ascites

TABLE 5–4. CAUSES OF JAUNDICE

Medical Jaundice (Nonobstructive)		Surgical Jaundice (Obstructive)
Hepatocellular Disease—disturbance within the liver cells that interferes with the excretion of bilirubin Hepatitis Drug-induced cholestasis Fatty liver (most commonly caused by alcohol) Cirrhosis	Hemolytic Disease—an increase in red blood cell destruction; the hepatocytes cannot deal with the severe hemolysis efficiently with resulting increase in indirect bilirubin (nonobstructive jaundice) Sickle-cell anemia Cooley's anemia	Interference with flow of bile caused by obstruction of the biliary tract, typical course includes Choledocholithiasis Pancreatitis Pancreatic pseudocyst Mass in the head of pancreas Hepatoma Metastatic carcinoma Cholangiocarcinoma Mass in the portahepatis (enlarged lymph nodes)

TABLE 5–5. LIVER FUNCTION TESTS

1. Alkaline Phosphatase: Normally found in serum. Its level rises in liver and biliary tract disorders when excretion is impaired, as in obstructive jaundice, biliary cirrhosis, acute hepatitis, and granulomatous liver disease.

2. α-Fetoprotein (AFP): A protein produced by fetal liver, yolk sac, GI tract, and hepatocellular carcinoma (hepatoma) germ cell neoplasms and other cancers in adults. AFP level used to monitor chemotherapy treatment and prenatal diagnosis neural tube defects in fetus. Rarely positive in other cases.

3. Ammonia:
   Normally metabolized in the liver and excreted as urea
   Increased in hepatocellular disease

4. Bromsulfalein Retention (BSP):
   After IV rejection of the dye, BSP is bound to albumin and is removed from the blood by the liver
   If liver is not functioning properly, abnormal amounts of BSP remain in the blood
   Diseases with large retained amounts of BSP:
   Acute hepatitis (83%)
   Cirrhosis (87%)
   Extrahepatic obstruction (79%)
   Metastatic liver cancer (93–100%)
   Chronic congestion (88%)

5. Bilirubin:
   Derived from the breakdown of hemoglobin in red blood cells
   Excreted by the liver in the bile (main pigment)
   When destruction of red blood cells increases greatly or when the liver is unable to excrete normal amounts, the bilirubin concentration in the serum increases
   If increased too high, jaundice may occur
   Intrahepatic and extrahepatic obstruction may be determined by the levels of indirect and direct bilirubin
   Obstruction is indicated by the increase in direct bilirubin
   Increased red blood cell destruction/hemolysis is indicated by an increase in indirect bilirubin

6. Casoni Test: Blood test positive for eosinophilia, tapeworm echinococcal disease, hydatid cysts

7. Hematocrit: Volume percentage of erythrocytes in whole blood. A drop in hematocrit can indicate hematoma due to liver trauma.

8. Leukocytosis: A substantial increase in white blood cells above normal limits as in inflammatory lesions or abscess in liver.

9. Prothrombin Time:
   Prothrombin is converted to thrombin in the clotting process by action of vitamin K that is absorbed in the intestine and stored in the liver
   In obstructive liver disease, IV administration of vitamin K returns prothrombin time to normal
   In parenchymal tissue disease, vitamin K injection will not alter the prothrombin time
   Deficiency can cause uncontrolled hemorrhage

10. Aspartate Aminotransferase (AST), formerly Serum Glutamic Oxaloacetic Transaminase (SGOT):
    This enzyme is increased in liver cell necrosis due to:
    Viral hepatitis
    Toxic hepatitis
    Other acute forms of hepatitis
    Helpful in detecting acute hepatitis before jaundice occurs and in following the course of hepatitis
    No significant increase occurs in chronic liver disease such as cirrhosis or obstructive jaundice

11. Alanine Aminotransferase (ALT), formerly Serum Glutamic Pyruvic Transminase (SGPT):
    This enzyme is increased higher than SGOT in hepatitis
    It falls slowly and reaches normal levels in 2–3 months
    SGPT is especially valuable in assessing jaundice
    If jaundice is caused by liver cell disease
    >300 U
    If jaundice is due to a condition outside the liver
    <300 U

12. Urinary Bile and Bilirubin:
    There may be spillover into the blood in:
    Obstructive liver disease
    Excessive red blood cell destruction
    Bile pigments are found in urine when there is obstruction of the biliary tract
    Bilirubin is found alone when there is excessive breakdown of red blood cells
    Bile and bilirubin are not normally found in urine

13. Urinary Urobilinogen:
    This test differentiates between:
    Complete obstruction of the biliary tract
    Incomplete obstruction of the biliary tract
    Urobilinogen is a product of hemoglobin breakdown and may be elevated in:
    Hemolytic diseases
    Liver damage
    Severe infections
    Urobilinogen does not increase or there is no excess amount found in urine in cases of complete obstructive jaundice

14. Fecal Urobilinogen:
    Considerable amounts are found in the feces but an increase or decrease in normal amounts may indicate hepatic digestive abnormalities
    Decrease with complete obstruction of biliary tree
    Increase may suggest an increase in hemolysis

Nuclear Medicine Tests

Planar Liver Scan: Radioactive isotope is injected—an area that does not take up the radiopharmaceutical (cold spot) will signify abscess, tumor, necrotic/abnormal tissue, or a cirrhotic liver
SPECT Liver Scan: Used for ruling out hemangiomas and is more precise in locating and resolving space-occupying lesions

---

directions owing to pressure gradients. Physiologically, the gallbladder contracts in response to cholecystokinin, the release of which is stimulated by food in the gut.

Congenital anomalies of the gallbladder are rare, though a gallbladder may be intrahepatic or may have septations or folds. When the fundus of the gallbladder is sharply bent over itself, it is termed a phrygian cap, a fold or kink between the body and infundibulum of the gallbladder, also termed a junctional fold.

The gallbladder is a thin-walled structure having a maximum wall thickness of 3 mm. Table 5–7 outlines causes of gallbladder wall thickness.

TABLE 5–6. SUMMARY OF LABORATORY TESTS IN SPECIFIC LIVER DIAGNOSES

	Hematological Disease	Hepatitis	Cirrhosis	Obstructive Jaundice	Carcinoma
SGOT		++	+	+	+
SGPT		+++	+	+	+
Alkaline Phosphatase		+	+	+++	++
α-Fetoprotein					+++
Bilirubin					
Indirect	+++				
Direct		+++	+++	+++	
Ammonia		+++			

Symbols: + = increase; ++ = marked increase; +++ = very marked increase.

Causes of a Large Gallbladder

A large gallbladder can be caused by prolonged fasting; IV hyperalimentation; obstruction of the cystic duct (hydrops of the gallbladder); and obstruction of the distal common bile duct (the gallbladder will enlarge before the biliary tree because it has the greatest surface). Therefore, if one encounters a patient with an enlarged gallbladder and slightly dilated common bile duct with an increase in serum bilirubin, one should suspect a common duct obstruction.

Other causes of a large gallbladder include a Courvoisier gallbladder, which constitutes any enlarged gallbladder due to any malignancy affecting the distal common bile duct (pancreatic carcinoma, common duct carcinoma, or duodenal carcinoma; diabetes (long-standing insulin diabetes), and postvagotomy.

Causes of a Small Gallbladder

A small gallbladder usually presents after the patient has eaten. It can also be caused by congenital hypoplasia (extremely rare); chronic cholecystitis (the gallbladder becomes chronically scarred); biliary obstruction (at the

level of the common hepatic duct, before the entry of the cystic duct—bile is not going to pass the obstruction and will not be able to fill the gallbladder); and hepatitis (bile production down).

Gallbladder Disease

Cholelithiasis—Intraluminal Echoes with Shadowing. Gallstones have 100% confidence if you demonstrate three criteria:

1. echogenic focus—echogenic due to the acoustic mismatch between stones and bile
2. acoustic shadow—most of the sound is absorbed with very little sound going through, producing a shadow
3. gravity dependent—put patient in decubitus position; the stones should be gravity dependent and fall to the gallbladder (GB) fundus

Beware. Causes of acoustic shadowing in the area of the GB are:

- spiral valves of Heister—folds in the neck of GB

TABLE 5–7. GALLBLADDER WALL THICKENING

Causes of Gallbladder Wall Thickening >3 mm	Sonographic Features
1. Contracted normal gallbladder 2. Inappropriate TGC and/or gain 3. Ascites } The gallbladder wall will appear thickened	
4. Hypoproteinemia (hypoalbuminemia): patient has inadequate amount of serum protein. Patients will have thickened bowel and gallbladder walls	Diffuse thickening of the gallbladder wall
5. Congestive heart failure (CHF): patient will have thickened bowel and gallbladder wall	
6. Acute hepatitis—sympathetic infection: gallbladder responds to the infection in the liver	
7. Carcinoma—primary or secondary: gallbladder wall irregularly thickened, associated with cholelithiasis	Irregular thickening of the gallbladder wall with cholelithiasis
8. Cholecystitis—acute or chronic: any inflammation will cause edema of the walls	Thickening of the gallbladder wall with associated cholelithiasis
9. Adenomyomatosis–noninflammatory gallbladder disease	An outpouching of the surface epithelium into the gallbladder wall and hypertrophy of the muscular layer of the wall; present in 25% of all patients, yet only 5% have symptoms; is associated with cholelithiasis
10. AIDS	Thickening of the gallbladder wall[44]

- edge effect—in any cystic structure, you might get refraction at the fluid, with the solid surface producing a shadow at the periphery due to refraction of sound. This will be seen especially on transverse sections of the GB
- junctional fold—normal fold between neck and body
- loop of duodenum

Intraluminal Echoes Without Shadowing/With Motility. The causes of intraluminal echoes with shadowing and with motility are viscous bile, sludge, blood, or pus. Sludge is made up of cholesterol crystals and bilirubin precipitate. Sludge is of no clinical significance, and not all sludge goes on to develop stones. Sludge will be present in:

- people who have been fasting for long periods of time will develop sludge owing to hypotonic gallbladder
- alcoholics have sludge for unknown reasons
- patients with biliary obstruction—the GB cannot empty well owing to the obstruction and stasis of bile ensues
- patients on IV hyperalimentation

Important Differential. If the patient is febrile, toxic, and hypotensive with extreme right upper quadrant pain and the GB is visualized filled with multiple intraluminal echoes, thickened wall, or with stones, this may represent hemorrhage or pus in a gangrenous or emphysematous GB.

Intraluminal Echoes Without Shadowing and Without Motility. The causes of intraluminal echoes without shadowing and without motility are:

- polyps
- GB carcinoma (CA)—the most common primary malignancy of the biliary tree. Pancreatic CA is the most common CA to *obstruct* the biliary tree

Gallbladder carcinoma presents in many ways:
- solid mass in the head of the GB fossa with no bile filling the lumen
- diffusely irregular GB, with thickened wall and a small lumen
- symmetrically thickened
- soft tissue mass that casts shadow but is not gravity dependent
- GB carcinoma associated with stones
- chronic cholecystitis may lead to GB carcinoma
- artifacts, eg, partial volume
- mucosal folds, eg, junctional fold at the junction of the GB body and neck
- cholesterosis—strawberry GB (multiple fixed mural plaques)
- adenomyomatosis—Rokitansky-Aschoff sinuses

Sonographic Nonvisualization of the Gallbladder. The reasons for nonvisualization of the GB sonographically are: patient is not NPO and is physiologically contracted; duodenal gas or gas in the hepatic flexure; if the

patient has had a cholecystectomy; ectopic GB; chronic cholecystitis with stones filling the lumen; and solid mass obliterating the GB. If you do not see the GB at all, but you see highly reflective shadows coming from where the GB should be, follow main lobar fissure from right portal vein to the GB fossa. It may be a completely contracted GB.

Beware. Causes of shadow simulators are:

- bowel, not a clear shadow
- high-level echoes within the liver
- air in the biliary tree from surgery. When you connect the common bile duct (CBD) to the jejunum (Whipple procedure), the sphincter of Oddi that normally blocks objects from going into biliary tree is now open
- sphincter of Oddi becomes fibrotic owing to the constant passage of stones and remains open
- fistula in GB or ducts allows air in
- porcelain GB—calcium in the wall of the GB; 20% of patients with porcelain GB will develop CA, and this is an indicator for cholecystectomy

Cholecystitis—Inflammation of the Gallbladder. Acute cholecystitis is inflammation of the GB wall, promoted by an obstruction of the cystic duct, usually by a stone. The problem with cholecystitis is that it sometimes presents as a calculus without stones or halo effect.

Chronic cholecystitis is the most common form of symptomatic GB disease and is associated with gallstones in 90% of the cases.

Table 5–8 outlines the sonographic and clinical findings for acute and chronic cholecystitis.

Complications of Cholecystitis. Emphysematous GB, porcelain GB, and carcinoma of the GB are complications of cholecystitis.

Emphysematous Gallbladder

- more common in males than in females
- occurs as a result of anaerobic infection (clostridia)
- signs and symptoms—right upper quadrant (RUQ) pain, fever and leukocytosis
- sonographic finding is the appearance of gas in the GB wall
- cholelithiasis in only 50%
- gangrene in 75%; perforation in 20%

Porcelain Gallbladder

- calcification of the GB wall
- associated cancer 10–20%
- frequently associated with cholelithiasis 95% of the time
- three sonographic patterns:
  1. echogenic line in GB fossa with posterior shadowing
  2. echogenic near and far walls with some shadowing
  3. irregular clumps of wall echoes with shadowing

TABLE 5–8. ACUTE VERSUS CHRONIC CHOLECYSTITIS

Etiology	Clinical Findings	Sonographic Findings
Acute Cholecystitis		
1. Obstruction of cystic duct by calculi 80–95% 2. Bacterial infection within biliary tract 3. Pancreatic reflux	1. RUQ pain, especially postprandial 2. Vomiting 3. Positive Murphy's sign 4. Leukocytosis	1. Enlarged gallbladder 2. Thickened gallbladder wall >3 mm (usually >5 mm) 3. Halo sign suggesting subserosal edema 4. Sludge or stone 5. Occasionally, one can see bizarre echoes in the gallbladder wall suggestive of necrosis, as in acute gangrene
Chronic Cholecystitis—Recurrent Inflammatory Changes		
1. Gallbladder mucosa scarred and inflamed due to previous infections 2. Long-standing intermittent presence of stones impacting cystic duct	1. Gallbladder usually is nontender	1. Stones 2. Generally small or normal gallbladder 3. Thickened gallbladder wall 4. Double arc and shadowing. The first arc is the gallbladder wall and the second is the stone followed by the shadow that represents contracted gallbladder with stone—WES sign: W = wall of gallbladder; E = echo of calculi; S = shadow of calculi

Carcinoma of the gallbladder

- more common in women than men
- etiology: gallbladder stones?
- signs and symptoms—RUQ pain, obstructive jaundice, cholangitis
- sonographically, thickened GB walls, poorly defined mass in the RUQ, and gallstones always exist

Benign Tumors of the Gallbladder. Polyps, hyperplastic cholecystoses, and adenomas are benign GB tumors.

Polyps. Most of polyps are not true neoplasms but rather cholesterol polyps. They do not shadow and do not move as the patient moves.

Hyperplastic Cholecystoses (Adenomyomatosis). This is characterized by:

- hyperplasia of epithelial and muscular elements of GB wall
- epithelial lined intramural diverticula (Rokitansky-Aschoff sinuses)
- localized, annular and diffuse varieties
- most common in fundus
- ultrasound demonstrates:
  1. nonspecific wall thickening; Rokitansky-Aschoff sinuses add specificity
  2. Rokitansky-Aschoff sinuses may be filled with bile, sludge, or calculi and thus vary from anechoic to echogenic with distal shadow or reverberation

3. segmental disease may appear as focal wall thickening or bandlike constriction

Adenomas (pedunculated adenomatous polyps). These have been associated with CA in certain situations. They do not shadow and do not move.

Causes of pericholecystic fluid are acute cholecystitis, pericholecystic abscess, ascites, pancreatitis, peritonitis, and acquired immunodeficiency syndrome (AIDS).

Causes of gallstones in children are hemolysis, e.g., sickle cell disease, cystic fibrosis, malabsorption syndrome (Crohn's disease), hepatitis, and congenital biliary anomalies (choledochal cyst, biliary atresia).

BILE DUCTS

Intrahepatic radicles in the liver converge to form the main right and left hepatic ducts at the porta hepatis. The right and left hepatic ducts unite to form the common hepatic duct.

The common hepatic duct joins with the cystic duct to form the common bile duct (Fig. 5–3). The common bile duct travels along the hepatoduodenal ligament (ligament between the liver and duodenum), behind the duodenal bulb and posterior aspect of the pancreatic head to enter the second portion of the duodenum. The common bile duct joins with the pancreatic duct at the ampulla of Vater.

The extrahepatic biliary tree or common duct is always anterior to the portal vein.

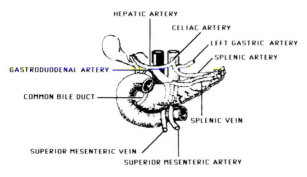

Figure 5-3. The common bile duct and surrounding vasculature.

The normal common bile duct measures ≤8 mm in luminal diameter, not including the wall. In older patients who are not jaundiced and have no pain, a common bile duct of 10–12 mm may be considered normal. This is due to the common bile duct becoming ectatic with age.

An enlarged common bile duct after a cholecystomy is normal, but one must rule out retained stones in the common bile duct or postoperative stricture.

The portion of the duct that is seen anterior to the right portal vein is the common hepatic duct. The common hepatic duct measures ≤4 or 5 mm.

The cystic duct is not seen sonographically, and intrahepatic biliary radicles are not visualized unless dilated.

Improper functioning of the bile duct and/or liver malfunction can cause jaundice (Table 5–4).

Sonographic Criteria for Biliary Tree Dilatation—Intrahepatic[31]

1. The bile duct runs anterior to the portal veins. When dilated, the sonographer will see the parallel channel sign (double-barrel shotgun sign)
2. Too many tubular structures are visible in the periphery of the liver
3. Stellate formation of the tubes near the porta hepatis
4. Enhancement of echoes distal to the ducts

Sonographic Criteria for Biliary Tree Dilatation—Extrahepatic[31]

1. Common bile duct lumen is larger than 6 mm
2. False-negative obstruction. If obstruction happens within 12 to 24 hours prior to sonography, the ducts may not yet be dilated
3. False-positive obstruction. The dilated common bile duct might be present, but no stone is present because the patient will have passed the stone

Table 5–9 outlines how to locate bile duct obstruction.

TABLE 5–9. LOCATING THE POINT OF COMMON BILE DUCT OBSTRUCTION

Remember—the ducts dilate proximal to the site of obstruction.

Intrahepatic biliary dilatation Common bile duct (normal) Gallbladder (normal)	1. Look for bile duct tumors, ie, cholangiocarcinoma, Klatskin tumor. Suspect stone in common hepatic duct. If biliary dilatation is confined to one lobe or another, suspect stone in right or left hepatic duct 2. Sclerosing cholangitis—inflammation and fibrosis of bile duct, with intrahepatic calculi a common complication. 3. Metastatic involvement and enlargement of porta hepatis lymph nodes 4. Biliary atresia is the most common and fatal liver disorder in children in the United States. Jaundice is the most common symptom. 5. Choledochal cyst—fusiform dilatation of the bile duct. Bile ducts are dilated above that point
Intrahepatic biliary dilatation Common bile duct dilatation Gallbladder enlarged	1. Stones in the common bile duct 2. Pseudocyst obstructing common bile duct 3. Acute pancreatitis—swollen pancreatic head will lead to obstructed bile flow 4. Chronic pancreatitis—fibrotic and shrunken pancreas will lead to obstructed bile flow 5. Carcinoma of the pancreatic head
Intrahepatic biliary dilatation Common bile duct dilatation Gallbladder small	Chronic cholecystitis

Congenital Anomalies of the Bile Ducts

The Jaundiced Infant

Biliary Atresia. This is the most common fatal liver disorder in children in the United States. In atresia of *intrahepatic radicles,* there is *no sonographic evidence of biliary* radicles. The condition is *untreatable.*

In atresia of *extrahepatic radicles,* there is an anastomosis of the biliary tree to the jejunum; in this case, you will see dilated intrahepatic radicles.

The Jaundiced Child

Choledochal Cyst. Cystic dilation and outpouching of the wall, involving *the common duct.* Classic triad is patient with jaundice, RUQ pain, RUQ mass.[26] Diagnosed sonographically by demonstrating common duct or biliary radicles going into the cystic mass. This will help in the diagnosis of choledochal cyst. Also, the sonographer must see GB separate from the cyst.

Caroli's Disease. Caroli's disease is an inherited trait characterized by a segmental saccular dilatation of the *intrahepatic ducts.* It may be associated with cystic kidney disease, in particular renal tubular ectasia. Caroli's disease leads to bile stasis, stones, bacterial growth, abscesses, cholangitis, and decreased liver function due to compression of hepatocytes.

Sonographically, Caroli's disease presents as multiple liver cysts continuous with the biliary tree; stones and echoes may appear within the biliary ducts.

Cholangitis

Inflammation of the bile ducts caused by bacterial infection of the biliary tract is almost always associated with obstruction; eg, choledocholithiosis, biliary stricture, and neoplasms. The signs and symptoms are Charcot's triad (biliary colic), jaundice, and chills and fever. Laboratory tests show leukocytosis, increased serum bilirubin, increased alkaline phosphatase, and bacteremia.

Choledocholithiasis

Calculi in the common bile duct is usually caused by GB stones. The signs and symptoms are biliary colic, jaundice, episodes of cholangitis, and GB stones. Laboratory tests show increased serum bilirubin and increased serum alkaline phosphatase. Sonographically, stones can be seen in the duct.

Acquired Immunodeficiency Syndrome (AIDS)

In AIDS, dilated ducts may be seen in the context of right upper quadrant (RUQ) pain, increased liver function tests, and jaundice. These signs and symptoms are thought to be secondary to papillary inflammation and edema. The probable cause is cytomegalovirus, *Cryptospordium,* or *Mycobacterium avium intracellulare.* A sclerosing cholangitislike pattern may develop with irregular areas of dilatation and duct wall thickening.[44]

Malignant Tumors of the Biliary Tree

Adenocarcinoma and Squamous Cell Carcinoma. Signs and symptoms are anorexia, weight loss, right upper quadrant pain, and jaundice. Predisposing factors associated with carcinoma of the biliary tree are inflammation, cholelithiasis and chronic ulcerative colitis.[24] All branches of the biliary tree may be affected, from the common bile duct to the smallest biliary radicle. A *Klatskin tumor* is the name given to carcinoma arising at the confluence of the hepatic ducts. This location offers the worst prognosis for it allows considerable obstruction to occur before the tumor attains a significant size to be diagnosed.[24]

Sonographic Appearance of Klatskin Tumor. Dilatation of the intrahepatic ducts but not the extrahepatic ducts is seen. The tumor usually occurs at union of the right and left hepatic ducts. It presents as a small, solid mass of the hepatic hilum. Lymphadenopathy is commonly associated with Klatskin tumor.

Nuclear Medicine Test

Hepato Biliary Scan. To rule out cystic and/or common bile duct obstruction, fat-soluble radionuclide is injected. If both the cystic duct and common bile duct are patent, the radionuclide will appear in the GB and bowel within a half hour postinjection.

PANCREAS

The pancreas lies transversely in the body within the retroperitoneal cavity. The gland is divided into head, body, and tail (from right to left). The boundaries of the pancreas are arbitrary, relating to its surrounding anatomy. The size and shape of the pancreas can be variable, and it is relatively larger in children than in adults. Approximate normal measurements are, head—2.5 cm, body—2.0 cm, and tail—2.0 cm in anteroposterior dimension.

The head of the pancreas is anterior to the inferior vena cava and right renal vein and medial to the second portion of the duodenum. The common bile duct can be seen on the posterolateral margin of the pancreatic head. The gastroduodenal artery is located on the anterolateral surface. Both will appear as sonolucent circular structures within the head of the pancreas.

The pancreatic body is the largest part of the gland. It lies anterior to the superior mesenteric vein, superior mesenteric artery, splenic vein, and aorta. Posterior to the superior mesenteric artery and anterior to the aorta, one also can visualize the left renal vein.

The pancreatic tail lies anterior to the left kidney and medial to the splenic hilum. The splenic artery forms the superior border and the splenic vein the posterior border.

Extending the entire length of the gland is the pancreatic duct. The primary duct is called Wirsung's duct. It enters the second part of the duodenum at the ampulla of Vater along with the common bile duct. The secondary duct is called Santorini's duct. It enters the second part of the duodenum separately, approximately 2 cm proximal to the ampulla of Vater.

Fig. 5–4 demonstrates the pancreas and its related landmarks.

The echogenicity pattern of the pancreas consists of fine homogeneous echoes equal to, or more echogenic than, the normal liver. Since the pancreas has no true capsule, it tends to blend in with the surrounding retroperitoneal fat. The pancreatic duct can be commonly seen as a cystic tubular structure running from the head to the tail of the pancreas. Its normal caliber is 2–3 mm, being largest in the head, and decreasing in size to the tail where it is smallest.

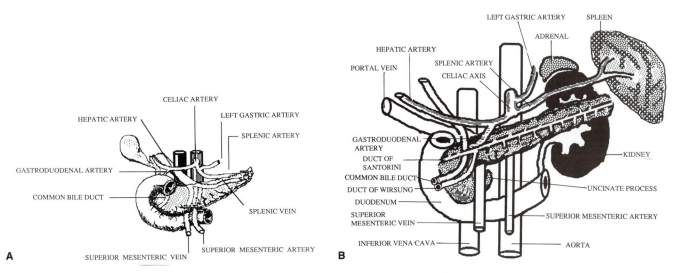

Figure 5–4. (A) Structures related to the pancreas; **(B)** Vascular anatomy related to the pancreas. *(Reprinted with permission from Fleischer AC, James AE. Diagnostic Sonography: Principles and Clinical Applications. Philadelphia: Saunders, 1989.)*

The endocrine function of the pancreas is to secrete insulin via the islets of Langerhans. The three exocrine enzymes are trypsin, lipase, and amylase.

Pancreatic Diseases (Table 5–10)

Pancreatitis: Inflammation of the Pancreas. Causes
of pancreatitis in older patients include alcohol—most common in men, biliary tract disease—most common in women, trauma, surgery, perforated peptic ulcer disease, and drugs.

Causes in younger patients include infectious agents—mumps, mononucleosis; hereditary—cystic fibrosis; and congenital pancreatitis (rare).

Pancreatitis can be generalized into two discrete forms, acute (edematous and hemorrhagic), and chronic (recurrent and calcific).

Acute Pancreatitis

Edematous. The pancreas goes through inflammatory changes and interstitial edema. The gland enlarges and swells; consequently a less echogenic pancreas will be noted. Acute pancreatitis may also be associated with intraperitoneal or retroperitoneal fluid.

Hemorrhagic. There is rapid progression of the disease due to the autodigestion of pancreatic tissue. Frequently, areas of fresh blood (hence the name) and fat necrosis are seen. It is the least common form of pancreatitis but the more urgent. Sonographically, the pancreas will have a very varied appearance from heterogeneous to hypoechoic. The pancreatic duct may be enlarged larger than 2 mm, and peripancreatic fluid may be present.

Chronic Pancreatitis. There is continued destruction of
pancreatic parenchyma, usually associated with chronic alcoholism and biliary tract disease. The pancreas will appear smaller and more echogenic.

Pancreatic Carcinoma. Pancreatic carcinoma can be
subdivided generally into adenocarcinoma, cystadenocarcinoma, and endocrine-active tumors such as islet cell carcinoma. Adenocarcinoma is the most common and is usually located within the head. Sonographically, the pancreatic borders are irregular, the parenchymal pattern changes, and the gland enlarges. Dilatation of the pancreatic duct may be seen, and one should also look for dilatation of the common bile duct secondary to enlargement of the pancreatic head.

Cystadenocarcinoma is visualized sonographically as an irregular cystic lobulated tumor with thick walls. It is more commonly seen in the body or tail.

Islet cell carcinomas are usually small and well circumscribed. Seventy-five percent cause endocrine hypersecretion and are usually found in the pancreatic tail. They are visualized sonographically as solid masses with cystic degeneration.

With any type of pancreatic carcinoma, clinically one can see an increase in alkaline phosphatase and bilirubin secondary to obstruction leading to jaundice and liver metastasis. Lymphadenopathy may also be seen.

Benign Tumors. Benign pancreatic tumors that are so-
nographically visualized include islet cell tumors, cystadenoma, papilloma of the duct, and duct cell adenoma. It is also possible to visualize pancreatic cysts, abscesses, metastatic diseases (to the pancreas), and lymphomas, all of which have the same sonographic appearances as when seen in other areas of the body (Table 5–11).

TABLE 5–10. PANCREATIC DISEASE

	Acute Pancreatitis	Chronic Pancreatitis	Adenocarcinomas	Islet Cell Tumors
Etiology	In males—Alcoholism increases gastric secretions, causes constriction of ampulla of Vater causing back-up of pancreatic secretions		The risk of pancreatic CA is increased in smokers, diabetics, and coffee drinkers	Develops from B cells of islet of Langerhans; 30% of these tumors are malignant
Clinical Findings				
Presentation	1. Abdominal pain characteristically in epigastrum or periumbilical, usually radiating to the back 2. Nausea and vomiting 3. Abdominal distension due to a decrease in gastric and intestinal motility and chemical peritonitis	1. May present with symptoms identical to acute pancreatitis or may have no pain 2. Pain increases with consumption of alcohol and fatty foods 3. Weight loss 4. Abnormal stools	1. Pain is the most common sympton 2. Jaundice 3. Weight loss 4. Palpable gallbladder (Courvoisier's sign)	1. Hypoglycemia 2. Elevated plasma insulin levels
Size	Enlarged (swollen)	Normal to small	Irregular, nodular Focal enlargement	Focal enlargement Small 1–2 cm Well encapsulated Maybe multiple
Usual site in gland	Entire gland	Entire gland (but may be focal)	Usually in the head	Body and tail
Sonographic findings				
Texture (compared to normal pancreas)	Generalized decrease in echogenicity of the entire gland	Generalized increase in echogenicity (focal or diffuse) of gland	Generalized decrease in echogenicity	Homogeneous and solid, frequently hypoechoic, whereas some may be echogenic
Attenuation (compared to normal pancreas)	Decreased	Increased	Decreased	
Shape	Generalized enlargement of the gland with smooth contours	Normal to small in size with irregular contours	Borders of mass are irregular	Borders of mass are smooth
Calcification	None	Yes	No	No
Associated sonographic findings	1. Dilatation of the biliary tree and calculi 2. Pancreatic pseudocyst	1. Dilatation of the pancreatic duct, possibly with stones 2. Pancreatic pseudocyst 3. Calcification of the gland in 50% of patients with malabsorption syndromes 4. Dilated common bile duct	1. Dilatation of the pancreatic duct 2. Biliary dilatation—jaundice if mass is in pancreatic head 3. Lymph nodes 4. Portal venous system involvement 5. Ascites	
Laboratory values	Serum amylase increased in 24 h Serum lipase increased in 72–94 h	Serum amylase (the pancreas must be intact to synthesize amylase and release, so in chronic pancreatitis serum amylase may not be elevated) Serum lipase	Increased bilirubin ⎫ Increased alkaline ⎬ Due to biliary obstruction phosphatase ⎭ Increased amylase Increased lipase	Decrease in the 2-hour postprandial (PP) blood sugar

TABLE 5–11. PANCREATIC MASSES

Pancreatic Growths	Sonographic Anatomy	Clinical Pathology
Cysts		
True Cyst	Sonographic features of a true cyst—smooth walls, echo free, good through transmission	True cysts have an epithelial lining and are usually found continuous with the pancreatic duct and/or arising from within the gland; most commonly found in the head
Pseudocyst	Pseudocysts generally take on the contour of the available space and may present as more than one "cyst." They are usually well defined with thick and echogenic borders. Internally they are anechoic, but debris may be seen on the dependent portion. Increased through transmission can also be seen posteriorly.	Pancreatic enzymes found outside of pancreatic duct. These enzymes can track anywhere. Sequelae in 2–60% of pancreatitis, usually appears 7 to 10 days after presenting symptoms; most commonly seen in alcoholic pancreatitis. If pseudocyst ruptures, can lead to pancreatic ascites
Benign Tumors		
Islet Cell Tumors	Well-circumscribed lesions of predominantly low-level echoes (may resemble an adenocarcinoma)	Most frequent benign tumor found within the pancreatic body and tail and presents as a small, solid mass with areas of cystic degeneration; 75% cause endocrine hypersecretion; 25% are nonfunctioning; 10% undergo malignant changes
Cystadenoma	The pancreas is lobulated with predominantly cystic areas, cannot be differentiated from malignant counterpart cystadenocarcinoma	Rare benign tumor arising from pancreatic duct, usually in tail
Malignant Tumor		
Adenocarcinoma	The pancreas demonstrates focal enlargement and is less echogenic than normal with ill-defined borders	Fourth or fifth most common cause of cancer death. Malignant solid tumor commonly found within the pancreatic head. Tumor becomes quite large. Patient presents with pain, weight loss, and jaundice
Associated Findings	Pancreatic duct dilatation Biliary tract dilatation Liver metastases Nodal metastases Portal venous system involvement Compression of inferior vena cava Large gallbladder (Courvoisier's sign) Laboratory values: Increased alkaline phosphatase (liver metastases), increased SGOT, increased serum amylase, increased bilirubin	Ascites; superior mesenteric vessel displacement posteriorly; a tumor of the uncinate process can cause anterior displacement of this vessel
Cystadenocarcinoma	The pancreas is lobulated with predominantly cystic areas. Can have similar appearance to pseudocyst	Rare malignant solid tumor commonly found within the tail and body. It presents as a cystic mass with solid components

SPLEEN

The spleen is the largest mass of reticuloendothelial tissue in the body. It normally measures about 12–14 cm in length, 7 cm in width, and 3 cm in anteroposterior dimension. It is situated in the left hypochondriac region, inferior to the diaphragm and posterolateral to the stomach. The left kidney, left adrenal gland, tail of the pancreas, and left colic flexure are all related to the visceral surface of the spleen.

Note that the spleen may be ectopic in location and/or accessory spleens may be present (usually in the area of the splenic hilum). Asplenia (congenital) is rare and often associated with congenital heart disease.

A fibroelastic capsule covers the spleen, the framework being composed of small fibrous bands that penetrate throughout the spleen. The capsule in turn is surrounded by peritoneum (thus the spleen is intraperitoneal).

The spleen is not essential to life, but it has important functions, particularly as the main component of the reticuloendothelial system. It is important because it functions in the breakdown of hemoglobin and formation of bile pigment; the filtration of organisms or other foreign material from the blood stream; the formation of antibodies and immunity; as a reservoir for blood; and blood formation in the fetus or where there is severe anemia.

Tumors of the Spleen

In general, primary tumors of the spleen, either benign or malignant, are rare.

Malignant Tumors of the Spleen. These may be *primary* and arise from the capsule (sarcoma) or from the splenic tissue (lymphoma). *Secondary* malignant tumors of the spleen are metastatic from breast, malignant melanoma, or ovaries.

Benign Tumors of the Spleen. These include congenital cysts, cysts associated with polycystic disease, hemangioma (most common primary tumor of the spleen), and lymphangioma.

Rupture of the spleen is common with trauma. Spontaneous rupture can also occur in certain disease states when the spleen is enlarged and soft.

Sonographically, the spleen can be imaged by placing the patient supine, left lateral oblique, and prone. The spleen should appear as fine homogeneous low-level echoes as seen within the liver.

The pathological sonographic appearances of the spleen can be divided into two categories, focal and diffuse.

It is important to remember that the stage at which the sonographer sees the patient during the course of the illness will influence the echogenicity of the spleen (Table 5–12).

Splenic Enlargement (Splenomegaly)

Size and Mass. The size of the spleen varies with energy and nutritional state of the person. It also varies at different states in life—at birth, it has the same proportion to total body weight as in the adult. What is really important is the relationship of the spleen to body size and nutritional state of the individual.

The approximate "normal" mass of the spleen in the adult is length—12–14 cm; width—7 cm; anteroposterior—4 cm.

Rule of thumb for splenomegaly is that if the anterior margin of the spleen extends more anteriorly than the anterior wall of the abdominal aorta on a transverse section, and the patient is in the supine position, this represents splenomegaly. Note that this may be seen in a very thin patient without being pathologically enlarged (eyeball technique most commonly used) (Table 5–13).

KIDNEY

The paired kidneys and ureters are retroperitoneal, lying against the deep muscles of the back. The kidney is covered by a fibrous capsule that is closely applied but not adherent to the renal parenchyma.

The capsule is seen by sonography as a strong continuous specular reflector surrounding the cortex.

Surrounding the encapsulated kidney is a collection of fat in the perinephric space. Located superior, anterior, and medial to each kidney is the adrenal gland. Enclosing the kidney, perinephric fat, and adrenal is a fibrous sheath known as Gerota's fascia.

TABLE 5–12. SONOGRAPHIC APPEARANCE OF THE SPLEEN

Focal		Diffuse	
Sonolucencies	Echogenic	Decreased Echogenicity	Increased Echogenicity
Splenic cysts		Congestion	Leukemia
Abscess		Multiple myeloma	Lymphoma
Lymphoma		Lymphopoiesis	
Metastases	Metastases	Granulocytopoiesis (eg, acute or chronic infection)	
		Erythropoiesis (as in sickle-cell disease, hemolytic anemia, thalassemia)	

TABLE 5–13. CAUSES OF SPLENIC ENLARGEMENT AND SHRINKAGE

Minimal	Moderate	Massive
Enlargement		
1. Acute splenitis	1. Acute leukemia	1. Chronic leukemia
2. Acute splenic congestion	2. Infectious mononucleosis	2. Lymphoma
3. Acute febrile disorders	3. Cirrhosis with portal hypertension	3. Hodgkin's disease
Bacteremic states	4. Chronic splenitis	4. Parasitic infections
Systemic toxemias	5. Tuberculosis	5. Primary tumors of the spleen
Systemic lupus erythematosus	6. Sarcoid tumor	
Intra-abdominal infections	7. Chronic congestive splenomegaly	
	8. Cancer	
	9. Iron deficiency anemias	
	10. Hemolytic anemias	
Shrinkage		
1. Myelofibrosis		The spleen *shrinks* and becomes strongly reflective
2. Sickle-cell disease		

The kidney parenchyma has two distinct areas: the outer cortex and the inner medullary pyramids, which surround the renal sinus. The renal parenchyma is measured from the margin of the renal sinus to the surface of the kidney. Renal size varies with the body size, age, and sex of the individual. Average adult size is 11.5 cm in length, 6 cm in width, and 3.5 cm in thickness.

Sonographically, the parenchyma can be resolved into cortex and medullary pyramids. The cortex is usually composed of uniform, closely spaced, relatively low-level echoes of an intensity less than that of either the normal liver or spleen parenchyma. The medullary pyramids are displayed as round or blunted hypoechoic zones between the cortex and renal sinus. These are separated from each other by bands of cortical tissue called columns of Bertin that also extend inward to the renal sinus. Intense specular echoes may be seen at the boundary between cortex and medulla. These represent the arcuate vessels.

The inner echogenic portion of the kidney consists of the renal sinus. The renal sinus contains fat, calyces, infundibula, renal pelvis, connective tissue, renal vessels, and lymphatics. The entrance to this sinus is termed the hilum and through it passes various blood vessels, nerves, lymphatic vessels, and the ureter.

The superior end of the ureter is expanded to form a funnel-shaped sac called the renal pelvis, which is located inside the renal sinus. The pelvis is divided into two or three tubes called major calyces, and they in turn are divided into 8 to 18 minor calyces. Each minor calyx is indented by the apex of a medullary pyramid called the renal papilla.

In a fluid-restricted subject, the infundibula (the major and minor calyces) are collapsed and not distinguishable within the echo-dense renal sinus fat. During diuresis, these structures can often be identified as narrow channels traversing the sinus. When the renal pelvis is partially extrarenal in location, it may be seen as a fluid-filled structure medial to the kidney.

Maternal pyelocalietasis without mechanical obstruction is commonly observed during pregnancy and involves the right kidney more than the left. Fetal pyelectasis is also common in utero.

ANTERIOR TO THE RIGHT KIDNEY	ANTERIOR TO THE LEFT KIDNEY	POSTERIOR TO THE KIDNEYS
Right adrenal	Left adrenal	Diaphragm
Liver	Stomach	Quadratus lumborum muscles
Duodenum	Spleen	
Right colic (hepatic) flexure	Pancreas	Psoas muscle
Small intestine	Jejunum	

Functions of the Kidneys

The kidneys serve in the excretion of inorganic compounds, eg, Na^+, K^+, Ca^{++}; excretion of organic compounds, eg, creatinine; blood pressure regulation; erythrocyte volume regulation; and vitamin D and Ca^{++} metabolism.

The ultimate goals of kidney functions are to (1) maintain salt and water balance, (2) regulate the fluid volume in the body, (3) maintain acid base balance.

Renal Congenital Anomalies

Renal congenital anomalies include incorrect position, number, and shape.

Position. Embryologically, the kidneys form in the pelvis in an anteroposterior orientation. They then ascend and rotate to the adult position, so that the upper pole of each kidney is more medial than the lower pole. Their ascension is usually completed by the fifth to sixth year of life. Incomplete ascension leads to ectopic kidneys.

Number. Anomalies of kidney number would include a solitary kidney (single functioning kidney with the other atrophied), unilateral renal agenesis (absence of one kidney and ureter), and a supranumary kidney (duplication of the kidney, pelvis, and ureter).

Unilateral renal agenesis is frequently associated with other anomalies; eg, bicornuate uterus, unicornuate uterus, uterine and vaginal septations.

Bilateral renal agenesis (Potter's syndrome) is associated with oligohydramnies and pulmonary hypoplasia, and it is fatal soon after birth.

Shape. Anomalies of kidney shape include hypertrophied columns of Bertin, fetal lobulation, dromedary humps, renunculus and fusion of the kidneys (ie, horseshoe-shaped kidneys and lump kidneys). Also included in this category are the congenital cystic diseases that distort the shape of the kidney, infantile polycystic disease, adult polycystic disease, and multicystic disease.

Multicystic Dysplastic Kidney (Potter 2). This is the most common cause of an abdominal mass in the newborn. It is usually unilateral, with the kidney presenting with cysts of various shapes and sizes owing to atresia of the ureter, pelvis, or both.

Polycystic Diseases. Polycystic disease may be present at birth or may not manifest until adult life.

Infantile Polycystic Disease. This is the least common and most fatal of the three anomalies of kidney shape. It is inherited as an autosomal recessive trait and is more common in females (2:1). Sonographically, it presents as bilateral, echogenic, enlarged kidneys (the cysts classically are too small to be resolved). If survival past infancy occurs, hepatic fibrosis becomes a complication with death resulting from hepatic failure and/or bleeding from esophageal varices (Potter 1).

Adult Polycystic Disease. This is inherited as autosomal dominant and occurs relatively frequently. The disease may be latent for many years and then manifest itself for unknown reasons. Sonographically, adult polycystic disease presents as bilateral, randomly distributed cortical cysts of various sizes. Associated findings include cysts in the liver, pancreas, and spleen. Destruction of the residual renal tissue in advanced stages leads to renal failure (Potter 3).

Medullary Cystic Disease. This is inherited with both dominant and recessive modes of transmission. Clinically, patients present with renal failure. Sonographically, there are small cysts confined to the medullary portion of both kidneys.

Renal Transplants

The transplanted kidney is placed within the ileopelvic region. A baseline sonogram should be obtained following the transplant to determine its exact location, size, and texture.

Acute failure of the transplanted kidney may be produced by acute rejection, acute tubular necrosis, or arterial obstruction. It is important to differentiate between these complications for correct treatment to be administered.

Acute rejection sonographically appears as enlarged kidney with increased cortical echogenicity (58%); decreased renal sinus echogenicity; irregular sonolucent areas in the cortex (47%); enlarged and decreased echogenicity of the pyramids; distortion of the renal outline; and indistinct corticomedullary junction.

Rejection due to **acute tubular necrosis** usually results in a normal sonogram. In rejection due to **acute renal arterial occlusion,** the sonographic anatomy remains grossly normal. However, duplex Doppler studies may reveal an absence of reduction of diastolic flow.

Perinephric fluid collections commonly associated with the transplanted kidneys are lymphocele, urinoma, abscess, and hematoma (Table 5–14).

Hydronephrosis

There are two major classifications of hydronephrosis, intrinsic and extrinsic.

Intrinsic Hydronephrosis. This may occur as a result of:

- stricture
- renal calculi
- renal neoplasm
- bleeding and blood clot
- ureterocele
- pyelonephrosis
- tuberculosis

Extrinsic Hydronephrosis. This may be the result of:

- pregnancy (usually right-sided)
- pelvic masses
- bladder neck obstruction
- neurogenic bladder
- trauma
- retroperitoneal fibrosis

TABLE 5–14. PERINEPHRIC FLUID COLLECTIONS[a]

Type	Sonographic Findings	Clinical Findings
Abscess (Renal carbuncle is a confluence of several small abscesses)	Usually echogenic with irregular thickened walls; gas may be encountered within an abscess and will be highly reflective resulting in shadowing	High white blood cell count and flank pain; patient is febrile
Hematoma	May resemble an abscess depending upon the degree of clot/liquification	Drop in hematocrit
Urinoma	Usually appears anechoic if not superimposed with infection	An encapsulated collection of extravasated urine
Lymphocele	Anechoic, but may contain echoes if superimposed by hemorrhage	Collection of lymphatic fluid

[a] Abscess, hematoma, urinoma, and lymphocele are commonly associated with renal transplantation, although it is not exclusive.

- prostatic hypertrophy
- urethritis
- inflammatory lesions—pelvic, gastrointestinal, retroperitoneal

Congenital Hydronephrosis. This is present at and existing from the time of birth. It may present as:

- UPJ obstruction
- ectopic ureterocele
- retrocaval ureter
- posterior urethral valves

False-Positive Hydronephrosis. This denotes a test result that wrongly *assigns* an individual to a diagnosis or category. In other words, the following list may mimic hydronephrosis.

- normal diuresis
- overdistended bladder
- parapelvic cyst
- renal sinus lipomatosis
- extra renal pelvis
- reflux—vesicoureteral
- diabetes insipidus

False-Negative Hydronephrosis. This denotes a test result that wrongly *excludes* an individual from a diagnosis or other category, in other words, patients suffering from severe dehydration or intermittent obstruction may indeed have hydronephrosis.

• severe dehydration
• nephrolithiasis with intermittent obstruction

Table 5–15 outlines clinical and sonographic findings associated with different renal masses.

Nephrolithiasis

Nephrolithiasis sonographically appears as a highly reflective echogenic foci with posterior shadowing. Nephrolithiasis may be composed of uric acid, cystine, or calcium, all of which sonographically appear the same. Staghorn calculi are large stones located in the center of the kidney.

Laboratory Values. In chronic obstruction, there is an increase in serum creatinine and BUN. In acute obstruction, there are no specific lab values. Urine may show hematuria and/or bacteria.

TABLE 5–15. RENAL MASSES

	Clinical Findings	Sonographic Findings
Cystic Masses		
Simple renal cyst	1. Seen in 50% of all patients over the age of 55 2. Usually originates in the renal cortex 3. Generally asymptomatic unless very large and obstructing the collecting system 4. Unilocular	1. Totally anechoic 2. Smooth, round border 3. Good through transmission
Atypical renal cyst	1. Septated or multilocular 2. The septation has no pathological significance	1. Fulfills all criteria for a cyst but, in addition, will have echogenic line or lines, ie, septations
Parapelvic cysts	Cysts located in the renal hilum developing from lymphatics or other nonparenchymal tissues in the renal hilar area	Similar to a simple cyst but located within the renal pelvis
Inflammatory cysts	1. Simple renal cysts that have become infected 2. An increase in leukocytosis	1. Complex pattern of internal echoes from inflammatory debris 2. Slightly thickened walls but not as thick as chronic abscess
Hemorrhagic cysts	6% of all renal cysts will hemorrhage	Complex echo pattern dependent upon state of hemorrhage (acute), hemorrhage (echogenic), chronic hemorrhage (more echogenic)
Calcified cysts	2% of all renal cysts will tend to have calcified walls	1. Anechoic 2. Smooth round borders that are highly echogenic or have echogenic foci 3. The calcified walls attenuate ultrasound, making it very hard to visualize
Renal abscess (carbuncle)[a]	1. May contain debris 2. Fever, chills, and flank pain 3. Elevated white blood cell count	1. Complex echo pattern due to debris 2. Walls are thickened and irregular 3. Gas may produce shadowing
Hydronephrosis	Obstruction 　a. *Intrinsic* within the collecting system either by a stone or stricture 　b. *Extrinsic,* a mass compresses the ureter or bladder outlet	The calices, infundibula, and pelvis dilate owing to the obstruction of urine flow. The sonographic picture may go from minor dilatation of the calices producing a cystic cauliflower effect to the gross dilatation of the pelvis and calices producing one large cystic area with little renal parenchyma
Pyonephrosis	Pus in the dilated collecting system complication of hydronephrosis that occurs secondary to urinary stasis and infection	Dilated pelvocaliceal system filled with internal echoes, shifting urine-debris level, may have shadowing due to gas-forming organisms
Renal Sinus Disease		
Renal sinus lipomatosis	More common in older patients; may be a sequelae to chronic calculous disease and inflammation. The renal sinus is replaced by fatty tissue	In replacement lipomatosis, the kidney is enlarged, the renal sinus appearing hypoechoic owing to the fat (one of the few times that fat will appear echo free rather than echogenic)

(continued)

TABLE 5–15. (Continued)

	Clinical Findings	Sonographic Findings
Benign Solid Tumor		
Angiomyolipoma, also called renal hamartoma (tumor composed of fat, muscle, and blood vessels)	More common in women than men (2:1). Symptoms are flank pain, hematuria, and hypertension	Discrete mass and highly echogenic
Adenomas (benign counterpart of renal cell carcinoma)	Asymptomatic, usually small and commonly found incidentally at autopsy	
Connective tissue tumors Hemangiomas Fibromas Myomas Lipomas	Gross hematuria	These tumors present as homogeneous echogenic lesions relating to their vascularity and fat content
Malignant Solid Tumor		
Hypernephroma (also known as adenocarcinoma, renal cell carcinoma, von Grawitz tumor)	1. Unilateral, solitary, and encapsulated 2. Affects males (2:1) more than females, most commonly after the age of 50 3. Hematuria 4. Metastases via the blood stream affecting the renal vein, inferior vena cava, contralateral kidney, ureter, peritoneum, liver, spleen, bone, heart, and brain 5. An arteriogram of the kidney demonstrates a mass with increased vascular supply and irregular branching	The tumor itself is well encapsulated and non-homogeneous, ranging in echogenicity from hyperechoic to hypoechoic. Look for tumor thrombus infiltrating the inferior vena cava and renal vein
Transitional cell carcinoma (affects the urothelium and may be located anywhere within the urinary collecting system)	1. Occurs in the central portion of the kidney, the renal pelvis. Known to be invasive 2. Occasionally seen as a bulky discrete mass 3. Hematuria	Invasive tumor not well defined or encapsulated within the renal pelvis
Renal lymphoma	1. Relatively common in patients with widely disseminated lymphomatous malignancy 2. Overall kidney enlargement	Solid mass with very soft internal echoes. May appear similar to renal cysts but will demonstrate no through transmission
Wilms' tumor (nephroblastoma)	1. Most common malignancy of renal origin in children 2. Presenting symptoms are abdominal mass, hypertension, nausea, hematuria	1. Well encapsulated 2. The sonographic pattern varies according to the amount of necrosis and/or hemorrhage

a May appear as a solid mass early in their course.

Renal Failure

Renal failure occurs as a result of deterioration of renal function, which may be acute or chronic. Laboratory findings are increased serum BUN and serum creatinine levels.

Etiology

Prerenal Causes. Renal hypoperfusion secondary to a systemic cause can occur as a result of *vascular disorders* leading to renal failure and includes the following conditions.

Nephrosclerosis. Arteriosclerosis of the renal arteries, resulting in ischemia of the kidney. Nephrosclerosis develops rapidly in patients with severe hypertension.

Infarction. This may result from occlusion or stenosis of the renal artery.

Congestive Heart Failure. This may cause renal hypoperfusion secondary to the heart failure.

Sonography. Doppler is employed to detect arterial blood flow patterns.

Renal Parenchymal Disease—Infection and Inflammatory Disease

Acute Tubular Necrosis (ATN). Of the renal medical diseases, this is the most common cause of acute renal failure. The destruction of the tubular epithelial cells of the proximal and distal convoluted tubules may occur as a result of ingestion or inhalation of toxic agents, ischemia due to trauma, hemorrhage, acute interstitial nephritis, cortical necrosis, and diseases of the glomeruli.

Pyelonephritis. Infection is the most *common* disease of the urinary tract, and the combination of parenchymal, caliceal, and pelvic inflammation constitutes pyelonephritis. Infection of the kidney is usually caused by bacteria ascending from the bladder or adjacent lymph nodes to the kidney.

Immunological Injuries. The nephrotic syndrome, glomerulonephritis, and lupus erythematosus are immunologic disorders involving the kidney.

Nephrotic syndrome is caused by deposition of antigen-antibody complexes on the glomerulus accompanied by proteinuria, hypoalbumenia, hyperlipidemia, and edema.

The etiology of *glomerulonephritis* is unknown, but it frequently follows other infections.

Systemic lupus erythematosus is an autoimmune disease. The echogenicity of the kidney will increase with increasing severity.

Metabolic Disorders. Diabetes mellitus, amyloidosis, gout, and nephrocalcinosis—deposition of calcium within the kidneys—are metabolic disorders associated with renal failure.

Chronic Nephrotoxicity. This is caused by exposure to radiation, heavy metals, industrial solvents, and drugs.

Sonography. In acute renal failure, the kidney may be normal sized or *enlarged*. In chronic renal failure, the kidney may be normal sized or *small*. As the case progresses from acute to chronic, the echogenicity of the kidney will increase. There is no definite correlation between the echogenicity of the kidney, kidney size, and degree of decreased renal function.

Postrenal Causes. These include urinary tract obstruction—hydronephrosis—which may be congenital or acquired intrinsically and extrinsically.

Sonography. There are varying degrees of dilatation of the renal sinus, calyces, infundibulum, and pelvis.

Renal Medical Disease (Table 5–16)

Type I. There are increased cortical echogenicity and an increase in corticomedullary differentiation. Type I diseases are those due to glomerular infiltrate such as acute and chronic glomerulonephritis, acute lupus nephritis, nephrosclerosis, any type of nephritis, and renal transplant rejection. All these disorders can increase the echo amplitude of the renal cortex to be more than that of liver and spleen. As the disease becomes more chronic, the kidney becomes smaller, the cortex has increased echogenicity, and eventually the medulla will become equally echogenic.

Type II. There is distortion of normal anatomy involving cortex and medullary pyramids, therefore, increased corticomedullary differentiation in either a focal or diffuse manner. The type II pattern is seen with focal lesions such as cysts, abscesses, hematomas, bacterial nephritis (lobar nephronia), infantile polycystic disease, adult polycystic disease, chronic pyelonephritis, and chronic glomerulonephritis.

BLADDER

The urinary bladder is located immediately behind the pubic bone. The apex of the bladder points anteriorly and is connected to the umbilicus by the median umbilical ligament, the remains of the fetal urachus. The ureters, enter at a superolateral angle, and the urethra extends from the bladder neck to the exterior of the body.

When distended with fluid, a normal bladder is seen as a symmetrical anechoic structure. It has a "sausage" shape on longitudinal scan, with a somewhat rounded appearance on a transverse scan. The bladder wall is seen as a thin, smooth, uniform echogenic line that usually measures from 3 to 6 mm in thickness. The normal bladder volume reaches 500 mL without major discomfort.

During an ultrasound examination of the bladder, wall thickness, irregularities of the wall, and bladder shape should be addressed. Table 5–17 reviews abnormalities that will distort the wall and shape of the bladder.

Ureters

Ureters lie on the anterior surface of the psoas near its medial edge. In the pelvis, they cross anterior to the common iliac vessels.

Congenital Anomalies of the Ureters. These include double or bifid ureters, narrowing, strictures, diverticuli, and hydroureter due to a congenital defect, as in polycystic kidney, or acquired as in a low ureteral obstruction.

Megaureter in Childhood

Primary—Nonobstructive, Nonrefluxing Megaureter. This includes *prune belly syndrome* (Eagle-Barrett syndrome), deficiency of the abdominal musculature, and urinary tract abnormalities; and *retroperitoneal fibrosis*, which fixes the ureters and prevents peristalsis leading to functional obstruction.

Secondary Megaureter. This is due to reflux of urine or obstruction.

Ureteral abnormalities are reviewed in Table 5–18.

ADRENAL GLANDS

The adrenal glands are triangular shaped structures situated superior and anteromedial to the upper pole of the kidneys. They measure $1 \times 3 \times 5$ cm, but at birth are

TABLE 5–16. RENAL MEDICAL DISEASES

	Clinical Findings	Ultrasound Findings
Acute Pyelonephritis	Ninety percent of the patients are female; dysuria, frequency, fever, leukocytosis, bacteruria	Normal to enlarged kidney may have mild hydronephrosis. The corticomedullary area is enlarged and less echodense than usual. These low-level echoes may be produced by multiple small abscesses and areas of necrosis in the cortex and medulla
Chronic Pyelonephritis (urinary tract infection)	Affects males and females; occurs due to recurrent urinary tract infection or inadequately treated pyelonephritis proteinuria	Normal to small kidney parenchymal thinning; increased echogenicity due to fibrosis
Acute Lobar Nephronia (acute focal bacterial nephritis)	Inflammatory mass without drainable pus results from gram-negative bacteria that ascends from ureteral reflux, fever, chills, flank pain	Poorly defined cystic mass containing echoes that may disrupt the corticomedullary junction. Cannot be differentiated from an abscess
Xanthogranulomatous Pyelonephritis	Rare form of inflammatory disease found in patients with long-standing renal calculi	Renal enlargement with multiple anechoic to hypoechoic areas
Glomerulonephritis	Glomerular disease results from an immunological reaction in which antigen-antibody complexes in the circulation are trapped in the glomeruli. It is the most common cause of chronic renal failure. In the acute stage, will present with oliguria, edema, increased BUN, increased creatinine, increased serum K. In the chronic stage, the patient presents with polyuria and proteinuria to such a high extent that 50% of patients develop nephrotic syndrome	Increases the echo amplitude of the renal cortex with a decrease in kidney size as the disease progresses
Acute Tubular Necrosis (ATN)	The most common cause of acute renal failure may result from ischemia and the interruption or impairment of blood flow in and out of the kidney. This may be due to trauma/surgery. It is the most comon cause of renal failure in the postrenal transplant patient and toxin induced	Increase in kidney size, especially in the anteroposterior diameter; normal renal parenchyma; the medullary pyramids will appear more prominent and anechoic

proportionately much larger. Gerota's fascia encloses the kidneys, adrenals, and the perinephric fat.

The right gland lies posterior to the inferior vena cava and anterior to the right crus of the diaphragm.

The left gland lies between the spleen and the aorta, posterior to the tail of the pancreas. Sonographically, the normal adrenal glands in adults are difficult to visualize owing to their small size and their echo texture being similar to the surrounding retroperitoneal fat. The recommended modality for evaluation of the adrenals is computed tomography (CT). Occasionally, an adrenal tumor will be found on sonography. Therefore, to rule out adrenal pathology with sonography, one should observe displacement and/or compression of adjacent organs.

Right adrenal pathology will displace—

ANTERIORLY	POSTERIORLY
The retroperitoneal fat line	The right kidney
The inferior vena cava	
The right renal vein	

Left adrenal pathology will displace—

ANTERIORLY	POSTERIORLY AND INFERIORLY
Splenic vein	The left kidney

The adrenal gland consists of two distinct endocrine organs, the cortex and the medulla.

Adrenal Cortex

The adrenal cortex, which produces steroid hormones, is further subdivided into three zones: (1) zona glomerulosa, which produces mineralocorticoids (to regulate electrolyte metabolism); (2) zona fasiculata; and (3) the zona reticularis, which produces glucocorticoids (for regulation of carbohydrate metabolism) and androgens (for regulation of the secretion of androgens and estrogens, which are the sex hormones of an individual).

The adrenal cortical hormones are regulated by the adrenocorticotropic hormones (ACTH) of the anterior pituitary. A *decrease* in adrenal cortical function leads to an increased ACTH which then stimulates the adrenal cor-

TABLE 5–17. BLADDER ABNORMALITIES

Abnormality	Clinical Findings	Ultrasound Findings
Urachal Cyst: The urachus connects the apex of the bladder with the allantois (an embryological structure with no function in humans) through the umbilical cord. Normally, it fibroses at birth, but it may, in part or in whole, remain patent. The urachus lies in the space of Retzius.	A urachal cyst remains clinically silent until an infection develops, then there is vague abdominal pain and/or urinary complaints	A urachal cyst is seen as an echo-free tubular structure in the lower mid-abdominal anterior wall. The upper pole may extend from the umbilicus to the bladder
Diverticuli of the bladder: Pouchlike envaginations of the bladder wall	The diverticula constitute a site of urinary stasis that tends to become infected	Diverticula vary greatly in size and appear separate from the bladder. They are round, well-defined, thin-walled cystic masses. To help delineate it from an adnexal mass, have the patient void; it should disappear.
Reduplication: Complete reduplication of the bladder is rare	Unilateral reflex, obstruction or infection	One would visualize two separate bladders separated by a peritoneal fold
Reflux: Vesicoureteral reflex is a common urinary tract abnormality in children secondary to anomalies such as ectopia, posterior urethral valves, prune belly, neurogenic bladder, and primary congenital abnormalities of the bladder	Reflux may be a cause of chronic renal failure with scarring and atrophic changes in the kidney	Cysto-Conray (20%) is injected into the bladder. Each kidney is scanned while the contrast is injected. With each increasing grade of reflux, there is increasing kidney dilation
Bladder Neck Obstruction: The lower portion continuous with the urethra, is called the neck	In the male bladder, neck obstruction commonly is secondary to benign prostatic hypertrophy or carcinoma. With prolonged obstruction, the bladder will become thickened and trabeculate	Ultrasound demonstrates a thickened and irregular-walled bladder
Cystitis: Infection or inflammation of the bladder	Secondary to diverticula, urethral obstruction, fistulas, cystocele, bladder neoplasm, pyelonephritis, neurogenic dysfunction	When it is long standing, the bladder walls may show inflammatory changes and thickening. With a neurogenic bladder a pus-urine fluid level may be seen
Primary Benign Tumor: papilloma, epithelial	There may be papillary growths, nodular infiltrating	Small to massive solid tumors are seen projecting from the bladder wall, some may invaginate the bladder wall, and may be smooth or irregular in contour. May mimic benign prostatic hypertrophy or cystitis
Primary Malignant Tumor: 95% are transitional cell carcinoma; 5% are squamous cell carcinoma	Invasive growths, with 40% having metastases to lymph nodes and invasion of the prostate and seminal vesicles	

TABLE 5–18. URETERAL ABNORMALITIES

Abnormality	Clinical Findings	Ultrasound Findings
Posterior Urethral Valves	Posterior urethral valves are the most common cause of urinary obstruction in the male infant and are the second most common cause of hydronephrosis in the neonate. This obstruction is related to a flap of mucosa that has a slitlike opening in the area of the prostatic urethra.	Distended bladder with a thickened wall dilated; ureters medial and posterior to the bladder
Ureterocele	A ureterocele is a cystic dilatation of the submucosa of the intravesicular ureter (that portion of the ureter that enters the bladder)with narrowing of the ureteric orifice. This may cause obstruction of the ipsilateral ureter and can obstruct the bladder neck.	An anechoic thin-walled structure of variable size and shape projecting into the bladder
"Ureteral Jets" (not an abnormality but only appearing as one)	The term *ureteral jets* is used to describe the appearance of urine entering the bladder. These jets are seen during bladder filling and are not visible when the bladder is full. They are seen at regular intervals, each jet lasting from a fraction of 1–3 seconds.[36]	The urinary jet starts in the area of the ureter and flows toward the center of the bladder. Doppler may be used because the ureteral jet will cause a Doppler shift due to the continued changes in the turbulent flow of the urine

tex. An *increase* in concentration of adrenal hormones leads to a drop in ACTH secretion, which in turn leads to a drop in the activity of the adrenal cortex.

The adrenal cortex may be affected either by lesions that produce an excess of steroid hormones or by lesions that produce a deficiency. Be aware that adrenocortical hormones may be altered as a result of an overproduction or underproduction of ACTH that is a result of a pituitary tumor. Table 5–19 outlines possible adrenal gland malfunctions.

Adrenal Medulla

The adrenal medulla produces epinephrine (adrenalin) and norepinephrine. These hormones have a wide range of effect.

Epinephrine dilates the coronary vessels and constricts the skin and kidney vessels. It increases coronary output, raises oxygen consumption, and causes hyperglycemia.

Norepinephrine constricts all arterial vessels except the coronary arteries (which dilate). It is an essential regulator of blood pressure.

Epinephrine, in particular, is responsible for the fight-or-flight reaction. It stimulates the metabolic rate, allowing more available energy.

TABLE 5–19. ADRENAL GLAND MALFUNCTIONS

	Clinical Findings	Sonographic Findings
Adrenal Cortex		
Adrenocortical Hyperfunction		
Cushing's syndrome	Prolonged exposure to elevated plasma cortico-steroids produces truncal obesity, rounded faces, mild hypertension, cardiac enlargement, and edema	May be solid, cystic, or complex appearing with focal zones of necrosis
Conn's syndrome	Hyperaldosteronism due to the increased secretion of aldosterone producing sodium retention, which leads to essential hypertension	
Adrenogenital syndrome	Exclusive oversecretion of androgens leading to virilism or masculinization in a female. Hypersecretion of estrogens (in the male) produces the feminizing syndrome	
Adrenocortical Hypofunction		
Addison's disease	Hypotension, small hearts, malaise, and weight loss, skin pigmentation, loss of body hair, and menstrual irregularity. 60% are due to idiopathic destruction, probably autoimmune in nature	
Adrenal Medulla		
Pheochromocytoma	Paroxysmal or sustained hypertension, angina, cardiac arrhythmias, and headaches. These features are due to the concentration of catecholamines released into the circulation	May grow to be quite large, may appear cystic, solid, or solid with calcific components
Neuroblastoma	Termed a nonfunctioning tumor (ie, tumors that do not produce epinephrine and norepinephrine) and arises from sympathetic nervous tissue. Most children are asymptomatic presenting with a palpable abdominal mass	The tumor appears echogenic and may be quite large
Adrenal Metastases	Most commonly from bronchogenic CA, lung adenocarcinoma, breast or stomach carcinoma	Metastases to the adrenals vary in size and echogenicity
Adrenal Cysts	None—patient may be asymptomatic	Strong back wall, no internal echoes, good through transmission. Adrenal cysts have the tendency to become calcified, which may appear as an echo-free structure, with an echogenic back wall but with poor through transmission.
Adrenal Hematomas	Especially encountered in infants	Varies from cystic to complex depending upon the age of the hematoma, ending in calcification

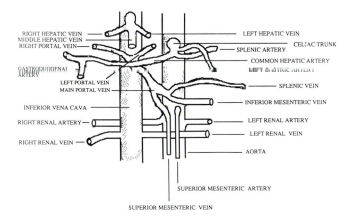

RIGHT HEPATIC VEIN
MIDDLE HEPATIC VEIN
RIGHT PORTAL VEIN
LEFT HEPATIC VEIN
SPLENIC ARTERY — CELIAC TRUNK
COMMON HEPATIC ARTERY
LEFT GASTRIC ARTERY
GASTRODUODENAL ARTERY
LEFT PORTAL VEIN
MAIN PORTAL VEIN
SPLENIC VEIN
INFERIOR VENA CAVA
INFERIOR MESENTERIC VEIN
RIGHT RENAL ARTERY
LEFT RENAL ARTERY
LEFT RENAL VEIN
RIGHT RENAL VEIN
AORTA
SUPERIOR MESENTERIC ARTERY
SUPERIOR MESENTERIC VEIN

Figure 5–5. Prevertebral vessels. *(Reprinted with permission from Hagen-Ansert S. Textbook of Diagnostic Ultrasonography, 2nd ed. St. Louis: CV Mosby, 1983, p 113.)*

MAJOR LANDMARK VESSELS

Knowledge of the prevertebral vessels (Fig. 5–5) is extremely important, for they are the road maps and guideposts in helping to identify both normal anatomy and pathology.

Aorta

The aorta lies anterior to the spine and posterior to the pancreatic body. On sagittal scans, the superior aspect is most posterior.

Ventral Branches of the Aorta

Celiac. The celiac is only 2–3 cm long and has three branches:

1. Splenic artery—runs superior to the pancreas on its way to the spleen.
2. Left gastric artery
3. Hepatic artery—enters the porta hepatis with the portal vein. The gastroduodenal artery, a branch of the hepatic artery, delineates the anteriolateral aspect of the pancreatic head.

Superior Mesenteric Artery. The superior mesenteric artery (SMA) lies posterior to the body of the pancreas.

Inferior Mesenteric Artery. Originates from the abdominal aorta close to the umbilicus and is rarely seen on ultrasound.

Lateral Branches of the Aorta

Renal Arteries. There are two renal arteries, the left renal artery and the right renal artery. The right renal artery is the only vessel that runs posterior to the inferior vena cava.

Anatomy and Measurement. The aorta enters the abdomen at the first lumbar vertebra (L1) and follows the curvature of the spine to bifurcate at L4. If there is a separation between the aorta and the spine, adenopathy, fibrosis, or hematoma should be ruled out.

The normal AP dimension of the aortic lumen should be < 3 cm

- thoracic: 2.5 cm
- diaphragm: 2.5–3.0 cm
- mid-abdomen: 2.0–2.5 cm
- renals: 1.8–2.0 cm
- bifurcation: 1.5–1.7 cm
- iliac: 1.0–1.3 cm

Aortic aneurysms—increased aortic diameter greater than 3 cm.

- aneurysm: 3–6 cm
- signifant: > 5 cm
- surgical emergency: > 6 cm
- 50% survival of 1 year: > 6 cm
- 75% risk of fatal rupture: > 7 cm

Classification of Aneurysms. Aortic aneurysms may be true, dissecting, or false.

True Aneurysms. The three layers of the vessel (aorta) are dilated to form the aneurysm. They may be caused by: arteriosclerosis with hypertension; Marfan's syndrome is associated with aneurysm of the first portion of the aorta that usually extends to affect the aortic valve leading to aortic insufficiency; infections, especially as a result of bacterial endocarditis; trauma; congenital; and syphilis.

Clinical Findings: The clinical findings in true aortic aneurysms are pulsatile abdominal mass, back pain—most aneurysms start below renal arteries and extend down to common iliac arteries.

Types

- fusiform: gradual, spindle-shaped dilation of the vascular lumen, usually occurring below renal arteries to the bifurcation
- cylindrical: uniform dilation within the longitudinal diameter producing lengthening of the expanded vessel
- saccular: localized, spherical outpouching of the vessel wall, often containing thrombus; it is the least common type
- berry: small spherical aneurysm, 1–1.5 cm usually within cerebral circulation (middle cerebral artery)

Sonographic Findings. Generally, the vessel will show irregularities, tortuosities, and aortic wall calcification. An accurate measurement of the anteroposterior diameter should be performed.

Dissecting Aneurysm. Intima (inner wall) of aorta dissects and pulls away from other two walls; hemorrhage occurs between walls. Seventy percent begin in ascending aorta. They may be caused by cystic aneurysms, as in Marfan's syndrome, hemorrhage of vasa vasorum, and spontaneous rupture of the intima.[21]

Clinical Findings. Severe pain that mimicks myocardial infarction; the site of the pain may indicate the site of the aneurysm. Most severe type of aneurysm occurs most frequently in males and patients with hypertension.

Sonographic Findings. Demonstration of the intimal flap, which moves with aortic pulsation; differentiation between the true and false lumen is difficult.

False Aneurysm. An injury to the vessel wall and extravasation occurs; the extravasated blood is retained and walled off by the surrounding tissues, so the wall of the false aneurysm is not the vessel wall. False aneurysms mimic a true aneurysm. Trauma is the most common cause.

Sonographic Findings. A mass is adjacent to the vessel; usually has variable echogenicity.

Inferior Vena Cava

The inferior vena cava (IVC) lies to the right of the aorta and posterior to the pancreatic head. It extends from the union of the common iliac arteries to the right of L5 and travels cephalad. It then curves *anterior* to enter the right atrium.

The IVC normally contracts on exhalation and expands on inhalation or the Valsalva maneuver. The IVC remains dilated with hepatomegaly, pulmonary hypertension, congestive heart disease, constrictive pericarditis, right atrial myxoma, atherosclerotic heart disease, and right ventricular failure.

The most common tumor to involve the IVC is renal cell carcinoma and is usually on the right because of the close proximity to the IVC. Venous tumors may be seen as intraluminal echogenic nodules or thrombi and can cause generalized IVC dilation and innumerable diffuse low-amplitude echoes coming from the lumen. It may even extend to the renal artery. Wilm's tumor in children is similar to renal cell carcinoma.

Causes of IVC Displacement

- mass in posterior, caudate, or right hepatic lobe
- right renal artery aneurysm
- lymphadenopathy
- tortuous aorta
- right renal masses
- right adrenal masses; eg, pheochromocytoma
- retroperitoneal liposarcoma ⎫
- leiomyosarcoma ⎬ retroperitonal
- osteosarcoma ⎬ tumors
- rhabdomyosarcoma ⎭

Hepatic Veins. There are three hepatic veins, right, middle, and left, which drain into the inferior vena cava.

Renal Veins. There are two renal veins, the right renal vein and the left renal vein. The left renal vein runs anterior to the aorta but posterior to the SMA.

Portal System

Portal Vein. The portal vein is formed by the confluence of the superior mesenteric vein and the splenic vein in the region of the neck of the pancreas.

Splenic Vein. The splenic vein runs posterior to the pancreatic body and tail.

Superior Mesenteric Vein. The superior mesenteric vein lies posterior to the body of the pancreas but anterior to the uncinate process.

THYROID

The thyroid has two lobes connected anteriorly by a narrow band of tissue referred to as the isthmus.

The common carotid artery and the internal jugular vein lie posterior and lateral, defining the posterolateral margins of the thyroid. The "strap muscles" lie anterior to the lateral aspect of the pancreas defining the anterolateral margins of the pancreas.

Sonographically, the thyroid has a homogeneous echogenicity that is greater than the strap muscles.

Size

LOBES	ISTHMUS
Length: 4–6 cm	Length: 2 cm
Width: 1.5–2 cm	Width: 2 cm
Height: 2–3 cm	Height: 2–6 mm

Table 5–20 outlines pathologies of the thyroid that can be seen sonographically.

SCROTUM

The scrotum is a sac that is divided by a septum, the median raphe. Each space contains a testis, an epididymis, a portion of spermatic cord, and the ductus deferens (Fig. 5–6). The innermost wall of the scrotum is lined by a thin, double layer of peritoneum, the tunica vaginalis. This double layer of peritoneum normally contains a small amount of fluid.

The testicles are ovoid glands that measure about 4–5 cm in length. A dense white fibrous capsule, called the tunica albiguina, encases each testicle and then enters the gland, separating the testes into approximately 200 cone-shaped lobules. Within these lobules, two primary functions occur: spermatogenesis (the production of spermatozoa) and the secretion of testosterone by the interstitial cells (Leydig cells).

The secretions are carried through the lobules to the rete testis. A series of ducts, called efferent ductules, drain the rete testis, piercing the tunica albuginea and entering the head of the epididymis.

The epididymis consists of a single tightly coiled duct

TABLE 5–20. THYROID PATHOLOGY

Pathology Observable by Sonography	Sonographic Characteristics
Adenomas (benign). Most common nodule occurring in the thyroid. May be singular or multiple	Measures 5–30 mm. Varied sonographic appearance ranging from very echogenic to a solid homogeneous mass with few internal echoes, resembling a cyst. Most frequently it will present as a solid mass, often having an anechoic halo created by blood and edematous tissue compressing the surrounding parenchyma
Simple cyst. Usually developmental, such as thyroglosal duct and brachial cleft	No internal echoes, smooth walls, good sound transmission
Hemorrhagic cysts	Well-defined cysts, mass with irregular borders, and multiple septations
Acute thyroiditis	Diffuse enlargement and decreased echogenicity of lobes. One lobe, usually the right one, might be larger
Subacute thyroiditis	Diffuse enlargement with decreased echogenicity
Hashimoto's thyroiditis	Diffusely abnormal pattern, multiple small, low-level echoes with a decrease in the overall echogenicity of the gland
Goiter	Gland usually enlarged in its initial stages and may have normal echo pattern. In later stages, may have multiple discrete nodules (50%), diffusely nodular in homogeneous gland with no normal tissue (50%), nodules may display cystic degeneration and calcification
Graves' disease	Diffusely enlarged lobes and isthmus, homogeneous echo pattern as in normal gland or heterogeneous echo pattern. Only one lobe might be enlarged
Carcinoma—80% are papillary	May be as small as 2 mm or as large as 10 cm. Masses are usually singular and hypoechoic. Cystic degeneration and specks of calcification may be present

that drapes the posterior aspect of the testis. The most superior aspect of the epididymis is the head, followed by the body and tail. This duct continues as the ductus deferens (vas deferens), leaving the pelvis via the inguinal canal with the testicular artery, the draining veins of the scrotum, nerves, and lymphatics, to form the spermatic cord. Each spermatic cord now extends over the top and

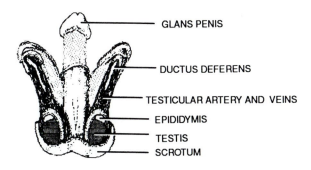

Figure 5–6. The male reproductive system.

down the posterior surface of the bladder, coming together to join with the duct from the seminal vesicle to form the ejaculatory ducts. The ejaculatory ducts pass through the prostate gland to terminate in the urethra.

Normal Sonographic Anatomy of the Scrotum

The normal testicle exhibits a homogeneous echo pattern of medium-level echogenicity. Posteriorly and superiorly capping the testis, the epididymial head is clearly distinguished owing to its coarser, more echogenic pattern. The body of the epididymis is harder to differentiate because of its posterior position and the tail is rarely seen. A brightly echogenic band, representing the mediastinum testis, is occasionally seen in the superior aspect.

On a transverse scan of the right side, the mediastinum testis is seen in the 9 o'clock position; on the left side, it is seen in the 3 o'clock position. Between the layer of the tunica vaginalis, a small amount of fluid is normally found.

The testicular artery and veins of the pampiniform plexus, which run along the posterior aspect of the testicle in the region of the epididymis, are not normally seen.

Scanning the testis transversely, comparing each testis and epididymis as to size and echogenicity, is the best guide for detecting lesions or enlargement.

Table 5–21 outlines scrotal pathology and associated sonographic and clinical findings.

DIAPHRAGM

The diaphragm is a dome-shaped muscle separating the thorax from the abdominal cavity. The diaphragm covers the superior border of the liver (and spleen) and sonographically can be identified as a curvilinear interface between the lungs and liver (spleen).

The *subphrenic space* is between the liver (or spleen) and the diaphragm and is a common site for abscess formation.

Crura of the Diaphragm

The diaphragmatic crura are right and left fibromuscular bundles that attach to the lumbar vertebra L3 on the right and L1 on the left and act as anchors to the diaphragm.

TABLE 5–21. SCROTAL PATHOLOGY

	Sonographic Anatomy	Clinical Pathology
Epididymis		
Acute epididymitis	The epididymis is enlarged and more hypoechoic	Specific epididymitis stemming from gonorrhea, syphilis, mumps, and/or tuberculosis
Chronic epididymitis	The epididymis is thickened, very echogenic, and may contain calcification	Nonspecific epididymitis is usually the result of a urinary tract infection
		Traumatic epididymitis due to strenuous exercise
Spermatocele	A cystic structure found superior to the testis, may be loculated and contain low-level echoes	A cystic mass of the epididymis containing spermatozoa
Testis		
Orchitis	The testis is enlarged and is less echogenic than the normal testis. An abscess of the testis appears as a localized area of inhomogeneity	Inflammation of a testis due to trauma, metastasis, mumps, or infection elsewhere in the body
Seminoma	Is usually hypoechoic compared to the rest of the testis but well circumscribed	Most common malignant tumor of patients between 30 and 40 years of age. Patients have elevated follicle-stimulating hormone levels
Teratoma	Areas of hemorrhage and necrosis are seen within this poorly circumscribed tumor	This tumor runs the spectrum from complete simple growth (benign) to the most malignant
Testicular torsion	An enlarged testicle is seen due to the edema. May have areas of infarcts and necrosis	Usually occurs in prepubertal boys. There is torsion of the spermatic cord, which causes strangulation of the blood supply to the testis, which in turn causes edema
Intratesticular hemorrhage	Appears as echogenic areas	
Pampiniform Plexus		
Varicocele	Numerous anechoic tortuous structures lying posterior to the testis and extending superiorly past the epididymis. May enlarge when patient is scanned in the upright position	Enlargement of the veins of the spermatic cord, commonly occurring on the left side
Scrotum		
Hydrocele	An accumulation of serous fluid between the parietal and visceral layers of the tunica vaginalis of the scrotum. Usually the result of inflammation of the epididymis or testis	The testis and the epididymis are surrounded by fluid
Inguinal hernia	Peristalsis of the mass will be visualized sonographically	Herniation of the abdominal contents into the scrotal sac
	Echogenic foci that represent air within the loops of bowel will be noted	

The crura can be visualized anterior to the aorta above the level of the celiac artery. Below the celiac artery, the crura extend along the lateral aspects of the vertebral columns.

Sonography of Right Crus

Longitudinal Scans. The entire right crus can be seen as a solid hypoechoic longitudinally oriented structure immediately *posterior* and *parallel* to the inferior vena cava. It should not be confused with the right renal artery, which will appear as a circular structure crossing anterior to the crus and posterior to the IVC.

The right crus is also noted as a hypoechoic longitudinal structure *anterior and parallel to the aorta,* ending cephalically near the esophagogastric (EG) junction. This represents the anterior decussation of the crus.

Transverse Scans. The right crus is seen posterior to the IVC, extending between the IVC and aorta, until it reaches anterior to the aorta. The right adrenal and right kidney are posterolateral to the right crus.

Sonography of Left Crus

Longitudinal Scan. The left crus cannot be visualized longitudinally.

Transverse Scans. The left crus can be seen as a hypoechoic structure running anterior and lateral to the aorta.

It is closely associated with the left adrenal, splenic vasculature, and esophagogastric junction.

FLUID COLLECTIONS

Ascites

Ascites is an abnormal collection of serous fluid in the peritoneum. It may be:

- transudative—anechoic/freely mobile usually benign, free-floating bowel in the abdomen
- exudative—internal echos/loculated—associated with infection and malignancy
- bowel matted or fixed to posterior abdominal wall—associated with malignancy
- nonmobile fluid associated with coagulated hematoma (trauma)

Pathology Associated with Ascites

- Congestive heart failure
- Infection (inflammatory process)
- Kidney failure
- Liver failure/disease—end-stage fatty liver, cirrhosis
- Malignancy
- Ruptured aneurysm
- Pyogenic peritonitis
- Tuberculosis
- Portal venous system obstruction
- Obstruction of lymph nodes/vessels
- Acute cholecystitis
- Ectopic gestation
- Postoperative

Clinical Presentation. The clinical presentation of ascites is that of an enlarged abdomen.

Sonographic Findings. Accumulations occur (supine position) in the following order:

1. inferior tip—right lobe liver
2. superior portion—right flank
3. pelvic cul-de-sac
4. right paracolic gutter—lateral and anterior to liver
5. Morison's pouch

- ascites is found inferior to the diaphragm
- gross (massive) ascites—extrahepatic portion of falciform ligament seen attaching liver to anterior abdominal wall
- ascites may cause upward displacement of liver
- may cause gallbladder wall to appear thickened
- liver may appear more echogenic
- may see patent umbilical vein
- changing patient's position to observe fluid movement may be useful
- disproportional accumulations in lesser sac suggestive of adjacent organ pathology (ie, acute pancreatitis, pancreatic CA)

Abscess

An abscess is a circumscribed collection of pus (acute/chronic). A cavity formed by liquefactive necrosis within solid tissue.

Pathology Associated with Abscesses

- Penetrating trauma (wounds)
- Postsurgical procedures
- Retained products of conception
- Pelvic inflammatory disease (PID)
- Chronic bladder disease
- Sepsis—blood-borne bacterial infection
- Long-standing hematoma
- Postcholecystectomy—site of GB
- GI tract—peptic ulcer perforation; bowel spill during surgery (peritonitis)
- Urinary tract infection (UTI)
- Infected ascites with septa/debris
- Amebic abscess—may be densely echogenic

Clinical Presentation. Pain, spiking fever, chills, elevated white blood cell count, solitary or multiple sites, tenderness.

Hepatic Abscess

Intrahepatic. Abscess associated with sepsis; penetrating trauma to liver.

- location: within liver parenchyma
- differential diagnosis: solid tumor, usually round lesion with scattered internal echoes, variable through transmission

Subhepatic. Abscess associated with cholecystectomy.

- location: inferior to liver; fluid collection anterior to right kidney (Morrison's pouch); bed of GB (postcholecystectomy)

Subphrenic. Abscess associated with bacterial spill into peritoneum during surgical procedure; bowel rupture; peptic ulcer perforation; trauma.

- location: fluid collection above liver, inferior to diaphragm; transmission variable; gas (dirty shadowing)

General Sonographic Findings. A variable, complex, solid, cystic lesion with septa, debris, and scattered echoes; through transmission may be good; mass/cyst with shaggy/thick irregular walls; mass displacing surrounding structures; complex mass with dirty gas shadowing from within. *Presence of gas within a mass demonstrates an abscess.*

General Differential Diagnosis. Necrosing tumor with fluid center (these usually have thicker walls and *no gas*).

Ascites Versus Abscess

A localized area of ascites may be mistaken for an abscess. Place the patient in the erect or Trendelenburg position; ascites will shift but an abscess will not.

Pleural Effusion

Pleural effusions are a nonspecific reaction to an underlying pulmonary or systemic disease such as cirrhosis. Obtaining fluid for analysis may allow a more specific diagnosis.

Sonographic appearance shows a pleural effusion to be a usually echo-free, wedge-shaped area that lies posteromedial to the liver and posterior to the diaphragm. Occasionally, pleural effusions contain internal echoes, sometimes indicating the presence of a neoplasm. These echoes may be due to blood or pus (empyema), especially when the collection is loculated. Loculated effusions do not necessarily lie adjacent to the diaphragm and may be loculated anywhere on the chest wall. Sometimes effusions lie between the lung and the diaphragm and are known as subpulmonic. Right-sided pleural effusions can be easily assessed on a view looking through the diaphragm and the liver. Effusions on the left are more difficult to see in the supine position but sometimes can be seen with an oblique scan through the spleen.

RETROPERITONEUM

The retroperitoneum is the area between the posterior portion of the parietal peritoneum and the posterior abdominal wall, extending from the diaphragm to the pelvis.

Divisions

The retroperitoneum is divided into three areas by the renal fascia (Gerota's fascia): Fig. 5–7 demonstrates the division of the retroperitoneum into anterior pararenal and posterior pararenal spaces.[43]

1. The anterior pararenal space contains the retroperitoneal portion of the intestines and the pancreas

□ Ant. Pararenal Space
▨ Perirenal Space
▩ Post. Pararenal Space

Figure 5–7. (A) Anatomy of the retroperitoneal compartments. Diagram of a right parasagittal view demonstrates the lumbar and iliac fossae. The lumbar fossa extends from the diaphragm (1) to the ilium (10). The anterior pararenal space is limited anteriorly by the peritoneum (15) and posteriorly by the anterior renal fascia (4). The perirenal space is contained between the anterior (4) and posterior (8) renal fascia. The posterior pararenal space lies between the posterior renal fascia (8) and the transversalis fascia (14) that continues about the entire abdomen. The retrofascial muscles (quadratus lumborum [7], psoas [12], and iliacus [13]) also are demonstrated. Note that the lumbar compartments are open inferiorly and merge as they enter the iliac fossa. 2 = liver, 3 = bare area of liver, 5 = kidney, 6 = duodenum, 9 = ascending colon, 11 = retrocecal appendix, 16 = ureter, 17 = iliac vessels. **(B)** Lumbar fossa of the retroperitoneum. Transverse sectional diagram viewed from below shows the relations between the retroperitoneal compartments on either side. The anterior pararenal space, bounded by the peritoneum (2) and anterior renal fascia (7), is continuous across the midline. The common bile duct (4), retroperitoneal portions of the duodenum (5, 13), ascending (6) and descending (18) colon, superior mesenteric vessels (14), and pancreas (16) are included in this space. The bilateral perirenal spaces are effectively separated from one another by the connective tissue sheaths surrounding the inferior vena cava (3) and aorta (15). The lateroconal fascia (8) is formed by the lateral fusion of the anterior (7) and posterior (10) renal fasciae. The transversalis fascia (1) lies behind the posterior pararenal space, forming the anterior boundary of the retrofascial spaces that include the quadratus lumborum (11) and psoas (12) muscles at this level. 9 = right kidney, 17 = right ureter, 19 = left kidney. *(Reprinted with permission from Koenigsberg M. Sonographic evaluation of the retroperitoneum. Semin Ultrasound 3:2, 1982.)*

2. The perirenal space contains the kidneys, ureters, adrenal glands, aorta, IVC, and retroperitoneal nodes
3. The posterior pararenal space contains the posterior abdominal wall, iliopsoas muscle, and quadratus lumborum muscle

Pathology

The retroperitoneal area is subject to infection, bleeding, inflammation, and tumors.

Anterior Pararenal Space. Pancreatic pathology, carcinoma of the duodenum, ascending and descending colon causing bowel thickening or infiltration resulting in a "bullseye" or inverted "bagel sign."

Perirenal Space. Kidney diseases, adrenal diseases, invasion or displacement of IVC, aortic aneurysms, ureteral abnormalities, sarcoma, liposarcoma, aortic, and retroperitoneal adenopathy.

Posterior Pararenal Space. Renal transplantation is usually performed in this extraperitoneal space within the iliac fossa, using the iliac vessels for anastomosis.

Primary Retroperitoneal Tumors

Primary retroperitoneal tumors are mostly malignant, rapidly growing, and the larger tumors are more likely to show evidence of necrosis and hemorrhage. Concurrence of mass with ascites indicates invasion of peritoneal surfaces.

Liposarcoma. Originates from fat. Liposarcoma has a complex echogenic pattern with thick walls.

Fibrosarcoma. Originates from connective tissue. Fibrosarcoma has a complex mostly sonolucent pattern, invading surrounding tissues.

Rhabdomyosarcoma. Originates from muscle. It occurs as a solid, complex or homogeneous echogenic mass, invading surrounding tissues.

Leiomyosarcoma. Originates from smooth muscle. It occurs as a complex echodense mass that may have areas of necrosis and cystic degeneration.

Teratoma. Originates from all three germ layers. Most teratomas occur in the vicinity of the upper pole of the left kidney. Ninety percent are benign. They are heterogeneously mixed echodense and cystic areas. Fifty percent occur in children.

Neurogenic Tumors. Originates from nerve tissue and occur mostly in the paravertebral region. They are heterogeneous and echodense.

Secondary Retroperitoneal Tumors

Secondary retroperitoneal tumors are primary recurrences from previously resected tumors or recurrent masses from previous renal carcinoma.

Ascitic fluid along with a retroperitoneal tumor usually indicates seeding or invasion of the peritoneal surface. Evaluation of the para-aortic region should be made for extension to the lymph nodes. The liver should also be evaluated for metastatic involvement.

Retroperitoneal Fibrosis

Retroperitoneal fibrosis is the formation of thick sheets of connective tissue extending from the perirenal space to the dome of the bladder. It encases, rather than displaces, the great vessels, ureters, and lymph channels, causing obstruction. Severe uropathy may ensue. The etiology of retroperitoneal fibrosis is usually idiopathic, but it may sometimes be associated with aortic aneurysm, the use of methysergide for vascular headaches, or retroperitoneal neoplasm.

Clinical Findings. The clinical findings in retroperitoneal fibrosis include hydronephrosis, hypertension, anuria, fever, leukocytosis, anemia, nausea and vomiting, weight loss, malaise, palpable abdominal or rectal mass, and abdominal, back, or flank pain. It is more frequent in males than females and is most common at ages 50 through the 60s.

Sonographic Findings. Retroperitoneal fibrosis appears as thick masses anterior and lateral to the aorta and IVC, extending from the renal vessels to the sacral promontory. The anechoic to hypoechoic sheets have smooth, well-defined anterior margins and irregular, poorly defined posterior margins. The differential diagnosis includes lymphoma, nodal metastases, and retroperitoneal sarcoma or hematoma.

Retroperitoneal Fluid Collections

Collections of fluids in the retroperitoneum include abscesses, hematomas, urinomas, lymphoceles, and cysts.

LYMPHATIC SYSTEM

The lymphatic system arises from veins in the developing embryo and is closely associated with veins throughout most parts of the body. Lymphatic vessels assist veins in their function by draining many of the body tissues and thus increasing the amount of fluid returning to the heart. The lymph vascular network does not form a closed-loop system like the blood vascular system. Lymph vessels begin as tiny, colorless, unconnected capillaries in the connective tissues. These merge to form progressively larger vessels that are interrupted at various sites by small filtering stations called lymph nodes. Lymph vessels ultimately drain into two principal lymph vessels: thoracic and right lymph ducts. These ducts, which have the appearance of small veins, pour about 2 L of lymph into the

Questions

1. All of the following statements about the kidneys are true *except*

   (A) the kidneys are intraperitoneal in location
   (B) the average adult kidneys measure approximately 11–12 cm in length
   (C) the kidneys may move with respiration
   (D) the anteroposterior thickness of the normal adult kidneys are approximately 4–5 cm

2. The renal sinus echoes are produced by

   (A) pelvis and calyces, renal vessels, fat, and areolar tissue
   (B) perinephric fat
   (C) renal parenchyma
   (D) all of the above

3. The renal parenchyma is separated into cortex and medulla by the

   (A) glomeruli
   (B) renal fat
   (C) arcuate vessels
   (D) renal pelvis

4. The best approach for the evaluation of the left kidney is

   (A) supine
   (B) prone
   (C) RAO
   (D) coronal

5. All of the following statements about infantile hypertrophic pyloric stenosis are true *except*

   (A) it causes projectile vomiting
   (B) it is predominantly a disorder of male infants
   (C) the hypertrophied pyloric muscle measures less than 3 mm
   (D) it appears sonographically as a target-shaped lesion

6. To fulfill the criteria of a cyst, one must demonstrate sonographically

   (A) an anechoic structure
   (B) distal acoustic enhancement
   (C) smooth walls
   (D) all of the above

7. While performing an ultrasound examination, the sonographer finds that both kidneys measure 5 cm in length. They are very echogenic. One should consider the possibility of all of the following *except*

   (A) chronic glomerulonephritis
   (B) chronic pyelonephritis
   (C) renal vascular disease
   (D) renal vein thrombosis

8. Columns of Bertin may be confused with a pseudotumor. These may be found

   (A) in the cortex surrounding and separating the renal pyramids and are unusually large
   (B) in the major calyces as a rudimentary ureter
   (C) in the minor calyces as a rudimentary calix
   (D) outside the renal capsule

9. In the fasting patient, what is a common cause for sonographic nonvisualization of the gallbladder?

   (A) contraction of the gallbladder due to chronic cholecystitis
   (B) biliary sludge
   (C) mobile stone
   (D) the ingestion of oral contrast medium used in x-rays of the gallbladder prior to sonographic examination

10. In cases of renal trauma, sonography may be helpful in identifying a hematoma within the renal parenchyma. A hematoma typically presents as

    (A) a sonolucent mass
    (B) an echogenic mass
    (C) a semicystic, semisolid mass
    (D) all of the above

Questions

1. All of the following statements about the kidneys are true *except*

   (A) the kidneys are intraperitoneal in location
   (B) the average adult kidneys measure approximately 11–12 cm in length
   (C) the kidneys may move with respiration
   (D) the anteroposterior thickness of the normal adult kidneys are approximately 4–5 cm

2. The renal sinus echoes are produced by

   (A) pelvis and calyces, renal vessels, fat, and areolar tissue
   (B) perinephric fat
   (C) renal parenchyma
   (D) all of the above

3. The renal parenchyma is separated into cortex and medulla by the

   (A) glomeruli
   (B) renal fat
   (C) arcuate vessels
   (D) renal pelvis

4. The best approach for the evaluation of the left kidney is

   (A) supine
   (B) prone
   (C) RAO
   (D) coronal

5. All of the following statements about infantile hypertrophic pyloric stenosis are true *except*

   (A) it causes projectile vomiting
   (B) it is predominantly a disorder of male infants
   (C) the hypertrophied pyloric muscle measures less than 3 mm
   (D) it appears sonographically as a target-shaped lesion

6. To fulfill the criteria of a cyst, one must demonstrate sonographically

   (A) an anechoic structure
   (B) distal acoustic enhancement
   (C) smooth walls
   (D) all of the above

7. While performing an ultrasound examination, the sonographer finds that both kidneys measure 5 cm in length. They are very echogenic. One should consider the possibility of all of the following *except*

   (A) chronic glomerulonephritis
   (B) chronic pyelonephritis
   (C) renal vascular disease
   (D) renal vein thrombosis

8. Columns of Bertin may be confused with a pseudotumor. These may be found

   (A) in the cortex surrounding and separating the renal pyramids and are unusually large
   (B) in the major calyces as a rudimentary ureter
   (C) in the minor calyces as a rudimentary calix
   (D) outside the renal capsule

9. In the fasting patient, what is a common cause for sonographic nonvisualization of the gallbladder?

   (A) contraction of the gallbladder due to chronic cholecystitis
   (B) biliary sludge
   (C) mobile stone
   (D) the ingestion of oral contrast medium used in x-rays of the gallbladder prior to sonographic examination

10. In cases of renal trauma, sonography may be helpful in identifying a hematoma within the renal parenchyma. A hematoma typically presents as

   (A) a sonolucent mass
   (B) an echogenic mass
   (C) a semicystic, semisolid mass
   (D) all of the above

Gastrointestinal Lymphoma. Fifteen percent of non-Hodgkin's lymphomas may present with gastrointestinal involvement. Sonographic features include a relatively hypoechoic mass with central sonodensity. Such findings are not specific for lymphomatous involvement, as gastric carcinoma or gastric wall edema may have a similar appearance.

Pancreatic Lymphoma. Ten percent of non-Hodgkin's patients present with pancreatic involvement—portions of tissue represented by focal hypoechoic or anechoic masses.

Thyroid Lymphoma. Lymphomatous thyroid masses also present in the same manner.

Inflammatory Conditions

There are three inflammatory conditions of the lymphatic system: acute and chronic lymphadentitis and infectious mononucleosis.

Common primary tumors with metastases to lymph are those of the breast, lung, melanoma, prostate, cervix, and uterus.

Sonographic Pitfalls

1. enlarged nodes can mimic an aortic aneurysm at lower gain settings on longitudinal scans; always scan in transverse to differentiate
2. aneurysms enlarge fairly symmetrically, whereas enlarged nodes tend to drape over prevertebral vessels
3. bowel can mimic enlarged nodes so check for peristalsis; nodes are reproducible, bowel is *not*

RETROPERITONEAL VERSUS INTRAPERITONEAL MASSES

The retroperitoneal location of a mass is confirmed when there is:

- anterior renal displacement
- anterior displacement of dilated ureters
- anterior displacement of the retroperitoneal fat pad—retroperitoneal lesions displace the fat pad ventrally and often cranially, whereas hepatic and subhepatic lesions produce inferior and posterior displacement. The vector of displacement may permit diagnosis of the anatomical origin of right upper quadrant masses.
- anterior vascular displacement—aorta, IVC, splenic vein, superior mesenteric vein

brachiocephalic veins every 24 hours. The lymph vascular system has no pump of its own to push the lymph forward as the heart does blood. Therefore, lymph flow largely depends upon the kneading action of neighboring skeletal muscles alternately contracting and relaxing.

This lymphatic network has tremendous clinical significance. Interruption of lymph drainage in an area generally creates considerable swelling (edema) owing to the accumulation of fluids. In addition, the lymph vessels offer a variety of routes for cancer cells to move from one site to another (metastasis).

Lymph Nodes

Lymph nodes contain lymphocytes and reticulum cells, their function being one of filtration and production of lymphocytes and antibodies. All the lymph passes through nodes, which act as filters not only for bacteria but also for cancer cells. Enlargement of lymph nodes is a usual sign of an ongoing bacterial or carcinogenic process. Normal lymph nodes measure less than 1 cm in size. Sonographically, we can evaluate lymph nodes in the pelvis, retroperitoneum, portahepatis, perirenal, and prevertebral vasculature.

Function. The lymph nodes function in (1) the formation of lymphocytes, (2) the production of antibodies, and (3) the filtration of lymph.

Sonographic Appearance. In order to visualize lymph nodes they must be at least 2 cm in size. They are very homogeneous. Lymph nodes are typically hypoechoic but there is no through transmission. Lymphomas have a nonspecific appearance but in general:

- adenopathy secondary to lymphoma are usually sonolucent
- adenopathy secondary to metastatic disease is usually complex
- posttherapy enlarged nodes are usually very echogenic but may develop cystic areas secondary to necrosis

Periaortic nodes have specific characteristics: They may drape the great vessels anteriorly (obscuring sharp anterior vascular border); may have a lobular, smooth, or scalloped appearance; and with mesenteric involvement, they may fill most of the abdomen in an irregular complex pattern.

Sonographic Technique. Concentrate on prevertebral vessels, aorta, IVC; portahepatis (can produce *biliary* obstruction); spleen size; iliopsoas muscles; urinary bladder contour; perirenal; retroperitoneum; and pelvis.

Para-aortic lymph nodes are involved with lymphoma in 25% of cases and 40% with Hodgkin's disease. The sonographic appearance of these lymphomatous nodes varies from hypoechoic to anechoic with good thorough transmission. Occasionally, anechoic nodal masses may resemble cystic structures. Nodal enlargement secondary to other neoplasms or inflammatory processes, such as retroperitoneal fibrosis, may be indistinguishable from lymphomatous lymphadenopathy. Para-aortic or para-caval nodes frequently obscure the sharp anterior vascular border or compress the aorta or inferior vena cava. Decubitus viewing of the aorta and IVC facilitates sonographic imaging of the retroperitoneal area down to the aortic bifurcation.

Tumors of Lymphoid Tissue

Lymphomas (Tumors of Lymphoid Tissue). *Hodgkin's disease* (40%) is a malignant condition characterized by generalized lymphoid tissue enlargement (eg, enlarged lymph nodes and spleen). Twice as many males as females are affected. It usually occurs between the ages of 15 and 34 or after age 50. Histopathologic classification: Reed Sternberg cells and multinucleated cells are present.

Non-Hodgkin's (60%) *disease* is further subdivided into nodular and diffuse histopathologies. It is a heterogeneous group of diseases that consist of neoplastic proliferation of lymphoid cells that usually disseminate throughout the body. It occurs in all age groups with the incidence increasing with age.

Mesenteric nodal involvement is less than 4% in patients with Hodgkin's disease but more than 50% in non-Hodgkin's patients. Lymphomatous cellular infiltration of the greater omentum may be seen as a uniformly thick, hypoechoic band-shaped structure. The appearance of mesenteric nodes can resemble that of retroperitoneal nodes. Mesenteric masses may also appear as multiple cystic or separated masses that may resemble fluid-filled bowel loops. Perihepatic nodes, celiac axis nodes, splenichilar, and renal-hilar nodes may also be demonstrated sonographically. Although most are hypoechoic to anechoic, inhomogenous areas of increased echogenicity can be found in areas of focal necrosis within large nodes. Nodes can encase or invade adjacent organs and produce significant organ displacement, whereas portal nodes can produce biliary obstruction.

Extranodal Lymphoma. The liver, kidneys, GI tract, pancreas, and thyroid may show lymphomatous involvement.

Hepatic Lymphoma. Hepatic lymphomatous involvement presents as multiple hypoechoic or anechoic focal parenchymal defects. Although these anechoic lesions may resemble cystic structures, they rarely demonstrate enhanced posterior acoustic transmission or peripheral refractory shadowing. Hepatic abscesses, metastases from sarcomas or melanomas, focal areas of cholangitis, radiation fibrosis, and extensive hemosiderosis have presented with findings sonographically indistinguishable from hepatic lymphoma.

Renal Lymphoma. Less than 3% of all non-Hodgkin's lymphomas present with renal involvement, mainly Burkitt's lymphoma or diffuse histiocytic lymphomas.

2. The perirenal space contains the kidneys, ureters, adrenal glands, aorta, IVC, and retroperitoneal nodes
3. The posterior pararenal space contains the posterior abdominal wall, iliopsoas muscle, and quadratus lumborum muscle

Pathology

The retroperitoneal area is subject to infection, bleeding, inflammation, and tumors.

Anterior Pararenal Space. Pancreatic pathology, carcinoma of the duodenum, ascending and descending colon causing bowel thickening or infiltration resulting in a "bullseye" or inverted "bagel sign."

Perirenal Space. Kidney diseases, adrenal diseases, invasion or displacement of IVC, aortic aneurysms, ureteral abnormalities, sarcoma, liposarcoma, aortic, and retroperitoneal adenopathy.

Posterior Pararenal Space. Renal transplantation is usually performed in this extraperitoneal space within the iliac fossa, using the iliac vessels for anastomosis.

Primary Retroperitoneal Tumors

Primary retroperitoneal tumors are mostly malignant, rapidly growing, and the larger tumors are more likely to show evidence of necrosis and hemorrhage. Concurrence of mass with ascites indicates invasion of peritoneal surfaces.

Liposarcoma. Originates from fat. Liposarcoma has a complex echogenic pattern with thick walls.

Fibrosarcoma. Originates from connective tissue. Fibrosarcoma has a complex mostly sonolucent pattern, invading surrounding tissues.

Rhabdomyosarcoma. Originates from muscle. It occurs as a solid, complex or homogeneous echogenic mass, invading surrounding tissues.

Leiomyosarcoma. Originates from smooth muscle. It occurs as a complex echodense mass that may have areas of necrosis and cystic degeneration.

Teratoma. Originates from all three germ layers. Most teratomas occur in the vicinity of the upper pole of the left kidney. Ninety percent are benign. They are heterogeneously mixed echodense and cystic areas. Fifty percent occur in children.

Neurogenic Tumors. Originates from nerve tissue and occur mostly in the paravertebral region. They are heterogeneous and echodense.

Secondary Retroperitoneal Tumors

Secondary retroperitoneal tumors are primary recurrences from previously resected tumors or recurrent masses from previous renal carcinoma.

Ascitic fluid along with a retroperitoneal tumor usually indicates seeding or invasion of the peritoneal surface. Evaluation of the para-aortic region should be made for extension to the lymph nodes. The liver should also be evaluated for metastatic involvement.

Retroperitoneal Fibrosis

Retroperitoneal fibrosis is the formation of thick sheets of connective tissue extending from the perirenal space to the dome of the bladder. It encases, rather than displaces, the great vessels, ureters, and lymph channels, causing obstruction. Severe uropathy may ensue. The etiology of retroperitoneal fibrosis is usually idiopathic, but it may sometimes be associated with aortic aneurysm, the use of methysergide for vascular headaches, or retroperitoneal neoplasm.

Clinical Findings. The clinical findings in retroperitoneal fibrosis include hydronephrosis, hypertension, anuria, fever, leukocytosis, anemia, nausea and vomiting, weight loss, malaise, palpable abdominal or rectal mass, and abdominal, back, or flank pain. It is more frequent in males than females and is most common at ages 50 through the 60s.

Sonographic Findings. Retroperitoneal fibrosis appears as thick masses anterior and lateral to the aorta and IVC, extending from the renal vessels to the sacral promontory. The anechoic to hypoechoic sheets have smooth, well-defined anterior margins and irregular, poorly defined posterior margins. The differential diagnosis includes lymphoma, nodal metastases, and retroperitoneal sarcoma or hematoma.

Retroperitoneal Fluid Collections

Collections of fluids in the retroperitoneum include abscesses, hematomas, urinomas, lymphoceles, and cysts.

LYMPHATIC SYSTEM

The lymphatic system arises from veins in the developing embryo and is closely associated with veins throughout most parts of the body. Lymphatic vessels assist veins in their function by draining many of the body tissues and thus increasing the amount of fluid returning to the heart. The lymph vascular network does not form a closed-loop system like the blood vascular system. Lymph vessels begin as tiny, colorless, unconnected capillaries in the connective tissues. These merge to form progressively larger vessels that are interrupted at various sites by small filtering stations called lymph nodes. Lymph vessels ultimately drain into two principal lymph vessels: thoracic and right lymph ducts. These ducts, which have the appearance of small veins, pour about 2 L of lymph into the

11. Extravasation of urine into the perinephric space (urinoma) may be found in cases of

(A) renal injuries
(B) renal transplants
(C) patients who have passed a renal stone
(D) all of the above

12. Hydronephrosis may be best demonstrated sonographically by which of the following patterns?

(A) distorted shape of the kidney outline
(B) multiple cystic masses throughout the renal parenchyma
(C) fluid-filled pelvocaliceal collecting system
(D) hyperechoic pelvocaliceal collecting system

13. Hydronephrosis may be caused by

(A) prostatic enlargement
(B) calculi
(C) congenital and/or inflammatory stricture
(D) pregnancy
(E) tumors
(F) all of the above

14. A 3-year-old boy presents with hematuria and a palpable left flank mass. Sonography depicts a solid renal mass. This finding would *most* likely represent

(A) hypernephroma
(B) Wilms' tumor
(C) neuroblastoma
(D) infantile polycystic kidney disease

15. A patient presents with right upper quadrant pain, fever, and elevated white blood cell count. The gallbladder appears enlarged with echogenic debris. This *most* probably represents

(A) porcelain gallbladder
(B) hydropic gallbladder
(C) empyema of the gallbladder
(D) carcinoma of the gallbladder

16. Acute cholecystitis is associated with

(A) right upper quadrant pain
(B) Murphy's sign
(C) stone impacted within the cystic duct
(D) fever and an elevated white blood cell count
(E) all of the above

17. A patient presents with ampulla of Vater obstruction, distension of the gallbladder, and painless jaundice. This is associated with

(A) hydrops of the gallbladder
(B) choledochal cyst
(C) Courvoisier's sign
(D) Hartmann's pouch

18. Gallbladder wall thickening may be due to

(A) ascites
(B) hypoproteinema
(C) right-sided congestive cardiac failure
(D) hepatitis
(E) acute cholecystitis
(F) chronic cholecystitis
(G) all of the above

19. Long-standing cystic duct obstruction will give rise to

(A) porcelain gallbladder
(B) hydropic gallbladder
(C) septated gallbladder
(D) gallbladder kink

20. The upper limits of the normal intraluminal diameter of the common duct should not exceed

(A) 4 mm
(B) 7 cm
(C) 7 mm
(D) 10 mm

21. In the normal adult, with gallbladder in place, the luminal diameter of the proximal common hepatic duct is less than or equal to

(A) 3–4 mm
(B) 5–6 mm
(C) 7–8 mm

22. Within the renal sinus, the following can be found *except*

(A) renal pyramids
(B) minor calyces
(C) major calyces
(D) the renal pelvis
(E) vessels
(F) lymphatics

23. The renal cortex contains one of the following

(A) Bowman's capsule and convoluted tubules
(B) renal pyramids
(C) major calyces
(D) minor calyces
(E) all of the above

24. Elevation of the following laboratory data may indicate renal failure *except* for

(A) blood urea nitrogen (BUN)
(B) alkaline phosphatase
(C) creatinine
(D) protein

25. A congenital abnormality in which both kidneys are united at their lower poles is termed a

    (A) column of Bertin
    (B) dromedary hump
    (C) horseshoe kidney

26. Adult polycystic disease may be characterized by all of the following *except*

    (A) it is a latent disease until the third or fourth decade
    (B) it is an autosomal dominant disease
    (C) it may have associated cysts in the liver, pancreas, and spleen
    (D) the involved kidneys are small and extremely echogenic

27. Staghorn calculus refers to a large stone within the

    (A) pancreas
    (B) urinary bladder
    (C) pelvis of the kidney
    (D) common bile duct

28. Thickening of the gallbladder wall is a common feature in

    (A) hypoalbuminemia
    (B) cholecystitis—acute or chronic
    (C) adenomyomatosis
    (D) carcinoma of the gallbladder
    (E) all of the above

29. Hypernephroma (renal adenocarcinoma) is characterized by

    (A) the most common renal cell tumor representing three quarters of all adult renal malignancies
    (B) irregular in shape but well-marginated solid mass
    (C) tumor growth so large that it replaces the renal volume
    (D) all of the above

30. Horseshoe kidneys may be confused sonographically with which of the following entities?

    (A) carcinoma of the head of the pancreas
    (B) lymphadenopathy
    (C) hypernephroma

31. The pancreatic head lies

    (A) caudad to the portal vein and medial to the superior mesenteric vein
    (B) cephalad to the portal vein and medial to the superior mesenteric vein
    (C) caudad to the portal vein and anterior to the inferior vena cava
    (D) cephalad to the portal vein and anterior to the inferior vena cava

32. The liver is covered by a thick membrane of collagenous fibers intermixed with elastic elements. This membrane is called

    (A) Glisson's capsule
    (B) Gerota's fascia
    (C) Bowman's capsule

33. The splenic vein is identified as

    (A) anterior to the aorta
    (B) anterior to the superior mesenteric artery
    (C) caudad to the celiac axis
    (D) all of the above

34. The proximal aorta is more posteriorly placed than the distal aorta with

    (A) a gradual increase in size as it proceeds distally in the abdomen
    (B) a generally horizontal course
    (C) it decreases in size as it proceeds distally in the abdomen

35. Hepatic veins can be differentiated from portal veins because

    (A) hepatic veins are not surrounded by bright acoustical reflections
    (B) hepatic veins increase in caliber as the vessel approaches the diaphragm
    (C) the angle formed by the branching of hepatic venous radicles will point superiorly to superomedially
    (D) hepatic veins drain dorsomedially toward the inferior vena cava
    (E) all of the above

36. The celiac trunk originates within the first 2 cm from the diaphragm and immediately branches into all of the following *except*

    (A) common hepatic artery
    (B) left gastric artery
    (C) gastroduodenal artery
    (D) splenic artery

37. The superior mesenteric artery arises 1 cm below the celiac trunk and runs

    (A) anterior to the pancreas and posterior to the uncinate process
    (B) cephalad to the pancreas and caudal to the uncinate process
    (C) posterior to the pancreas and anterior to the uncinate process

38. The division into anatomic left and right lobes of the liver is along the line of attachment of the

    (A) major hepatic fissure and middle hepatic vein
    (B) ligamentum venosum

(C) falciform ligament
(D) middle hepatic duct

39. Which of the following is *not* true about pleural fluid?

(A) it can be anechoic
(B) it can be loculated
(C) it can be seen superior to the diaphragm
(D) it can be seen inferior to the diaphragm

40. In acute renal disease, the kidney size is

(A) generally enlarged
(B) generally small
(C) not affected

41. When the gallbladder fundus is folded over on itself, this is referred to as a

(A) junctional fold
(B) Hartmann's pouch
(C) phrygian cap

42. On a transverse sonogram, the common bile duct is located _____ to the head of the pancreas and lies _____ to the inferior vena cava

(A) anterior; medial
(B) posterior; posterior
(C) posterior; anterior

43. Which of the following statements regarding the spleen are *false?*

(A) a prominent bulge along the medial surface of the spleen can be seen in normal patients
(B) the normal-sized spleen should not extend caudal to the midportion of the left kidney
(C) the spleen is a retroperitoneal organ
(D) the sonographic texture of the normal spleen is homogeneous

44. Which statement about the kidneys is *false?*

(A) the kidneys are rigidly fixed on the abdominal wall
(B) the kidneys consist of an internal medullary and external cortical substance
(C) the kidneys rest on the psoas and quadratus lumborum muscles
(D) renal pyramids are found within the medullary region

45. Gallbladder carcinoma has a strong association with

(A) calculi and chronic mechanical irritation
(B) polypoid mass
(C) jaundice with weight loss
(D) bile duct obstruction
(E) chronic cholecystitis

(F) porcelain gallbladder
(G) all of the above

46. The inferior vena cava forms at the confluence of the

(A) right and left carotid veins
(B) right and left lumbar veins
(C) right and left common iliac veins

47. All of the following describe the inferior vena cava *except*

(A) Valsalva maneuver results in a change in the diameter of the inferior vena cava
(B) it lies immediately anterior to the surface of the spine, to the right of the aorta
(C) the caliber of the inferior vena cava increases as it courses cephalad
(D) it passes through the caval hiatus of the diaphragm to enter the left atrium

48. To distinguish dilated bile ducts from portal veins, all of these criteria can be used *except*

(A) distal acoustic enhancement
(B) echogenic walls
(C) parallel channel sign
(D) stellate pattern of the ducts near the porta hepatis
(E) numerous tubular structures within the periphery of the liver

49. A congenital dilation of the biliary tree is called

(A) sclerosing cholangitis
(B) Courvoisier gallbladder
(C) choledochal cyst

50. A fluid-filled mass anterior to the pancreas may be all of the following *except*

(A) pseudocyst
(B) loculated ascites
(C) aortic aneurysm
(D) fluid-filled stomach

51. The left renal vein runs

(A) between the aorta and the superior mesenteric artery
(B) posterior to the aorta
(C) posterior to the inferior vena cava
(D) parallel to the portal vein

52. The superior mesenteric vein

    (A) enters the inferior vena cava at the level of the renal vein
    (B) runs upward to the right of the superior mesenteric artery
    (C) runs medially to enter the posterior and lateral aspect of the inferior vena cava
    (D) none of the above

53. Throughout its course, the splenic vein relates to the

    (A) anterior surface of the pancreatic body and tail
    (B) anterior surface of the uncinate process
    (C) posterior surface of the pancreatic body and tail

54. If on sonographic examination, one finds a patient with intrahepatic dilated ducts and a small gallbladder, this may indicate that the level of obstruction is

    (A) at the common bile duct
    (B) above the cystic duct
    (C) below the cystic duct

55. The normal thickness of the gallbladder wall is

    (A) 15 mm
    (B) 7 mm
    (C) 10 mm
    (D) 3 mm
    (E) 5 mm

56. Adenomyomatosis of the gallbladder is

    (A) a disease of childbearing years
    (B) an inflammation of the gallbladder
    (C) associated with Murphy's sign
    (D) a benign proliferation and thickening of the muscle and glandular layer

57. Strong specular reflections arising from the liver are the result of

    (A) liver parenchyma
    (B) Glisson's capsule
    (C) portal veins
    (D) hepatic arteries

58. An increase in parenchymal echogenicity within the liver may be due to

    (A) alcohol abuse
    (B) diabetes
    (C) chemotherapy
    (D) toxic substances
    (E) all of the above

59. Hydronephrosis frequently occurs in

    (A) renal hypoplasia
    (B) duplication of ureters in a duplicated kidney collecting system
    (C) horseshoe kidney

60. A patient presents with a dilated interhepatic duct, dilated gallbladder, and a dilated common bile duct. The level of obstruction should be at the

    (A) proximal common bile duct
    (B) distal common bile duct
    (C) common hepatic duct

61. Sonographically, the gastroesophageal junction can be visualized

    (A) anterior to the inferior vena cava
    (B) anterior to the aorta and posterior to the left lobe of the liver
    (C) it cannot be recognized sonographically

62. In cases of acute viral hepatitis, the liver parenchyma appears

    (A) hyperechoic
    (B) echogenic
    (C) normal

63. The gallbladder contracts in response to gastrointestinal peptide hormones, chiefly

    (A) gastrin
    (B) peptine
    (C) lipase
    (D) cholecystokinin
    (E) alkaline phosphatase

64. Diffuse thickening of the gallbladder wall an be seen with all of the following except

    (A) acute cholecystitis
    (B) hepatitis
    (C) congestive heart failure
    (D) elevated portal pressure

65. The best sonographic window to the left hemidiaphragm is the

    (A) spleen
    (B) kidney
    (C) stomach
    (D) left lung

66. The most frequent benign tumor of the pancreas is

    (A) adenoma
    (B) islet cell tumor
    (C) cystadenoma

67. The most common primary neoplasm of the pancreas is adenocarcinoma. This

(A) is usually found in the head of the pancreas
(B) is accompanied by weight loss and painless jaundice
(C) is accompanied by a dilated gallbladder
(D) causes enlargement of the gland with irregular nodular border
(E) causes enlargement of the common duct
(F) all of the above

68. The portion of the pancreas that lies posterior to the superior mesenteric artery and vein is the

(A) head
(B) uncinate process
(C) body
(D) tail

69. High levels of serum amylase may be a result of all of the following *except*

(A) liver disease
(B) acute pancreatitis
(C) blockage of the pancreatic duct by a stone within the common bile duct

70. The pancreas produces all of the following *except*

(A) insulin
(B) glucagon
(C) bile
(D) lipase

71. On the medial border of each kidney is the renal hilum that contains

(A) the renal vein
(B) the renal artery
(C) the proximal ureter
(D) all of the above

72. The kidneys, the perinephric fat, and the adrenal glands are all covered by

(A) a true capsule
(B) Gerota's fascia
(C) peritoneum
(D) Glisson's capsule

73. The normal adult kidneys measure

(A) 6–9 cm in length and 4–5 cm in thickness
(B) 12–15 cm in length and 4–5 cm in thickness
(C) 10–12 cm in length and 4–5 cm in thickness

74. If a heavy deposition of fat (sinus lipomatosis) is found within the kidney on renal sonography, the renal sinus will appear

(A) enlarged
(B) mostly echo free

(C) mostly echogenic
(D) all of the above

75. If one does renal sonogram and finds a solid mass, one should

(A) end the examination and document what was found
(B) continue the examination and look at the pancreas for metastasis
(C) continue the examination and check the inferior vena cava and renal vein for tumor extension as well as the retroperitoneum for nodes
(D) continue the examination and check the aorta for tumor extension

76. Chronic pancreatitis may be associated with which of the following sonographic patterns?

(A) usually hyperechoic, with echogenicity greater than the liver
(B) a generalized decrease in the size of the pancreas
(C) occasionally one may see bright discrete echoes of calcification with a dilated pancreatic duct
(D) all of the above

77. Which of the following does *not* describe the pancreas?

(A) it lies within the peritoneal space
(B) it is a retroperitoneal structure
(C) it is nonencapsulated
(D) it is a multilobulated gland
(E) it is approximately 15 cm in length

78. One of the most frequent complications of pancreatitis is pseudocyst formation. Uncomplicated pseudocysts are usually

(A) echogenic with irregular walls and good ultrasound transmission distally
(B) echogenic with smooth walls and poor ultrasound transmission distally
(C) anechoic with smooth walls and good ultrasound transmission distally

79. Occasionally, a pseudocyst may have internal echoes and be confused with an abscess. To distinguish the two, one should look for

(A) calcification
(B) fluid in the pouch of Douglas
(C) gas

80. A pancreatic pseudocyst

(A) must be treated surgically
(B) may regress spontaneously
(C) must be treated with a diet of liquid lipase

81. Pancreatic pseudocysts are usually found in the area of the lesser sac. On occasion, a pancreatic pseudocyst may be found in the

    (A) groin
    (B) mediastinum
    (C) the porta hepatis area
    (D) pelvis
    (E) all of the above

82. The pancreas is both an exocrine and endocrine gland. The endocrine function is to produce

    (A) insulin
    (B) lipase
    (C) amylase
    (D) carboxypeptide
    (E) trypsin
    (F) chymotrypsin

83. The exocrine products of the pancreas are carried within the

    (A) blood stream
    (B) acinar cells
    (C) pancreatic duct

84. The maximum inner diameter of the pancreatic duct in young adults is

    (A) 5 mm
    (B) 2 mm
    (C) 3 mm
    (D) 4 mm

85. It is very important to image the duct within the substance of the pancreas. Structures that may be confused with the duct are

    (A) collapsed stomach wall anteriorly
    (B) portal vein posteriorly
    (C) splenic vein posteriorly
    (D) all of the above

86. The most common primary carcinoma of the pancreas is

    (A) leiomyosarcoma
    (B) adenocarcinoma
    (C) lymphoma
    (D) all of the above

87. All of the following statements pertaining to adenocarcinoma of the pancreas are *true except* that it is

    (A) imaged as a solid, focally enlarged lobulated mass with low-level echoes
    (B) usually found in the head of the pancreas
    (C) associated with biliary obstruction
    (D) not associated with biliary obstruction
    (E) associated with pancreatic duct obstruction

88. If a mass in the area of the pancreatic head is found, special attention should be directed to which of the following areas?

    (A) the portal vein
    (B) the liver (for "fatty" changes)
    (C) the common bile duct
    (D) the spleen
    (E) the kidney

89. When a pancreatic mass is imaged, raising the possibility of carcinoma, what other findings may lead to a diagnosis of malignancy?

    (A) liver masses
    (B) lymphadenopathic masses
    (C) venous obstruction
    (D) ascites
    (E) inferior vena cava compression
    (F) all of the above

90. The most common sonographic appearance of acute pancreatitis is

    (A) usually hyperechoic, with echogenicity greater than the liver and irregular in shape
    (B) the pancreas is enlarged with smooth contours, uniformly hypoechoic, demonstrating a decrease in ultrasound absorption, and an increase in through transmission
    (C) the pancreas is enlarged with smooth contours, uniformly hypoechoic, demonstrating an increase in ultrasound absorption and a decrease in through transmission

91. What structure may be mistaken for a mass in the head of the pancreas?

    (A) duodenum
    (B) portal vein
    (C) Riedel's lobe
    (D) quadrate lobe

92. The liver's exocrine function includes producing

    (A) glycogen
    (B) urea
    (C) heparin
    (D) bile

93. The accessory duct of the pancreas is termed

    (A) Wirsung's duct
    (B) Santorini's duct
    (C) Müllerian duct

94. The uncinate process of the pancreas extends

    (A) lateral to the inferior vena cava and posterior to the superior mesenteric artery
    (B) medial to the inferior vena cava and anterior to the portal vein

(C) medial to the inferior vena cava and posterior to the superior mesenteric vein

95. The extrahepatic portion of the falciform ligament

(A) runs between the inferior vena cava and the gallbladder

(B) is seen with ascites

(C) connects the liver to a lesser sac

96. The portion of the liver that is not covered by the peritoneum is termed

(A) quadrate lobe

(B) caudate lobe

(C) Riedel's lobe

(D) bare area

97. The right and left hepatic ducts unite to form the common hepatic duct most commonly

(A) in the porta hepatis

(B) within the hepatic parenchyma

(C) at the level of the pancreas

98. A patient with known carcinoma of the breast reveals unequivocal signs of biliary tree dilatation. However, the gallbladder is small and the common bile duct is normal. The sonographic findings that could be found include which of the following?

(A) stone in the cystic duct

(B) stone in the right hepatic duct

(C) enlarged lymph nodes in the porta hepatis

99. The main pancreatic duct is

(A) Santorini's duct

(B) Wirsung's duct

(C) Hirschsprung's duct

100. The ligamentum venosum is all of the following *except*

(A) a remnant of the umbilical vein

(B) a remnant of the ductus venosus

(C) a remnant of the fetal circulation, in which shunted oxygenated blood from the umbilical vein to the inferior vena cava bypasses the liver

(D) defines caudate lobe from left lobe of liver

101. Sonography is helpful in the evaluation of the transplanted kidney. Anechoic masses that occur around a renal transplant include

(A) urinoma

(B) lymphocele

(C) hematoma

(D) abscess

(E) all of the above

102. All of the following are causes of hydronephrosis *except*

(A) posterior urethral valves

(B) acute glomerulonephritis

(C) cancer of the ovary

(D) retroperitoneal tumor

(E) retroperitoneal fibrosis

103. A retroperitoneal abscess may *not* be found within

(A) the rectus abdominus muscle

(B) the psoas muscle

(C) the iliacus muscle

(D) the quadratus lumborum muscle

(E) none of the above

104. Which of the following is *not* retroperitoneal?

(A) kidney

(B) aorta

(C) psoas muscle

(D) spleen

105. Renal vein thrombosis is characterized sonographically by

(A) an enlarged kidney with decreased cortical echogenicity

(B) a normal-sized kidney with an increase in echogenicity

(C) decreased renal size with loss of corticomedullary definition

(D) all of the above may signify acute or chronic conditions

106. Dilatation of the intrahepatic biliary tree without dilatation of the extrahepatic duct includes all of the following *except*

(A) Klatskin tumor

(B) enlarged portal lymph nodes

(C) cholangiocarcinoma

(D) pancreatic carcinoma

107. The gastroduodenal artery

(A) is the first branch of the common hepatic artery

(B) proceeds caudally along the right anterolateral margin of the pancreatic head

(C) is seen in the transverse views directly anterior to the common bile duct

(D) all of the above

108. The liver may be divided segmentally with the right lobe, left lobe, and caudate lobe. The right lobe may be divided further into anterior and posterior segments and the left lobe into medial and lateral segments. The quadrate lobe is part of the

    (A) lateral segment of the left lobe
    (B) lateral segment of the right lobe
    (C) medial segment of the left lobe
    (D) posterior segment of the left lobe

109. The caudate lobe occupies much of the

    (A) anteroinferior surface of the liver
    (B) posteroinferior surface of the liver
    (C) anterosuperior surface of the liver
    (D) posterosuperior surface of the liver

110. The lobes of the liver are clearly defined by the hepatic veins that course between them to form the boundaries of the various hepatic segments and lobes. The hepatic veins are

    (A) right and left
    (B) right, left, and middle
    (C) right, left, middle, and lateral

111. Within the liver there are three ligaments of primary importance to ultrasound. They are ligamentum teres, ligamentum venosum, and falciform ligaments. The ligamentum teres

    (A) resides in the left intersegmental fissure
    (B) is a remnant of the umbilical vein
    (C) recannalizes in severe cirrhosis of the ligament
    (D) is an echogenic spot on transverse scans
    (E) is always seen above the portal vein
    (F) all of the above

112. A dilated common bile duct without the presence of dilated intrahepatic biliary radicles suggests all of the following *except*

    (A) acute obstruction of the common bile duct
    (B) may appear in the presence of chronic infiltrative liver disease
    (C) ascending cholangitis may be present
    (D) a mass in the head of the pancreas

113. Cystic lesions within the liver include

    (A) congenital cysts
    (B) polycystic liver disease
    (C) Caroli's disease
    (D) all of the above

114. Shadowing from the area of the gallbladder fossa can be a source of confusion and error in ruling out cholithiasis. Sources of shadowing include

    (A) spiral valve of Heister
    (B) calcification within the liver

    (C) air in the biliary tree
    (D) all of the above

115. Complex lesions within the liver include

    (A) biliary cystadenoma
    (B) echinococcal cyst
    (C) large cavernous hemangioma
    (D) hematoma
    (E) all of the above

116. The most common cause of pancreatitis in adults in the United States is

    (A) biliary tract disease
    (B) alcohol abuse
    (C) trauma

117. Impaired fat digestion is an important indicator of pancreatic dysfunction. This is due to the reduction of

    (A) insulin
    (B) lipase
    (C) amylase
    (D) carboxypeptide
    (E) trypsin

118. Which of the following is *least* likely to be associated with acute pancreatitis?

    (A) ileus
    (B) jaundice
    (C) the pancreas becomes edematous
    (D) the pancreas becomes diffusely enlarged
    (E) anterior compression of the inferior vena cava

119. Which of the following is *least* likely to be associated with chronic pancreatitis?

    (A) jaundice
    (B) the pancreas becomes edematous
    (C) the pancreatic duct may dilate and contain calculi
    (D) the pancreas becomes fibrotic
    (E) pseudocyst formation

120. Several techniques for imaging the pancreas are

    (A) prone scan
    (B) ingestion of fluid
    (C) positioning the patient erect or sitting up
    (D) positioning the patient right side up
    (E) all of the above

121. The tail of the pancreas extends to the left and has all of the following relationships *except*

    (A) the lesser sac lies anterior
    (B) the left adrenal gland is anterior
    (C) it lies in close relationship to the splenic hilum
    (D) it lies anterior to the left kidney

Figure 5–8. Diagram of the pancreas and other adjacent structures.

Questions 122 through 139: Identify the structures in Fig. 5–8 with the list of terms given in Column B.

COLUMN A

122. _____
123. _____
124. _____
125. _____
126. _____
127. _____
128. _____
129. _____
130. _____
131. _____
132. _____
133. _____
134. _____
135. _____
136. _____
137. _____
138. _____
139. _____

COLUMN B

(A) spleen
(B) gastroduodenal artery
(C) kidney
(D) inferior vena cava
(E) splenic artery
(F) left gastric artery
(G) adrenal
(H) superior mesenteric artery
(I) superior mesenteric vein
(J) celiac axis
(K) common bile duct
(L) portal vein
(M) aorta
(N) duodenum
(O) Santorini's duct
(P) Wirsung's duct
(Q) uncinate process
(R) hepatic artery

140. After cholecystectomy, the luminal diameter of proximal bile duct in normal individuals (ie, individuals with no current bile duct obstruction) is more than 5 mm in a significant (more than 10%) proportion of patients and may be up to 10 mm to be considered within normal limits.

(A) true
(B) false

141. Compare the echogenicities of the following structures and place them in decreasing echogenic order.

(A) pancreas > renal sinus > liver > spleen > renal parenchyma
(B) renal sinus > pancreas > liver > spleen > renal parenchyma

(C) renal sinus > renal parenchyma > pancreas > liver > spleen
(D) pancreas > renal sinus > renal parenchyma > liver > spleen

142. Splenomegaly may be the result of all of the following *except*

(A) an inflammatory process
(B) a left subphrenic abscess
(C) metastic disease to the spleen
(D) polycythemia vera
(E) chronic leukemia and lymphomas

143. With respect to thickening of the bowel wall

(A) the upper limit of normal is 5 mm when non-distended
(B) both inflammation and neoplasm can produce thickening
(C) the bowel wall itself is hypoechoic
(D) diminished or absent peristalsis on real-time is helpful in identifying a disease segment
(E) all of the above

144. A retroperitoneal sarcoma may displace

(A) the kidney posteriorly
(B) the spleen anteriorly
(C) the pancreas posteriorly
(D) the diaphragm inferiorly

145. An adrenal mass may displace the splenic vein

(A) anteriorly
(B) posteriorly
(C) medially

146. A fluid collection located between the diaphragm and the spleen may represent

(A) a pleural effusion
(B) a subcapsular hematoma
(C) a subphrenic abscess

147. At its maximum diameter, the normal adult adrenal rarely measures more than

(A) 2 cm
(B) 2 mm
(C) 3 cm
(D) 3 mm

148. The causes of a large gallbladder include all of the following *except*

(A) adenomyomatosis
(B) cystic duct obstruction
(C) pancreatic carcinoma
(D) diabetes mellitus
(E) a fasting patient
(F) common duct obstruction

149. Patients with right-sided heart failure and elevated systemic venous pressure may develop

    (A) fatty liver
    (B) portal-systemic anastomoses
    (C) marked dilatation of the intrahepatic veins
    (D) nonfocal liver disease

150. The body of the pancreas is bound on its anterior surface by

    (A) the dorsum of the stomach
    (B) the greater sac
    (C) the splenic vein
    (D) all of the above

151. Which of the following is associated with the pancreatic body?

    (A) splenic vein lying posteriorly to the body
    (B) splenic vein lying anteriorly to the body
    (C) gastroduodenal artery
    (D) common bile duct

152. The landmarks associated with the pancreatic head are

    (A) the inferior vena cava lying posteriorly to the head
    (B) the gastroduodenal artery outlining the anterolateral margin of the head of the pancreas
    (C) the common bile duct marking the posterolateral margin of the head of the pancreas
    (D) all of the above

153. Which landmark is most associated with the pancreatic neck?

    (A) hepatic artery
    (B) superior mesenteric vein
    (C) porta hepatis
    (D) superior mesenteric artery

154. Which of the following is *not* a true statement concerning the pancreas?

    (A) the pancreas is a retroperitoneal organ
    (B) the neck and body of the pancreas lies anterior to the superior mesenteric vein and superior mesenteric artery, respectively, and is usually found at the midline
    (C) the pancreas has a true capsule
    (D) the normal anteroposterior dimensions are 2.5 cm for the head, 2.0 cm for the body, and 2.0 cm for the tail
    (E) the upper limits of the pancreatic duct are 3 mm
    (F) the right renal vein lies posterior to the pancreatic head

155. Which of the following is *least* likely to be confused with hydronephrosis?

    (A) an angiomyolipoma
    (B) a multicystic kidney
    (C) sinus lipomatosis
    (D) a central renal cyst

156. The common bile duct is joined by the pancreatic duct as they enter the

    (A) transverse portion of the duodenum
    (B) first portion of the duodenum
    (C) third portion of the duodenum
    (D) second portion of the duodenum

157. On a sagittal scan, the portal vein is seen as a circular anechoic structure

    (A) anterior to the inferior vena cava
    (B) posterior to the aorta
    (C) medial to the head of the pancreas
    (D) inferior to the head of the pancreas

158. The prostate lies

    (A) posterior to the symphysis pubis
    (B) inferior to the urinary bladder
    (C) inferior to the seminal vesicles
    (D) all of the above

159. When performing transverse scans of the pelvis, to best visualize the prostate sonographically, one should

    (A) angle the transducer 20° cephalad
    (B) scan, angling the transducer 15° caudad
    (C) scan, with 0° angulation
    (D) scan, angling the transducer 15° cephalad

160. If the prostate is found to be enlarged, one should also check the

    (A) spleen for enlargement
    (B) scrotum for hydroceles
    (C) kidneys for hydronephrosis
    (D) liver for metastases

161. A 48-year-old female presents postcholecystectomy with right-upper quadrant pain, an elevated serum bilirubin (mainly conjugated), and bilirubin in her urine. It is true that

    (A) she probably has hepatitis
    (B) she probably has a stone, tumor, or stricture obstructing the bile duct
    (C) the common duct will probably be less than 5 mm in internal diameter
    (D) alkaline phosphatase will be normal

162. Acute prostatitis may be due to or complicated by all the following *except*

    (A) hematogenous spread of infection to the prostate

(B) ascending or descending urinary infection

(C) acute cystitis and acute urinary retention

(D) trauma

163. The *most* common prostatic neoplasm is

(A) adenocarcinoma

(B) acute prostatitis

(C) benign cystic teratoma

(D) seminoma

164. A mirror-image artifact within the liver

(A) will appear as high-amplitude parallel lines occurring at regular periodic intervals

(B) will cause the gallbladder to fill in with echoes

(C) may result in a supradiaphragmatic projection of an infradiaphragmatic mass

165. The normal sonographic texture of the spleen is

(A) moderately echogenic but less echogenic than the liver

(B) hypoechoic

(C) strongly echogenic but more echogenic than the liver

(D) hyperechoic

166. The spleen is

(A) center for hematopoietic activity

(B) the largest organ of the reticuloendothelial system

(C) not a part of the reticuloendothelial system

(D) can contribute to the production of alkaline phosphatase

167. Which statement describes the correct anatomic location of structures adjacent to the spleen?

(A) the diaphragm is anterior, lateral, and inferior to the spleen

(B) the fundus of the stomach and lesser sac are medial and posterior to the splenic hilum

(C) the left kidney lies inferior and medial to the spleen

168. Benign ascites may be associated with

(A) peritoneal implants

(B) bowel that is matted posteriorly

(C) floating bowel loops

169. Malignant ascites may be associated with

(A) ascites that are anechoic and freely mobile

(B) bowels that are matted posteriorly

(C) floating bowel loops

170. The scrotum is an extraperitoneal sac that is divided by a septum into two compartments by the median raphe. Each compartment contains all of the following *except*

(A) a testis

(B) glomerulus

(C) an epididymis

(D) a portion of spermatic cord

(E) ductus deferens

171. Hematoceles are complicated hydroceles. The sonographic findings that accompany this abnormality include

(A) a cyst along the course of the vas deferens

(B) blood filling the sac that surrounds the testicle, secondary to trauma or surgery

(C) dilated veins caused by obstruction of the venous return

(D) a condition in which the testicles have not descended

172. Obstructive jaundice may be diagnosed sonographically by demonstrating

(A) a mass on the head of the pancreas with a dilated common bile duct

(B) an enlarged liver

(C) a fibrotic and shrunken liver

(D) cholangitis

173. In patients with uncomplicated acute epididymitis

(A) there is enlargement of the scrotum with focal or generalized thickening of the epididymis

(B) the epididymis is uniformly enlarged and more anechoic than usual

(C) a loculated fluid collection often containing low-level echoes appears cephalad to the testis

174. Acute hydroceles are *not* a result of

(A) trauma

(B) testicular torsion

(C) tumor

(D) infection of the testis or epididymis

175. The sonographic texture of the normal testis is

(A) heterogeneous with high-intensity echoes

(B) homogeneous with low-level echogenicity

(C) homogeneous with medium-level echogenicity

(D) variable echo pattern

176. Which of the following are benign lesions of the thyroid?

(A) adenomas

(B) diffuse nontoxic goiter

(C) adenomatous hyperplasia (multinodular goiter)

(D) thyroiditis

(E) thyroglossal duct cyst

(F) all of the above

177. When scanning a 22-year-old patient to rule out cholelithiasis, a single echogenic lesion is seen within the liver. This most probably represents

    (A) a cavernous hemangioma
    (B) a hematoma
    (C) a hepatic cyst
    (D) an abscess

178. Hyperthyroidism associated with a diffuse goiter is associated with

    (A) papillary carcinoma
    (B) Graves' disease
    (C) Hashimoto's thyroiditis
    (D) adenoma

179. Anatomic landmarks associated with the thyroid are the

    (A) trachea medially, longus colli muscle laterally, carotid artery and strap muscles posteriorly
    (B) trachea medially, longus colli muscles posteriorly, carotid artery and internal jugular vein laterally, strap muscles medially
    (C) trachea medially, longus colli muscle posteriorly, carotid artery and internal jugular vein laterally, strap muscles anterolaterally
    (D) trachea and strap muscles medially, longus colli muscle posteriorly, carotid artery inferiorly

180. If the sonogram suggests a mass in the head of the pancreas, the sonographer should

    (A) examine the biliary radicles, common bile duct, and gallbladder to determine whether they are dilated
    (B) outline the hepatic artery and splenic arteries to determine whether they are dilated
    (C) scan the pancreas using the left kidney as a window, then end the examination
    (D) examine both kidneys carefully to exclude a mass

181. The common carotid arteries can be differentiated from the internal jugular veins by all of the following except

    (A) the jugular veins have a greater diameter than the carotids
    (B) the jugular veins lie lateral to the carotids
    (C) the trachea and esophagus lie medial to the common carotid arteries
    (D) the jugular veins lie directly posterior to the thyroid lobes

182. The transducer of choice when scanning the thyroid gland should be

    (A) a 5-MHz or higher short focus transducer if using the direct contact method
    (B) a 5-MHz or higher medium focus transducer if using the direct contact method
    (C) a 7.5-MHz short internal focus transducer if using a water bath technique
    (D) none of the above

183. Which of the following is highly suspicious for prostatic carcinoma?

    (A) a large cystic mass located within the prostate
    (B) an enlarged prostate
    (C) a well-encapsulated solid mass located within the prostate
    (D) an uneven echo pattern and ill-defined borders
    (E) none of the above; sonography cannot detect changes in the prostate due to prostatic carcinoma because the lesions are usually less than 1 mm.

184. Altered echogenicity within the prostate may indicate

    (A) benign prostatic hypertrophy
    (B) prostatic calculi
    (C) prostatic neoplasm
    (D) all of the above

185. The position of the parathyroid glands are variable. Most often they are located

    (A) posterior to the thyroid lobes and medial to the common carotid arteries
    (B) posterior to the thyroid lobes and anterior to the strap muscles
    (C) anterior to the thyroid lobes and lateral to the anterior scalene muscles
    (D) lateral to the thyroid lobes
    (E) anterior to the trachea and within the isthmus of the thyroid

186. All of the following can mimic a parathyroid adenoma except

    (A) minor neurovascular bundle
    (B) longus colli muscle
    (C) left lateral border of the esophagus
    (D) intrathyroidal adenoma
    (E) goiter

187. Normal measurements of the thyroid gland are

    (A) there are no known normal measurements
    (B) 3–4 cm in anteroposterior dimensions and in length
    (C) 1–2 cm in anteroposterior dimensions and 4–6 cm in length
    (D) 4–6 cm in anteroposterior dimensions and 1–2 cm in length

188. Thyroiditis will usually appear sonographically as

    (A) multiple cysts within the thyroid
    (B) diffusely enlarged thyroid lobes with decreased echogenicity
    (C) diffusely enlarged thyroid lobes with no change in echogenicity
    (D) small, echogenic thyroid

189. The halo sign as it pertains to thyroid masses is defined as a rim of sonolucency surrounding an intrathyroidal mass. It is most commonly encountered in

    (A) cyst
    (B) adenoma
    (C) carcinoma
    (D) thyroiditis

190. All of the following findings could suggest malignant neoplasm of the prostate *except*

    (A) hypoechoic focal lesions
    (B) uneven echo pattern, with irregular border
    (C) an elevation of acid phosphatase
    (D) overall enlargement of the gland with homogeneous echoes

191. The spermatic cord is composed of

    (A) internal spermatic artery, vas deferens, testicular vessels, and nerves
    (B) vas deferens, testicular vessels, nerves, and sperm
    (C) vas deferens, testicular vessels, nerves, and efferent ductules
    (D) vas deferens, testicular vessels, nerves, sperm, and efferent ductules
    (E) vas deferens and its surrounding muscle

192. A varicocele is an

    (A) abnormal dilatation of the draining veins of the scrotum seen in association with epididymitis
    (B) abnormal dilatation of the draining veins of the scrotum seen in approximately 35–40% of infertile and subfertile men
    (C) abnormal dilatation of the draining veins of the scrotum seen only with a malignant condition
    (D) abnormal dilatation of the draining veins of the scrotum that cannot be sonographically differentiated from spermatoceles and epididymal cysts
    (E) all of the above

193. Which of the following would sonographically appear as cystic fluid surrounding a testicle?

    (A) tumor
    (B) orchitis
    (C) epididymitis
    (D) hydrocele

194. All of the following disease states will cause upward displacement of the liver *except*

    (A) excessive dilatation of the colon
    (B) ascites
    (C) abdominal tumor
    (D) subphrenic abscess

195. Budd-Chiari syndrome is

    (A) relative enlargement of the caudate lobe due to hepatic vein thrombosis
    (B) relative shrinking of the caudate lobe due to hepatic vein thrombosis
    (C) relative enlargement of the quadrate lobe due to hepatic vein thrombosis
    (D) relative shrinking of all the lobes of the liver due to hepatic vein thrombosis
    (E) metastatic disease of the liver from the gastrointestinal tract

196. The pyramidal lobe is a normal variant of the thyroid gland. Which of the following is its correct location?

    (A) inferior extension of the right lobe
    (B) superior extension of the isthmus
    (C) inferior extension of the isthmus
    (D) lateral extension of the isthmus

197. Ultrasonography of the urinary bladder is helpful in detecting

    (A) bladder masses
    (B) bladder calculi
    (C) foreign bodies
    (D) bladder diverticula
    (E) all of the above

198. Epididymitis appears sonographically as a(n)

    (A) enlarged prostate
    (B) hypoechoic epididymis with diffuse enlargement of the gland
    (C) hyperechoic epididymis with focal enlargement of the organ
    (D) hydrocele that cannot be differentiated from it

199. On sonographic examination, a seminoma of the testicle may appear as a

    (A) solid, homogeneous mass
    (B) large, multilocular cystic mass
    (C) small, simple cyst
    (D) cannot be detected sonographically

200. Crytorchidism is a condition in which

(A) there is congenital agenesis of the testis
(B) the testicles have not descended and lie either in the abdomen or in the groin
(C) there is a benign enlargement of the testis
(D) the testicles do not produce the hormones that produce masculine features

201. The seminal vesicles

(A) produce sperm located within the prostate
(B) produce sperm located posterior to the bladder
(C) are the reservoir for sperm and are located posterior to the bladder
(D) are the reservoir for sperm and are located between the mediastinum testes and the pampiniform plexus

202. Infarcted testicle following testicular torsion will appear sonographically

(A) in the acute stage, indistinguishable from a hypoechoic tumor occupying the entire organ; in its chronic stage, small and echogenic
(B) in the acute stage, small and echogenic; in its chronic stage, indistinguishable from a hypoechoic tumor occupying the entire organ
(C) in its acute and chronic stages, indistinguishable from a hypoechoic tumor occupying the entire organ

203. The best way to distinguish hepatic veins from portal veins is by

(A) size, the hepatic veins are much smaller than the portal veins
(B) tracing them to their point of origin
(C) visualizing the pulsations of the hepatic veins
(D) visualizing the wall thickness of the vessels knowing that hepatic veins have thicker walls

204. The fundus of the stomach has the following anatomical relationship to the left lobe of the liver

(A) posteromedial
(B) anterolateral
(C) posterolateral
(D) anteromedial
(E) directly superior

205. Fatty infiltration of the liver may be due to all of the following except

(A) cardiac failure
(B) obesity
(C) alcoholic liver disease
(D) renal failure
(E) none of the above

206. Which of the following laboratory values may be elevated in the presence of liver metastases?

(A) blood urea nitrogen
(B) white blood count
(C) α-fetoprotein
(D) alkaline phosphatase
(E) none of the above

207. Metastatic lesions in the liver may appear sonographically as

(A) a target lesion ("bull's eye")
(B) echogenic
(C) anechoic
(D) complex
(E) none of the above

208. A cyst within a cyst (daughter cysts) is a classic example of which of the following liver masses?

(A) polycystic liver disease
(B) echinococcal (hydatid) cyst
(C) hepatoma
(D) hemangiomas
(E) pseudocysts

209. Riedel's lobe is a normal liver variant defined as a(n)

(A) elongated left lobe of the liver
(B) tonguelike extension of the caudate lobe
(C) tonguelike extension of the right lobe of the liver
(D) extra lobe of the liver visualized in some of the population

210. All of the following laboratory tests can be used for liver evaluation except

(A) bilirubin
(B) serum protein
(C) prothrombin time
(D) fetal antigen
(E) amylase
(F) SGOT

211. Given the clinical findings of a fever, right upper quadrant pain, and elevated white blood cell count, what should one expect to find in the patient's liver?

(A) abscess
(B) hepatoma
(C) hemangioma
(D) hematoma
(E) metastasis

212. Subphrenic abscess will

(A) push the liver up toward the diaphragm
(B) depress the liver away from the diaphragm
(C) enlarge the liver size
(D) never effect the liver; it is a separate entity
(E) none of the above

213. Portal vein size can be affected by

(A) Valsalva maneuver
(B) respiratory changes
(C) portal venous hypertension
(D) all of the above

214. Which of the following procedures would aid in distinguishing regenerating liver nodules from tumor masses?

(A) biopsy
(B) angiography
(C) isotope scan
(D) all of the above

215. Which of the following statements about the right crus of the diaphragm is *not* true?

(A) it is posterior to the right kidney
(B) it is anterior to the inferior vena cava
(C) it is posterior to the inferior vena cava
(D) it is posterior to the right adrenal gland

216. Structures that commonly alter the liver shape are

(A) diaphragm
(B) right kidney
(C) abdominal lymph nodes
(D) pancreas
(E) gallbladder
(F) all of the above except one

217. Lymphoma (Hodgkin's and non-Hodgkin's) can appear sonographically as

(A) echogenic
(B) anechoic
(C) focal lesion
(D) all of the above

218. Obstruction of lymph vessels can produce

(A) ascites
(B) effusion
(C) edema
(D) all of the above

219. Normal lymph nodes are no longer than

(A) 1 mm
(B) 1 cm
(C) 3 cm
(D) 4 cm
(E) dependent upon body habitus

220. When scanning a patient for lymphadenopathy, one should check the

(A) pelvis
(B) porta hepatis
(C) retroperitoneum
(D) perirenal area

(E) around the major blood vessels and their tributaries
(F) all of the above

221. In order to differentiate enlarged nodes from an aneurysm, one should

(A) have the patient perform the Valsalva maneuver
(B) scan the patient left anterior oblique
(C) know that aneurysms enlarge fairly symmetrically, whereas large nodes tend to drape over prevertebral vessels
(D) raise the overall gain
(E) decrease the overall gain

222. What is the approximate size at which lymph nodes can be depicted sonographically?

(A) 3 mm
(B) 10 mm
(C) 1.5 cm
(D) 3 cm

223. Sonographically, enlarged lymph nodes typically appear as

(A) solid masses
(B) complex masses
(C) anechoic masses with no demonstration of through transmission
(D) cystic masses with demonstration of through transmission

224. Which of the following will cause anterior displacement of the inferior vena cava?

(A) splenomegaly
(B) hydronephrosis
(C) enlarged lymph nodes
(D) pancreatitis

225. Which of the following can be potentially confused with the normal right adrenal gland?

(A) crus of the diaphragm
(B) bowel gas
(C) renal cyst
(D) aorta

226. To optimally scan the right adrenal, one should position the patient

(A) right anterior oblique
(B) left lateral decubitus
(C) right lateral decubitus
(D) erect

227. All of the following are functions of the spleen *except*

    (A) production of plasma cells
    (B) production of lymphocytes
    (C) destruction of red blood cells
    (D) destruction of white blood cells
    (E) all of the above

228. Which of the following infectious diseases are associated with splenomegaly

    (A) infective endocarditis
    (B) tuberculosis
    (C) syphilis
    (D) schistosomiasis
    (E) all the above

229. Which of the following vessels can be seen posterior to the inferior vena cava?

    (A) right renal vein
    (B) right renal artery
    (C) left renal vein
    (D) left renal artery
    (E) no vessels course posterior to the inferior vena cava

230. A 35-year-old alcoholic male presented with epigastric pain. Sonography demonstrated a moderately enlarged gallbladder with a round, fluffy, nonshadowing mobile echo. This finding suggests

    (A) a gallstone
    (B) carcinoma of the gallbladder
    (C) choledochal cysts
    (D) a sludge ball

231. Cysts of the spleen are

    (A) rare
    (B) common
    (C) of no clinical significance
    (D) usually congenital

232. Metastases to the spleen occur more frequently with

    (A) breast carcinoma
    (B) colon carcinoma
    (C) hepatitis
    (D) leiomyoma

233. Metastases to the spleen

    (A) are common
    (B) only appear when the primary lesion has disseminated widely
    (C) are usually the first sign of carcinoma
    (D) are not known to occur

234. A spleen with overall decreased echogenicity is seen with all of the following *except*

    (A) lymphopoiesis
    (B) multiple myeloma
    (C) congestion
    (D) metastasis

235. The most common cause of splenomegaly in the United States is

    (A) malaria
    (B) portal hypertension
    (C) syphilis
    (D) mononucleosis

236. The retroperitoneal space is defined as the area between the

    (A) posterior portion of the parietal peritoneum and the posterior abdominal wall muscles
    (B) anterior portion of the parietal peritoneum and the posterior abdominal wall muscles
    (C) anterior portion of the parietal peritoneum and the posterior portion of the visceral peritoneum
    (D) posterior portion of the parietal peritoneum and the anterior portion of the visceral peritoneum
    (E) none of the above

237. When assessing the upper retroperitoneum (ie, para-aortic lymph nodes) the best patient position for optimum visualization is

    (A) prone
    (B) supine
    (C) RAO
    (D) LAO

238. Primary retroperitoneal tumors are generally

    (A) benign
    (B) malignant
    (C) very large
    (D) none of the above

239. Urinomas are known to develop after

    (A) urinary tract surgery
    (B) subacute urinary obstruction
    (C) chronic urinary obstruction
    (D) trauma
    (E) all of the above

240. The etiology of retroperitoneal fibrosis is

    (A) iatrogenic
    (B) unknown
    (C) infectious
    (D) blood borne

241. If retroperitoneal fibrosis is suspected, one should also check the

    (A) kidneys for hydronephrosis
    (B) liver for metastasis

(C) spleen for enlargement
(D) bladder for urinomas

242. The renal arteries are best seen on

(A) oblique sonogram
(B) transverse sonogram
(C) longitudinal sonogram
(D) they are not visualized

243. The largest major visceral branch of the inferior vena cava is the

(A) portal vein
(B) hepatic veins
(C) inferior mesenteric vein
(D) splenic vein

244. The spleen is variable in size, but it is considered to be which of the following?

(A) concave superiorly and inferiorly
(B) convex superiorly and concave inferiorly
(C) concave superiorly and convex inferiorly
(D) convex superiorly and inferiorly

245. When accessory spleens are present, they are usually located

(A) at the inferior margin of the spleen
(B) on the posterior aspect of the spleen
(C) near the hilum of the spleen
(D) near the kidney
(E) none of the above

246. Which of the following diseases would result in splenic atrophy?

(A) infectious mononucleosis
(B) typhoid fever
(C) splenitis
(D) sickle-cell anemia

247. The most common benign tumor of the spleen is

(A) fibroma
(B) osteoma
(C) chondroma
(D) cavernous hemangioma
(E) none of the above

248. When the spleen enlarges, it does so by extending

(A) inferomedially in an anterior position
(B) superomedially in an anterior position
(C) inferolaterally in a posterior position
(D) inferomedially in a posterior position

249. Which of the following vessels is *most* likely to appear round on a transverse sonogram?

(A) portal vein
(B) inferior vena cava

(C) right renal artery
(D) superior mesenteric artery

250. Alkaline phosphatase produced by cells lining the biliary tree is increased in all of the following *except*

(A) biliary obstruction
(B) pancreatic carcinoma
(C) hepatocellular disease
(D) presence of mass lesions in the liver

251. A hematoma in the posterior pararenal space will

(A) be located posteromedially and extend above and well below the level of the kidney
(B) be located posterior to the kidney and extend medially into the region of the pancreas
(C) be located posterior to the kidney, and extend laterally, to displace the kidney posteriorly
(D) extend up the lateral walls of the abdomen and displace the kidney anteriorly

252. A retroperitoneal sarcoma will displace which of the following organs anteriorly?

(A) kidney
(B) spleen
(C) pancreas
(D) all of the above

253. A hypertrophied column of Bertin is a

(A) benign tumor of the kidney
(B) malignant tumor of the kidney
(C) normal renal variant
(D) benign tumor of adrenal origin

254. If the patient has hydronephrosis, one may find all of the following *except*

(A) a renal calculus
(B) prostatic hypertrophy in a male or fibroid uterus in a female
(C) ureterocele
(D) renal vein thrombosis

255. An angiomyolipoma is

(A) rare
(B) benign tumor
(C) fatty tumor
(D) usually seen in middle-aged women
(E) all of the above

256. A hypernephroma is a solid renal mass. It is known as all of the following *except*

(A) renal cell carcinoma
(B) von Grawitz tumor
(C) adenocarcinoma of the kidney
(D) transitional cell carcinoma

257. All of the following will cause a false-positive abnormal intravenous pyleography *except*

(A) malrotated kidneys
(B) enlarged spleen or liver compressing the kidney
(C) dromedary hump
(D) renal vein thrombosis

258. With any renal tumor, one should also check for

(A) para-aortic nodes
(B) liver metastases
(C) tumor invasion of the inferior vena cava
(D) all of the above

259. The most common cause of nonvisualization of a kidney (unilateral) on intravenous pyelography is

(A) hydronephrosis
(B) renal calculus
(C) polycystic kidney disease
(D) pyelonephritis
(E) none of the above

260. All of the following will cause nonvisualization of the kidney on an intravenous pyelography *except*

(A) renal vein thrombosis
(B) renal artery occlusion
(C) pyonephrosis
(D) end-stage kidney disease
(E) all of the above

261. A pelvic kidney has a(n)

(A) abnormal appearance in a normal location
(B) normal appearance in an abnormal location
(C) normal appearance in a normal location
(D) all of the above

262. Ascites can be caused by all of the following *except*

(A) malignancy
(B) nephrotic syndrome
(C) congestive heart failure
(D) tuberculosis
(E) liver disease
(F) adenomyomatosis

263. Loculations within ascites are most commonly found in

(A) malignancy
(B) infection
(C) benign conditions
(D) A and B
(E) B and C

264. Internal echoes in ascitic fluid are suggestive of

(A) malignancy
(B) infection
(C) a benign condition
(D) A and B
(E) B and C

265. Acute pancreatitis may lead to all of the following *except*

(A) gallstones
(B) pancreatic pseudocyst
(C) pancreatic ascites
(D) common bile duct obstruction
(E) pancreatic abscess

266. Pancreatic pseudocyst may be found in the

(A) liver
(B) spleen
(C) mediastinum
(D) mesentary
(E) lesser sac
(F) all of the above

267. To best visualize the pancreatic tail, one should position the patient

(A) prone
(B) supine
(C) right anterior oblique
(D) left lateral decubitus

268. At times, what vessel can be confused with the pancreatic duct?

(A) superior mesenteric artery
(B) superior mesenteric vein
(C) splenic artery
(D) left renal artery

269. The splenic artery is located

(A) posterior to the body of the pancreas
(B) medial to the pancreas
(C) superior margin of the pancreas (body and tail)
(D) lateral to the uncinate process

270. Which of the following statements is true?

(A) the right kidney lies slightly higher than the left
(B) the right kidney lies slightly lower than the left
(C) both kidneys always lie at the same level
(D) none of the above

271. Signs of renal disease include all of the following *except*

(A) oliguria
(B) palpable flank mass
(C) generalized edema
(D) polyuria
(E) Murphy's sign

272. What percentage of the functioning renal parenchyma if lost will lead to the elevation of either blood urea nitrogen (BUN) or creatinine?

(A) 10%
(B) 20%
(C) 30%
(D) 40%
(E) 50%
(F) over 60%

273. The term *supernumerary kidney* refers to

(A) a pseudokidney in the renal fossa
(B) a double-collecting system
(C) the complete duplication of the renal system
(D) a pelvic kidney

274. To best evaluate the internal composition of a cyst, one should change

(A) the gain setting (TGC)
(B) the overall gain (power)
(C) the transducer to a higher frequency
(D) all of the above

275. Clinical symptoms associated with inflammatory renal masses include all of the following *except*

(A) fever
(B) chills
(C) flank pain
(D) hypoglycemia

276. The best way of delineating a dissecting aneurysm on sonography is to

(A) begin scanning in the transverse and record serial scans
(B) show an intimal flap vibration with the flow of blood
(C) have the patient lie left side down, so as to better visualize the lateral walls
(D) have the patient perform a Valsalva maneuver to dilate the aorta

277. Which of the following disorders may *not* produce a complex sonographic pattern?

(A) infected cyst
(B) hemorrhagic cyst
(C) hematomas
(D) congenital cyst
(E) abscesses

278. The abdominal aorta can be distinguished from the inferior vena cava by all of the following *except*

(A) change in gain setting
(B) anterior-posterior course
(C) left-right location
(D) Valsalva maneuver

279. With advanced chronological age, the pancreas

(A) becomes less echogenic and grossly enlarged
(B) decreases in size with increased echogenicity
(C) increases in size with no change in echogenicity
(D) increases in size with decrease in echogenicity

280. Which of the following are anatomically correct?

(A) the lesser sac is anterior and superior to the pancreas
(B) the greater sac is anterior and inferior to the pancreas
(C) the lesser sac is anterior and inferior to the pancreas
(D) A and B
(E) B and C

281. In comparison to the normal adult, the pancreas in children will be relatively

(A) more echogenic
(B) less echogenic
(C) the same echogenicity
(D) larger and less echogenic
(E) the same size and less echogenic

282. Compare the echogenicities of the following structures and place them in increasing echogenic order.

(A) renal sinus < pancreas < liver < spleen < renal parenchyma
(B) renal sinus < liver < spleen < pancreas < renal parenchyma
(C) pancreas < liver < spleen < renal sinus < renal parenchyma
(D) renal parenchyma < liver < spleen < pancreas < renal sinus

283. On a longitudinal scan, the pancreatic head can be seen

(A) anterior to the inferior vena cava
(B) caudad to the portal vein
(C) cephalad to the duodenum
(D) all of the above

284. The most common sonographic properties of a lymphoma are

(A) anechoic cystic mass with good through transmission and little ultrasound absorption
(B) relatively hypoechoic, solid mass with some decrease in through transmission and some increase in ultrasound absorption
(C) complex, predominantly cystic mass with internal debris; through transmission is increased and ultrasound absorption is decreased
(D) relatively hypoechoic solid mass with some increase in through transmission and some decrease in ultrasound absorption

285. Islet cell tumors of the pancreas are most likely to be located

   (A) in the head, never in the body or tail
   (B) frequently in the head, rarely in the body or tail
   (C) never in the head, frequently in the body or tail
   (D) rarely in the head, frequently in the body or tail

286. The normal right adrenal gland is located

   (A) medial to the left kidney, inferior to the spleen
   (B) superior to the right kidney, medial to the liver
   (C) medial to the right kidney and liver
   (D) anterior to the inferior vena cava

287. Addison's disease is a syndrome that results from

   (A) chronic adrenal hypofunction
   (B) thyroid hypofunction
   (C) parathyroid hypofunction
   (D) goiter

288. Anatomic landmarks helpful in locating the left adrenal gland are

   (A) aorta, spleen, and left kidney
   (B) gastric antrum, left kidney, and inferior vena cava
   (C) left kidney, spleen, and inferior vena cava
   (D) left kidney, left psoas muscle, and left hemidiaphragm

289. Adrenal hemorrhage sonographically appears

   (A) echogenic
   (B) anechoic
   (C) complex
   (D) all of the above

290. The spiral valves of Heister

   (A) are located within the cystic duct
   (B) may simulate a polypoid tumor
   (C) may cause shadowing, therefore, simulating a stone
   (D) all of the above

291. Landmarks for the right adrenal gland include

   (A) liver, inferior vena cava, and right crus of diaphragm
   (B) liver, right kidney, and aorta
   (C) liver, right kidney, and right psoas muscle
   (D) liver, inferior vena cava, and fourth part of duodenum

292. Which of the following masses are adrenal in origin and secrete hormones?

   (A) adenoma
   (B) teratoma
   (C) pheochromocytoma
   (D) neuroblastoma
   (E) none of the above

293. Anterior displacement of the splenic vein can be caused by

   (A) pancreatitis
   (B) pseudocysts
   (C) left adrenal hyperplasia
   (D) aneurysm

294. Which of the following syndromes are associated with an adrenal mass?

   (A) Frohlich's syndrome
   (B) Cushing's syndrome
   (C) Graves' syndrome

295. The vessel that originates from the celiac axis and is very tortuous is

   (A) splenic artery
   (B) proper hepatic artery
   (C) right gastric artery
   (D) none of the above

296. In reference to the gallbladder, a phrygian cap and Hartmann's pouch are

   (A) two names for an enlarged gallbladder
   (B) a fold at the gallbladder fundus and neck, respectively
   (C) two names for the fold in the gallbladder neck
   (D) two names for fold in the gallbladder fundus

297. Nonshadowing, nonmobile, echogenic foci seen within the gallbladder are most likely

   (A) polyps
   (B) calculi
   (C) biliary gravel
   (D) sludge balls

298. Echogenic bile within the gallbladder lumen may be caused by all of the following except

   (A) hemobilia
   (B) empyema
   (C) long-standing cystic duct obstruction
   (D) prolonged fasting
   (E) all of the above can cause echogenic bile

299. The celiac axis is _____ to the origin of the superior mesenteric artery.

   (A) caudal
   (B) cephalad
   (C) ventral
   (D) medial

300. The inferior vena cava increases in diameter superior to the entrance of the

(A) renal vein
(B) portal vein
(C) superior mesenteric vein
(D) splenic vein

Question 301: Select the letter indicating the appropriate numbered choice(s).

301. Sonography is helpful in the evaluation of the dilated common bile duct. List the physiologic events given below in order of occurrence that lead to this phenomenon.

1. intrahepatic bile duct dilatation
2. common bile duct larger than 5 mm
3. stellate formation of the ducts near the porta hepatis
4. double-barrel shotgun sign

(A) 4, 2, 1, 3
(B) 2, 1, 4, 3
(C) 1, 3, 2, 4
(D) 1, 4, 3, 2

302. Jaundice in a pediatric patient is most probably due to

(A) hepatitis
(B) fatty infiltration
(C) biliary atresia
(D) cirrhosis

303. If a patient is in the right decubitus position, this means

(A) right side up and left side on the table
(B) left side up and right side on the table
(C) the patient is in a 45° angle
(D) the patient is being scanned coronally

304. Large gallbladders are detected in patients with

(A) diabetes
(B) hepatitis
(C) lymphoma
(D) cirrhosis

305. A patient presents with empyema of the gallbladder; the sonographer should expect to find

(A) pus within the gallbladder
(B) common bile duct obstruction
(C) stones within the gallbladder
(D) abscess surrounding the gallbladder

306. Which of the following laboratory values is higher with biliary obstruction than with liver disease?

(A) serum alkaline phosphatase
(B) serum glutamic oxaloacetic transaminase (SGOT)

(C) serum glutamic pyruvic transaminase (SGPT)
(D) lactic acid dehydrogenase (LDH)

307. The basic mechanisms in which jaundice occurs are all of the following *except*

(A) obstruction of intra- or extrahepatic ducts
(B) hepatocellular disease
(C) red blood cell destruction
(D) white blood cell destruction

308. Acute cholecystitis is associated with all of the following *except*

(A) gallbladder wall thickening greater than 3 mm
(B) obstruction of the cystic duct
(C) jaundice
(D) episode of right upper quadrant pain
(E) tender enlarged gallbladder (Murphy's sign)
(F) sonographic halo effect

309. Which of the following laboratory values is specific for a hepatoma of the liver?

(A) α-fetoprotein
(B) alkaline phosphatase
(C) bilirubin
(D) blood urea nitrogen (BUN)

310. Enlarged lymph nodes will usually appear sonographically as a

(A) heterogeneous mass with poor through transmission
(B) homogeneous mass with poor through transmission
(C) homogeneous mass with excellent through transmission

311. All of the following statements concerning the patterns periaortic nodes will follow are correct *except*

(A) they may drape or mantle the great vessels anteriorly
(B) they may displace the superior mesenteric artery posteriorly
(C) they may displace the great vessels anteriorly
(D) they may have lobular, smooth, or scalloped appearance
(E) as mesenteric involvement occurs, the adenopathy may fill most of the abdomen in an irregular complex pattern

312. A primary retroperitoneal tumor is one that originates independently within the retroperitoneal space. Most are malignant and may exhibit a variety of sonographic patterns. An example of a primary tumor that is retroperitoneal is

(A) hepatoma
(B) hypernephroma
(C) leiomyosarcoma
(D) adenocarcinoma

313. Retroperitoneal fluid collections may be

(A) urinoma
(B) hemorrhage
(C) abscess
(D) lymphocele
(E) all of the above

314. All of the following are characteristics for dilated intrahepatic bile ducts *except*

(A) the parallel channel sign
(B) irregular borders to dilated bile ducts
(C) echo enhancement behind dilated ducts
(D) decreasing size as they course toward the porta hepatis

315. The superior mesenteric artery is

(A) posterior to the body of the pancreas
(B) anterior to the splenic vein
(C) posterior to the renal vein
(D) usually larger in caliber than the superior mesenteric vein

316. Which of the following is *not* a remnant of the fetal circulation?

(A) ligamentum teres
(B) ligamentum venosum
(C) coronary ligament

317. A subhepatic abscess would be located

(A) superior to the liver
(B) inferior to the liver, anterior to the right kidney
(C) inferior to the liver, posterior to the right kidney

318. All of the following mass lesions are benign *except*

(A) hematoma
(B) hamartoma
(C) hepatic adenoma
(D) hepatoma
(E) hemangioma

319. If the ultrasound beam passes partially through bone where the speed of ultrasound is greater than in soft tissue, the transducer will register these echoes

(A) further away than they really are
(B) closer than they really are
(C) in their true position
(D) all of the above, depending upon which frequency transducer is used

320. If the ultrasound beam passes through a fatty tumor within the liver, and we know that the speed of sound in fat is lower than in soft tissue, where will this fatty tumor be placed?

(A) further away than it really is
(B) closer than it really is
(C) its true position
(D) all of the above, depending upon which frequency transducer is used

321. In which of the following ways does ascites sonographically affect the liver?

(A) there will be no effect
(B) the liver will appear more echogenic
(C) the ascites will attenuate the liver, resulting in decreased echoes

322. An obese patient has a known mass in the posterior aspect of the right lobe of the liver. Which transducer would help the most in visualizing it?

(A) 5-MHz short-focus transducer
(B) 3.5-MHz long-focus transducer
(C) 2.25-MHz long-focus transducer
(D) 2.25-MHz short-focus transducer

323. All of the following will cause jaundice *except*

(A) hemolytic disease
(B) obstructive disease
(C) hepatitis
(D) hepatocellular disease
(E) Reye's syndrome

324. The celiac artery arises from the ventral surface of the aorta. Its branches consist of the

(A) common hepatic, right gastric, splenic arteries
(B) common hepatic, left gastric, splenic arteries
(C) coronary, common hepatic, left gastric arteries
(D) splenic, right hepatic, right gastric arteries

325. A major branch of the common hepatic artery is the

(A) gastroduodenal artery
(B) coronary artery
(C) esophageal artery
(D) left gastric artery

326. The splenic artery

(A) originates from the anterior abdominal aorta
(B) lies posterior to the inferior aspect of the body of the pancreas
(C) is very tortuous and runs superior to the body and tail of the pancreas

327. Artifactual echoes may occur within cysts owing to each of the following *except*

(A) slice thickness artifacts
(B) side-lobe artifacts
(C) edge artifacts
(D) reverberation artifacts

328. Owing to the abrupt change in aortic caliber at the site of an aneurysm, laminar flow will be altered, thereby creating

   (A) areas of increased echogenicity that will be seen as a result of calcification
   (B) irregularities of flow that significantly increase the likelihood of clot formation and thrombus
   (C) blood flow will not be altered

329. To detect irregularities of blood flow, the following may be used?

   (A) A-mode
   (B) B-mode
   (C) Doppler sampling
   (D) real-time study

330. Cavernous hemangiomas would be *least* likely to appear sonographically

   (A) as an echogenic lesion
   (B) distinguishable from a hepatoma
   (C) as a smooth-walled, echo-free structure
   (D) as a single or multiple lesions

331. An abscess may appear sonographically

   (A) echo-free with smooth borders and good through transmission
   (B) solid with smooth borders and no through transmission
   (C) a variable echo texture with irregular borders and varied through transmission
   (D) all of the above

332. Patients with portal hypertension may have

   (A) dilated portal veins
   (B) potential anastomoses between the portal and systemic circulation
   (C) splenomegaly
   (D) all of the above

333. In portal hypertension, potential anastomoses between the systemic circulation may open and bypass the liver. Those that can be seen sonographically include

   (A) left umbilical vein
   (B) lienorenal anastomoses
   (C) anastomoses around the esophagus
   (D) all of the above

334. During an ultrasound examination, a sonographer identifies a patent lumen within the umbilical vein. This finding may be associated with

   (A) ascites
   (B) an abscess
   (C) portal hypertension
   (D) an incidental finding

335. The major node-bearing areas in the retroperitoneum are

   (A) the iliac nodes in the pelvis
   (B) the hypogastric nodes within the pelvis
   (C) para-aortic group in the upper retroperitoneum
   (D) all of the above

336. Indications for scrotal sonography include all of the following *except*

   (A) detection of testicular tumors
   (B) evaluation of an enlarged, painful scrotum
   (C) distinction between epididymitis and tumor involving the testicle
   (D) a primary method for diagnosis of testicular torsion

337. Lymph nodes may be confused with all of the following *except*

   (A) an abdominal aortic aneurysm
   (B) chronic pancreatitis
   (C) the crus of the diaphragm
   (D) bowel

338. Sonography is used often in the evaluation of suspected palpable breast masses. In which situations is sonography of the breast *least* helpful?

   (A) detection of microcalcifications associated with invasive ductal carcinoma
   (B) evaluation of cystic breast masses
   (C) in a patient concerned about irradiation exposure from radiographic mammographic examination
   (D) detection of breast masses in the radiographically dense breast

339. The superior mesenteric vein can be differentiated from the superior mesenteric artery by all of the following *except*

   (A) following the superior mesenteric vein into the portal vein
   (B) respiratory variations are seen in the superior mesenteric vein
   (C) on sagittal scan, the superior mesenteric artery angles away from the aorta and the superior mesenteric vein tends to parallel the aorta
   (D) the superior mesenteric vein is smaller in caliber than the superior mesenteric artery

340. If the outer-to-outer dimension of an aortic aneurysm is found to be 7 cm, what percentage may rupture?

   (A) 10–30%
   (B) 30–50%
   (C) 60–80%

341. Which vessel is not found posterior to the pancreas?

(A) splenic vein
(B) superior mesenteric artery
(C) superior mesenteric vein
(D) celiac trunk
(E) inferior vena cava

342. Which vessel is found anterior to the uncinate process?

(A) gastroduodenal artery
(B) superior mesenteric vein
(C) left gastric vein
(D) left renal vein

343. Which of the following statements are *true* if a patient has acute pancreatitis?

(A) amylase and BUN will both rise, but amylase remains higher for a longer period of time
(B) amylase and alkaline phosphatase will both rise, but amylase remains higher for a longer period of time
(C) amylase and lipase rise at the same rate, but lipase remains higher for a longer period of time

344. Acute hemorrhagic pancreatitis may occur from all of the following *except*

(A) alcoholism
(B) surgical trauma
(C) external trauma
(D) fibrocystic disease of the pancreas

345. One can determine if a lesion is cystic or solid within the liver by all of the following *except*

(A) posterior enhancement
(B) reverberation artifact
(C) through transmission
(D) amount of internal echoes
(E) well-defined borders

346. During a sonographic examination, a solid mass is found. The mass is seen superior to the left kidney, displacing the spleen anteriorly. The origin of this mass is most probably

(A) from the psoas muscle
(B) the stomach
(C) the tail of the pancreas

347. In the supine view, the spleen is considered enlarged if

(A) it crosses the medial aspect of the left kidney
(B) it displaces the stomach posteriorly
(C) its anterior border lies in front of the aorta and inferior vena cava
(D) it displaces the left kidney laterally

348. A pheochromocytoma is a benign hormone producing

(A) kidney tumor
(B) adrenal tumor
(C) splenic tumor
(D) pancreatic tumor

349. Enlarged lymph nodes are almost always anechoic and can be associated with fever of unknown origin. Lymphadenopathy can be found in

(A) the para-aortic area
(B) the celiac axis, displacing the pancreas anteriorly and involving the porta hepatis
(C) adjacent to the iliopsoas muscles in the pelvis
(D) all of the above

350. A 64-year-old male presents with renal failure with a BUN of 50 mg/dL and a creatinine of 1.5 mg/dL. The sonographer may expect to find

(A) hydronephrotic kidney
(B) small kidneys that are consistent with chronic glomerulonephritis
(C) normal kidneys that are consistent with acute pyelonephritis
(D) all of the above are consistent with renal failure

351. Optimal imaging of the left adrenal gland is achieved by the specific alignment of the

(A) left kidney to the aorta
(B) left kidney to the inferior vena cava
(C) superior mesenteric artery to the aorta
(D) tail of the pancreas to the aorta

352. The right adrenal is _____ to the kidney.

(A) lateral and superior
(B) anteromedial and inferior
(C) anteromedial and superior
(D) posterior and superior
(E) anterior and superior

353. The right adrenal gland tends to be located directly _____ to the inferior vena cava and _____ to the crus of the diaphragm.

(A) superior and posterior
(B) anterior and superior
(C) lateral and superior
(D) posterior and anterior

354. In children, a relatively common malignant tumor originating from the adrenal gland is called

(A) nephroblastoma
(B) hamartoma
(C) neuroblastoma
(D) cortical teratoma

355. The adrenal is an endocrine gland that can be divided into

    (A) pelvis and sinus
    (B) cortex and medulla
    (C) major and minor calices

356. Above the level of the celiac axis the diaphragm can be visualized

    (A) anterior to the inferior vena cava and posterior to the aorta
    (B) posterior to the inferior vena cava and anterior to the aorta
    (C) the crus of the diaphragm never crosses the aorta

357. The segments of the left lobe of the liver are

    (A) medial and lateral
    (B) anterior and posterior
    (C) cephalad and caudad
    (D) caudate and quadrate

358. A patent umbilical vein may be found in the

    (A) ligamentum
    (B) main lobar fissure
    (C) ligamentum teres
    (D) intersegmental fissure

359. A patient with ampullary carcinoma most likely will demonstrate all of the following *except*

    (A) dilated pancreatic duct
    (B) dilated common bile duct
    (C) dilated hepatic veins
    (D) dilated intrahepatic duct

360. The segments of the right lobe of the liver are

    (A) medial and lateral
    (B) anterior and posterior
    (C) cephalad and caudad
    (D) caudad and quadrate

361. In a dissecting aneurysm, the dissection is through

    (A) the adventia
    (B) the media
    (C) the intima
    (D) all three layers at once

362. Which of the following is *not* a type of aortic aneurysm?

    (A) congenital
    (B) mycotic
    (C) atherosclerotic
    (D) syphilitic
    (E) phlebitis

363. The minimum anterior-posterior diameter for the diagnosis of aortic aneurysm is

    (A) 1 cm
    (B) 2 cm
    (C) 3 cm
    (D) above 3 cm

364. Abdominal aortic aneurysms are usually arteriosclerotic in origin. The most common type of aneurysm is

    (A) dissecting
    (B) saccular
    (C) fusiform

365. What echo-poor linear structure may be visualized anterior to the aorta above the level of the celiac artery?

    (A) superior mesenteric artery
    (B) left renal vein
    (C) crus of diaphragm
    (D) none of the above

366. The inferior vena cava may be compressed and displaced anteriorly by

    (A) mass lesion in the caudate lobe of the liver
    (B) right renal artery aneurysm
    (C) a tumor in the head of the pancreas
    (D) right renal vein thrombosis

367. Dilatation of the inferior vena cava can be seen in which of the following pathologic conditions?

    (A) hepatitis
    (B) Valsalva maneuver
    (C) right ventricular heart failure
    (D) hydronephrosis

368. An 80-year-old male with dysuria and fatigue has an elevated serum acid phosphatase. Elevated acid phosphatases may be seen in

    (A) acute pancreatitis
    (B) acute cholecystitis
    (C) hepatitis
    (D) prostatic carcinoma
    (E) hypernephroma

369. Artifactual echoes seen within the lumen of the aorta could be a result of all of the following *except*

    (A) improper TGC (too high)
    (B) poor lateral resolution
    (C) thrombus
    (D) improper overall gain (too high)

370. The gastroduodenal artery supplies the

    (A) duodenum, parts of the stomach, and the head of the pancreas and arises from the common hepatic artery
    (B) small bowel, the duodenum, the head of the pancreas and arises from the splenic artery
    (C) duodenum, part of the stomach, the head of the pancreas and arises directly off the celiac axis
    (D) stomach and the duodenum and arises from the superior mesenteric artery

371. Sonographically, one may recognize fatty infiltration of the liver by all of the following *except*

    (A) hepatomegaly
    (B) parenchymal echoes are brighter
    (C) decreased vascular structures
    (D) decreased through transmission
    (E) a focal hyperechoic mass

372. End-stage fatty liver, like severe cirrhosis, may present with all of the following *except*

    (A) ascites
    (B) small shrunken liver
    (C) biliary dilatation
    (D) portal hypertension
    (E) irregular liver borders due to liver nodules

373. The head of the pancreas is located anterior to the

    (A) inferior vena cava
    (B) aorta
    (C) superior mesenteric artery
    (D) splenic vein

374. The lesser sac is located between the

    (A) pancreas and the inferior vena cava
    (B) stomach and the pancreas
    (C) abdominal wall and the stomach

375. Common bile duct obstruction is associated with

    (A) a predominant increase in direct bilirubin
    (B) a predominant increase in indirect bilirubin
    (C) neither A nor B; the common bile duct is not in the liver

376. The renal pyramids are found in the

    (A) cortex
    (B) medulla
    (C) renal sinus
    (D) renal pelvis

377. Urine formation involves

    (A) tubular reabsorption
    (B) tubular secretion
    (C) filtration
    (D) all of the above

378. Urine passes, in the order given, through which of the following structures?

    (A) glomerulus, urethra, bladder, ureter
    (B) hilum, bladder, ureter
    (C) renal pelvis, ureter, bladder, urethra
    (D) hilum, urethra, bladder, ureter

379. Which of the following statements is true?

    (A) Bowman's capsule is the fibrous capsule around the kidney
    (B) a glomerulus, Bowman's capsule, and renal tubules together constitute a nephron
    (C) nephrons are about the only structures, if not the only ones, in which active transport of substances through cell membranes does not occur
    (D) the renal cortex secretes hormones called corticoids

380. A 34-year-old male presents with right-upper quadrant pain and recurrent attacks of pancreatitis. His laboratory values could indicate a(n)

    (A) increase in blood urea nitrogen (BUN)
    (B) decrease in serum amylase
    (C) increase in lipase
    (D) increase in indirect bilirubin

381. A jaundiced male child with a hemolytic disorder may be found to have

    (A) a predominant increase in direct bilirubin
    (B) a predominant increase in indirect bilirubin
    (C) bilirubin generally does not increase in childhood

382. If a 68-year-old male is found to have choledocholithiasis on ultrasound, this may result in

    (A) an increase in indirect bilirubin
    (B) an increase in direct and a slight increase in indirect bilirubin
    (C) bilirubin is not elevated in choledocholithiasis

383. A common anatomical variant is a bulge off the lateral border of the left kidney. This is termed a

    (A) vascular pedicle
    (B) Glisson's capsule
    (C) dromedary hump

384. The most common intrascrotal inflammation is

    (A) varicocele
    (B) seminoma
    (C) spermatocele
    (D) epididymitis

385. On a longitudinal scan of the scrotum, a normal testicle is seen. Located superior to the testis is the

(A) ductus deferens
(B) rete testis
(C) head of the epididymis
(D) tunica albuginea

386. When measuring the diameter of the extrahepatic bile duct on ultrasound examination, which one(s) of the following statements is(are) true?

(A) one measures the luminal diameter (i.e., excludes the wall thickness)
(B) one measures the diameter from the outside of the wall (ie, includes wall thickness)
(C) one measures from the outside of one wall to the inside of the other

387. Which of the following is posterior to the spleen?

(A) right kidney
(B) left kidney
(C) stomach
(D) tail of pancreas

388. The stomach is located _____ to the spleen.

(A) anterior
(B) posterior
(C) lateral
(D) inferior

389. If a testicular tumor is found, one should also check

(A) the kidney for hydronephrosis
(B) the renal hilum for possible nodal metastases
(C) the abdominal cavity for ascites
(D) do nothing else; no further evaluation is necessary

390. The average dimensions of the testes are

(A) 6–7 cm long and 4–5 cm wide
(B) 4–5 cm long and 4–5 cm wide
(C) 4–5 cm long and 2.5–3 cm wide
(D) 3–4 cm long and 5–6 cm wide
(E) dependent on body habitus

391. The testes are considered to be

(A) endocrine glands
(B) exocrine glands
(C) both endocrine and exocrine glands
(D) neither an endocrine nor exocrine gland

392. Primary tumors found in childhood are

(A) hepatoblastoma found in the liver
(B) Wilms' tumor found in the pancreas
(C) neuroblastoma found in the kidneys

393. Hydroceles can be defined as serous fluid accumulated between the

(A) two layers of the tunica vaginalis
(B) tunica vaginalis and the tunica albuginea
(C) two layers of the tunica albuginea
(D) tunica albuginea and the testicle

394. Testicular malignancy is most often a disease affecting which of the following age groups?

(A) 80 years and above
(B) between 60 and 80 years
(C) between 40 and 60 years
(D) between 20 and 40 years
(E) between 10 and 20 years

395. Which one of the following statements is true?

(A) all neoplasms are benign
(B) all neoplasms are malignant
(C) a neoplasm is any new growth and therefore may be benign or malignant

Questions 396 through 403: Identify the structures in Fig. 5–9A with the list of terms in Column B.

COLUMN A	COLUMN B
396. _____	(A) gallbladder
397. _____	(B) left lobe
398. _____	(C) falciform ligament
399. _____	(D) right lobe
400. _____	(E) inferior vena cava
401. _____	(F) ligamentum teres
402. _____	(G) portal vein
403. _____	(H) hepatic artery

Figure 5–9A. Anterior projection of the liver.

Figure 5–9B. Posterior projection of the liver.

Questions 404 through 415: Identify the structures in Fig. 5–9B with the list of terms in Column B.

COLUMN A

404. _____
405. _____
406. _____
407. _____
408. _____
409. _____
410. _____
411. _____
412. _____
413. _____
414. _____
415. _____

COLUMN B

(A) gallbladder
(B) left lobe
(C) falciform ligament
(D) right lobe
(E) inferior vena cava
(F) ligamentum teres
(G) portal vein
(H) hepatic artery
(I) fissure for ligamentum venosum
(J) common bile duct
(K) caudate lobe
(L) quadrate lobe (medial aspect of the left lobe)

Questions 416 through 426: Identify the structures in Fig. 5–10 with the list of terms in Column B.

COLUMN A

416. _____
417. _____
418. _____
419. _____
420. _____

COLUMN B

(A) cystic duct
(B) ampulla of Vater
(C) duodenum
(D) fundus of the gallbladder
(E) common hepatic duct

Figure 5–10. Extrahepatic biliary system.

Figure 5–11. Kidney.

421. _____
422. _____
423. _____
424. _____
425. _____
426. _____

(F) left hepatic duct
(G) body of the gallbladder
(H) right hepatic duct
(I) neck of the gallbladder
(J) infundibulum of the gallbladder (Hartmann's pouch)
(K) common bile duct

Questions 427 through 435: Identify the structures in Fig. 5–11 with the list of terms in Column B.

COLUMN A

427. _____
428. _____
429. _____
430. _____

COLUMN B

(A) renal papilla
(B) minor calyx
(C) renal capsule
(D) renal artery

Figure 5–12. Prevertebral vessels.

431. _____
432. _____
433. _____
434. _____
435. _____

(E) ureter
(F) renal pelvis
(G) renal vein
(H) pyramid
(I) cortex

Questions 436 through 456: Match the numbered structures in Fig. 5–12 with the list of terms in Column B.

COLUMN A

436. _____
437. _____
438. _____
439. _____
440. _____
441. _____
442. _____
443. _____
444. _____
445. _____
446. _____
447. _____
448. _____
449. _____
450. _____
451. _____
452. _____
453. _____
454. _____
455. _____
456. _____

COLUMN B

(A) superior mesenteric artery
(B) splenic vein
(C) aorta
(D) middle hepatic vein
(E) celiac trunk
(F) right hepatic vein
(G) left hepatic vein
(H) inferior vena cava
(I) right renal vein
(J) left renal artery
(K) left renal vein
(L) right renal artery
(M) right portal vein
(N) splenic artery
(O) gastroduodenal artery
(P) left portal vein
(Q) inferior mesenteric vein
(R) common hepatic artery
(S) main portal vein
(T) superior mesenteric vein
(U) left gastric artery

Questions 457 through 466: Identify the structures in Fig. 5–13 with the list of terms in Column B.

COLUMN A

457. _____
458. _____
459. _____
460. _____
461. _____
462. _____
463. _____
464. _____
465. _____
466. _____

COLUMN B

(A) vertebral body
(B) trachea
(C) common carotid artery
(D) internal jugular vein
(E) thyroid gland
(F) strap muscles
(G) esophagus
(H) sternocleidomastoid muscle
(I) parathyroid gland
(J) longus colli muscle

Questions 467 through 473: Identify the structures in Fig. 5–14 with the list of terms in Column B.

COLUMN A

467. _____
468. _____
469. _____
470. _____
471. _____
472. _____
473. _____

COLUMN B

(A) testis
(B) rete testis
(C) epididymis body
(D) septa
(E) epididymis tail
(F) epididymis head
(G) seminiferous tubules

Figure 5–13. Cross-section of the thyroid.

Figure 5–14. Longitudinal section of the testis.

474. In acute renal vein thrombosis, the kidney sono-graphically will *not* appear

(A) hydonephrotic
(B) enlarged
(C) more sonolucent

475. A 50-year-old female with a long history of alcohol-ism presents with increased abdominal girth. An ultrasound examination is performed and the most probable finding is

(A) liver metastases
(B) massive ascites with cirrhosis
(C) hepatoma

476. A known heroin addict presents with high fever and right flank pain. Ultrasound examination reveals expansion of the upper pole of the kidney by a mass with low-level echoes and a fluid level. This most probably represents

(A) a hypernephroma
(B) an abscess
(C) metastatic spread to the kidney
(D) hematoma

477. SGOT (serum glutamic oxalocetic transaminase) and SGPT (serum glutamic pyruvic transaminase) are highest in

(A) obstructive disease
(B) viral hepatitis and toxic hepatitis
(C) chronic cholecystitis

478. Which of the following laboratory values when ele-vated proportionally greater than the rest is an ex-cellent indication of biliary obstruction?

(A) SGOT (serum glutamic oxalocetic transami-nase)
(B) SGPT (serum glutamic pyruvic transaminase)
(C) prothrombin time
(D) alkaline phosphate
(E) serum amylase

479. A 1-week-old male infant presents with a left flank mass. An IVP demonstrates a normal right kidney but fails to demonstrate the left kidney. The ultra-sound examination demonstrates many noncom-municating spherical cystic structures in the left renal fossa, the largest of which is located laterally. No true renal parenchyma is identified. The right kidney is normal sonographically. This most proba-bly represents

(A) severe hydronephrosis
(B) polycystic kidneys
(C) a multicystic kidney
(D) nephroblastoma

480. A 6-year-old female child presents with recurrent fever, right upper quadrant pain, and jaundice. She has had similar episodes in the past. An oral cholecystogram fails to visualize the gallbladder. A sonogram is performed and the liver and gallblad-der are normal. A 2-cm cyst is found medial and separate from the gallbladder but communicating with the common bile duct. This cystic structure most probably represents

(A) a choledochal cyst
(B) a pseudocyst
(C) an aortic aneurysm
(D) a mucocele

481. Ascites is usually due to

(A) obstruction of the portal venous system
(B) lymphoma
(C) severe colitis

482. A phlebolith is a

(A) venous calculus
(B) common bile duct calculus
(C) renal calculus
(D) arterial calculus

483. Chronic active hepatitis is a progressive destructive liver disease that eventually leads to

(A) liver cysts
(B) hepatoma
(C) cirrhosis
(D) pancreatitis

484. The term *fatty liver* is usually associated with which of the following conditions?

(A) diabetes
(B) chronic alcoholism
(C) obesity
(D) ulcerative colitis

485. Aneurysms of the popliteal arteries are

(A) usually arteriosclerotic
(B) found posterior to the knee joint
(C) associated with partially calcified walls
(D) all of the above

486. Chronic renal disease is associated with

(A) an enlarged kidney
(B) unilateral hydronephrosis
(C) dense, small echogenic kidneys
(D) a renal carbuncle

487. Gallstones may *not* produce symptoms; however, they can produce injury by

- (A) the chronic irritation of calculi that may be a factor in the development of carcinoma of the gallbladder
- (B) inducing inflammation (acute or chronic cholecystitis)
- (C) causing obstruction at the neck of the gall-bladder or in the bile ducts
- (D) all of the above

Question 488: Select the letter indicating the appropriate numbered choice(s).

488. Sonography is helpful in evaluation of a solitary, hypofunctioning thyroid nodule (a cold nodule) that is initially encountered on a thyroid scintigram. List in order of greatest to least incidence the types of masses that can manifest as a solitary, hypofunctioning thyroid nodule.

1. cyst (such as a colloid cyst)
2. solid mass, malignant (such as follicular-papillary carcinoma)
3. solid mass, benign (such as an adenoma)

- (A) 1, 2, 3
- (B) 3, 2, 1
- (C) 3, 1, 2

489. Obstruction of the common duct by pressure from outside the biliary tract is termed

- (A) Courvoisier's law
- (B) Raynaud's phenomenon
- (C) Franconi's syndrome
- (D) the Bernoulli effect

490. When performing a gallbladder examination, the patient is asked to be NPO (nothing by mouth) for approximately 12 hours before the examination because this will

- (A) eliminate any gas that may collect in the bowel
- (B) dehydrate the patient
- (C) cause bile to collect within the gallbladder lumen

491. Sonography of a normally functioning transplanted kidney will appear

- (A) more echogenic than usual
- (B) with the renal cortex thinned, whereas the medullary pyramids increase in size
- (C) not any different than a kidney found within the renal fossa
- (D) with the renal sinus echoes occupying more space

492. Obstruction of the common bile duct by a mass in the head of the pancreas will lead to

- (A) dilated gallbladder with dilated biliary radicles

- (B) contracted gallbladder with dilated biliary radicles
- (C) dilated biliary radicles with normal or shrunken gallbladder

493. A kidney can appear sonographically smaller than it actually is due to

- (A) TGC (time gain compensation)
- (B) gain
- (C) scanning technique, imaging the kidney in an oblique rather than true long axis

494. Transplanted kidneys are usually placed

- (A) within the kidney fossa
- (B) in the pelvis along the iliopsoas margin
- (C) in the pelvis posterior to the quadratus lumborum muscle

495. The membrane that lines the abdominal cavity is the

- (A) visceral peritoneum
- (B) parietal peritoneum
- (C) pleura
- (D) endometrial lining
- (E) serosal lining

Questions 496 through 498: Refer to Fig. 5–15.

496. The echogenic line (*B*) represents the ligamentum venosum.

- (A) true
- (B) false

497. Echogenic foci (*A*) represents the ligamentum teres.

- (A) true
- (B) false

498. The portion of the liver between the inferior vena cava (IVC) and *B* is the caudate lobe.

- (A) true
- (B) false

Figure 5–15. Schematic transverse scan of the liver.

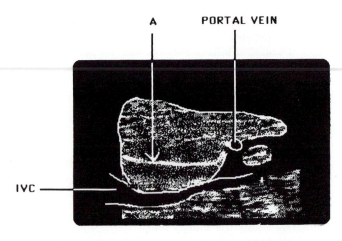

Figure 5–16. Schematic sagittal scan of the liver.

Figure 5–17. Sagittal sonogram taken through the right upper quadrant of a child.

Questions 499 through 501: Refer to Fig. 5–16.

499. The arrow is pointing to the ligamentum teres.

(A) true
(B) false

500. The caudate lobe is cephalad to the portal vein.

(A) true
(B) false

501. The head of the pancreas is caudal to the portal vein.

(A) true
(B) false

502. When hypertrophic pyloric stenosis is delineated in short axis the abnormally hypertrophied muscle wall usually measures

(A) 5 mm or more
(B) more than 5 cm
(C) less than 2 mm
(D) about 5 mm

503. The sonographic findings of hydronephrosis may present with

(A) the calices and pelvis so grossly dilated that only a single large sac is seen
(B) multiple cystic areas within the kidney sinus
(C) very little renal parenchyma that can be visualized owing to the obstructing calices
(D) all of the above

504. To localize a dilated ureter, it is most helpful to

(A) place the patient in a supine position and scan the abdomen
(B) place the patient in a prone position and scan the abdomen

(C) scan the pelvis with a full bladder and evaluate the area posterior to the bladder
(D) all of the above

505. The abnormal sonographic findings in Fig. 5–17 include

(A) a mass within the right kidney
(B) a large complex mass within the liver
(C) no abnormality
(D) pleural effusion

506. The most common liver mass found in children is

(A) hepatoblastoma
(B) metastatic disease
(C) polycystic liver and kidney disease
(D) hepatic fibrosis

Figure 5–18. Sagittal sonogram through the right upper quadrant of a 9-hour-old neonate who failed to produce urine.

507. The abnormal sonographic findings in Fig. 5–18 include

(A) abnormal sonographic appearance of the right kidney suggestive of adult-type polycystic kidney disease

(B) abnormal sonographic appearance of the right kidney, highly suggestive of infantile polycystic disease

(C) abnormal sonographic appearance of the right kidney, most consistent with multicystic disease

(D) none of the above

508. In infantile polycystic disease

(A) cysts can be seen on sonography

(B) cysts are not seen because they are microscopic

(C) only a portion of the kidney is affected

(D) the other kidney appears normal because it is usually only unilateral

509. The abnormal sonographic findings in Figs. 5–19A and B include a

(A) simple cortical cyst in the upper pole of the right kidney

(B) distended upper pole moiety of a duplex collecting system because the cystic mass seems to be contiguous with a distended ureter to the upper pole

(C) renal tumor

(D) large arteriovenous malformation

510. Typically, with a duplex collecting system, the upper pole moiety (Figs. 5–19A and B) is

(A) hydronephrotic due to reflux

(B) hydronephrotic due to obstruction from a ureterocele

(C) usually the least affected

(D) none of the above

511. The positive sonographic findings in Fig. 5–20 include

(A) cyst arising from the lateral aspect of the right kidney

(B) a 1-cm cyst seen lateral to an enlarged and flattened adrenal

(C) metastases in the liver

(D) none of the above

512. In renal agenesis, the adrenal

(A) has no abnormal shape and may mimic a kidney

(B) is also not present

(C) both A and B

(D) none of the above

A

B

Figures 5–19. (A) and (B) Sagittal sonograms taken through the right upper abdomen. Figure 5–19A is lateral to Figure 5–19B.

Figure 5–20. Transverse sonogram of the right upper abdomen in an anuric neonate.

Figure 5–21. Coronal sonogram of the left kidney.

Figure 5–22. Long axis image of a renal transplant.

513. The positive sonographic findings in Fig. 5–21 include

(A) a solid tumor in the lower pole
(B) multiple cysts of various sizes, highly suggestive of adult-type polycystic disease
(C) marked hydronephrosis
(D) none of the above

514. In adult-type polycystic kidney disease, cysts may be found in

(A) the liver
(B) the pancreas
(C) the spleen
(D) any of the above

515. The abnormal sonographic findings in Fig. 5–22 include

(A) hydronephrosis
(B) the transplanted kidney appears normal
(C) very prominent medullary pyramids, consistent with acute rejection
(D) a large cyst in the upper pole of the transplanted kidney

516. Sonography is very helpful in evaluation of renal transplants that have impaired function. This is because

(A) sonography can differentiate obstructive causes from rejection
(B) sonography is helpful because it can detect early rejection earlier and more reliably than the renal scintigram
(C) sonography is only helpful in detection of masses that can be treated surgically
(D) both A and C

517. The arrow in Fig. 5–23 points to

(A) a medullary pyramid
(B) the renal cortex
(C) a parapelvic cyst
(D) none of the above

518. The size of the kidney in normal adults is

(A) 10–12 cm in long axis, 5–6 cm in width, and 3–4 cm in anterior-posterior and transverse dimensions

Figure 5–23. Sagittal sonogram through the right upper abdomen.

(B) there is too much variation and a normal range cannot be established

(C) the renal parenchyma (medulla and cortex) should measure at least 1 cm

(D) both A and B

519. The abnormal sonographic findings in Figs. 5–24A and B include

(A) gallbladder wall thickening

(B) viscid bile or sludge in the gallbladder

(C) a tumor within the gallbladder wall

(D) both A and B

520. Viscid bile within the gallbladder indicates

(A) the gallbladder has not been completely emptied, allowing viscid bile to build up within the lumen

(B) a normal finding that can be encountered in any patient

(C) that viscid bile typically is the precursor to small calculi and should be removed percutaneously

(D) both A and C

521. The abnormal sonographic findings in Fig. 5–25 include

(A) the pancreas as very echogenic; highly suggestive of chronic pancreatitis

(B) the pancreas is echogenic; but in older patients, it may normally be this echogenic

(C) both A and B

(D) none of the above

522. Sonography can be used intraoperatively in detecting pancreatic tumors. Most pancreatic tumors appear

(A) as hypoechoic focal lesions within the pancreas

(B) as echogenic lesions within the pancreas

(C) sonography is not useful in intraoperative pancreatic cases

(D) none of the above

A

B

Figure 5–24. (A) Long axis view of the gallbladder. **(B)** Short axis view of the gallbladder.

Figure 5–25. Transverse sonogram of the upper abdomen.

Figure 5–26. Sagittal sonogram taken through the midabdomen.

523. Sonographic findings in Fig. 5–26 include

(A) an abnormal mass in the upper abdomen most likely within the liver
(B) a structure that has a target configuration
(C) both A and B
(D) none of the above

524. The halo around the mass (Fig. 5–26) probably represents

(A) edema around a tumor
(B) the wall of the stomach
(C) both A and B
(D) none of the above

525. The anechoic structure immediately posterior to the gallbladder neck, as shown in Fig. 5–27, is probably

(A) a cystic tumor arising from the right adrenal
(B) a fluid-filled loop of bowel, probably transverse colon
(C) a fluid-filled loop of duodenum
(D) either B or C, but not A

526. Another maneuver to evaluate the gallbladder and the presence or absence of calculi within its lumen includes

(A) an upright view looking for stones to drop into the fundus
(B) a Trendelenburg view to see if the stone is impacted in the neck of the gallbladder
(C) both A and B
(D) none of the above

527. The structure depicted in Fig. 5–28 is the

(A) gallbladder
(B) stomach
(C) liver
(D) hydronephrotic right kidney

528. The malformation variant in the gallbladder that involves an acutely angulated pouch of the fundus is termed

(A) phrygian cap
(B) duplication of the gallbladder
(C) megagallbladder
(D) Smurf's cap

Figure 5–27. Sagittal sonogram of the right upper abdomen.

Figure 5–28. Sagittal sonogram of the right upper abdomen.

Figure 5–29. Transverse sonogram of the upper abdomen.

529. The vascular structures depicted in Fig. 5–29 include

    (A) the aorta and superior mesenteric artery
    (B) the aorta and celiac axis
    (C) the aorta and splenic artery only
    (D) none of the above

530. The normal celiac axis includes

    (A) the common hepatic artery, splenic artery, and left gastric artery
    (B) the superior mesenteric artery only
    (C) A and B
    (D) none of the above

531. Structures identified in Fig. 5–30 include

    (A) the abdominal aorta
    (B) the left lobe of the liver
    (C) the right kidney
    (D) both A and B

532. The most frequent cause of abdominal aortic aneurysm is

    (A) atherosclerosis
    (B) mycosis
    (C) trauma
    (D) none of the above

533. The arrows in Fig. 5–31 delineate

    (A) a hypertrophied pyloric muscle
    (B) a normal pyloric muscle
    (C) a lesion within the liver that obstructs the stomach
    (D) none of the above

534. Hypertrophic pyloric stenosis can be diagnosed when

    (A) the pyloric muscle is greater than 4 mm in thickness
    (B) when the lumen of the pyloris remains totally open allowing reflux
    (C) A and B
    (D) none of the above

Figure 5–30. Sagittal image of the upper abdomen.

Figure 5–31. Transverse sonogram of a 2-week-old infant with excessive vomiting.

Figure 5–32. Sagittal sonogram obtained through the right upper abdomen.

535. The abnormalities in Fig. 5–32 include

    (A) the liver parenchyma is very echogenic when compared to the kidney

    (B) there are no abnormalities

    (C) there are metastases throughout the liver

    (D) there are multiple masses in the kidney

536. Fatty metamorphosis of the liver can be assessed sonographically by noting

    (A) increased echogenicity when compared with normal kidney

    (B) normal vessels being identified throughout the liver

    (C) A and B

    (D) none of the above

537. The echogenic focus within the testicle (Fig. 5–33) represents

    (A) a "burnt out" germ cell tumor

    (B) the mediastinum of the testis

    (C) an infarct

    (D) none of the above

538. In testicular torsion

    (A) the testes have a nonhomogeneous texture due to areas of hemorrhagic infarction

    (B) the testes appear normal

    (C) only after 2 weeks do the testes have an abnormal appearance

    (D) none of the above

Figure 5–33. Transverse sonogram through the left hemiscrotum.

539. The abnormal sonographic features in Fig. 5–34 include

    (A) marked hydronephrosis

    (B) a calculus within the midpolar region

    (C) a tumor in the upper pole

    (D) all of the above

540. Sonography can occasionally detect renal calculi not seen on excretory urography or plain film radiography.

    (A) true

    (B) false

Figure 5–34. Transverse sonogram of the right kidney.

Figure 5–35. Long axis sonogram of the gallbladder.

541. The abnormal sonographic findings in Fig. 5–35 include

(A) a calculus within the gallbladder neck
(B) viscid bile within the gallbladder lumen
(C) A and B
(D) none of the above

542. The presence of intraluminal calculus indicates that there is cholecystitis.

(A) true
(B) false

543. The abnormal sonographic findings in Fig. 5–36 include

(A) a cortical cyst within the right kidney
(B) echogenic foci throughout the kidney probably representing a staghorn calculus
(C) focally echogenic medulla and cortex
(D) A and C

544. Disorders associated with this sonographic appearance (Fig. 5–36) include

(A) renal tubular acidosis
(B) medullary sponge kidney
(C) papillary necrosis
(D) all of the above

545. The abnormal sonographic findings in Fig. 5–37 include

(A) a renal tumor filling the renal pelvis
(B) a large renal calculus
(C) massive hydronephrosis
(D) all of the above

546. The type of renal calculi that may be nonopaque radiographically but appear as echogenic foci on sonography includes

(A) a calcium oxalate
(B) calcium bilirubinate
(C) cholesterol
(D) none of the above

547. The sonographic findings in Fig. 5–38 include

(A) massive splenomegaly
(B) a subphrenic abscess
(C) metastasis within the spleen
(D) normal-appearing spleen

Figure 5–36. Sagittal sonogram through the liver and right kidney.

Figure 5–37. Transverse or short axis image of the left kidney. Plain film radiograph failed to reveal any abnormal calcifications.

Figure 5–38. Coronal image through the left upper quadrant.

548. Splenomegaly can be encountered in

(A) chronic myelogenous leukemia
(B) portal hypertension
(C) sickle-cell crisis
(D) A and B

549. Fig. 5–39 depicts which of the following structures?

(A) the common hepatic duct
(B) a normal common bile duct
(C) the main portal vein
(D) all of the above

Figure 5–40. Coronal sonogram of the left kidney.

550. The common bile duct is formed by

(A) the right and left hepatic ducts joining the cystic duct
(B) the cystic duct joining the right hepatic duct
(C) the common hepatic duct joining the cystic duct
(D) none of the above

551. The abnormal sonographic findings in Fig. 5–40 include

(A) a solid mass in the lower pole
(B) a simple cyst in the lower pole
(C) hydronephrosis
(D) all of the above

Figure 5–39. Magnified sagittal sonogram of the porta hepatis area.

Figure 5–41. Sagittal image of the right upper quadrant.

Figure 5–42. Transverse sonogram of the right upper quadrant.

Figure 5–44. Transverse sonogram of the liver.

552. Cortical cysts are relatively common in adults 45 years of age and over.

    (A) true
    (B) false

553. Figs. 5–41 and 5–42 are long and short axes sonograms of the right upper quadrant of the abdomen, respectively. The abnormality is (are)

    (A) marked thickening of the gallbladder wall
    (B) gallstones
    (C) sludge
    (D) A and C

554. Causes of gallbladder wall thickening include

    (A) cholecystitis
    (B) nondistension
    (C) hepatitis
    (D) all of the above

555. Elicitation of pain while scanning over the gallbladder fundus is termed

    (A) Chandelier's sign
    (B) Murphy's sign
    (C) Murphy's law
    (D) Courvoisier gallbladder

556. Figs. 5–43, 5–44, and 5–45 were obtained during an abdominal sonogram performed on a 50-year-old man. The arrow in Fig. 5–43 points to

    (A) the left portal vein
    (B) a dilated intrahepatic duct in the left lobe
    (C) an hepatic vein
    (D) none of the above

557. The arrow in Fig. 5–45 points to

    (A) a dilated common bile duct with a rat-tail deformity
    (B) the main portal vein
    (C) a hepatic vein
    (D) hepatic artery

Figure 5–43. Sagittal image slightly left of midline.

Figure 5–45. Sagittal image of the right upper quadrant.

Figure 5–46. Transverse sonogram throughout the right hepatic lobe.

Figure 5–47. Midline longitudinal scan of the abdomen.

558. The most likely diagnosis is

(A) biliary obstruction due to cholelithiasis
(B) biliary obstruction due to pancreatitis
(C) distended portal vein due to portal hypertension
(D) distended hepatic vein due to chronic congestive heart failure
(E) obstruction of the distal common bile duct due to pancreatic tumor

559. Dilated intrahepatic ducts tend to be readily delineated in the left lobe because

(A) they are first affected by obstruction
(B) they course transversely in the left lobe
(C) they are bigger in the left lobe than in the right lobe
(D) none of the above

560. Fig. 5–46 is a transverse sonogram throughout the right hepatic lobe. The abnormality is

(A) an echogenic mass
(B) absence of portal vein
(C) a left-sided gallbladder
(D) none of the above

561. The most likely diagnosis is

(A) hemangioma
(B) metastases
(C) A or B
(D) neither

562. Hemangiomas can be diagnosed by

(A) needle biopsy
(B) a tagged red blood cell liver scan
(C) a computed tomographic (CT) scan
(D) an magnetic resonance imaging scan
(E) all of the above

563. Fig. 5–47 is a midline longitudinal scan of the abdomen. The abnormality is

(A) an ectopic gallbladder
(B) aneurysmal dilatation of the distal abdominal aorta
(C) total occlusion of the abdominal aorta by thrombus
(D) none of the above

564. An aneurysm is usually the result of

(A) degenerative joint disease
(B) atherosclerosis
(C) hypertension
(D) diabetes

565. Other arteries that may be affected by an aneurysm include

(A) the coronary arteries
(B) the carotids
(C) popliteal arteries
(D) all of the above

566. Fig. 5–48 is a midline sagittal transrectal sonogram of the prostate. The abnormality is

(A) dilatation of the prostatic urethra
(B) tumor within the transitional zone
(C) both A and B
(D) none of the above

567. The most likely diagnosis in the patient in Fig. 5–48 is

(A) carcinoma of the prostate stage A
(B) carcinoma of the prostate stage C
(C) idiopathic dilatation of the urethra
(D) iatrogenic dilatation of the urethra
(E) A and D

Figure 5–48. Midline sagittal transrectal sonogram of the prostate.

Figure 5–50. Long axis sonogram of the right hemiscrotum.

568. The prostatic-specific antigen (PSA) in the patient in Fig. 5–48 would most likely be

(A) normal
(B) elevated
(C) subnormal

569. Fig. 5–49 is an abdominal sonogram obtained through the right upper quadrant. The abnormality is

(A) an echogenic kidney
(B) hypoechogenic liver
(C) both A and B
(D) neither

570. The most likely diagnosis in the patient in Fig. 5–49 is

(A) a colonic tumor
(B) severe renal parenchymal disease
(C) a liver infarct
(D) none of the above

571. Normally, the liver is slightly more echogenic than the renal parenchyma because

(A) it has fibrous septa within the hepatic lobule
(B) the kidney has more water content
(C) the liver has more water content
(D) none of the above

572. Fig. 5–50 is a long axis sonogram of the right hemiscrotum. The abnormality is

(A) a diffusely abnormal testis
(B) enlarged and echogenic head of the epididymis
(C) a hydrocele
(D) none of the above

573. The most likely diagnosis in the patient in Fig. 5–50 is

(A) testicular tumor
(B) testicular torsion
(C) epididymitis
(D) A and C

574. The presenting symptom of a testicular tumor can be

(A) para-aortic lymphadenopathy
(B) mediastinum lymphadenopathy
(C) retroperitoneal lymphadenopathy
(D) all of the above

575. Fig. 5–51 is a parasagittal transrectal sonogram of the prostate rotated slightly from the midline. The abnormality is

(A) a small prostate
(B) absence of the seminal vesicle
(C) a hypoechoic lesion in the peripheral zone
(D) both B and C

Figure 5–49. Sagittal sonogram obtained through the right upper quadrant.

Figure 5–51. Parasagittal transrectal sonogram of the prostate rotated slightly from the midline.

576. The next procedure for definitive diagnosis after the sonogram would be

(A) useless—this finding is diagnostic
(B) transperineal biopsy
(C) transrectal biopsy
(D) either B or C

577. The approximate chance that a hypoechoic lesion in the peripheral zone is carcinoma is

(A) 2%
(B) 20%
(C) 50%
(D) 80%

578. The relative advantage of transrectal biopsy over transperineal biopsy includes

(A) an increased chance of infection in transperineal biopsy
(B) an increased chance of infection in transrectal biopsy
(C) increased incidence of hematospermia with transrectal biopsy
(D) none of the above

579. Fig. 5–52 is a long axis sonogram of the common bile duct. The abnormality is

(A) thrombosed portal vein
(B) a dilated common bile duct
(C) aneurysm or dilatation of the hepatic artery
(D) A and B

580. The most likely cause of the abnormality shown in Fig. 5–52 is

(A) cholelithiasis
(B) tumor in the pancreatic head
(C) A or B
(D) neither

581. The common bile duct may distend with age and measure 7 mm or greater

(A) true
(B) false

582. Fig. 5–53 is a transverse sonogram of the left lobe of the liver. The arrow points to

(A) hepatic vessels
(B) hypoechoic lesions
(C) portal sinuses
(D) none of the above

583. Diagnostic possibilities in the findings in Fig. 5–53 include

(A) metastases
(B) hemangiomas
(C) infection foci
(D) A or C

584. The next step in the evaluation of the liver lesions seen in Fig. 5–53 would be

(A) a red blood cell liver scan
(B) liver–spleen scan

Figure 5–52. Long axis sonogram of the common bile duct.

Figure 5–53. Transverse sonogram of the left lobe of the liver.

Figure 5-54. Duplex Doppler sonogram obtained in the upper hemiscrotum.

(C) computed tomography (CT) or magnetic resonance imaging (MRI) of the liver
(D) fine needle aspiration

585. Fig. 5-54 is a duplex Doppler sonogram obtained in the upper hemiscrotum. The abnormality is

(A) dilated spermatic duct
(B) dilated vessels near the head of the epididymis
(C) vascular tumor of the testes
(D) B or C

586. The waveform of a varicocele indicates

(A) increased flow within the varicocele
(B) decreased flow within the varicocele
(C) no change in flow after varicocele

587. The most likely diagnosis from the findings in Fig. 5-54 is

(A) varicocele
(B) testicular tumor
(C) testicular torsion
(D) A and C

588. Fig. 5-55 is a long axis sonogram of the right upper quadrant of the abdomen. The abnormality is (are):

(A) contracted gallbladder filled with stones
(B) contracted gallbladder without stones
(C) cyst in the liver
(D) nothing, the patient is status/postcholecystectomy

589. The most likely diagnosis in the patient in Fig. 5-55 is

(A) calculus cholecystitis
(B) hepatitis
(C) A and B
(D) neither

590. The patient in Fig. 5-55 is a good candidate for lithotripsy.

(A) true
(B) false

591. Fig. 5-56 is a longitudinal sonogram of the left kidney obtained in the prone position. The abnormality is

(A) a renal tumor affecting the upper pole
(B) distension of the renal pelvis and proximal ureter
(C) parapelvic cyst
(D) none of the above

592. The most likely diagnosis in the patient in Fig. 5-56 is

(A) vesicourethral reflex
(B) ureteropelvic junction obstruction
(C) pyelonephrosis
(D) ureterovesical junction obstruction
(E) A or D

Figure 5-55. Long axis sonogram of the right upper quadrant.

Figure 5-56. Longitudinal sonogram of the left kidney obtained in the prone position.

Figure 5–57. Transverse sonogram obtained through the urinary bladder.

Figure 5–58. Longitudinal sonogram of the right upper quadrant.

593. In xanthogranulomatous pyelonephritis, there is

    (A) a calculus usually obstructing the renal collecting system
    (B) parenchymal changes within the kidney secondary to infection
    (C) multiple transitional cell tumors
    (D) renal cell carcinomas
    (E) A and B

594. Fig. 5–57 is a transverse sonogram obtained through the urinary bladder. The abnormality is

    (A) a thickened bladder wall, particularly in the posterior portion of the wall
    (B) bilateral ureteroceles
    (C) A and B
    (D) none of the above

595. The most likely diagnosis in the patient in Fig. 5–57 is

    (A) bladder tumor (transitional carcioma)
    (B) focal cystitis
    (C) A or B
    (D) none of the above

596. In a child, cystitis may be associated with

    (A) chemotherapy
    (B) frequent and painful urination
    (C) renal infection
    (D) all of the above

597. Fig. 5–58 is a longitudinal scan of the right upper quadrant. The abnormality is

    (A) a hypoechoic texture to the renal parenchyma
    (B) an echogenic texture to the liver
    (C) no abnormality—this is a normal study
    (D) none of the above

598. Diagnostic possibilities in the patient in Fig. 5–58 include

    (A) glycogen storage disease
    (B) fatty metamorphosis
    (C) hemochromatosis
    (D) all of the above

599. A disorder associated with glycogen storage disease is

    (A) multiple hepatic adenomata
    (B) multiple hepatic tumors
    (C) A and B
    (D) none of the above

600. Fig. 5–59 is a transverse scan obtained through the right upper quadrant of a neonate. The abnormality is

    (A) the absence of a right kidney
    (B) an abnormal right adrenal

Figure 5–59. Transverse scan obtained through the right upper quadrant of a neonate.

(C) an abnormality of the right kidney with reduced parenchyma

(D) none of the above

601. Assuming that the findings are similar on the left side of the patient, the most likely diagnosis in the patient in Fig. 5–59 is

(A) chronic leiomyonephritis

(B) horseshoe kidney

(C) bilateral renal agenesis

(D) none of the above

602. In renal agenesis, the adrenal

(A) can appear elongated

(B) also is absent

(C) can contain multiple tumors

(D) none of the above

603. Fig. 5–60 is a long axis image of the gallbladder. The abnormality is

(A) a distended gallbladder with a markedly thickened wall

(B) multiple floating calculi

(C) an hydropic gallbladder

(D) none of the above

604. The most likely diagnosis in the patient in Fig. 5–60 is

(A) gallbladder hydrops probably secondary to obstruction

(B) cholelithiasis

(C) acalculus cholelithiasis

(D) none of the above

605. Hydrops of the gallbladder may be secondary to

(A) cholelithiasis

(B) obstruction of the distal common bile duct by pancreatic tumor

(C) obstruction of the distal common bile duct secondary to ampullary tumor

(D) obstruction of the cystic duct due to an anomalous portal vein

(E) all of the above

606. Fig. 5–61 is a long axis image of the gallbladder. The abnormality is

(A) diffuse thickening of the gallbladder wall

(B) difficult to determine because the gallbladder is not fully distended

(C) both A and B

(D) cholelithiasis

607. The most likely diagnosis in the patient in Fig. 5–61 is

(A) normal, nondistended gallbladder

(B) hyperplastic cholecystitis

(C) cholecystitis

(D) none of the above

608. Conditions that may be associated with gallbladder wall thickening include

(A) cholecystitis

(B) nondistension

(C) ascites

(D) right upper quadrant inflammatory bowel disease

(E) all of the above

Figure 5–60. Long axis image of the gallbladder.

Figure 5–61. Long axis image of the gallbladder.

Figure 5–62. Long axis image of the left kidney obtained in the sagittal plane in the patient who is in a prone position.

609. Fig. 5–62 is a long axis image of the left kidney obtained in the sagittal plane in the patient in the prone position. The abnormality is

(A) large tumor involving the lower pole of the left kidney
(B) hydronephrosis
(C) adrenal tumor
(D) none of the above

610. Diagnostic possibilities in the patient in Fig. 5–62 include

(A) renal cell tumor
(B) angiomyolipoma
(C) transitional cell tumor
(D) A or B

611. Angiomyolipomas may be encountered in

(A) patients with tuberous sclerosis
(B) postmenopausal women
(C) prepubertal boys
(D) prepubertal girls
(E) A and B

612. Fig. 5–63 is a coronal image through the left upper quadrant of the abdomen. The arrow points to

(A) a small shrunken kidney
(B) the normal left adrenal
(C) a loop of bowel
(D) the splenic flexure

613. The most likely diagnosis in the patient in Fig. 5–63 is

(A) hepatic tumor
(B) splenic tumor
(C) normal left adrenal
(D) atrophic left kidney

614. A condition that may affect the adrenal is

(A) neonatal hypotension
(B) severe fulminant tuberculosis infection
(C) malignant lung carcinoma
(D) all of the above

615. Fig. 5–64 is a transverse image obtained in the upper abdomen. The cursors (+s) indicate

(A) an ectatic main pancreatic duct in an elderly patient
(B) a distended main pancreatic duct in a child
(C) the pancreatic duct appears to be in normal limits
(D) A or B

616. Given that this is a scan (Fig. 5–64) of a child the most likely diagnosis is

(A) hereditary pancreatitis
(B) chronic pancreatitis
(C) acute pancreatitis
(D) A or B

Figure 5–63. Coronal image through the left upper quadrant.

Figure 5–64. Transverse image obtained in the upper abdomen.

Figure 5–65. Parasagittal scan obtained through the liver.

Figure 5–66. Transverse scan obtained through the abdomen of a child with a palpable mass.

617. Pancreatic duct dilatation can be seen in

(A) pancreatic tumors
(B) chronic pancreatitis
(C) a normal ectatic duct in an elderly patient
(D) all of the above

618. Fig. 5–65 is a parasagittal scan obtained through the liver. The abnormality is

(A) a distended gallbladder
(B) a cystic mass related to the common bile duct
(C) a liver cyst
(D) none of the above

619. The most likely diagnosis in the patient in Fig. 5–65 is

(A) hydropic gallbladder
(B) choledochal cyst
(C) liver cyst
(D) none of the above

620. The types of choledochal cysts include

(A) type I—aneurysmal dilatation of the common bile duct
(B) type II—cystic diverticulum arising from common bile duct
(C) type III-choledochocele within the duodenum wall
(D) type IV—aneurysmal dilatation of the intra-hepatic bile ducts
(E) all of the above

621. Factors that may contribute to development of a choledochal cyst include

(A) abnormal angulation of distal common bile duct and pancreatic duct
(B) abnormal fusion of the two tissues that fuse to form the pancreas
(C) retrograde secretion of pancreatic digestive juices in the wall of the pancreatic duct
(D) A and B
(E) none of the above

622. Fig. 5–66 is a transverse scan obtained through the abdomen of a child with a palpable mass. The abnormality is

(A) a cystic mass with several septations
(B) a cystic mass which appears to displace bowel and mesentery
(C) free fluid within the abdomen
(D) none of the above

623. The most likely diagnosis in the patient in Fig. 5–66 is

(A) mesenteric cyst
(B) complicated ascites
(C) ovarian carcinoma
(D) none of the above

Figure 5–67. Longitudinal image through the gastric antrum of a child.

624. Figs. 5–67 and 5–68 are long and short axes sonograms through the gastric antrum of a child. The abnormality is

    (A) thickened antrum wall
    (B) shortened antrum
    (C) lengthened pyloric canal
    (D) A and C

625. The most likely diagnosis in the patient in Figs. 5–67 and 5–68 is

    (A) normal stomach
    (B) hypertrophic pyloric stenosis
    (C) duodenal tumor
    (D) none of the above

626. Criteria used for diagnosis of hypertrophic pyloric stenosis include

    (A) a wall greater than 3 mm
    (B) a wall less than 3 mm
    (C) length greater than 14 mm
    (D) length less than 14 mm
    (E) A and C
    (F) B and D

Figure 5–68. Transverse scan through the gastric antrum of a child.

Figure 5–69. Transverse sonogram through the upper abdomen.

627. Fig. 5–69 is a transverse sonogram through the upper abdomen. The abnormality is

    (A) enlarged and thickened pancreas
    (B) dilatation of the main pancreatic duct
    (C) dilatation of the duodenal bulb
    (D) aneurysmal dilatation of the superior mesentery vein
    (E) none of the above

628. The most likely diagnosis in the patient in Fig. 5–69 is

    (A) pancreatitis
    (B) normal
    (C) gastric outlet obstruction
    (D) portal hypertension

629. Fig. 5–70 is a long axis image in the upper outer quadrant of the right breast. The abnormality is

Figure 5–70. Long axis sonogram of the upper outer quadrant of the right breast.

(A) a cystic lesion within the breast
(B) a solid lesion with well-circumscribed borders
(C) a solid lesion with irregular borders
(D) none of the above

630. The most likely diagnosis in the patient in Fig. 5–70 is

(A) cyst
(B) fibroadenoma
(C) carcinoma
(D) mastitis

631. The sonographic findings in breast lesions are usually definitive and do not require future evaluation by biopsy or fine needle aspiration.

(A) true
(B) false

632. Fig. 5–71 is a transverse image in the right side of the neck at the level of the common carotid artery The abnormality is

(A) thrombosis of the common carotid artery
(B) a parathyroid mass
(C) a thyroid mass
(D) a mass within the strap muscles

633. The most likely diagnosis in the patient in Fig. 5–71 is

(A) parathyroid adenoma
(B) thyroid adenoma
(C) lymph node
(D) cannot tell

634. Parathyroid adenomas may be associated with

(A) hypercalcemia
(B) hypertension
(C) bloating
(D) headaches

Figure 5–72. An upright coronal image of the lower left hemithorax of a 12-year-old child with fever and cough.

635. Fig. 5–72 is an upright coronal image of the lower left hemithorax of a 12-year-old child with fever and cough. The abnormality is

(A) loculated pleural effusion
(B) nonloculated pleural effusion
(C) hydronephrotic kidney
(D) none of the above

636. The most likely diagnosis in the patient in Fig. 5–72 is

(A) simple effusion
(B) cystic lung mass
(C) empyema
(D) none of the above

637. One of the findings useful in determining whether a fluid collection within the thorax will be successfully aspirated includes

(A) if there is deformation of shape with breathing
(B) how close it is to the chest
(C) if it has echogenic material within it
(D) all of the above

638. Regarding sonography of the appendix

(A) it is a clinically useful test for the diagnosis of acute appendicitis
(B) it is not a clinically useful test for the diagnosis of acute appendicitis
(C) it cannot be performed because the patient is usually too tender to tolerate adequate compression of the right lower quadrant
(D) bowel gas always obscures visualization in this region

Figure 5–71. Transverse image of the right side of the neck at the level of the common carotid artery.

Figure 5–73. Sonogram of the right lower quadrant of the abdomen. *(Courtesy of John Worrell, M.D.)*

Figure 5–74. Sonogram of the right lower quadrant of the abdomen. *(Courtesy of John Worrell, M.D.)*

Figure 5–75. Sonogram of the right lower quadrant of the abdomen. *(Courtesy of John Worrell, M.D.)*

Figure 5–76. Longitudinal sonogram of the right upper quadrant.

639. Sonographic parameters used for diagnosis of an abnormal appendix include

(A) wall greater than 3 cm
(B) inability to compress completely with transabdominal pressure
(C) length of more than 1 cm
(D) presence of an appendicolith
(E) B and D

640. Figs. 5–73, 5–74, and 5–75 are sonograms of the right lower quadrant of the abdomen. The correct statements concerning these figures include

(A) Fig. 5–73 represents a normal appendix
(B) Fig. 5–74 represents a normal appendix
(C) Fig. 5–75 represents a normal appendix
(D) none of the above

641. The findings in Fig. 5–76 are consistent with

(A) pancreatic carcinoma
(B) cholelithiasis
(C) choledocholithiasis
(D) portal hypertension

Figure 5–77. Sagittal sonogram of the right upper abdomen.

Figure 5–78. Longitudinal scan of the right upper quadrant.

Figure 5–80. Transverse scan of the liver.

642. The findings in Fig. 5–77 are consistent with

(A) recanalized umbilical vein
(B) dilated common bile duct
(C) normal hepatic veins
(D) normal portal veins

643. The findings shown in Fig. 5–78 are consistent with

(A) chronic cholecystitis with cholelithiasis
(B) adenomyomatosis
(C) postprandial gallbladder contraction
(D) duodenal bulb

644. The arrow in Fig. 5–79 is pointing to

(A) main portal vein
(B) left portal vein
(C) hepatic duct
(D) hepatic artery

645. The arrow in Fig. 5–80 is pointing to

(A) dilated bile duct
(B) endothelioma
(C) mesenchymal hamartoma
(D) hepatocellular carcinoma
(E) ligamentum teres

646. The findings in Fig. 5–81 are associated with the following *except*

(A) alkaline phosphatase
(B) serum glutamic-oxaloacetic transaminase
(C) direct bilirubin
(D) α-fetoprotein
(E) jaundice

Figure 5–79. Transverse scan of the liver.

Figure 5–81. Longitudinal scan of the gallbladder.

Figure 5–82. Longitudinal scan of the liver.

647. The findings in Fig. 5–82 are associated with a(n)

(A) decrease in direct bilirubin
(B) increase in indirect bilirubin
(C) increase in alkaline phosphatase
(D) increase in α-fetoprotein

648. The findings in Fig. 5–83 are associated with

(A) hypoproteinemia
(B) congestive heart failure
(C) acute hepatitis
(D) cholecystitis
(E) choledocholithiasis

649. The arrow in Fig. 5–84 is pointing to

(A) major lobar fissure
(B) ligamentum teres
(C) stone in the common bile duct
(D) stone within the cystic duct

Figure 5–83. Magnified view of the gallbladder.

Figure 5–85. Longitudinal scan of the liver.

Figure 5–84. Longitudinal scan of the right upper quadrant.

Figure 5–86. Transverse scan of the liver.

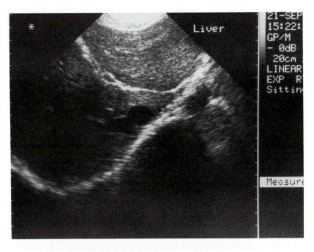

Figure 5–87. Transverse scan of the liver.

Figure 5–89. Longitudinal scan of the right upper quadrant.

650. The findings in Fig. 5–85 are suggestive of

(A) metastastic disease of the liver
(B) acute hepatitis
(C) fatty liver
(D) cirrhosis

651. The findings in Fig. 5–86 are representative of

(A) portal hypertension
(B) congestive heart failure
(C) cirrhosis
(D) normal scan

652. Which of the following ligaments are visualized in Fig. 5–87

(A) main lobar fissure
(B) ligamentum venosum
(C) coronary ligament
(D) ligamentum teres

653. The findings in Fig. 5–88 represent

(A) gallbladder carcinoma
(B) adenomyomatosis
(C) cholecystitis
(D) gallbladder papilloma

654. The findings in Fig. 5–89 are consistent with

(A) pancreatic carcinoma
(B) hydrops
(C) ascites
(D) normal duodenum

655. A patient presents with right upper quadrent pain, fever, nausea, and leukocytosis. The findings in Fig. 5–90 are most consistent with

(A) chronic cholecystitis
(B) gallbladder carcinoma
(C) adenomyomatosis
(D) acute cholecystitis

Figure 5–88. Longitudinal scan of the gallbladder.

Figure 5–90. Longitudinal scan of the gallbladder.

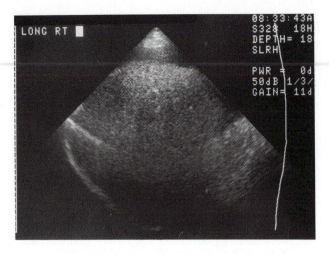

Figure 5–91. Longitudinal scan of the liver.

Figure 5–94. Coronal scan of the mid-abdomen.

Figure 5–92. Longitudinal scan of the liver.

656. The findings in Fig. 5–91 are suggestive of

(A) liver metastases
(B) hepatoma
(C) cirrhosis
(D) fatty liver

657. A patient presents with an increase in direct bilirubin, SGOT, and alkaline phosphatase. The findings in Fig. 5–92 are suggestive of

(A) liver metastases
(B) hepatoma
(C) cirrhosis
(D) fatty liver

Figure 5–93. Transverse scan of the liver.

Figure 5–95. Longitudinal scan of the gallbladder.

Figure 5–96. Longitudinal scan of the liver and gallbladder.

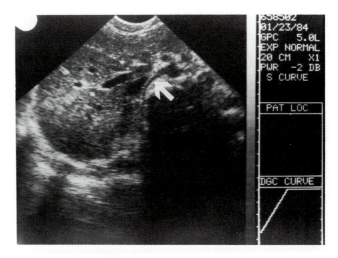

Figure 5–98. Transverse scan of the abdomen.

658. The hemangioma in Fig. 5–93 is located in

   (A) posterior segment of the right lobe
   (B) anterior segment of the right lobe
   (C) anterior segment of the left lobe
   (D) medial segment of the right lobe
   (E) medial segment of the left lobe

659. Which vessels are visualized in Fig. 5–94?

   (A) inferior vena cava, portal vein, left renal
       vein, right renal vein
   (B) inferior vena cava, aorta, right hepatic artery,
       splenic vein
   (C) inferior vena cava, aorta, left renal vein,
       right renal vein
   (D) inferior vena cava, aorta, right renal artery,
       left renal artery

660. A patient with known pancreatic carcinoma presents with the findings in Fig. 5–95, which most
   likely represent

   (A) cholilithiasis
   (B) tumefactive biliary sludge
   (C) carcinoma of the gallbladder
   (D) cholidocholithiasis

661. A 53-year-old man with a history of liver cirrhosis
   presents with increased abdominal girth. Fig. 5–96
   demonstrates a thickened gallbladder wall, which
   is most probably due to

   (A) acalculus cholecystitis
   (B) associated pancreatitis
   (C) cirrhosis and the adjacent ascites
   (D) cirrhosis
   (E) the associated ascites

662. The findings in Fig. 5–97 are consistent with

   (A) cholecystitis
   (B) aortic aneurysm
   (C) pancreatic carcinoma
   (D) a normal pancreas

663. The arrow in Fig. 5–98 is pointing to

   (A) the right crus of the diaphragm
   (B) the right renal artery
   (C) the right portal vein
   (D) the right renal vein

Figure 5–97. Transverse scan of the pancreas.

Figure 5–99. Longitudinal scan of the aorta.

Figure 5–101. Longitudinal scan of the gallbladder.

664. The arrow in Fig. 5–99 is pointing to

    (A) the inferior vena cava
    (B) the superior mesenteric artery
    (C) the celiac
    (D) the right crus of the diaphragm

665. The arrowhead in Fig. 5–99 is pointing to

    (A) esophagogastric junction
    (B) hepatic artery
    (C) portal vein
    (D) superior mesenteric vein

666. The arrow in Fig. 5–100 is pointing to

    (A) inferior vena cava
    (B) superior mesenteric artery
    (C) celiac artery
    (D) right crus of the diaphragm

667. The arrowhead in Fig. 5–100 is pointing to

    (A) right renal artery
    (B) right renal vein
    (C) left renal artery
    (D) left renal vein

668. The shadowing from the region of the gallbladder in Fig. 5–101 is most likely due to

    (A) stones impacted in Hartmann's pouch
    (B) cystic duct stone
    (C) choledocholithiasis
    (D) refraction artifact

669. There seem to be two hemangiomas in Fig. 5–102, one located superior and the other inferior to the diaphram, which are most probably due to

    (A) slice-thickness artifact
    (B) reflection
    (C) mirror-image artifact
    (D) refraction

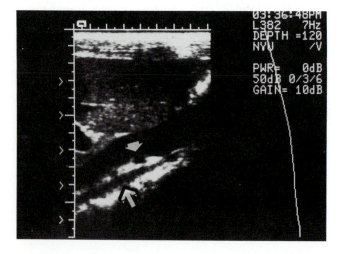

Figure 5–100. Longitudinal scan of the inferior vena cava.

Figure 5–102. Longitudinal scan of the right upper quadrant.

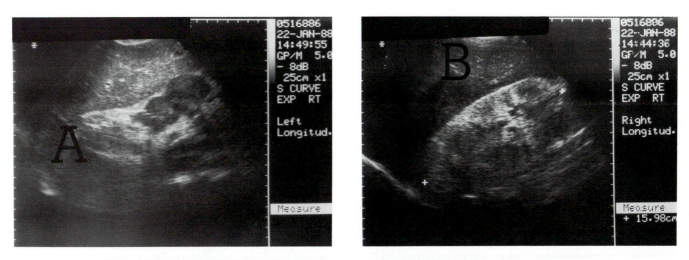

Figure 5–103. (A) Sagittal scan of the right upper quadrant. **(B)** Sagittal scan through the right kidney.

670. A 38-year-old man, who is an intravenous drug abuser, with a known mediastinal mass is seen in Fig. 5–103A and B. Fig. 5–103A demonstrates

(A) a mass near the head of the pancreas
(B) periportal lymphadenopathy
(C) chronic cholecystitis
(D) Klatzkin tumor

671. Fig. 5–103B demonstrates

(A) a normal kidney
(B) a kidney consistent with acute renal insufficiency
(C) a kidney consistent with chronic renal insufficiency
(D) renal cell carcinoma

672. The 32-year-old woman shown in Fig. 5–104 has a history of pancreatic carcinoma. The scan most likely represents

(A) celiac nodes
(B) an aortic aneurysm
(C) a horseshoe kidney
(D) a normal scan

673. Fig. 5–105 demonstrates

(A) a fusiform aneurysm
(B) a saccular aneurysm
(C) a cylindrical aneurysm
(D) a normal aneurysm

Figure 5–104. Transverse scan of the abdomen.

Figure 5–105. Longitudinal scan through the abdominal aorta.

Figure 5–106. Longitudinal scan through the abdominal aorta.

Figure 5–107. Sagittal scan through the right upper quadrant.

Figure 5–108. Sagittal scan through the right upper quadrant.

674. The arrow in Fig. 5–106 is pointing to

    (A) right renal artery
    (B) right renal vein
    (C) left renal artery
    (D) left renal vein

675. The arrow in Fig. 5–107 is pointing to

    (A) head of the pancreas
    (B) body of the pancreas
    (C) caudate lobe of the liver
    (D) quadrate lobe (medial aspect of the left lobe) of the liver

676. The thin black arrow in Fig. 5–108 is pointing to

    (A) celiac artery
    (B) superior mesenteric artery
    (C) portal vein
    (D) left gastric artery

677. The white arrowhead in Fig. 5–108 is pointing to

    (A) celiac artery
    (B) superior mesenteric artery
    (C) portal vein
    (D) left gastric artery

678. The larger black arrow in Fig. 5–108 is pointing to

    (A) splenic vein
    (B) portal vein
    (C) inferior mesenteric vein
    (D) left gastric artery

Figure 5–109. Longitudinal scan through the right kidney.

Figure 5–111. Transverse scan through the pancreas.

679. The arrow in Fig. 5–109 is pointing to

    (A) levator ani muscle
    (B) quadratus lumborum muscle
    (C) psoas muscle
    (D) internal oblique muscle

680. The patient in Fig. 5–110 presented with massive ascites. The arrow is pointing to

    (A) ligamentum teres
    (B) ligamentum venosum
    (C) falciform ligament
    (D) coronary ligament

681. The arrow in Fig. 5–111 is pointing to

    (A) normal head
    (B) normal body
    (C) acute pancreatitis
    (D) chronic pancreatitis
    (E) adenocarcinoma

682. The arrow in Fig. 5–112 is pointing to

    (A) normal body
    (B) normal tail
    (C) acute pancreatitis
    (D) chronic pancreatitis
    (E) adenocarcinoma

Figure 5–110. Transverse scan through the liver.

Figure 5–112. Transverse sonogram through the pancreas.

Figure 5–113. Transverse sonogram through the pancreas.

Figure 5–115. Longitudinal scan of the inferior vena cava.

683. The arrow in Fig. 5–113 is pointing to

    (A) gastroduodenal artery
    (B) common bile duct
    (C) portal vein
    (D) superior mesenteric vein
    (E) hepatic artery

684. Fig. 5–114 is consistent with

    (A) acute pancreatitis
    (B) chronic pancreatitis
    (C) adenocarcinoma
    (D) islet cell tumor
    (E) normal scan

685. The arrow in Fig. 5–115 is pointing to

    (A) gastric antrum
    (B) head of pancreas
    (C) caudate lobe of liver
    (D) body of pancreas
    (E) adrenal gland

686. A 37-year-old man with a past history of repeated episodes of pancreatitis due to alcoholism presents with an epigastric mass. Fig. 5–116 suggests

    (A) negative study
    (B) pancreatic pseudocyst
    (C) acute pancreatitis
    (D) chronic pancreatitis
    (E) adenocarcinoma

Figure 5–114. Transverse sonogram through the pancreas.

Figure 5–116. Transverse scan through the pancreas.

A

B

C

Figure 5–117. (A) Sagittal scan through the head of the pancreas. **(B)** Sagittal scan through the liver. **(C)** Sagittal scan through the gallbladder.

687. A 70-year-old man presents with a history of weight loss, abdominal pain, and anorexia. Figs. 5–117A–C suggest

(A) negative study
(B) pancreatic pseudocyst
(C) acute pancreatitis
(D) chronic pancreatitis
(E) pancreatic adenocarcinoma

688. In Fig. 5–118, the structures visualized within the liver are

(A) normal bile ducts
(B) dilated bile ducts
(C) hepatic arteries
(D) hepatic veins
(E) portal veins

Figure 5–118. Sagittal scan through the liver.

Figure 5–119. Transverse scan through the pancreas.

Figure 5–121. Longitudinal scan through the kidney.

689. The arrow in Fig. 5–119 is pointing to

   (A) normal pancreas
   (B) acute pancreatitis
   (C) chronic pancreatitis
   (D) adenocarcinoma
   (E) islet cell tumor

690. As an incidental finding, this sagittal scan in Fig. 5–120 demonstrated two cystic structures within the liver. This is *most* likely

   (A) liver metastases
   (B) hydatid disease
   (C) simple benign hepatic cysts
   (D) lymphoma
   (E) polycystic liver disease

691. The renal transplant patient in Fig. 5–121 was referred for a sonogram. The perirenal fluid collec-

tion may be associated with all of the following *except*

   (A) abscess
   (B) hematoma
   (C) ascites
   (D) urinoma
   (E) lymphocele

692. Fig. 5–122 shows a 38-year-old man with a distended bladder and enuresis. The sonogram depicts

   (A) an enlarged prostate
   (B) a normal scan
   (C) diffuse bladder wall thickening
   (D) bladder neck obstruction
   (E) endometriosis of the bladder

Figure 5–120. Longitudinal scan through the right upper quadrant.

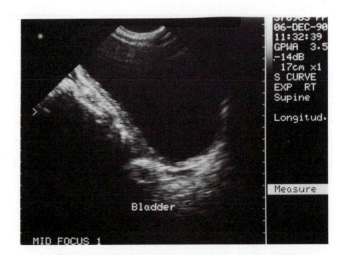

Figure 5–122. Longitudinal scan of a male pelvis.

Figure 5–123. Longitudinal scan of the right kidney.

Figure 5–125. Transverse scan of the right kidney.

693. Which of the following laboratory values would you expect to be elevated in the patient in Fig. 5–123?

(A) serum glutamic oxaloacetic transaminase (SGOT) and serum glutamic pyruvic transaminase (SGPT)
(B) alkaline phosphatase and bilirubin
(C) amylase and lipase
(D) creatinine and blood urea nitrogen (BUN)
(E) acid phosphatase

694. Internal echoes inside the simple renal cyst shown in Fig. 5–124 may be due to all of the following *except*

(A) reverberation
(B) beam width artifact
(C) refraction
(D) attenuation
(E) side lobe artifact

695. This transverse scan of the right kidney (Fig. 5–125) shows findings *most* consistent with

(A) parapelvic cysts
(B) chronic renal failure
(C) hydronephrosis
(D) adult polycystic kidney disease
(E) juvenile polycystic kidney disease

696. The newborn in Fig. 5–126 presented with a palpable abdominal mass. The sonogram suggests

(A) multicystic dysplastic kidney
(B) hydronephrosis
(C) infantile polycystic disease
(D) peripelvic cysts
(E) multiple renal cortical cysts

Figure 5–124. Longitudinal scan of the right kidney.

Figure 5–126. Transverse scan of the left kidney of a newborn baby.

Figure 5–127. Longitudinal scan of the right kidney.

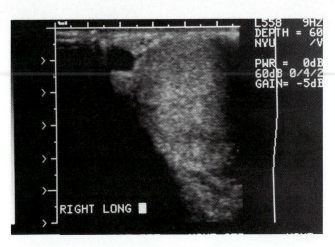

Figure 5–129. Longitudinal scan through the right testis.

697. Fig. 5–127 suggests that this patient may have all of the following *except*

(A) a normal scan
(B) benign prostatic enlargement
(C) prostatitis
(D) calculi
(E) retroperitoneal fibrosis
(F) pyelonephritis

698. The most obvious cause of hydronephrosis in the patient in Fig. 5–128 is

(A) angiomyolipoma
(B) vesicoureteral reflux
(C) tuberous sclerosis
(D) parapelvic cysts
(E) staghorn calculus

699. A scrotal ultrasound was performed on the 69-year-old man in Fig. 5–129. The findings are consistent with

(A) spermatocele
(B) epididymal cyst
(C) seminoma
(D) varicocele
(E) may be two of the above

700. A scrotal ultrasound was performed on the 78-year-old man in Fig. 5–130. The arrow is pointing to

(A) a fractured testicle
(B) normal head of epididymis
(C) the mediastinum
(D) seminoma
(E) testicular torsion

Figure 5–128. Coronal scan of the right kidney.

Figure 5–130. Magnified longitudinal scan of the right testis.

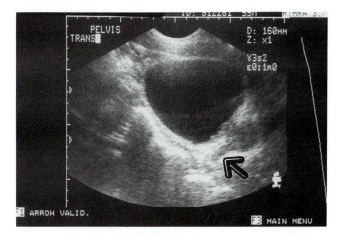

Figure 5–131. Longitudinal scan through a normal male pelvis.

Figure 5–133. Longitudinal scan through the right kidney.

701. Fig. 5–131 is a scan of a male pelvis. The arrow is pointing to

(A) prostate
(B) seminal vesicle
(C) prostatic urethra
(D) membranous urethra
(E) urethra

702. In Fig. 5–132, the arrow is pointing to

(A) spermatocele
(B) epididymal cyst
(C) cryptorchidism
(D) varicocele
(E) mediastinum testis

703. Fig. 5–133 is most consistent with

(A) acute pyelonephritis
(B) acute tubular necrosis
(C) tubular sclerosis
(D) chronic glomerulonephritis
(E) medullary nephrocalcinosis

704. Fig. 5–134 is consistent with

(A) acute pyelonephritis
(B) acute tubular necrosis
(C) tubular sclerosis
(D) acute focal bacterial nephritis
(E) an angiomyolipoma
(F) two of the above

Figure 5–132. Longitudinal scan through the right testis.

Figure 5–134. Coronal scan of the right kidney.

Figure 5–135. Transverse scan of the abdomen.

Figure 5–137. Coronal scan of the left kidney.

705. This sonogram (Fig. 5–135) of a 43-year-old man with a palpable abdominal mass suggests

(A) adenopathy
(B) aortic aneurysm
(C) horseshoe kidney
(D) dilated loop of bowel

706. The arrow in Fig. 5–136, showing a 14-day-old baby boy born 2 weeks prematurely, is pointing to

(A) normal adrenal
(B) perirenal hemorrhage
(C) retroperitoneal fat
(D) neuroblastoma
(E) pheochromocytoma

707. This is a scan (Fig. 5–137) of the left kidney. It suggests

(A) a parapelvic cyst
(B) hydronephrosis
(C) pyonephrosis
(D) urinoma
(E) renal infarction

708. The thin black arrow in Fig. 5–138 is pointing to

(A) the renal sinus
(B) arcuate arteries
(C) pyramids
(D) simple renal cysts
(E) the major calyx

709. The open arrowhead in Fig. 5–138 is pointing to

(A) the renal sinus
(B) arcuate arteries
(C) pyramids
(D) simple renal cyst
(E) renal stones

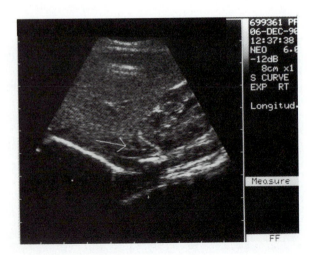

Figure 5–136. Longitudinal sonogram of a neonate through the area of the right kidney.

Figure 5–138. Longitudinal scan of the right kidney.

710. The larger black arrow in Fig. 5–138 is pointing to

  (A) renal column of Bertin
  (B) an angiomyolipoma
  (C) dromedary hump
  (D) bifid collecting system
  (E) the renal pelvis

711. A patient presents with the sonogram reproduced in Fig. 5–139. The findings may be initiated by all of the following *except*

  (A) stone in the common bile duct
  (B) mass in the head of the pancreas
  (C) ampullary carcinoma
  (D) diffuse metastatic disease of the liver
  (E) cirrhosis

712. A patient presents with the sonogram reproduced in Fig. 5–140. The findings may be initiated by all of the following *except*

  (A) lymphoma
  (B) portal hypertension
  (C) infectious diseases
  (D) myeloproliferative disorders
  (E) neuroblastoma

713. The best position to place the patient to evaluate renal size and function is

  (A) prone
  (B) supine
  (C) decubitus coronal
  (D) transverse

Question 714: The following statements are either true or false.

714. Acute tubular necrosis is associated with

  (A) increased renal size T _____ F _____

Figure 5–139. Longitudinal scan of the liver.

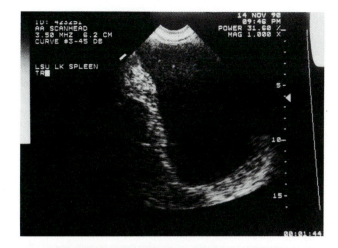

Figure 5–140. Longitudinal scan of the spleen.

  (B) the medullary pyramids are prominent and anechoic T _____ F _____
  (C) acute renal failure, of which acute tubular necrosis is the most common cause T _____ F _____
  (D) a rise in serum creatinine of greater than 2.5 mg/dL T _____ F _____
  (E) in renal transplantation, the most common cause of failure in the immediate posttransplant period is acute tubular necrosis T _____ F _____

715. The valves of Heister are located in

  (A) common bile duct
  (B) cystic duct
  (C) gallbladder
  (D) common hepatic duct

716. Chronic cholecystitis is associated with

  (A) pancreatic pseudocyst
  (B) gallbladder polyps
  (C) gallbladder carcinoma
  (D) increased α-fetoprotein levels

717. One may find associated with biliary dilatation all of the following *except*

  (A) jaundice
  (B) right upper quadrant pain
  (C) increased alkaline phosphatase
  (D) elevated amylase
  (E) elevated acid phosphatase

718. People with diabetes may present with

  (A) hypotonic and paralytic intestines
  (B) renal insufficiency
  (C) chronic distension of the gallbladder
  (D) pancreatic phlegmon

719. If a patient presents with weight loss and jaundice, one would expect to find all of the below *except*

    (A) liver metastasis
    (B) dilated common bile duct
    (C) hepatoma
    (D) mass in the head of the pancreas
    (E) hemangioma

720. Choledochal cyst is a

    (A) cyst within the gallbladder
    (B) focal dilatation of the biliary tree
    (C) complication of a pseudocyst
    (D) associated with adenomyomatosis

721. Carcinoma of the gallbladder would most likely appear as

    (A) thin-walled enlarged gallbladder
    (B) small gallbladder with thickened walls
    (C) large gallbladder with a halo effect
    (D) a diffusely thickened gallbladder with gallstones

Answers and Explanations

At the end of each explained answer there is a number combination in parentheses. The first number identifies the reference source; the second number or set of numbers indicates the page or pages on which the relevant information can be found.

1. **(A)** The kidneys are *not* intraperitoneal in location. They lie behind the parietal peritoneum; therefore, they are referred to as a retroperitoneal structure. *(2:308–309)*

2. **(A)** The renal sinus echoes are produced by the renal pelvis and calyces, renal vessels, fat, and areolar tissue. *(2:310)*

3. **(C)** Arcuate vessels separate the renal parenchyma into cortex and medulla. Sonographically, they may be visualized as bright echoes within this corticomedullary junction. *(2:310)*

4. **(D)** The best approach for evaluation of the left kidney is coronal. Satisfactory images of the left kidney are usually not obtainable in the supine and RAO positions due to overlying bowel gas. In patients with well-developed psoas muscles, the prone views may be of little value. *(2:318)*

5. **(C)** The normal pyloric muscle is 3 mm, and should measure less than 15 mm in total diameter. In the presence of pyloric stenosis, the muscle increases in size and measures more than 5 mm in thickness. *(34:1024)*

6. **(D)** All of the above. To fulfill the criteria of a cyst anywhere within the body, one must show an anechoic (echo-free) structure with good through transmission, distal acoustic enhancement, and well-defined smooth walls. *(1:109)*

7. **(D)** Renal vein thrombosis is associated with large kidneys. Small kidneys are associated with end-stage renal disease. (The normal adult kidneys range from 9 to 12 cm in length.) The renal parenchyma is normally less echogenic when compared to the liver parenchyma. However, in the presence of end-stage renal disease, the kidneys become more echogenic. End-stage renal disease may be due to chronic glomerulonephritis, chronic pylonephritis, and renal vascular disease. *(2:309; 10:60)*

8. **(A)** The columns of Bertin are the inward extensions of the cortex, surrounding and separating the renal pyramids of the medulla. At times, they may be confused with a pseudotumor. *(2:344; 10:52)*

9. **(A)** In the fasting patient, the most common cause for sonographic nonvisualization of the gallbladder is contraction of the gallbladder due to chronic cholecystitis. The contrast medium used to visualize the gallbladder in x-ray does not prevent ultrasound visualization. *(34:559)*

10. **(D)** All of the above. A hematoma may appear either sonolucent, echogenic, or as a semicystic, semisolid mass, depending on how soon after injury the patient is examined. A new hematoma will appear echo free, whereas old blood will appear quite echogenic. *(2:359)*

11. **(D)** All of the above. Urinomas often accompany renal injuries, renal transplants, and patients who have passed a renal stone. *(2:264, 362)*

12. **(C)** Fluid-filled pelvocaliceal collecting system. Sonographically, hydronephrosis presents with a spectrum of ultrasound appearances from a ring-shaped echo-free area in the region of the renal pelvis to a totally distended pelvocaliceal collecting system. Later, with progressive distention, large cystic areas are seen within the kidney with very little renal tissue identified. *(2:362)*

13. **(F)** All of the above. Hydronephrosis is a dilatation of the renal pelvis with associated atrophy of renal tissue resulting from an obstruction to the flow of urine. Possible causes may be prostatic enlargement, calculi, congenital and/or inflammatory strictures, pregnancy, and tumors, all of which can compress or block the outward flow of urine. *(4:363)*

14. **(B)** Wilms' tumor. This is a rapidly developing malignant tumor of the kidneys, usually affecting children before 5 years of age.   *(4:372)*

15. **(C)** Empyema is a complication of acute cholecystitis with the development of purulent material within the gallbladder lumen. Since this is essentially an abscess, the patient is ill with fever and has local tenderness. Sonographically, the appearance is similar to acute cholecystitis with echogenic debris.   *(1:252)*

16. **(E)** All of the above. Acute cholecystitis is associated with right upper quadrant pain, Murphy's sign, a stone impacted within the cystic duct, and in severe cases fever and an elevated blood count.   *(2:124)*

17. **(C)** Courvoisier's sign. Courvoisier's law states that obstruction of the *common bile duct* by pressure from the *outside,* ie, by a carcinoma of the pancreas, produces a *distended* gallbladder. Obstruction by a stone from *within* produces *little* or *no distension* of the gallbladder. The gallbladder is thickened and contracted as a result of the inflammation, and the inflow of bile into the gallbladder is impeded. Classically, patients with a tumor in the head of the pancreas present with painless jaundice and a palpable Courvoisier gallbladder.   *(2:127; 4:462)*

18. **(G)** All of the above. Causes of gallbladder wall thickening may include ascites, hypoproteinemia, right-sided congestive cardiac failure, hepatitis, and acute and chronic cholecystitis. In addition, carcinoma, primary or secondary adenomyomatosis, and a normal contracted gallbladder present with thickened walls.   *(2:143)*

19. **(B)** Hydropic gallbladder. Complete obstruction of the neck of the gallbladder or the cystic duct leads to hydrops or mucocele of the gallbladder. In this condition, the bile within the gallbladder is absorbed and replaced by a mucoid secretion from the lining of the gallbladder.   *(2:146)*

20. **(C)** The upper limits of the intraluminal diameter of the common duct should not exceed 7 mm. The term *common duct* was adopted in sonography to describe either the common hepatic or the common bile duct. The origin of the common duct, which is the anatomical point at which the cystic duct communicates with the common hepatic to form the common bile duct, cannot be visualized and/or differentiated sonographically; therefore one cannot recognize with surety if one sees the common hepatic or common bile, hence the term *common duct.* If one can visualize the duct at the level of the pancreas, at that point one can safely say it is the common bile duct.   *(2:150)*

21. **(A)** In the adult, the luminal diameter of the proximal common hepatic duct should be less than or equal to 3–4 mm.   *(3:157)*

22. **(A)** The renal pyramids are found within the medulla of the kidney not within the renal sinus.   *(2:310; 3:194)*

23. **(A)** Bowman's capsule and the convoluted tubules are found within the renal cortex.   *(3:194)*

24. **(B)** Alkaline phosphatase is elevated in hepatobiliary disease not in renal failure. Laboratory data that may indicate renal failure consists of an elevated blood urea nitrogen (BUN), creatinine, and increased protein in the urine.   *(3:194)*

25. **(C)** Horseshoe kidney. This congenital abnormality occurs during fetal development with fusion of the upper or lower poles of the kidney.   *(3:197)*

26. **(D)** The involved kidneys will be moderately to extremely enlarged resulting from an increase in the size of the individual cysts rather than an increase in their number.   *(4:367)*

27. **(C)** A staghorn calculus is a large stone located within the pelvis of the kidney.   *(3:207)*

28. **(E)** All of the above. Hypoalbuminemia, cholecystitis—acute or chronic, adenomyomatosis, and carcinoma of the gallbladder are all associated with thickening of the gallbladder wall.   *(1:248)*

29. **(D)** All of the above. A hypernephroma, also known as a renal cell carcinoma, adenocarcinoma, or Grawitz's tumor, is the most common malignant renal tumor in adults. The tumor is an irregular in shape but well-marginated solid mass and may grow so large as to replace the renal volume.   *(4:370)*

30. **(B)** Lymphadenopathy. Horseshoe kidneys occur during fetal development with fusion of the upper or lower poles of the kidney. The fused poles and the isthmus drape over the spine and may be confused with lymphadenopathy.   *(3:197)*

31. **(C)** The pancreatic head lies caudad to the portal vein and anterior to the inferior vena cava.   *(2:167)*

32. **(A)** Glisson's capsule is a dense fibrous membrane that surrounds the liver and encloses the portal vein, hepatic artery, and bile ducts within the liver.   *(2:83)*

33. **(D)** All of the above. The splenic vein runs anterior to the aorta and superior mesenteric artery and caudad to the celiac axis to join with the superior mesenteric vein to become the portal vein.   *(8:37)*

34. **(C)** In the normal individual, the abdominal aorta shows a gradual tapering of its luminal dimensions as it proceeds distally to its bifurcation. *(3:117–120)*

35. **(E)** All of the above. To distinguish hepatic veins from portal veins, all of the given anatomical considerations should be recognized. *(3:116)*

36. **(C)** The celiac trunk does *not* branch into the gastroduodenal artery. It does branch into the left gastric, splenic, and common hepatic arteries. *(3:118)*

37. **(C)** The superior mesenteric artery runs posterior to the neck of the pancreas, then emerges and crosses anterior to the uncinate process. *(3:120)*

38. **(A)** The division into anatomic right and left lobes of the liver is along the line of the major hepatic fissure and middle hepatic vein. *(3:130)*

39. **(D)** The pleural fluid may be anechoic to loculated and is found superior to the diaphragm. *(8:305)*

40. **(A)** In acute renal disease, the kidneys are enlarged and swollen. *(8:139)*

41. **(C)** When the gallbladder fundus is folded over on itself, this variation is termed a phrygian cap. *(1:228)*

42. **(C)** On transverse sonogram, the common bile duct is located anterior to the inferior vena cava and posterior to the head of the pancreas. The common bile duct will define the posterolateral aspect of the pancreatic head. *(1:260)*

43. **(C)** The spleen is *not* a retroperitoneal organ. It is an intraperitoneal organ, thus it is covered on both its anterior and posterior surfaces by the peritoneum. *(1:331)*

44. **(A)** The kidneys are *not* rigidly fixed on the abdominal wall. They may move downward during inspiration by as much as 2.5 cm. *(3:192)*

45. **(G)** Gallbladder carcinoma has a strong association with calculi and chronic mechanical irritation. It initially may begin as a polypoid mass eventually progressing to bile duct obstruction, jaundice, and weight loss. *(1:256)*

46. **(C)** The inferior vena cava forms at the confluence of the right and left common iliac veins. *(3:111)*

47. **(D)** The inferior vena cava passes through the caval hiatus of the diaphragm to enter the right, not the left, atrium. *(3:111)*

48. **(B)** Both bile ducts and portal veins have echogenic walls, therefore, this cannot be used as ultrasound criteria. *(1:260)*

49. **(C)** A choledochal cyst is not a true cyst but a congenital outpouching of the common duct that may cause obstructive jaundice in children. *(1:259)*

50. **(C)** A pancreatic pseudocyst, loculated ascites, and a fluid-filled stomach will all be found anterior to the pancreas. An aortic aneurysm is found posterior to the pancreas. *(5:175)*

51. **(A)** The left renal vein runs between the aorta and the superior mesenteric artery. *(3:116)*

52. **(B)** The superior mesenteric vein, a tributary of the portal vein, runs upward to the right of the superior mesenteric artery. *(3:114)*

53. **(C)** After leaving the spleen, the splenic vein courses along the posterior surface of the pancreatic body and tail. *(3:114)*

54. **(B)** If on sonographic examination one finds dilated intrahepatic ducts and a small gallbladder, the obstruction should be at the level of the common hepatic duct above the entry of the cystic duct. Bile is not going to pass the obstruction to fill the gallbladder. *(2:155)*

55. **(D)** The normal thickness of the gallbladder wall is 3 mm. Thicker walls suggest a pathological condition. *(1:248)*

56. **(D)** Adenomyomatosis is a benign proliferation and thickening of the muscle and glandular layer of the gallbladder with the formation of intramural diverticula. It is most common in the fundus where it appears as a focal mass. *(7:163)*

57. **(B)** Glisson's capsule is a strong specular reflector, having a large, smooth interface. The dimensions are much greater than the ultrasonic wavelength. *(2:83)*

58. **(E)** All of the above. An increase in the parenchymal echogenicity of the liver giving rise to a "fatty liver" may be due to alcohol abuse (most common), diabetes, chemotherapy, or toxic substances. *(2:102)*

59. **(B)** Hydronephrosis frequently occurs in a duplicated kidney collecting system. *(2:365)*

60. **(B)** If on sonographic examination, a patient is found to have dilated interhepatic ducts, a dilated common bile duct, and a dilated gallbladder (the

gallbladder enlarging before the biliary tree because it has the greatest surface area), one should expect obstruction at the distal common duct.

(2:155)

61. **(B)** The gastroesophageal junction can sonographically be visualized anterior to the aorta and posterior to the left lobe of the liver. *(1:33)*

62. **(C)** In acute viral hepatitis, the liver parenchyma appears normal. *(2:103)*

63. **(D)** Cholecystokinin, a hormone released by the intestinal mucosa, stimulates the ejection of bile from the gallbladder. *(1:226)*

64. **(D)** Diffuse thickening of the gallbladder wall is a nonspecific finding and frequently is not a result of primary gallbladder disease. It can be seen with acute cholecystitis but may also be associated with hepatitis, congestive heart failure, and severe hypoalbumenic state. However, elevated portal pressure is *not* a recognized cause for diffuse gallbladder wall thickening. *(3:162)*

65. **(A)** The best sonographic window to the left hemidiaphragm is the spleen. *(8:302)*

66. **(B)** An islet cell tumor is the most common benign tumor of the pancreas. These tumors are usually small, well encapsulated, and most commonly found in the tail. Sonographically, they are very difficult to image owing to their small size. *(3:186)*

67. **(F)** All of the above. Adenocarcinoma is the most malignant tumor of the pancreas. These tumors may be quite large with irregular nodular borders and are commonly found within the pancreatic head. The enlarged gland causes obstruction of the common bile duct and possibly the pancreatic duct. Dilated bile ducts, an enlarged gallbladder (a Courvoisier gallbladder), weight loss, and painless jaundice are associated findings. *(3:186)*

68. **(B)** The uncinate process of the pancreas lies posterior to the superior mesenteric artery and vein.

(3:174)

69. **(A)** High levels of serum amylase can be due to pancreatitis. One of the most common causes of pancreatitis is cholelithiasis. *(4:465)*

70. **(C)** Bile is produced within the liver *not* the pancreas. Lipase is an exocrine function and insulin and glucagon are endocrine functions of the pancreas. *(4:472)*

71. **(D)** All of the above. The renal hilum on the medial border of each kidney contains the renal vein, two branches of the renal artery, and the proximal ureter. *(3:192)*

72. **(B)** The kidneys, the perinephric fat, and the adrenal glands are covered by Gerota's fascia but not by a true capsule. *(3:192)*

73. **(C)** The normal adult kidneys measure 10–12 cm in length and 4–5 cm in thickness. *(2:309; 3:192)*

74. **(D)** Fat can sonographically present as either anechoic or echogenic depending upon its composition and location. In renal sinus lipomatosis, the renal sinus will be enlarged and its fat content runs the spectrum from echo-free to echogenic. *(5:318–319)*

75. **(C)** If one finds a solid renal mass, one should continue the examination and check the inferior vena cava and renal vein for tumor extension as well as the retroperitoneum for nodes. *(2:344)*

76. **(D)** All of the above. In the case of chronic pancreatitis, as the pancreas becomes more fibrotic, it will decrease in size and will appear more echogenic with an irregular outline. Dilatation of the pancreatic duct (over 2 mm) with calculi is a sequela of ductal obstruction. *(8:54)*

77. **(A)** The pancreas *does not* lie in the peritoneal space. It is a retroperitoneal organ. It is approximately 10–15 cm in length. The gland is multilobulated and nonencapsulated. Because there is no capsule, it is hard to visualize sonographically.

(3:174; 2:163)

78. **(C)** Pseudocyst formation is a frequent complication of pancreatitis. Pseudocysts are usually located around the pancreas but may dissect through the retroperitoneum and be located anywhere in the body. An uncomplicated pseudocyst is one without any internal debris. Sonographically, it will appear anechoic, have smooth walls, and good ultrasound transmission distally. *(2:192)*

79. **(C)** The presence of gas within a mass confirms the diagnosis of an abscess. An abscess usually has a more irregular appearance than a pseudocyst and contains more internal echoes. *(2:192)*

80. **(B)** A pancreatic pseudocyst may regress spontaneously by draining into the communicating pancreatic duct and then into the bowel. *(2:192)*

81. **(E)** Pancreatic pseudocysts contain strong pancreatic enzymes. These enzymes can dissect into the porta hepatis area, or they can dissect through the esophageal or aortic hiatus to be found in the mediastinum. A pseudocyst may dissect into the retro-

peritoneal area and may extend into the pelvis and groin. *(2:197)*

82. **(A)** The endocrine function of the pancreas is to produce insulin. The exocrine function of the pancreas is to produce lipase, amylase, carboxypeptidase, trypsin, and chymotrypsin. *(3:175)*

83. **(C)** The acinar cells of the pancreas are the exocrine secretory cells. These cells secrete enzymes, which are carried by the pancreatic duct. *(3:175)*

84. **(B)** The maximum inner diameter of the pancreatic duct in young adults measures 2 mm. *(2:177)*

85. **(D)** All of the above. By visualizing pancreatic tissue on both sides of the pancreatic duct, one can avoid confusion between the pancreatic duct and the splenic or portal vein posteriorly. Confusion of the collapsed stomach wall anteriorly is best avoided by having the patient drink fluid. The splenic artery is located anteriorly and pulsations should be noted to avoid confusion. *(2:177)*

86. **(B)** Adenocarcinoma is the most common primary carcinoma of the pancreas. The clinical symptoms are weight loss, painless jaundice, nausea, vomiting, and changes in stool. *(3:186)*

87. **(D)** Adenocarcinoma of the pancreas is imaged as a solid focally enlarged lobulated mass with low-level echoes. It most commonly occurs in the pancreatic head, which in turn may lead to pancreatic duct obstruction or biliary duct obstruction. *(2:178)*

88. **(C)** When a mass is visualized in the area of the pancreatic head, one should check the liver for metastasis and dilation of the intrahepatic ducts. The common bile duct and the pancreatic duct should be checked for enlargement secondary to obstruction. *(2:177)*

89. **(F)** All of the above. Nodal masses, compression of the inferior vena cava, splenic vein, or portal vein posteriorly, and ascites are associated findings of pancreatic carcinoma. *(2:183)*

90. **(B)** In acute pancreatitis, the pancreas is enlarged and edematous demonstrating a decrease in ultrasound absorption. It is secondary to this that sonographically the pancreas becomes uniformly hypoechoic, with an increase in through transmission. *(2:183)*

91. **(A)** To delineate the duodenum from the pancreatic head, have the patient drink water and then scan a few minutes later. *(8:53)*

92. **(D)** Bile is an example of an exocrine function of the liver (the releasing of secretions via a duct). *(3:132)*

93. **(B)** Wirsung's duct is the main pancreatic duct and Santorini's duct is an accessory duct. *(1:275)*

94. **(C)** The head of the pancreas may extend medial to the inferior vena cava and posterior to the superior mesenteric vein. This extension is termed the uncinate process. *(3:174)*

95. **(B)** The extrahepatic portion of the falciform ligament can be visualized in ascites. It will appear as an echogenic band attaching the liver to the anterior abdominal wall. *(2:87)*

96. **(D)** The liver is considered to be an intraperitoneal structure. The portion of the liver that is devoid of peritoneum is termed the bare area. The bare area is located between the right and left triangular ligaments. *(2:85; 6:209)*

97. **(A)** The right and left hepatic ducts usually unite to form the common hepatic duct in the porta hepatis. Occasionally, they may unite within the hepatic parenchyma. *(1:228)*

98. **(C)** Lymphadenopathy is usually associated with carcinoma. A common site for enlarged nodes is in the porta hepatis. This in turn may cause dilatation of the intrahepatic ducts but will not affect the common bile duct or gallbladder because of the level of the obstruction. *(1:270)*

99. **(B)** The main pancreatic duct is Wirsung's duct. The duct starts at the tail of the pancreas, transverses the body, and courses to the head where it is largest in diameter. Normally, it should not exceed 2 mm in luminal diameter. *(2:176)*

100. **(A)** The ligamentum venosum is a remnant of the ductus venosus that shunts oxygenated blood from the umbilical vein to the inferior vena cava, bypassing the liver. In the adult, the ligamentum venosum is a landmark separating the caudate lobe from the left lobe of the liver. *(3:130; 6:211)*

101. **(E)** All of the above. All of the listed fluid collections are sonolucent masses that may occur around the renal transplant. To help differentiate between them, keep in mind the number of days or weeks at which they occur postoperatively. Abscesses usually occur immediately after surgery, hematomas appear early in the postoperative period, urinomas usually occur within the first 2 weeks, and lymphoceles occur between 2 weeks and 6 months. *(2:381)*

102. **(B)** Acute glomerulonephritis is *not* a cause of hydronephrosis. Posterior urethral valves obstruct the urethra directly and can lead to hydronephrosis. Ovarian cancer and retroperitoneal tumors may place extrinsic pressure on the ureters leading to hydronephrosis. Retroperitoneal fibrosis may encase and thereby obstruct the ureters also leading to hydronephrosis. *(2:415)*

103. **(A)** The rectus abdominus muscle is not considered to be retroperitoneal in location, therefore, a retroperitoneal abscess cannot be found there. *(3:231)*

104. **(D)** The spleen is an intraperitoneal organ. Retroperitoneal structures include the kidney, pancreas, aorta, vena cava, duodenum, and adrenal glands. *(3:231)*

105. **(D)** All of the above. Findings for renal vein thrombosis are determined by the stage of the disease. The order in which they appear (A, B, C) is from acute to chronic, respectively. *(2:373)*

106. **(D)** A Klatskin tumor is a ductal cancer at the bifurcation of the right and left hepatic ducts. *Cholangiocarcinoma* is a general term for ductal cancer. A Klatskin tumor, cholangiocarcinoma, and enlarged portal lymph nodes will only obstruct the intrahepatic biliary tree. Pancreatic carcinoma will first block the common duct before dilatation of the intrahepatic ducts can be seen. *(1:259; 2:144)*

107. **(D)** All of the above. The gastroduodenal artery is the first branch of the common hepatic artery. It proceeds caudally and is used as a landmark delineating the anterolateral aspect of the head of the pancreas. On transverse scans, it is seen as a round sonolucent structure anterior to the common bile duct. *(5:186)*

108. **(C)** The quadrate lobe is the medial segment of the left lobe. *(3:135)*

109. **(D)** The caudate lobe occupies much of the posterosuperior surface of the liver. It lies between the inferior vena cava and the ligamentum venosum. *(1:31)*

110. **(B)** There are three hepatic veins; right, left, and middle. They run intersegmentally and define the lobes of the liver. *(3:130)*

111. **(F)** The ligamentum teres is defined by all of the above and is an anatomic landmark which separates the caudal aspect of the left lobe of the liver into medial and lateral segments. *(3:130)*

112. **(D)** Acute obstruction of the common bile duct may not dilate the intrahepatic biliary radicles for a few days. In chronic infiltrative liver disease and cholangitis, the ducts cannot dilate easily due to secondary fibrotic narrowing. Given time, both of these circumstances will eventually lead to dilated intrahepatic biliary radicles to some degree. *(1:259)*

113. **(D)** Caroli's disease is cavernous ectasia of the biliary tree and may appear as focal cystic collections throughout the liver. Polycystic liver disease and congenital cysts are cystic lesions within the liver. *(2:108)*

114. **(D)** All of the terms given may lead to shadowing from the area of the gallbladder fossa. *(2:107)*

115. **(E)** All of terms given are complex lesions within the liver. Biliary cystadenoma is a rare benign tumor of the bile ducts. An echinococcal cyst is classically multiseptated with daughter cysts. A large cavernous hemangioma can be visualized but is best diagnosed by angiography or CT. The appearance of a hematoma depends on the stage of clot formation. *(2:111)*

116. **(A)** The most common cause of pancreatitis in adults in the United States is biliary tract disease. Alcohol abuse is the second most common cause followed by trauma. *(3:183)*

117. **(B)** Lipase secreted by the pancreas accounts for 80% of all fat digestion. The other 20% is secreted by the small intestine. *(3:176)*

118. **(B)** Jaundice is generally not seen in acute pancreatitis. Sonographically, the swollen pancreas is enlarged, becoming less echogenic and possibly pressing on the inferior vena cava anteriorly. *(3:184)*

119. **(B)** In chronic pancreatitis, the patient is usually jaundiced. The pancreas becomes small and fibrotic and echogenic calcifications are noted. Pseudocysts are commonly seen in association with chronic pancreatitis. *(3:184)*

120. **(E)** All of the techniques given may be useful in imaging the pancreas. The prone position is helpful in visualizing the tail. *(2:175)*

121. **(B)** The left adrenal is posterior, not anterior, to the tail of the pancreas. *(2:164)*

122. **(L)** Portal vein. *(8:49–51)*

123. **(R)** Hepatic artery. *(8:49–51)*

124. **(K)** Common bile duct. *(8:49–51)*

125. **(F)** Left gastric artery. *(8:49–51)*

126. **(J)** Celiac axis.   *(8:49–51)*

127. **(E)** Splenic artery.   *(8:49–51)*

128. **(B)** Gastroduodenal artery.   *(8:49–51)*

129. **(A)** Spleen.   *(8:49–51)*

130. **(G)** Adrenal.   *(8:49–51)*

131. **(C)** Kidney.   *(8:49–51)*

132. **(M)** Aorta.   *(8:49–51)*

133. **(H)** Superior mesenteric artery.   *(8:49–51)*

134. **(D)** Inferior vena cava.   *(8:49–51)*

135. **(I)** Superior mesenteric vein.   *(8:49–51)*

136. **(N)** Duodenum.   *(8:49–51)*

137. **(P)** Duct of Wirsung.   *(8:49–51)*

138. **(O)** Duct of Santorini.   *(8:49–51)*

139. **(Q)** Uncinate process.   *(8:49–51)*

140. **(A)** True. In a significant proportion of patients after cholecystectomy, the luminal diameter of the normal proximal bile duct is more than 5 mm and may be up to 10 mm.   *(1:260)*

141. **(B)** In decreasing order of echogenicity is the renal sinus > pancreas > liver > spleen > renal parenchyma.   *(2:165; 8:108)*

142. **(B)** A subphrenic abscess will displace the spleen inferiorly, not enlarge it.   *(1:344)*

143. **(E)** All of the above. The thickening of the nondistended bowel wall greater than 5 mm whether due to inflammatory disease or a variety of neoplasm depends upon the amount of bowel wall infiltration. Absence of peristalsis on real-time and the bull's eye configuration will aid in the recognition of bowel abnormalities.   *(2:299)*

144. **(B)** If a mass is solid, displacement of adjacent organs will aid in helping to evaluate the origin of the mass. In a retroperitoneal sarcoma, the kidney, spleen, and pancreas would be displaced anteriorly.   *(8:110)*

145. **(A)** The splenic vein courses anteriorly to the left adrenal gland to join with the superior mesenteric vein to become the main portal vein. An adrenal mass may lead to anterior displacement of this vein.   *(8:271)*

146. **(C)** A fluid collection located between the diaphragm and the spleen may represent a subphrenic abscess.   *(8:110)*

147. **(C)** The normal adult adrenal rarely measures more than 3 cm at its maximum diameter.   *(2:396)*

148. **(A)** Adenomyomatosis is a benign infiltrative disease that will *not* lead to a large gallbladder but rather to an irregular thickening of the gallbladder wall.   *(3:152; 5:121)*

149. **(C)** Right-side heart failure will produce venous congestion of the liver, which in turn will lead to marked dilatation of the intrahepatic veins.   *(2:104)*

150. **(A)** The body of the pancreas is bound on its anterior surface by the dorsum of the stomach.   *(2:163)*

151. **(A)** The landmark associated with the pancreatic body is the splenic vein that lies posteriorly. The gastroduodenal artery defines the anterolateral and the common bile duct the posterolateral margins of the pancreatic head.   *(1:274)*

152. **(D)** All of the above. The landmarks for visualizing the pancreatic head are the inferior vena cava lying posteriorly, the gastroduodenal artery defining the anterolateral margin, and the common bile duct defining the posterolateral margin.   *(8:37)*

153. **(B)** The landmark most associated with the pancreatic neck is the superior mesenteric vein.   *(1:274)*

154. **(C)** The pancreas *does not* have a true capsule; therefore when there is inflammation and/or obstruction, pancreatic enzymes are released, forming a pseudocyst.   *(2:345–368)*

155. **(A)** Angiomyolipoma is least likely to be confused with hydronephrosis. It is a fatty tumor that is highly echogenic.   *(2:345–368)*

156. **(D)** The common bile duct merges with the pancreatic duct just before entering the second portion of the duodenum.   *(1:275)*

157. **(A)** On a sagittal scan the portal vein is seen as a circular structure anterior to the inferior vena cava and superior to the head of the pancreas.   *(3:181)*

158. **(D)** All of the above. The prostate lies posterior to the symphysis pubis and inferior to the urinary bladder and seminal vesicles.   *(8:159)*

159. **(B)** Owing to the prostate's posterior position, one must angle the transducer approximately 15° caudad to best visualize the gland.   *(8:159)*

160. **(C)** If the prostate is found to be enlarged, one should check the kidneys for hydronephrosis.
(8:162)

161. **(B)** The laboratory findings suggest obstructive jaundice; therefore, one must check for a stone or mass obstructing the bile duct. *(3:134)*

162. **(D)** Acute prostatitis is an infection and would not be caused by trauma. *(10:90)*

163. **(A)** Adenocarcinoma of the prostate is the most common prostatic neoplasm. *(10:91)*

164. **(C)** A mirror-image artifact occurs with highly reflective acoustic interfaces, such as the diaphragm and adjacent lung. This results in a supradiaphragmatic projection of an infradiaphragmatic mass. This artifact is noticed quite regularly when liver echoes are seen superior to the diaphragm. *(12:29)*

165. **(A)** The normal sonographic texture of the spleen is less echogenic than the liver but more echogenic than the cortex of the kidney. *(8:108)*

166. **(B)** The spleen is the largest organ of the reticuloendothelial system. *(10:76)*

167. **(C)** The left kidney lies inferior and medial to the spleen. The diaphragm is anterior, lateral, and superior to the spleen, and the stomach and lesser sac are anterior. *(5:245)*

168. **(C)** Benign ascites is generally anechoic and is freely mobile within the peritoneal cavity. The bowel is seen anteriorly floating. *(2:272; 5:425)*

169. **(B)** Malignant ascites may have echoes or septations. Matted bowel loops posteriorly and peritoneal implants may be seen. *(2:273; 5:437)*

170. **(B)** The glomerulus is part of the kidney *not* the scrotum. The scrotum contains the testes, epididymis, ductus deferens, and a portion of the spermatic cord. *(3:246)*

171. **(B)** Hematocele is a condition in which blood occupies the scrotal sac surrounding the testes as a result of trauma or surgery. *(8:295)*

172. **(A)** A mass in the head of the pancreas with a dilated common bile duct is most suggestive of obstructive jaundice. *(1:258)*

173. **(B)** The epididymis is uniformly enlarged and more anechoic than usual owing to the inflammatory process. On a sagittal sonogram, it will appear as a nonechogenic tubular structure along the underside of the testicle. *(5:388)*

174. **(B)** Acute hydroceles are a result of trauma, infection of the testicle or epididymis, and tumor. They are *not* caused by testicular torsion. *(3:247)*

175. **(C)** Sonographically, the testicles have a homogeneous texture of medium-level echogenicity. *(3:248)*

176. **(F)** All of the above. Adenomas (a true solitary thyroid nodule), diffuse nontoxic goiter (a compensatory enlargement of the thyroid due to thyroid hormone deficiency), adenomatous hyperplasia (multinodular goiter, most common), thyroiditis (as a result of infection or autoimmune disease), and thyroglossal duct cysts are all benign lesions of the thyroid. *(3:241)*

177. **(A)** A cavernous hemangioma is the most common benign hepatic lesion and presents as an echogenic, well-circumscribed tumor. *(3:241)*

178. **(B)** Hyperthyroidism associated with a diffuse goiter is known as Graves' disease. *(3:241)*

179. **(C)** The thyroid gland consists of two lobes, right and left, connected by a narrow isthmus. The trachea is medial to the lobes, the longus colli muscle lies posteriorly, the carotid artery and internal jugular vein laterally, and the strap muscles anterolaterally. *(11:38)*

180. **(A)** When there is extrinsic pressure and obstruction of the common bile duct (i.e., a mass in the head of the pancreas), the gallbladder, common bile duct, and biliary tree will be enlarged. *(1:260)*

181. **(D)** The jugular veins are lateral, not posterior, to the thyroid lobes. *(5:458)*

182. **(A)** Since the thyroid is a superficial structure, a 5-MHz or higher short focus transducer is appropriate (the higher the frequency, the better the resolution and the poorer the penetration). *(8:275)*

183. **(D)** Prostatic carcinoma presents sonographically as an enlarged prostate with ill-defined borders of uneven echogenicity. *(5:588)*

184. **(D)** All of the above. Prostatic neoplasm and prostatic calculi present with an uneven echo texture. Benign prostatic hypertrophy is an overall enlargement of the gland and may present with a heterogeneous echo pattern. *(8:162)*

185. **(A)** The four parathyroid glands, two on each side, lie posterior to the thyroid lobes and medial to the common carotid arteries. *(8:275)*

186. **(E)** A parathyroid adenoma is a discrete mass. A goiter is a diffuse enlargement of the thyroid.
(8:280)

187. **(C)** The normal thyroid gland measures 1–2 cm in anteroposterior dimension and 4 to 6 cm in length.
(5:454)

188. **(B)** Thyroiditis will present sonographically as diffusely enlarged thyroid lobes with decreased echogenicity, similar to other organs involved with diffuse inflammatory changes. *(5:476)*

189. **(B)** Most thyroid masses demonstrating a halo are adenomas. *(8:279)*

190. **(D)** Invasive prostatic carcinoma enlarges in an uneven fashion, with irregular and nondiscrete borders. An elevation of acid phosphatase is highly suggestive of prostate cancer. *(5:588)*

191. **(A)** The spermatic cord is composed of the internal spermatic artery, veins that drain the testis, nerves, and the vas deferens. All of these are enclosed by the cremaster muscle and layers of fascia. *(3:246)*

192. **(B)** Varicocele is a varicose dilatation of the veins of the pampiniform plexus, the draining veins of the scrotum, and is associated with infertility. *(2:469)*

193. **(D)** In a hydrocele, the testicle and the appendix epididymis are surrounded by serous fluid, which will appear cystic on ultrasound. *(8:299)*

194. **(D)** A subphrenic abscess will displace the liver inferiorly *not* upward. *(3:127)*

195. **(A)** Budd-Chiari syndrome is caused by hepatic venous congestion. There is relative enlargement of the caudate lobe due to hepatic vein thrombosis. *(1:44)*

196. **(B)** The pyramidal lobe is a superior extension of thyroid tissue arising from the isthmus. *(8:274)*

197. **(E)** All of the above. Sonography of the urinary bladder is extremely valuable in the diagnosis of foreign bodies, masses, calculi, and diverticula. *(3:297)*

198. **(B)** Epididymitis will appear sonographically as a diffuse enlargement of the gland with decreased echogenicity (hypoechoic). *(5:276; 10:42)*

199. **(A)** A seminoma is a solid malignant mass of the testicles that will appear sonographically homogeneous and well circumscribed. *(10:43)*

200. **(B)** Crytorchidism is a condition in which the testicles have not descended and lie either in the abdomen or in the groin. *(8:295)*

201. **(C)** The seminal vesicles are the reservoir for sperm and are located posterior to the bladder. *(8:295)*

202. **(A)** Owing to the interrupted blood supply, the acute infarcted testicle will appear sonographically indistinguishable from a hypoechoic tumor and in its *chronic* stage it will appear small and echogenic. *(8:300)*

203. **(B)** The best way to distinguish hepatic veins from portal veins is by tracing them from their point of origin. Hepatic veins may be traced into the inferior vena cava, whereas the portal system arises from the main portal vein. *(3:129)*

204. **(C)** The fundus of the stomach lies posterolateral to the left lobe of the liver. The remainder of the stomach is located inferior to the liver. *(3:130)*

205. **(D)** Fatty infiltration may be due to cardiac failure, obesity, and more commonly alcoholic liver disease. It is the damage to the hepatocytes that cause accumulation of fat within the liver cells. Renal failure does *not* cause fatty infiltration. *(3:139)*

206. **(C)** α-Fetoprotein and carcinoembryonic antigen are biochemical markers that indicate liver metastases. *(8:57)*

207. **(E)** None of the above. Metastatic lesions in the liver have no specific sonographic appearance. Liver metastases are usually suspected clinically by a palpable liver mass, an enlarged liver, and/or a sudden onset of ascites. *(1:146)*

208. **(B)** A daughter cyst is a classic example of an echinococcal (hydatid) cyst. Hydatid disease is caused by a parasite that enters through the digestive tract and is carried to the liver by the portal system. *(8:66)*

209. **(C)** Reidel's lobe is a normal liver variant. This tonguelike extension of the right lobe of the liver lies anterior to the right kidney. It may clinically lead to a palpable liver descending below the costal margin. *(8:71)*

210. **(E)** Bilirubin, serum protein, prothrombin time, fetal antigen, and SGOT are lab tests that may be used for evaluation of the liver. Serum amylase is elevated in acute pancreatitis. *(10:15)*

211. **(A)** There is no sonographic diagnostic appearance for a liver abscess due to the spectrum of appearances it may have. An abscess is suspected when sonographically one finds a liver mass, and clinically when the patient has an elevated white blood cell count, right-upper quadrant pain, and is febrile. *(5:65)*

212. **(B)** A subphrenic abscess lies between the diaphragm and liver therefore depressing the liver away from the diaphragm. *(5:66)*

213. **(D)** All of the above. The normal portal vein measures up to 1.5 cm in luminal diameter. Its size can be affected by Valsalva maneuver, respiratory changes, and portal venous hypertension. *(5:78)*

214. **(D)** All of the above. Regenerative nodules can be distinguished from tumor masses by biopsy, angiography, and isotope scan. Enlarged portal vein, ascites, recanalized umbilical vein, and esophageal and splenic varices are associated findings. *(5:66)*

215. **(B)** The right crus of the diaphragm extends posterior to the inferior vena cava and posterior to the right kidney and adrenal gland. *(8:33)*

216. **(F)** All but the pancreas. Structures that commonly alter the liver shape are the diaphragm, right kidney, abdominal lymph nodes, and the gallbladder. *(1:54)*

217. **(D)** Lymphoma (Hodgkin's and non-Hodgkin's) can appear sonographically as focal lesions, both anechoic and echogenic. *(2:103)*

218. **(D)** All of the above. The function of lymph vessels is to absorb lymph that has filtered out of the blood capillaries. If the lymph vessel is obstructed, it may lead to edema, ascites, or an effusion of the affected location. *(2:208)*

219. **(B)** Normal lymph nodes are no larger than 1 cm. Sonographically, to be visualized they must be larger than 3 cm. *(10:84)*

220. **(F)** All of the above. The lymph nodes are closely related to the aorta and form a preaortic and a right and left lateral aortic (para-aortic) chain. Therefore, when scanning a patient for lymphadenopathy, one should check the pelvis, porta hepatis, retroperitoneum, perirenal area, and around the major blood vessels and their tributaries. *(10:84)*

221. **(C)** Para-aortic nodes have characteristic sonographic appearances. They can be differentiated from an aortic aneurysm by shape. Aneurysms enlarge fairly symmetrically, whereas large nodes tend to drape over prevertebral vessels in lobular fashion. *(10:86)*

222. **(D)** Sonographically, for lymph nodes to be visualized they must be enlarged up to at least 3 cm. *(10:86)*

223. **(C)** Sonographically, enlarged nodes appear as anechoic masses with no demonstration of through transmission on account of its composition. *(5:368)*

224. **(C)** Enlarged lymph nodes being closely related to the aorta and forming preaortic and para-aortic nodes may displace the inferior vena cava anteriorly. The spleen, pancreas, and kidneys are situated anterior to lymph nodes, therefore these organs could not be displaced anteriorly. *(5:368)*

225. **(A)** The right adrenal gland lies directly anterior to the crus of the diaphragm. Both are posterior to the inferior vena cava and may be confused with one another. *(5:336)*

226. **(B)** To optimally scan the right adrenal gland, one should position the patient in the left lateral decubitus position (right side up) because of the adrenal gland's location between the right lobe of the liver and the crus of the diaphragm. *(3:216)*

227. **(D)** The functions of the spleen include the production of plasma cells, lymphocytes and antibodies, storage of iron, and breakdown of red blood cells. *(10:75)*

228. **(E)** All of the above. Splenomegaly occurs in a vast range of infectious diseases. Infective endocarditis, tuberculosis, syphilis, and schistomiasis are only a few infectious diseases that cause splenomegaly. *(10:76)*

229. **(B)** The right renal artery can be seen as a pulsatile circular structure posterior to the inferior vena cava on a longitudinal scan. *(3:120)*

230. **(D)** Virtually all gallstones demonstrate an acoustic shadow. Biliary sludge and sludge balls are mobile and do not demonstrate an acoustic shadow. *(2:136)*

231. **(A)** Splenic cysts are rare. Care must be taken not to confuse them with a pseudocyst or renal cyst. *(10:79)*

232. **(A)** Metastases to the spleen occur more frequently with breast carcinoma. *(10:79)*

233. **(B)** Metastases of the spleen is a late sign of a carcinoma. It only appears once the primary lesion has disseminated widely. *(10:79)*

234. **(D)** A spleen with overall decreased echogenicity is seen with lymphopoiesis, multiple myeloma, and congestion. Metastasis to the spleen will not effect its overall appearance, but will appear as a mass of lesions. *(10:81)*

235. **(B)** The most common cause of splenomegaly in the United States is portal hypertension. The spleen will appear to have an overall decrease in echogenicity owing to congestion.   *(2:234)*

236. **(A)** The retroperitoneal space is the area between the posterior portion of the parietal peritoneum and the posterior abdominal wall muscles.   *(3:231)*

237. **(B)** When assessing the upper retroperitoneum, ie, para-aortic lymph nodes, it is best visualized with the patient in the supine position. This is because of the location of such nodes along the lateral and anterior margins of the aorta.   *(3:231)*

238. **(B)** Primary tumors of the retroperitoneum are generally malignant. They can be cystic, solid, or complex depending upon their physical composition.   *(3:237)*

239. **(E)** All of the above. A urinoma is a collection of urine located outside the genitourinary tract. Urinomas are known to develop after urinary tract surgery, trauma, or subacute or chronic urinary obstruction.   *(3:237)*

240. **(B)** The etiology of retroperitoneal fibrosis is unknown. It is not an invasion of the body by pathogenic organisms (infections) or carried by the blood or physician induced (iatrogenic).   *(3:238)*

241. **(A)** If retroperitoneal fibrosis is suspected, one should also check the kidneys for hydronephrosis because it may encase the ureters and thereby obstruct them.   *(3:120)*

242. **(B)** The renal arteries are best seen on a transverse sonogram.   *(3:120)*

243. **(B)** The right, middle, and left hepatic veins originate in the liver and drain into the inferior vena cava at the level of the diaphragm. They are the largest major visceral branch of the inferior vena cava.   *(3:116)*

244. **(B)** The spleen is variable in size but is considered to be convex superiorly and concave inferiorly. When the spleen enlarges, it extends inferiorly and medially in an anterior position.   *(3:221)*

245. **(C)** Accessory spleens are a common congenital anomaly and are usually located near the splenic hilum.   *(3:221)*

246. **(D)** Sickle-cell anemia results in splenic atrophy. In its advanced stages, the spleen becomes small because of "autosplenectomy" from repeated infarcts.   *(3:222)*

247. **(D)** The most common benign tumor of the spleen is a cavernous hemangioma.   *(3:224)*

248. **(A)** Splenic size is variable with 14 cm in length being upper-normal. When the spleen enlarges, it does so inferomedially in an anterior position.   *(1:331)*

249. **(D)** The superior mesenteric artery will appear as a round sonolucent dot surrounded by an echogenic ring.   *(8:51)*

250. **(C)** Alkaline phosphatase is synthesized and excreted by hepatocytes. With obstruction, metastatic involvement and infiltrative disease, one sees a sharp rise in the production and synthesis of this enzyme. SGOT and SGPT are specific as indicators of hepatic function (hepatocellular disease).   *(3:133)*

251. **(D)** If it is located in the posterior pararenal space, a hematoma will extend up the lateral walls of the abdomen and displace the kidney anteriorly.   *(8:172)*

252. **(D)** All of the above. Solid masses tend to displace surrounding organs therefore indicating its place of origin. A retroperitoneal sarcoma will displace the kidney, pancreas, and spleen anteriorly.   *(8:110)*

253. **(C)** A hypertrophied column of Bertin is a normal renal variant in which there is hypertrophy (enlargement) of the cortex between two pyramids. It will appear sonographically as normal renal tissue.   *(8:133)*

254. **(D)** If a patient presents with hydronephrosis, one should look for the cause of the obstruction. This may include renal calculus, pelvic masses, prostatic hypertrophy, fibroid uterus, and ureteroceles. Renal vein thrombosis is *not* associated with hydronephrosis.   *(8:143)*

255. **(E)** All of the above. An angiomyolipoma is a rare benign renal tumor usually seen in middle-aged women. It is composed of mostly fat and can be associated with tuberous sclerosis.   *(8:145)*

256. **(D)** Hypernephroma is a malignant solid renal tumor also known as renal cell carcinoma, von Grawitz tumor, and adenocarcinoma of the kidney but *not* transitional cell carcinoma.   *(8:145)*

257. **(D)** Malrotated kidneys, enlarged spleen or liver compressing the kidneys, and the presence of a dromedary hump will cause a false-positive abnormal intravenous pyelogram. Renal vein thrombosis will lead to nonvisualization of the affected kidney and is a true abnormality.   *(8:150)*

258. **(D)** All of the above. Solid renal masses are considered malignant until proven otherwise. Therefore, one should also check for para-aortic nodes, liver metastases, and tumor invasion of the inferior vena cava.   *(8:153)*

259. **(A)** The most common cause of unilateral nonvisualization of a kidney on intravenous pyelography is hydronephrosis.   *(8:155)*

260. **(E)** All of the above. Renal vein thrombosis, renal artery occlusion, pyonephrosis, and end-stage renal disease will all lead to nonvisualization of the kidneys on intravenous pyelography. Other causes include hydronephrosis, a tumor large enough to involve the entire kidney, tumor obstructing the renal vein, multicystic kidney, and xanthogranulomatous pyelonephritis.   *(8:155)*

261. **(B)** A pelvic kidney is a normal kidney in size and shape but is located in an abnormal position. *(8:151)*

262. **(F)** Ascites is free fluid located within the peritoneal cavity. It can be caused by malignancy, nephrotic syndrome, congestive heart failure, tuberculosis, and/or liver disease but not adenomyomatosis.   *(8:120)*

263. **(D)** Loculations within ascites are more commonly found in malignancies and infections. Benign ascites tend to have no internal echoes or loculations.   *(8:130)*

264. **(D)** Internal echoes within ascites are most commonly found in malignancies and infections. Benign ascites tend to be anechoic with no internal debris.   *(8:130)*

265. **(A)** Acute pancreatitis may lead to pancreatic pseudocyst, pancreatic ascites, common bile duct obstruction, and/or chronic pancreatitis but not gallstones.   *(8:48)*

266. **(F)** All of the above. Pancreatic pseudocysts may be found in the liver, spleen, mediastinum, mesentary, and lesser sac. Owing to its composition of enzymes, pseudocysts are capable of tracking anywhere in the body.   *(8:48)*

267. **(A)** To best visualize the pancreatic tail, one should position the patient in prone position, using the left kidney as an acoustic window.   *(2:175)*

268. **(C)** The splenic artery may be confused with the pancreatic duct. In order to differentiate between the two, remember that the splenic artery pulsates and the pancreatic duct does not.   *(8:56)*

269. **(C)** The splenic artery courses along the superior margin of the pancreatic body and tail.   *(8:50)*

270. **(B)** The right kidney lies slightly lower than the left because the right lobe of the liver occupies more of the right upper quadrant.   *(3:192)*

271. **(E)** Signs of renal disease include oliguria, polyuria, palpable flank mass, generalized edema, pain, fever, and urgency but not Murphy's sign.   *(3:194)*

272. **(F)** Over 60% of functioning renal parenchyma must be lost in order to elevate either the blood urea nitrogen (BUN) or creatinine. Since the kidneys have a significant reserve, an elevation of these laboratory values shows an already severely impaired kidney.   *(3:194)*

273. **(C)** A supernumerary kidney is a complete duplication of the renal system. It is rare and generally found in the pelvis.   *(3:197)*

274. **(D)** All of the above. To best evaluate the internal composition of a cyst, one should change the gain setting, overall power, and/or transducer to a higher frequency. All of these will lead to better resolution of the cyst.   *(3:199)*

275. **(D)** Clinical symptoms associated with inflammatory renal masses include fever, chills, and flank pain but not hypoglycemia.   *(3:204)*

276. **(B)** Sonographically, the best way of delineating a dissecting aneurysm is by showing the intimal flap waving along with the pulsations of blood through the aorta.   *(2:55)*

277. **(D)** Lesions that produce complex echo patterns include infected cysts, hemorrhagic cysts, hematomas, and abscesses but not congenital cysts. Correlating the sonographic appearance with the clinical history may help to differentiate the pathology.   *(2:327)*

278. **(A)** The abdominal aorta courses anteriorly, whereas the inferior vena cava has a horizontal course. The aorta is to the left of the inferior vena cava and is not affected by Valsalva maneuvers.   *(8:35)*

279. **(B)** With advanced chronological age, the pancreas decreases in size with increased echogenicity.   *(1:278)*

280. **(D)** The lesser sac is located anterior and superior to the pancreas and the greater sac is located anterior and inferior to the pancreas. The origin of the transverse mesocolon is the dividing line.   *(1:275)*

281. **(B)** The pancreas in children will be relatively less echogenic. With increasing age and body fat deposition, there are increased amounts of fat within the parenchyma of the pancreas, accounting for an increase in its echogenicity.   *(1:278)*

282. **(D)** A series of relative echogenicity has been established. It is from least echogenic to most, renal parenchyma < liver < spleen < pancreas < renal sinus. *(2:165)*

283. **(D)** All of the above. Several landmarks can be helpful in identifying the pancreatic head on a longitudinal scan. The pancreatic head is visualized directly anterior to the inferior vena cava, caudad to the portal vein, and cephalad to the duodenum. *(2:167)*

284. **(B)** The sonographic appearance of lymphoma has been known to vary but it is most commonly seen as a solid mass that is relatively hypoechoic and has some decrease of through transmission with an increase in ultrasound absorption. *(2:179)*

285. **(D)** Islet cell tumors of the pancreas are well-circumscribed solid masses with low-level echoes and are frequently found in the body and tail and rarely in the head of the gland. *(2:179)*

286. **(B)** The normal right adrenal gland is located superior to the right kidney and medial to the liver, posterior to the inferior vena cava, and anterior to the crus of the diaphragm. *(5:338)*

287. **(A)** Addison's disease is a syndrome that results from chronic adrenal hypofunction. The decrease in function may be due to a primary adrenal tumor or secondary to metastases. *(3:218)*

288. **(A)** Anatomical landmarks helpful in locating the left adrenal gland are the aorta, spleen, left kidney, and left crus of the diaphragm. *(5:340)*

289. **(D)** All of the above. Adrenal hemorrhage sonographically may appear either echogenic, anechoic, or complex depending upon the stage of clot organization. *(5:272)*

290. **(D)** All of the above. The spiral valves of Heister are located within the cystic duct. They are very tortuous and may simulate a polypoid tumor or cause shadowing simulating a stone. Note that there is no valvular action by the spiral valves of Heister. Bile flow is dependent upon the pressure gradient between the gallbladder and cystic duct. *(1:226)*

291. **(A)** The right adrenal gland is located superior and anteromedial to the upper pole of the right kidney. Anatomic landmarks include the liver, inferior vena cava, and right crus of diaphragm. *(5:271)*

292. **(C)** A pheochromocytoma is an adrenal tumor that secretes hormones that in turn elevate blood pressure. *(8:265)*

293. **(C)** Left adrenal hyperplasia, for whatever reason, may cause anterior displacement of the splenic vein and posterolateral displacement of the left kidney. *(8:271)*

294. **(B)** Cushing's syndrome may be associated with an adrenal mass or be caused by a mass in the anterior pituitary. The syndrome is characterized by an increase in androgen production, hypertension, truncal obesity, and a moon-shaped face. *(3:218)*

295. **(A)** The celiac axis has three branches, the common hepatic artery, left gastric artery, and splenic artery. Sonographically, only a short section of the splenic artery can be seen owing to its tortuous course. *(1:66)*

296. **(B)** A phrygian cap is a fold near the fundus of the gallbladder. If a fold is visualized near the neck of the gallbladder, it is termed Hartmann's pouch. *(2:132)*

297. **(A)** Gallbladder polyps can be distinguished from stones by the absence of shadowing or movement. *(1:255)*

298. **(E)** Long-standing cystic duct obstruction and prolonged fasting will cause the gallbladder to retain sludge. Other examples of echogenic bile within the gallbladder may be due to hemobilia and empyema of the gallbladder. *(2:146)*

299. **(B)** The celiac axis is cephalad to the superior mesenteric artery. *(3:120)*

300. **(A)** Blood that is returning from the kidneys via the renal veins to the inferior vena cava accounts for this enlargement. *(3:116)*

301. **(B)** 2, 1, 4, 3. The biliary tree generally dilates in a routine fashion when obstructed. First the common bile duct will dilate (larger than 5 mm in luminal dimension). This is followed by dilatation of intrahepatic ducts. Next, one can see the double-barrel shotgun sign and with increased obstruction, the biliary tree continues to dilate in a stellate formation. *(1:260)*

302. **(C)** The most common cause of jaundice in the pediatric patient is biliary atresia, a narrowing and obstruction of the intrahepatic bile duct. *(8:87)*

303. **(B)** Right decubitus, left coronal, or left side up view indicates that the right side of the patient is on the table and the left side is up. *(8:31)*

304. **(A)** Large gallbladders are detected in patients with diabetes, prolonged fasting, status-postvagotomy,

or the use of anticholinergic drugs and other causes. *(3:152)*

305. **(A)** Empyema of the gallbladder is a complication of acute cholecystitis, whereby purulent exudate fills the cavity. Since the gallbladder contains gas due to the bacteria in the exudate, posterior shadowing will be noted, but it will not be a "clean" shadow. *(1:252)*

306. **(A)** SGOT, SGPT, LDH, and alkaline phosphatase are all liver enzymes released from damaged hepatic cells. SGOT, SGPT, and LDH tend to be higher with intrinsic liver disease, whereas alkaline phosphatase levels tend to be higher with biliary obstruction. *(8:87)*

307. **(D)** Three mechanisms of jaundice are red blood cell destruction, hepatocellular disease, and obstruction of intra- or extrahepatic ducts. Red blood cell destruction occurs with hemolytic anemias. Hepatocellular disease is most commonly due to alcoholic liver disease. Obstruction of intra- or extrahepatic ducts is most commonly caused by cholelithiasis, choledocholithiasis, pancreatic tumors, and/or ductal tumors. *(8:88)*

308. **(C)** Acute cholecystitis is characterized by an edematous wall (the halo sign) greater than 3 mm, acute pain over the gallbladder (Murphy's sign), and/or a stone impacted within the cystic duct. *(1:248)*

309. **(A)** α-Fetoprotein and carcinoembryonic antigen (CEA) are laboratory values that are elevated in hepatoma of the liver. *(2:116)*

310. **(B)** Enlarged lymph nodes will usually appear sonographically as a homogeneous anechoic mass with poor through transmission. *(3:232)*

311. **(B)** Periaortic nodes will displace the superior mesenteric artery anteriorly *not* posteriorly. *(3:237)*

312. **(C)** Examples of primary retroperitoneal tumors seen on sonography are leiomyosarcomas, neurogenic tumors, fibrosarcomas, rhabdomyosarcomas, and teratomatous tumors. *(3:237)*

313. **(E)** All of the above. Retroperitoneal fluid collections include urinoma, lymphocele, abscess, and hemorrhage. To help to distinguish among them, their sonographic appearance and clinical correlation are necessary. *(3:238)*

314. **(D)** The parallel channel sign, irregular borders to dilated ducts, and echo enhancement behind dilated ducts are all characteristic of dilated intrahepatic bile ducts. It is the common bile duct near the porta hepatis that is the first to dilate and is greatest in size. *(1:260)*

315. **(A)** The superior mesenteric artery can be seen on transverse scans as an anechoic circle with an echogenic wall posterior to the body of the pancreas. *(3:120)*

316. **(C)** The ligamentum venosum is a remnant of the fetal ductus venosus and the ligamentum teres is a remnant of the fetal umbilical vein. The coronary ligaments define the bare area of the liver. *(1:30)*

317. **(B)** A subhepatic abscess would be located inferior to the liver and anterior to the right kidney. Other common sites for abscesses are subphrenic, perinephric, intrarenal, intrahepatic, pelvic, and around incisions. *(3:141)*

318. **(D)** The primary malignant tumor of the liver is a hepatoma. Another name for a hepatoma is hepatocellular carcinoma. Eighty percent of hepatomas occur in livers with preexisting cirrhosis. *(1:146)*

319. **(B)** The ultrasound instrument assumes that the speed of sound in all tissues in its path is 1540 m/s. The speed of sound through bone is greater than that in the average soft tissue. This is what causes the registration error of the reflector to appear closer to the transducer than its actual distance. *(3:58)*

320. **(A)** All ultrasound equipment is calibrated at 1540 m/s, the speed of sound in soft tissue. When the ultrasound beam goes through a fatty tumor with a lower propagation speed, the tumor will appear *further* than its actual distance. *(3:58)*

321. **(B)** When ascites is present it acts as an acoustic window. Therefore, the liver will appear more echogenic. *(2:83)*

322. **(C)** As one *decreases* the frequency of the transducer, one *decreases* the resolution but *increases* the depth of penetration. With an obese patient, depth of penetration is important, especially if a mass is suspected deep in the posterior aspect of the right lobe of the liver; therefore one should use a 2.25-MHz long-focused transducer. *(8:6)*

323. **(E)** Reye's syndrome typically occurs in childhood and is associated with fatty changes in the liver and encephalopathy. Jaundice is *not* associated with this disease. *(4:438)*

324. **(B)** The three branches of the celiac artery are the common hepatic, left gastric, and splenic arteries. *(2:38)*

325. **(A)** The gastroduodenal artery is a major branch of the common hepatic artery. *(2:38)*

326. (C) The splenic artery originates from the celiac axis and runs superior to the body and tail of the pancreas throughout most of its course.   *(8:35)*

327. (C) Artifacts that cause spurious echoes result from a variety of sources including beam thickness and side-lobe artifacts, reverberation artifacts, electronic noise, and range ambiguity effects. Edge effects cause acoustic shadowing owing to reflection and refraction of sound.   *(14:31–37)*

328. (B) Irregularities of flow within a vessel greatly increase the likelihood of clot formation and thrombus.   *(2:48)*

329. (C) Doppler sampling across a vessel is utilized to detect irregularity of blood flow.   *(2:48)*

330. (C) Hepatic hemangiomas are least likely to be echo-free structures with smooth walls. They generally appear echogenic and may present as solitary or multiple lesions. Sonographically, they cannot be distinguished from a hepatoma.   *(10:17)*

331. (C) The sonographic appearance of an abscess has a variable echo texture from echo free to echogenic, with irregular borders, and varied through transmission. The sonographic appearance of an abscess is dependent upon the stage and age of the abscess.   *(2:250)*

332. (D) All of the above. Patients with portal hypertension may have a portal vein greater than 11 ± 2 mm in luminal dimension, splenomegaly, portal venous collaterals, and a patent umbilical vein.   *(2:66)*

333. (D) All of the above. Three main sites of potential anastomoses within the systemic circulation seen with ultrasound include the left umbilical vein, lienorenal anastomoses, and anastomoses around the esophagus. The most clinically significant anastomosis is esophageal varices.   *(1:218)*

334. (C) In response to the pressure changes associated with portal hypertension, the umbilical vein located within the ligamentum teres recanalizes.   *(1:221)*

335. (C) The para-aortic group is the major node-bearing region in the upper retroperitoneum. The major node-bearing regions in the pelvis are the iliac and hypogastric nodes.   *(3:231)*

336. (D) Acute torsion of the spermatic cord, whereby the arterial blood supply to the testis is disrupted, has no specific sonographic characteristics. Therefore, ultrasound is not used as the primary method of diagnosis.   *(2:474; 3:247)*

337. (B) Lymphocytes may be confused with an aortic aneurysm, the crus of the diaphragm, and bowel, because they are generally echo free, whereas chronic pancreatitis is echogenic.   *(3:232)*

338. (A) Sonographic evaluation of the breast is certainly helpful in those patients who are concerned about being exposed to irradiation. More specifically, sonography is helpful in evaluating those masses thought to be cystic in patients who have radiographically dense breasts. The radiographic appearance of these breasts occasionally impairs detection of surrounding breast masses. Cysts represent 25% of palpable and/or mammographically detected masses. Ultrasound can detect cysts as small as 2 mm. The detection of microcalcifications associated with invasive ductal carcinoma cannot be ruled out by ultrasound. One must remember that the detection of an exact "type" of tumor can only be determined by a histologic diagnosis.   *(3:268–269)*

339. (D) The superior mesenteric vein is larger, not smaller, in caliber than the superior mesenteric artery.   *(8:50)*

340. (C) An aortic aneurysm of 6 cm or greater is considered a surgical emergency. At 7 cm, 60–80% are said to rupture.   *(2:52)*

341. (D) The celiac trunk originates within the first 2 cm of the abdominal aorta; therefore, it is not found posterior to the pancreas.   *(2:38; 3:118)*

342. (B) Landmarks for the uncinate process are the superior mesenteric vein anteriorly and the inferior vena cava posteriorly.   *(2:163)*

343. (C) Amylase and lipase levels rise at the same rate, but lipase levels remain higher for a longer period of time. Amylase becomes elevated for many other reasons than acute pancreatitis; therefore, lipase is more consistent with, but not specific for, acute pancreatitis.   *(10:45)*

344. (D) Alcoholism and surgical and external trauma can all lead to acute hemorrhagic pancreatitis. Cystic fibrosis is the most common childhood congenital disease causing the pancreatic tissue to fibrose with ductal enlargement.   *(10:47)*

345. (B) A reverberation artifact results from a strong echo returning from a large acoustic interface to the transducer. This artifact appears in both cystic and solid masses and is not specific for delineating cystic structures.   *(8:29)*

346. **(C)** Pancreatic tail masses lie superior to the kidney and displace the spleen anteriorly.   *(8:110)*

347. **(C)** If the spleen is as thick as the normal kidney or thicker, and its anterior border crosses the aorta and inferior vena cava, it is considered to be enlarged.   *(8:109)*

348. **(B)** A pheochromocytoma is a benign adrenal tumor that secretes epinephrine and norepinephrine. These two hormones are responsible for the clinical symptom of intermittent hypertension associated with a pheochromocytoma.   *(3:218; 8:265)*

349. **(D)** All of the above. Common sites of lymphadenopathy include all of the listed possible answers. Other common sites include the left renal hilum and the porta hepatis.   *(8:104)*

350. **(D)** All of the above are consistent with renal failure. Sonographic appearance of the kidneys depends upon the stage of renal failure (acute or chronic) the patient is in. Acutely, the kidneys are normal-sized or enlarged. Chronically, they are small. Hydronephrosis may be the sole cause of the renal failure.   *(2:351; 8:133)*

351. **(A)** Optimal imaging of the left adrenal gland is achieved by the specific alignment of the left kidney to the aorta.   *(2:376)*

352. **(C)** Both adrenal glands are located superior and anteromedial to the upper pole of their respective kidney.   *(2:397; 8:267)*

353. **(D)** The right adrenal gland is located directly posterior to the inferior vena cava and anterior to the right crus of the diaphragm.   *(2:397; 8:267)*

354. **(C)** A neuroblastoma is a relatively common malignant adrenal tumor seen in children. Sonographically, it appears as an echogenic mass.   *(2:399)*

355. **(B)** The adrenal gland can be divided into cortex and medulla. The cortex secretes mineralocorticoids. The medulla secretes epinephrine and norepinephrine.   *(3:215)*

356. **(B)** Above the level of the celiac axis the diaphragm can be visualized posterior to the inferior vena cava and anterior to the aorta.   *(8:43)*

357. **(A)** The left hepatic vein separates the medial and lateral aspects of the left lobe of the liver.   *(8:42)*

358. **(C)** A patent umbilical vein may be found in the ligamentum teres and is associated with portal hypertension.   *(8:43)*

359. **(C)** Ampullary carcinoma is found within the ampulla of Vater, which is where the pancreatic duct and common bile duct enter the duodenum. The carcinoma will obstruct the pancreatic duct, leading to its dilatation, and obstruct the common bile duct, leading to its dilatation and progressive dilatation of the intrahepatic ducts.   *(5:222)*

360. **(B)** The right hepatic vein separates the anterior and posterior segments of the right lobe.   *(3:130)*

361. **(B)** A dissecting aneurysm is a hemorrhage into the aorta itself. The dissection is generally through the media of the aorta.   *(4:290)*

362. **(E)** Phlebitis is an inflammation of the veins and therefore, is not a type of aortic aneurysm.   *(4:290–293)*

363. **(D)** The minimum anterior-posterior diameter for the diagnosis of aortic aneurysm is above 3 cm.   *(2:47)*

364. **(C)** The most common type of arteriosclerotic, aortic aneurysm is fusiform. Generally, it arises below the origin of the renal arteries and may continue down into the iliac vessels.   *(2:47)*

365. **(C)** The crus of the diaphragm is visualized sonographically as an echo-poor linear structure. It runs anterior above the level of the celiac axis. Below that level, it extends along the lateral aspect of the vertebral column.   *(1:65)*

366. **(B)** A mass in the caudate lobe of the liver and head of the pancreas would displace the inferior vena cava posteriorly. The right renal vein lies lateral to the inferior vena cava. The right renal artery lies posteriorly and can cause anterior displacement with pathology.   *(3:120)*

367. **(C)** Dilatation of the inferior vena cava can be seen with right ventricular heart failure. The Valsalva maneuver will increase the size of the inferior vena cava but is not a pathologic condition.   *(7:112)*

368. **(D)** Acid phosphatase is usually increased in patients with carcinoma of the prostate gland, particularly when metastases are present.   *(4:385)*

369. **(C)** Thrombus will be visualized as echoes within the aorta but they are not artifactual.   *(3:118)*

370. **(A)** The gastroduodenal artery arises from the common hepatic artery and supplies the duodenum, parts of the stomach, and the head of the pancreas. Sonographically, it can be visualized as a circular anechoic structure located in the anterior portion of the head of the pancreas.   *(3:120)*

371. **(E)** Fatty infiltration of the liver usually causes a diffuse hyperechoic pattern not a focal mass. *(3:139)*

372. **(C)** Ascites, small liver portal hypertension, and irregular liver borders due to liver nodules may all be present with end-stage fatty liver as well as severe cirrhosis. The bile ducts do not dilate because of the fibrosis. *(3:139)*

373. **(A)** The head of the pancreas is located anterior to the inferior vena cava. *(3:181)*

374. **(B)** The lesser sac is located between the stomach and pancreas. *(3:78)*

375. **(A)** In biliary obstruction, the increase in direct bilirubin predominates, although the indirect bilirubin may also rise slightly. *(3:192)*

376. **(B)** The pyramids are located in the medulla of the kidney. *(3:192)*

377. **(D)** All of the above. The function of the kidneys is to excrete urine. Urine formation includes filtration in the glomeruli, tubular reabsorption, and tubular secretion, respectively. *(3:194)*

378. **(C)** Major calices of the kidney converge to form the renal pelvis located in the hilum of the kidney. The ureter emerges from the hilum and travels down to the urinary bladder entering it in its trigone. Urine is then stored in the bladder until it passes out of the body via the urethra. *(3:192)*

379. **(B)** Bowman's capsule and glomerulus together are termed the renal corpuscle or malpighian body. Extending from Bowman's capsule is a renal tubule. Each tubule has three sections: a proximal tubule, a descending limb, and an ascending limb. Together the Bowman's capsule, glomerulus, and renal tubules constitute a nephron. *(3:194)*

380. **(C)** A rise in lipase levels indicates acute pancreatitis or pancreatic carcinoma. Amylase levels will also rise with acute pancreatitis but are not as specific for this as the rise in lipase levels. *(3:176)*

381. **(B)** In hemolytic disease associated with abrupt breakdown of large amounts of red blood cells, the reticuloendothelial cells receive more bilirubin than it can detoxify. Therefore, one would present with an elevated indirect or unconjugated bilirubin. *(3:134)*

382. **(B)** With biliary obstruction at any level in the biliary tree, the direct bilirubin levels rise predominantly and the indirect bilirubin levels rise only slightly. *(3:134)*

383. **(C)** A dromedary hump is a common anatomical variant. It is visualized as a bulge off the lateral border of the left kidney consisting of normal renal tissue. *(3:134)*

384. **(D)** The most common intrascrotal inflammation is epididymitis. Acutely, the epididymis becomes enlarged and less echogenic. Chronically, the epididymis becomes very echogenic and may contain calcium. *(3:248)*

385. **(C)** The head of the epididymis is located superior to the testes. The rest of the epididymis courses along the posterior margin of the testicle inferiorly. *(2:461)*

386. **(A)** The sonographic diagnosis of ductal obstruction should be dependent upon the luminal diameter of the common bile duct at or below the porta hepatis. *(1:260)*

387. **(B)** The left kidney is located posterior to the spleen. *(10:74)*

388. **(A)** The stomach is located anterior to the spleen. *(10:74)*

389. **(B)** If a testicular tumor is found, one should also check the renal hilum for possible nodal metastases. Testicular tumors will not cause hydronephrosis or ascites. *(8:300)*

390. **(C)** The average dimensions of the testes are 4–5 cm long and 2.5–3 cm wide. Enlargement or atrophy is a sign of a pathological process. *(3:247)*

391. **(C)** The testes produce spermatozoa that travel via the spermatic cord; therefore, the testes are considered exocrine glands. They also are considered endocrine glands because they produce testosterone, a male sex hormone. *(3:246)*

392. **(A)** A hepatoblastoma is a primary malignant liver tumor found in childhood. Wilms' tumor is a childhood tumor found in the kidney. Neuroblastoma is the most common tumor of infancy and is adrenal in origin. *(3:143, 220, 320)*

393. **(A)** Hydroceles can be defined as serous fluid accumulated between the two layers of the tunica vaginalis. Sonographically, the testicle and epididymis are visualized surrounded by anechoic fluid. *(3:247)*

394. **(D)** Testicular malignancy usually affects men between 20 and 40 years of age. The most common type of testicular malignancy is a seminoma. Other types include embryonal carcinoma, choriocarcinoma, and teratomas. *(3:247)*

395. **(C)** A neoplasm is any new growth or development of abnormal tissue. The best way to know if a neoplasm is benign or malignant is to biopsy it. *(3:143)*

396. **(E)** Inferior vena cava.

397. **(D)** Right lobe.

398. **(A)** Gallbladder.

399. **(G)** Portal vein.

400. **(B)** Left lobe.

401. **(C)** Falciform ligament.

402. **(F)** Ligamentum teres.

403. **(H)** Hepatic artery.

404. **(D)** Right lobe.

405. **(A)** Gallbladder.

406. **(L)** Quadrate lobe (medial aspect of the left lobe).

407. **(E)** Inferior vena cava.

408. **(K)** Caudate lobe.

409. **(J)** Common bile duct.

410. **(B)** Left lobe.

411. **(C)** Falciform ligament.

412. **(I)** Fissure for ligamentum venosum.

413. **(H)** Hepatic artery.

414. **(F)** Ligamentum teres.

415. **(G)** Portal vein.

416. **(F)** Left hepatic duct.

417. **(E)** Common hepatic duct.

418. **(A)** Cystic duct.

419. **(K)** Common bile duct.

420. **(C)** Duodenum.

421. **(B)** Ampulla of Vater.

422. **(D)** Fundus of the gallbladder.

423. **(J)** Infundibulum of the gallbladder (Hartmann's pouch).

424. **(I)** Neck of the gallbladder.

425. **(H)** Right hepatic duct.

426. **(G)** Body of the gallbladder.

427. **(D)** Renal artery.

428. **(G)** Renal vein.

429. **(E)** Ureter.

430. **(H)** Pyramid.

431. **(F)** Renal pelvis.

432. **(C)** Renal capsule.

433. **(I)** Cortex.

434. **(B)** Minor calyx.

435. **(A)** Renal papilla.
(3:149,150,175,193,for answers 396–435)

436. **(F)** Right hepatic vein.

437. **(H)** Inferior vena cava.

438. **(L)** Right renal artery.

439. **(I)** Right renal vein.

440. **(E)** Celiac trunk.

441. **(G)** Left hepatic vein.

442. **(M)** Right portal vein.

443. **(N)** Splenic artery.

444. **(A)** Superior mesenteric artery.

445. **(Q)** Inferior mesenteric vein.

446. **(J)** Left renal artery.

447. **(K)** Left renal vein.

448. **(C)** Aorta.

449. **(P)** Left portal vein.

450. **(O)** Gastroduodenal artery.

451. (U) Left gastric artery.

452. (D) Middle hepatic vein.

453. (B) Splenic vein.

454. (R) Common hepatic artery.

455. (T) Superior mesenteric vein.

456. (S) Main portal vein.   *(3:113,177, for answers 436–456)*

457. (F) Strap muscle.

458. (H) Sternocleidomastoid muscle.

459. (E) Thyroid gland.

460. (J) Longus colli muscle.

461. (A) Vertebral body.

462. (G) Esophagus.

463. (C) Common carotid artery.

464. (D) Internal jugular vein.

465. (B) Trachea.

466. (I) Parathyroid gland.   *(3:240, for answers 457–466)*

467. (C) Epididymis body.

468. (E) Epididymis tail.

469. (A) Testis.

470. (G) Seminiferous tubules.

471. (D) Septula.

472. (B) Rete testis.

473. (F) Epididymis head.   *(3:246, for answers 467–473)*

474. (A) Renal vein thrombosis may be a cause of renal failure. In *acute* renal vein thrombosis, the kidney becomes edematous *not* hydronephrotic. Sonographically, there is decreased cortical echogenicity and an increase in renal size. Later, there is increased echogenicity due to cellular infiltration.
(2:373; 11:38)

475. (B) A long history of alcoholism implies cirrhosis with accompanying massive ascites.   *(8:120)*

476. (B) High fever is an indication of an abscess. An abscess will sonographically appear as a complex mass.   *(2:327)*

477. (B) SGOT and SGPT are enzymes that are released from damaged liver cells. High levels can be seen in an obstructive process but more commonly indicate intrinsic liver disease. Viral and toxic hepatitis are diseases intrinsic to the liver and will therefore lead to elevated levels of SGOT and SGPT.   *(8:87)*

478. (D) Marked elevation of alkaline phosphatase is typically associated with biliary obstruction. Other liver enzymes will also rise but not in the same proportion.   *(8:87)*

479. (C) A multicystic (dysplastic) kidney is a common cause of a neonatal mass. It is always a unilateral phenomenon.   *(3:200)*

480. (A) A choledochal cyst is a focal cystic dilatation of the common duct. It will cause relative obstruction secondary to the segment of the biliary tree affected. This entity is usually congenital and treated by surgery.   *(10:25)*

481. (A) Ascites is commonly associated with obstruction of the portal venous system, as in cirrhosis.
(4:484,572)

482. (A) A phlebolith is a small stone or calcification that may occur in an organized thrombus within a vein; ie, a venous calculus.   *(4:111)*

483. (C) Chronic active hepatitis may eventually lead to postnecrotic cirrhosis. The etiology of chronic active hepatitis is usually ideopathic but may be immunological or viral.   *(4:445)*

484. (B) In the early stages of alcoholic cirrhosis, the liver enlarges and undergoes severe fatty changes. This is followed by a fibrofatty change. Ultimately, the liver undergoes fibrosis and shrinks.   *(4:447)*

485. (D) All of the above. The popliteal artery is located posterior to the knee joint. Focal dilatation of this artery is usually due to atherosclerosis and is associated with partially calcified walls.   *(4:290; 8:293)*

486. (C) In chronic renal disease, both kidneys are dense, small, and echogenic.   *(5:314; 8:139)*

487. (D) Gallstones can produce injury by all of the listed alternative answers. Other possible complications include empyema of the gallbladder, ascending cholangitis, biliary cirrhosis of the liver, acute pancreatitis, and gallstone ileus.   *(4:462)*

488. (B and C) Sixty percent of all masses that appear as a hypofunctioning thyroid nodule (cold nodule) on a nuclear medicine thyroid scintigram are adenomas and/or benign thyroid nodules. The remaining 40% are cysts and malignant nodules.   *(3:242)*

489. (A) Courvoisier's law states that obstruction of the common bile duct by pressure from the outside (ie, mass in the pancreatic head) will produce a distended gallbladder. Obstruction by a stone (intrinsic pressure) will produce an inflamed contracted gallbladder.   *(2:132; 4:462)*

490. (C) When food containing fat enters the small intestines, cholecystokinin is released and activates the gallbladder to empty its bile. A contracted gallbladder is very difficult to visualize.   *(35:358–362)*

491. (C) A normally functioning transplanted kidney should not appear different from a normal kidney located within the renal fossa.   *(3:211)*

492. (A) As stated in Courvoisier's law, obstruction of the common bile duct due to pressure from the outside will lead to dilated gallbladder and biliary radicles.   *(4:462)*

493. (C) Time gain compensation (TGC) and gain cannot make an organ look larger or smaller. Imaging the kidney in an oblique view will shorten the kidney.   *(8:143)*

494. (B) Transplanted kidneys are usually placed in the pelvis along the iliopsoas margin. The ureter of the donor kidney is anastomosed to the bladder.   *(10:59)*

495. (B) The parietal peritoneum lines the abdominal cavity. Organs are said to be intraperitoneal if they are surrounded by peritoneum or retroperitoneal if they are only covered on their anterior surface.   *(2:244)*

496. (A) True.   *(1:45)*

497. (A) True.   *(1:45)*

498. (A) True.   *(1:45)*

499. (B) False.   *(1:45)*

500. (A) True.   *(1:45)*

501. (A) True.   *(1:45)*

502. (A) Wall thickness of an abnormal bowel has been reported to be from 5 to 30 mm, averaging 23 mm.   *(2:299)*

503. (D) All of the alternative answers are possible. The appearance of a hydronephrotic kidney is dependent on the severity of the hydronephrosis.   *(8:140)*

504. (C) To localize a dilated ureter, scanning the pelvis with a full bladder and evaluating the area posterior to it may be helpful. Localization of the ureter is usually very difficult owing to overlying bowel gas.   *(5:308)*

505. (B) There is a large complex mass within the liver. This mass is a hepatoblastoma.   *(13:313)*

506. (A) The most common liver tumor in children is hepatoblastoma.   *(13:313)*

507. (B) The renal architecture is disorganized and the kidney is enlarged indicating infantile polycystic kidney disease. In this disorder, the renal parenchyma appears echogenic and macroscopic cysts are not identified.   *(13:307)*

508. (B) Microscopic cysts are not identified in infantile polycystic kidney disease because the disorder involves ectasis of the distal collecting ducts.   *(13:307)*

509. (B) This cyst represents a dilated upper pole moiety in the duplex collecting system.   *(13:304–305)*

510. (B) The hydronephrotic upper moiety implants ectopically and is associated with a ureterocele.   *(13:304–305)*

511. (B) This structure is not a kidney because it does not have the typical configuration in transverse action. It represents the right adrenal that has an echogenic medulla in hypoechoic cortex. There is a cystic structure along its lateral aspect, which represents a remnant of dysplastic renal tissue.   *(13:307)*

512. (A) In renal agenesis, the adrenal has an abnormal shape because the kidneys are not present. The abnormally shaped adrenal may mimic, to some degree, the sonographic appearance of a kidney.   *(13:307)*

513. (B) This is a kidney in a patient affected by adult-onset polycystic kidney disease.   *(13:228)*

514. (D) Cysts can be found in any of the given structures.   *(13:214)*

515. (B) This is a normal renal transplant.   *(13:238)*

516. (D) Since sonography can detect masses that may be surgically treated, it has an important role in distinguishing surgically amenable causes of post-transplant poor renal function from those that occur as a result of rejection.   *(13:216)*

517. **(A)** The arrow points to a medullary pyramid.
(13:26)

518. **(D)** The size of the kidney in normal patients can be correlated with the patient's overall body height. Normal adult kidneys range from 10–12 cm in long axis, 5–6 cm in width, and 3–4 cm in anteroposterior dimension. The renal parenchyma (the medulla and cortex) ranges from 1.5–2.0 cm.   *(13:210)*

519. **(A)** There is gallbladder wall thickening.   *(13:184)*

520. **(D)** Viscid bile results from incomplete gallbladder emptying and represents the precursor to formation of calculi.   *(13:184)*

521. **(B)** The pancreas may be echogenic in older adults owing to deposition of fat within the pancreatic lobules.   *(13:194)*

522. **(A)** Most pancreatic lesions are hypoechoic.   *(2:179)*

523. **(B)** This is the appearance of a normal stomach with an echogenic center and a hypoechoic halo representing the wall; ie, it has a target configuration.   *(13:206)*

524. **(B)** The hypoechoic portion represents the wall of the stomach.   *(13:206)*

525. **(D)** Either a fluid-filled loop of bowel, probably transverse colon, or a fluid-filled loop of duodenum may have the appearance shown in Fig. 5–27.   *(13:178)*

526. **(A)** The upright view is helpful to detect any mobile calculi that move into the fundus when the patient stands upright.   *(13:160–162)*

527. **(A)** This structure is an unusually shaped gallbladder.   *(13:180)*

528. **(A)** The sonogram represents a phrygian cap, an anatomical variant.   *(13:180)*

529. **(B)** The sonogram represents the aorta and celiac axis.   *(13:202)*

530. **(A)** The common hepatic artery, splenic artery, and left gastric artery arise from the celiac axis.   *(13:202)*

531. **(D)** The abdominal aorta and the left lobe of the liver are shown.   *(13:202)*

532. **(A)** Atherosclerosis is the most common cause of abdominal aortic aneurysms.   *(13:169)*

533. **(A)** The arrows delineate a hypertrophied pyloric muscle.   *(13:323)*

534. **(A)** A muscle thickness of greater than 4 mm is diagnostic of hypertrophic pyloric stenosis.   *(13:172)*

535. **(A)** The liver parenchyma is very echogenic compared to the kidney.   *(13:199)*

536. **(C)** The hepatic parenchyma is more echogenic when compared with the kidney.   *(13:199)*

537. **(B)** The echogenic focus represents the mediastinum of the testes through which many of these central vessels and tubules arise.   *(18:112)*

538. **(A)** The testes appear as nonhomogeneous structures because interstitial hemorrhage associated with hemorrhagic infarction and testicular torsion is indicated.   *(19:527)*

539. **(B)** The abnormal sonographic findings indicate a calculus in the midpolar region of the kidney.
(20:191)

540. **(A)** True. Oxalate and uric acid stones are radiopaque but are echogenic on sonography.   *(20:191)*

541. **(C)** There is evidence of viscid bile and a large calculus within the gallbladder lumen.   *(22:499)*

542. **(B)** False. The presence of calculus within the gallbladder does not always indicate that there is active cholecystitis. However, there is a possible complication of perforation when cholelithiasis is associated with cholecystitis.   *(23:798)*

543. **(D)** There is focal echogenicity within the cortex and medulla and an incidental finding of a small cortical cyst.   *(13:199)*

544. **(D)** All of the suggested answers can be associated with echogenic medulla and cortex.   *(27:830)*

545. **(B)** Abnormal sonographic findings indicate a large renal calculus with an associated shadow in the medial portion of the kidney.   *(20:191)*

546. **(A)** Calcium oxalate stones may be radiopaque but are echogenic on sonography.   *(20:191)*

547. **(D)** The spleen appears normal.   *(28:537)*

548. **(D)** Splenomegaly is typically encountered in chronic myelogenous leukemia and portal hyper-

tension. In sickle-cell crisis, there is typically auto-infarction of the spleen producing a very small spleen. *(29:697)*

549. **(B)** The sonogram shows a normal common bile duct. *(30:703)*

550. **(C)** The common bile duct is formed from the confluence of the common hepatic duct and cystic duct. *(30:703)*

551. **(B)** Abnormal sonographic findings show that the mass has all the characteristics of a simple cyst in the lower pole of the kidney. *(32a:87)*

552. **(A)** Approximately one-third of normal adults over the age of 45 have cysts in their kidney. *(33:671)*

553. **(D)** The sonograms demonstrate marked gallbladder thickening with a small amount of intraluminal sludge. *(35:361)*

554. **(D)** All of the above. Gallbladder wall thickening (> 3.5) is associated with cholecystitis, hepatitis, ascites, alcoholic liver disease, hypoproteinemia, hypoalbuminemia, and a nondistended gallbladder. The patient has AIDS, and this pattern is consistent with cholecystitis associated with this disorder. *(35:361)*

555. **(B)** Murphy's sign *(35:361)*

556. **(B)** The sonogram demonstrates a dilated intra-hepatic duct in the left lobe. *(35:363)*

557. **(A)** The abnormal sonographic findings indicate a dilated common bile duct with a rat-tail deformity of the distal common bile duct usually associated with tumors in the head of the pancreas. *(35:363)*

558. **(E)** This is an example of biliary duct obstruction both intra- and extrahepatic due to a pancreatic tumor. *(35:363)*

559. **(B)** The intrahepatic bile ducts course in a transverse plane in the left lobe, therefore, they are more readily detected on a transverse scan of the left lobe than bile ducts occurring within the right lobe. *(35:363)*

560. **(A)** An echogenic mass is noted. *(35:383)*

561. **(A)** This is an echogenic focus within the liver most consistent with a hemangioma. *(35:383)*

562. **(B)** A tagged red blood cell liver/spleen scan is most definitive in the diagnosis of hemangioma. *(35:383)*

563. **(B)** This is a typical fusiform dilated aneurysm of the distal abdominal aorta. *(35:402)*

564. **(B)** Atherosclerosis is the most common cause of an aneurysm. *(35:402)*

565. **(D)** All of the above. Aneurysmal dilation of an artery may occur in any area of the body. *(35:402)*

566. **(B)** There is a hypoechoic tumor that was found during a transrectal sonogram. The hypoechoic tumor appears to extend into the transitional zone. *(35:486)*

567. **(A)** Carcinoma of the prostate stage A. *(35:486)*

568. **(B)** Elevated. *(35:486)*

569. **(A)** An echogenic kidney. *(35:445)*

570. **(B)** Normally, the liver parenchyma should be more echogenic than the renal cortex in chronic renal disease. The kidney is found to be small and echogenic. This kidney had severe parenchymal disease and is markedly more echogenic that the liver. *(35:445)*

571. **(A)** The liver appears more echogenic because of the fibrous septa within the hepatic lobules. *(35:445)*

572. **(A)** This testis has a diffusely abnormal pattern consistent with a testicular tumor or possible testicular torsion. *(35:501)*

573. **(A)** This scan is diagnostic of a testicular tumor. In testicular torsion, one usually observes enlargement of the head of the epididymis, which in this case is normal. *(35:501)*

574. **(D)** Lymphadenopathy may be a presenting symptom associated with a testicular tumor. *(35:512)*

575. **(C)** The transrectal sonogram demonstrates a hypoechoic lesion in the peripheral zone. *(35:499)*

576. **(C)** Biopsy of this lesion through the transrectal approach would be preferred owing to its proximity to the rectum. *(35:499)*

577. **(B)** This has approximately a 20% chance of being carcinoma. *(35:499)*

578. **(D)** Transperineal and transrectal biopsy are the most common routes of obtaining prostate tissue using ultrasound guidance. Transrectal biopsy is preferred because of its closer proximity to the prostate. *(35:499)*

579. (B) This sonogram demonstrates a dilated common bile duct. *(35:363)*

580. (C) The most likely cause of this includes pancreatic tumor or gallstone in the distal common bile duct. *(35:363)*

581. (A) With age, the common bile duct may distend and measure 7 mm or greater. *(35:363)*

582. (B) The arrow points to hypoechoic lesions within the left lobe of the liver. *(35:397)*

583. (C) These hypoechoic lesions are the results of infectious foci. It is very unusual to have metastases with hypoechoic texture. Occasionally, lymphoma may produce hypoechoic liver metastases. Hemangiomas are echogenic. *(35:397)*

584. (D) A fine needle aspiration would be the next step to evaluate the nature of these liver lesions. *(35:397)*

585. (B) This sonogram is diagnostic of a varicocele, dilated vessels, near the head of the epididymis. *(35:513)*

586. (A) Increase flow within the dilated vessels can be seen with a Valsalva maneuver. *(35:513)*

587. (A) A varicocele appears as tortuous vessels near the head of the epididymis, mostly occurring on the left. *(35:513)*

588. (A) This patient has a contracted gallbladder filled with stones. *(35:360)*

589. (A) The sonogram demonstrates calculus cholecystitis. *(35:360)*

590. (False) With this many stones, the patient would not be a candidate for biliary lithotripsy. *(35:434)*

591. (B) This sonogram shows distension of the renal pelvis and proximal ureter. *(35:444)*

592. (E) This may be secondary to reflux or ureterovesicle junction (UVJ) obstruction. Since the proximal ureter is dilated, ureteropelvic junction (UPJ) obstruction is unlikely. *(35:444)*

593. (E) Xanthogranulomatous pyelonephritis is an inflammatory process accompanied by calculi. Sonographically, the kidney appears as an enlarged hydronephrotic kidney with stones obstructing within the renal collecting system. *(35:454)*

594. (A) This sonogram shows thickening of the posterior bladder wall. *(35:562)*

595. (C) This may be secondary to cystitis or tumor. *(35:562)*

596. (D) Chemotherapy, renal infection, frequent and painful urination is associated with cystitis in a child. *(35:562)*

597. (B) This sonogram shows marked increased echogenicity of the liver compared with the kidney. *(35:581)*

598. (D) All of the above. In the adult, glycogen storage disease, fatty metamorphosis, cirrhosis, and hemochromatosis all present with an echogenic liver. In the child, this is frequently a complication of glycogen storage disease. *(35:581)*

599. (A) These children have a greater incidence of multiple hepatic adenomata and tumors. Portions of normal liver may appear hypoechoic relative to the abnormal echogenic liver. *(35:581)*

600. (A) The absence of a right kidney. *(35:577)*

601. (C) This sonogram shows a flattened and relatively large adrenal in a patient with bilateral renal agenesis. *(35:577)*

602. (A) In neonates affected by this disease, the adrenals may be relatively long and misshapen. *(35:577)*

603. (C) This sonogram shows a markedly hydropic gallbladder. *(35:587)*

604. (A) Hydrops of the gallbladder may be related to obstruction at the level of a cystic or distal common bile duct. *(35:587)*

605. (E) All of the above will lead to an hydropic gallbladder. In addition, in mucocutaneous lymph node syndrome (Kawasaki's disease), there may be gallbladder hydrops related to obstruction of the neck by lymph nodes. *(35:587)*

606. (B) Difficult to determine because the gallbladder is not fully distended, and as one can see from the centimeter marker on the side of the image, this gallbladder is perhaps only 3 cm in length and is nondistended. *(35:358)*

607. (A) When the gallbladder is nondistended, the wall may look thickened just because the gallbladder wall is not fully stretched as in the distended state. *(35:358)*

608. (E) All of the above. There are a variety of nonphysiological conditions that can be associated with gallbladder wall thickening. These include cardiac dysfunction, lymphadenophathy, right upper quadrant inflammatory process, and hyperplastic cholecystitis. *(35:358)*

609. **(A)** This sonogram shows a large mass in the lower pole of the left kidney. *(35:574)*

610. **(D)** In an adult, this would most likely represent a renal cell tumor; in a child, Wilms' tumor. Angiomyoneuromas may also have this appearance but typically have a more echogenic texture related to their fat content. *(35:574)*

611. **(E)** Angiomyolipomas are seen in patients with tuberous sclerosis and in postmenopausal women. *(35:574)*

612. **(B)** This sonogram shows the normal left adrenal. *(35:578)*

613. **(C)** Normal left adrenal. *(35:578)*

614. **(D)** All of the above are conditions that may affect the adrenal. *(35:578)*

615. **(D)** This sonogram demonstrates an ectatic or dilated main pancreatic duct. *(35:594)*

616. **(D)** Cystic fibrosis is a genetic disease affecting 1 in 2000 persons. The complications of cystic fibrosis are related to the increase in secretions of the exocrine glands. This leads to chronic pancreatitis and a small echogenic pancreas with a dilated duct. Hereditary pancreatitis is an autosomal dominant disease producing recurrent inflammation of the pancreas. Hereditary pancreatitis is not as common as cystic fibrosis. *(35:594)*

617. **(D)** Pancreatic tumors and chronic pancreatitis will lead to a dilated pancreatic duct. In elderly patients, the duct has lost its elasticity and will be ectatic and dilated. *(35:594)*

618. **(B)** This sonogram demonstrates a cystic mass contiguous with the common bile duct. *(35:591)*

619. **(B)** This is a choledochal cyst, of which there are at least three varieties. *(35:591)*

620. **(E)** All of the above are variations of choledochal cysts. *(35:591)*

621. **(E)** None of the above. A choledochal cyst occurs as a result of an anomalous insertion of the common bile duct into the pancreatic duct, permitting reflux of pancreatic juices into the bile duct leading to cholangitis, weakening, and dilatation. *(35:591)*

622. **(B)** A cystic mass that appears to displace the bowel and mesentery. *(35:600)*

623. **(A)** This is a mesenteric cyst. Bowel loops are displaced by the cyst and their mesentery is seen. Note how the cyst conforms closely to the contour of the anterior wall, pushing the bowel and mesentery posteriorly. An ovarian cyst and free fluid do not displace bowel posteriorly. *(35:600)*

624. **(D)** These sonograms demonstrate marked thickening and lengthening of the antral muscle (pyloric canal and muscle). *(35:604)*

625. **(B)** This is consistent with hypertrophic pyloric stenosis. *(35:604)*

626. **(E)** The criteria for this diagnosis include wall thickness greater than 3 mm and antral length greater than 14 mm. *(35:604)*

627. **(E)** None of the above. This transverse sonogram of the upper abdomen demonstrates a normal pancreas and duodenum. *(35:371)*

628. **(B)** Normal. *(35:371)*

629. **(C)** This real-time sonogram demonstrates a solid mass within irregular borders. *(35:737)*

630. **(C)** At biopsy, this was carcinoma. Fibroadenomas usually are well circumscribed, whereas carcinomas are not. *(35:737)*

631. **(B)** False. One cannot tell with an adequate degree of confidence whether a solid lesion is benign or malignant by its sonographic appearance. *(35:737)*

632. **(B)** A parathyroid mass. This is a large mass adjacent to the thyroid and right common carotid artery. *(35:737)*

633. **(A)** This represents a parathyroid adenoma or carcinoma. *(35:715)*

634. **(A)** Parathyroid adenoma may present with hypercalcemia. *(35:715)*

635. **(E)** None of the above. The chest radiograph demonstrates a large amount of fluid density in the left hemidiaphragm. *(35:744)*

636. **(C)** The sonogram demonstrates that this fluid density contains multiple loculations consistent with an empyema. *(35:744)*

637. **(A)** If the fluid seems to move with each breath, one can assume that it is nonloculated, simple effusion. *(35:744)*

638. (A) Sonography is useful in confirming the clinical impression of acute appendicitis. *(35:409)*

639. (E) The primary criteria for diagnosis of acute appendicitis is visualization of a noncompressible appendix. Other diagnostic criteria are muscular wall thickness greater than 3 mm, and the presence of an appendicolith. *(35:409)*

640. (C) 5–75 represents a normal appendix. *(35:409)*

641. (C) Choledocholithiasis. Ductal stones are identified by the presence of echogenic material within the duct. *(36:132)*

642. (B) The dilated common bile duct has an internal dimension if greater than 6 mm. Also note the "parallel channel" sign ("shotgun" sign), which represents the dilated hepatic duct and the portal vein. *(36:129)*

643. (A) In *chronic* cholecystitis, the gallbladder generally is contracted, with the walls being thickened, but rarely more than five times its size with associated cholelithiasis. Remember in *acute* cholecystitis, the gallbladder is *enlarged* with *thickened* walls and leukocytosis. *(36:107)*

644. (B) Main portal vein. It branches into left portal and right portal. The left portal vein proceeds cranially *vertically* along the anterior surface of the caudate lobe, whereas the right portal has a horizontal course. *(36:7, 9)*

645. (E) The ligamentum teres courses in the caudal aspect of the left intersegmental fissure and may be used as a landmark in dividing the left lobe into medial (quadrate) and lateral segments. Sonographically on a transverse scan, it appears as a round echogenic area. *(36:4)*

646. (D) In obstructive jaundice, alkaline phosphatase, and direct bilirubin will be markedly increased with SGOT also being increased. Keep in mind that SGOT also is markedly increased in hepatitis. *(38:172)*

647. (C) The sonogram demonstrates dilated biliary radicles. A serum alkaline phosphatase level greater than five times the upper limit of normal is characteristic of cholestatic hepatobiliary disease. *(40:369)*

648. (D) The sonogram suggests a *thickened* gallbladder wall (cholecystitis). A gallbladder wall greater than 3 mm is seen with hepatitis, ascites, alcoholic liver disease, hypoproteinemia, hypoalbuminemia, heart failure, systemic venous hypertension, and renal disease. *(36:107)*

649. (A) The major lobar fissure is seen on longitudinal scans as a linear echo coursing from the gallbladder to the porta hepatis. It divides the liver into left and right lobes. *(36:5)*

650. (A) Metastases are neoplastic involvement in the liver, causing liver enlargement with multiple nodules of varying sonographic patterns. Metastases have been described as hypoechoic, echogenic, bullseye, anechoic, and diffusely inhomogeneous. *(36:61)*

651. (B) The sonogram shows dilated hepatic veins and a dilated inferior vena cava. This is consistent with congestive heart failure. *(37:223)*

652. (B) The ligamentum venosum is noted here. The fissure for the ligamentum venosum contains the hepatogastric ligament, which is located between the caudate lobe and the left lobe of the liver. *(36:5)*

653. (B) This sonogram is suggestive of adenomyomatosis of the gallbladder. Sonographically, one should look for diffuse or segmental thickening of the gallbladder wall with intramural diverticula protruding into the lumen. *(36:19)*

654. (D) At the level of the gallbladder, one may see the fluid-filled second or descending portion of the duodenum, which runs along the right side of the inferior vena cava. *(36:611)*

655. (D) The clinical features of acute cholecystitis are *leukocytosis*, fever, nausea, vomiting, and referred shoulder pain if the inflammation irritates the diaphragm. Sonographically, the gallbladder is enlarged with a thickened wall greater than 5 mm. *(36:107)*

656. (C) The ultrasound findings in cirrhosis include increased echogenicity of the anterior portion of the liver, with decreasing echogenicity as one proceeds posteriorly owing to the difficulty of the beam to penetrate the cirrhotic liver. The echogenicity that is noted is much higher than that of the kidney. There may be associated ascites, splenomegaly, and portal hypertension. It is difficult to pinpoint when a liver changes from being a fatty to a cirrhotic but generally a fatty liver is homogeneously enlarged and echogenic. *(36:17)*

657. (A) This liver is enlarged and extremely heterogeneous consistent with metastatic disease. Metastatic patterns within the liver may vary from hypoechoic to echogenic. *(36:61)*

658. (B) The hemangioma is located between the right and middle hepatic veins; therefore it is in the anterior segment of the right lobe. The right hepatic vein separates the right lobe into anterior and posterior segments; the middle hepatic vein divides the liver into right and left lobes. *(36:5)*

659. **(D)** When scanning coronally left side down and placing the transducer longitudinally on the patient's right side, the aorta will be seen posterior to the inferior vena cava. Sometimes one may also be able to see the renal arteries arising off the aorta. This scan is very beneficial to rule out lymphadenopathy. *(36:444)*

660. **(B)** Owing to long-standing obstruction, tumefactive biliary sludge has been described as a Courvoisier gallbladder. Because of the stasis, the sludge eventually will become so thick as to attenuate enough sound to cause distal shadowing. Metastatic tumor to the gallbladder should be suspected in the presence of focal gallbladder wall thickening in association with nonshadowing intraluminal soft tissue masses. *(36:104, 125)*

661. **(C)** Cirrhosis is a chronic and progressive disease leading to liver cell failure, portal hypertension, and ascites. The thickened gallbladder wall is most likely related to hypoproteinemia and to the adjacent ascites that will make the gallbladder appear thickened. *(36:17)*

662. **(D)** This is a sonogram of a normal pancreas. With high-resolution ultrasound, the pancreatic duct is routinely visualized. The normal pancreatic duct should not measure more than 2 mm in its internal diameter. *(36:174)*

663. **(B)** The arrow is pointing to the right renal artery, which lies posterior to the inferior vena cava. *(36:443)*

664. **(D)** The crura of the diaphragm are extensions (tendinous fibers) of the diaphragm that attach to the vertebral process of L3 on the right and L1 on the left. The right crus appears as a hypoechoic linear structure and can be visualized as it runs from posterior to the inferior vena cava to anterior to the aorta. *(36:387)*

665. **(A)** The esophagogastric junction can be seen anterior to the aorta and posterior to the left lobe of the liver. *(36:387)*

666. **(D)** Here we see the right crus of the diaphragm posterior to the inferior vena cava. *(36:387)*

667. **(A)** The right renal artery runs posterior to the inferior vena cava and anterior to the right crus of the diaphragm. *(36:387)*

668. **(D)** When an ultrasound beam having an oblique incidence (not on a perpendicular angle) is directed at an interface and travels between two media (liver and gallbladder) of different propagation speeds, refraction of the ultrasound beam will occur (Snell's law). Here we can see the beam refracting off the curved surface of the gallbladder wall. *(41:161)*

669. **(C)** The echogenic foci sitting superior to the diaphragm (arrow) is a mirror-image artifact. A mirror-image artifact is a duplication artifact secondary to the sound beam bouncing off (reflecting off) a strong reflector in its path; ie, the diaphragm. This strong reflector acts as a mirror and the image will present as two reflected objects rather than one. *(41:151)*

670. **(B)** The sonogram demonstrates periportal lymphadenopathy, which is characterized by enlarged lymph nodes that are secondarily involved in almost all infections and neoplastic disorders. Lymph nodes consist of lymphocytes and reticulum cells, their function being filtration and production of lymphocytes. All the lymph passes through these nodes that act as filters, not only for bacteria but also for cancer cells. Sonographically, we can evaluate lymph nodes in the pelvis, retroperitoneum, porta hepatis, and perirenal and prevertebral vasculature. The ultrasound appearance of lymphomatous nodes varies from hypoechoic to anechoic with very good sound transmission. *(36:419)*

671. **(C)** There is no definite correlation between kidney size and echogenicity with the degree of renal failure. Generally, if the kidney parenchyma (cortex) is more echogenic than the liver, chronic renal insufficiency should be considered. *(36:290)*

672. **(C)** The sonogram demonstrates celiac nodes surrounding the celiac artery and its winglike configuration. Note the increased distance between the celiac artery and the aorta due to these masses. *(36:426)*

673. **(A)** This sonogram depicts a fusiform aneurysm. The fusiform type is a gradual dilatation of the vascular lumen. The saccular type is a discrete round structure and the cylindrial aneurysm is a dilatation longitudinally producing lengthening of the expanded vessel in a uniform diameter. The aorta is considered aneurysmal if it exceeds 3 cm; greater than 6 cm requires surgery. *(36:451)*

674. **(D)** The left renal vein courses between the aorta and the superior mesenteric artery. *(36:448)*

675. **(C)** The caudate lobe of the liver is seen posterior to the ligamentum venosum. *(36:4)*

676. **(A)** The celiac artery is the first anterior branch of the abdominal aorta.   *(36:445)*

677. **(B)** The superior mesenteric artery is the second branch of the abdominal aorta.   *(36:445)*

678. **(A)** The splenic vein is noted posterior to the body of the pancreas, and on a longitudinal scan can be seen between the celiac artery and the superior mesenteric artery.   *(36:445)*

679. **(B)** The kidney rests on the quadratus lumborum muscle that runs laterally to the psoas muscle.   *(36:396)*

680. **(C)** The falciform ligament extends from the umbilicus to the diaphragm and can only be seen sonographically in patients with ascites.   *(36:5)*

681. **(A)** Normal head, which lies anterior to the inferior vena cava.   *(35:372)*

682. **(B)** Normal tail, which lies anterior to the splenic vein.   *(35:371)*

683. **(B)** Common bile duct, which defines the posterolateral margin of the pancreas. In the head of the pancreas, the internal diameter should not be more than 4 cm.   *(36:168)*

684. **(B)** Chronic pancreatitis is associated with a normal to small pancreas, increased echogenicity due to fibrotic changes, calcification, and ductal dilation.   *(35:375)*

685. **(B)** The head of the pancreas lies anterior to the inferior vena cava.   *(36:167)*

686. **(B)** A pancreatic pseudocyst is a fluid collection that arises as a result of obstruction associated with pancreatitis. The pancreatic duct being obstructed increases in size until it can no longer dilate; it ruptures and allows pancreatic juices to escape. Blunt trauma is the most common cause of pseudocysts in children. Pseudocysts may track anywhere from the mediastinum to the pelvis.   *(36:184)*

687. **(E)** Adenocarcinoma is found most often in elderly males, in whom the pancreatic head is affected 70% of the time. As a rule the mass is hypoechoic, with irregular borders. (Fig. 5–117A). Associated findings include dilation of the pancreatic duct, biliary dilation (Fig. 5–117B), and an enlarged gallbladder (Courvoisier gallbladder) (Fig. 5–117C).   *(36:206)*

688. **(B)** There have been several ultrasound signs described for biliary dilatation. In this sonogram, we can recognize (1) tubular lucencies within the liver demonstrating acoustic enhancement—bile op-

posed to blood increases through transmission; (2) the tubules have a stellate (starlike with little points extending into the periphery) appearance as opposed to veins or arteries that are straight; (3) dilated ducts are generally seen running in pairs—as two tubular lucencies—normal bile ducts are not visualized within the liver.   *(36:129)*

689. **(C)** The arrow is pointing to an example of chronic pancreatitis. With chronic pancreatitis, the pancreas generally is diffusely smaller and more fibrotic than usual with areas of calcification and ductal dilatation. In acute pancreatitis, the pancreas is generally diffusely larger and *less* echogenic than normal. In adenocarcinoma and islet cell tumors, the pancreas is generally focally enlarged in the pancreatic head with the former and the tail in the latter.   *(36:196)*

690. **(C)** Because the patient was asymptomatic, this is most likely a simple benign hepatic cyst.   *(36:36)*

691. **(C)** The perirenal fluid collection may be associated with lymphocele, a collection lymph fluid caused by injury to lymphatic channels during transplantation; hematoma, a collection of blood; and abscess, which are all associated with renal transplantation. Unfortunately it is difficult to differentiate one from the other. Urinoma is a collection of urine due to a urinary leak of a uretero pelvic or ureteroureter anastomosis. Abscess is a collection of pus due to an inflammatory response. Ascites is not associated with a renal transplant.   *(36:335)*

692. **(C)** There is an irregular diffuse thickening of the bladder wall of unknown origin. The prostate is not enlarged, and there is no suggestion of a bladder neck obstruction that most commonly is secondary to benign prostatic hypertrophy or carcinoma. Endometrial tissue may be found penetrating the bladder wall and extending into the lumen in severe cases of endometriosis in premenopausal women.   *(36:349)*

693. **(D)** Serum creatinine and BUN (blood urea nitrogen) are elevated in kidney disease.   *(38:126)*

694. **(D)** Attenuation is the *decrease* in amplitude and intensity as a wave travels through a medium. On the contrary, one of the criteria for a cyst is the acoustic enhancement posterior to the cyst due to the nonattenuating characteristics of a cyst.   *(41:173)*

695. **(D)** Adult polycystic kidney disease is an inherited autosomal dominant disease that most often manifests in the fourth decade. It manifests by cystic dilatation of the proximal convoluted tubules, Bowman's capsule, and the collecting tubules. It is mostly a bilateral process, with associated cysts found in the liver (25–50%), pancreas, lungs, spleen, ovaries, and testes. Juvenile polycystic disease is part of the spectrum of infantile polycystic kidney diseases, whereby the kidney presents as enlarged and echogenic owing to the many *small* cystic interfaces found within the kidney   *(36:236)*

696. **(A)** Multicystic dysplastic kidney disease is the most common cause of an abdominal mass in the newborn. It is usually unilateral, although the other kidney may be associated with abnormalities, and the left kidney is affected more than the right. Sonographic criteria of this disease are cysts of varying size with the largest in the periphery, absence of connections between the cysts, absence of an identifiable renal sinus, and absence of renal parenchyma surrounding cysts.   *(36:232)*

697. **(A)** The sonogram is not normal. It depicts hydronephrosis. There are numerous causes for hydronephrosis: congenital anomolies, as in posterior urethral valves; bladder neck obstruction; acquired causes such as calculi; benign prostatic hypertrophy; tumors; inflammation; intrinsic causes such as calculi; pyelonephritis; and extrinsic causes such as neoplasm and retroperitoneal adenopathy.   *(36:252)*

698. **(E)** Staghorn calculus is a large calculi within the renal collecting system that leads to hyronephrosis. An angiomyolipoma (renal hamartoma) is a benign renal tumor that is highly echogenic because of its fat content. Vesicoureteral reflux is a common urinary tract abnormality in children and stems from several congenital anomalies such as ectopia, posterior urethral valves, and prune belly syndrome. The reflux will eventually reach the kidney and may progress to hydronephrosis, but the ureteral reflux is not due to obstruction in the kidney but rather is ureteral in origin. Tuberous sclerosis is an inherited neurocutaneous disorder and is associated with angiomyolipomas in 40–80% of cases. Parapelvic cysts do not communicate with the collecting system and are lymphatic in nature.   *(36:297, 298, 306)*

699. **(E)** The sonogram depicts an extratesticular mass. This may be a spermatocele (which is a cyst in the epididymis) containing spermatozoa or an epididymal cyst. A varicocele (enlargement of the veins of the spermatic cord) is also extratesticular but is found on the posterior surface, commonly occurring on the left, and sonographically appears tubular in shape. A seminoma is a malignant tumor within the testes.   *(35:512)*

700. **(B)** A normal head of the epididymis is noted.   *(35:506)*

701. **(B)** The arrow is pointing to the seminal vesicle, which is posterior to the bladder and superior to the prostate.   *(35:489)*

702. **(D)** Varicoceles are enlargements of the veins of the pampiniform plexus, which runs along the posterior aspect of testicle and is more prominent on the left. Spermatocele and epididymal cyst are found in the epididymis. The mediastinum testis is found within the testis and connects the rete testis with the epididymis. Cryptorchidism is another name for undescended testes.   *(35:503)*

703. **(D)** The sonogram depicts a small echogenic kidney with a loss of distinction between cortex medulla and renal sinus. This patient has chronic glomerulonephritis, which is the most common cause for chronic renal failure.   *(36:291)*

704. **(F)** An angiomyolipoma (renal hamartoma) is a benign fatty renal tumor that presents as a discrete hyperechoic lesion. Of patients with tuberous sclerosis, 40–80% have angiomyolipomas.   *(36:298, 306)*

705. **(C)** This is a sonogram of malrotated kidneys fused at the upper pole (horseshoe kidney) draped anterior to the vertebral vessels.   *(35:460)*

706. **(A)** The sonogram shows normal adrenals. At birth, the normal neonatal adrenal is relatively thick and prominent, being one-third the size of the kidney.   *(36:391)*

707. **(B)** This decubitus coronal sonogram depicts severe hydronephrosis, extending into the renal pelvis, with marked thinning of the renal parenchyma. Pyonephrosis is a collection of pus within the dilated collecting system due to the stasis of urine and would have internal echoes. The few echoes that are present within this hydronephrotic kidney are due to artifact.   *(35:252)*

708. **(C)** The arrow is pointing to the renal pyramids, which are in the medulla.   *(36:222)*

709. **(B)** The arcuate arteries, which are depicted as the small echogenic line above the pyramids are used as a landmark to differentiate the cortex from the medulla.   *(36:224)*

710. **(A)** The renal column of Bertin is composed of cortical tissue (cortex) that extends into the medullary area between the pyramids.   *(36:227)*

711. **(E)** The sonogram depicts dilated biliary radicles that are caused by obstructed bile ducts. This may be due to a stone, mass lesions in the area of the head of the pancreas, or tumor or metastatic lesions within the liver. Cirrhosis is related to "medical" jaundice and there will be no evidence of biliary dilatation.   *(8:99)*

712. **(E)** A neuroblastoma is an adrenal tumor found in children. It will not cause splenomegaly.   *(8:108)*

713. **(C)** The decubitus coronal position will provide the longest dimension to evaluate the kidney and will allow visualization of the renal pelvis extending into the renal hilum. *(36:222)*

714. **(T)** All of the answers are true. Acute tubular necrosis (ATN) is the most common cause of acute renal failure resulting in the accumulation of creatinine and nitrogenous wastes (BUN) in the body. ATN may be due to renal ischemia (the impairment of blood flow in and out of the body), trauma, toxin exposure, or a complication of surgery. Owing to the inflammatory changes, the kidney becomes edematous and congested; it therefore increases in size and the medullary pyramids appear more prominent and anechoic. *(36:287)*

715. **(B)** The valves of Heister are located within the cystic duct, at its junction with the neck of the gallbladder. *(37:228)*

716. **(C)** Gallbladder carcinoma is frequently associated with cholelithiasis, chronic cholecystitis, and/or calcification of the gallbladder wall. *(35:362;39:318)*

717. **(E)** Jaundice and right upper quandrant pain are associated with biliary obstruction. An increase in alkaline phosphatase is indicative of biliary obstruction, and one may see an increase in amylase if a tumor in the pancreatic head or pancreatitis is noted obstructing the common bile duct. Elevated acid phosphatase is associated with prostate carcinoma. *(38:185)*

718. **(D)** A large gallbladder, hypotonic intestines, and renal insufficiency are commonly seen in patients with diabetes. *(42:231)*

719. **(E)** Excessive weight loss is associated with carcinoma; therefore, liver metastases, dilated common bile duct (as may be present with adenocarcinoma within the pancreatic head), hepatoma, and pancreatic mass are correct. A hemangioma is the most common benign tumor of the liver. *(36:49)*

720. **(B)** Most commonly choledochal cyst is a cystic dilation of the common bile duct with the common hepatic duct being normal. Sonographically, one finds a large cystic mass in the porta hepatis with a dilated common hepatic or common bile duct entering the cyst. The gallbladder must be visualized as a separate structure. *(36:147)*

721. **(D)** A diffusely thickened gallbladder with localized infiltrating or fungating tumors protruding into the lumen. In 65–90% of cases, cholelithiasis is noted. *(36:119)*

REFERENCES

1. Cosgrove DO, McCready VR.: *Ultrasound Imaging: Liver, Spleen, Pancreas.* New York: Wiley, 1982.

2. Goldberg BB. *Abdominal Ultrasonography,* 2nd ed. New York: Wiley, 1984.

3. Hagen-Ansert SL. *Textbook of Diagnostic Ultrasonography.* 2nd ed. St. Louis: CV Mosby, 1983.

4. Anderson WAD, Scotti TM. *Synopsis of Pathology,* 10th ed. St. Louis: CV Mosby, 1980.

5. Sarti DA, Sample WF. *Diagnostic Ultrasound Text and Cases.* Boston: GK Hall, 1980.

6. Snell RS. *Clinical Anatomy for Medical Students.* Boston: Little, Brown, 1973.

7. Durrell C. Gallbladder ultrasonography in clinical context. Semin Ultrasound CT MR **5**(4):315, 1984.

8. Saunders RC, Campbell J, Guidi SM, et al. *Clinical Sonography: A Practical Guide.* Boston: Little, Brown, 1984.

9. Beeson PB, McDermott W, Wyngaarden JB. *Cecil's Textbook of Medicine,* 15th ed. Philadelphia: WB Saunders, 1979.

10. *SMDS Educational Outline Abdomen, Small Parts.* Vol. 2. Dallas: Society of Diagnostic Medical Sonographers, 1983.

11. *SMDS Educational Outline Abdomen, Small Parts.* Vol. 5. Dallas: Society of Diagnostic Medical Sonographers, 1983.

12. Lang FC. Commonly encountered artifacts in clinical Ultrasound. *Semin Ultrasound* **4**(1):22, 1983.

13. Fleischer AC, James AE: Real-Time Sonography. *Textbook with Accompanying Videotape.* Norwalk, CT: Appleton-Century-Crofts, 1984.

14. Hirsch J, Rogers J, Mack L. Real-time sonography of pleural opacities. *AJR* **136**:297, 1981.

15. Fleischer A, Winfield A, Page D. Synergistic use of sonomammography and x-ray mammography. *Postgrad Radiol* **5**:163, 1985.

16. Cole-Beuglet C, Sorino R, Kurtz A, et al. Fibroadenoma of the breast: Sonography correlate with pathology in 122 patients. *AJR* **140**:369, 1983.

17. Reading C, Carboneau J, James EM. *High resolution parathyroid sonography. AJR* **139**:539, 1982.

18. Hricak H, Filly R. Sonography of the scrotum. *Invest Radiol* **18**:112, 1983.

19. Bird K, Rosenfield A, Taylor K. Ultrasonography in testicular torsion. *Radiology* **147**:527, 1983.

20. King W, Kimme-Smith C, Winter J. Renal stone shadowing: An investigation of contributing factors. *Radiology* **154**:191, 1985.

21. Bernstein E, Chan E. Abdominal aortic aneurysm in high-risk patients. *Ann Surg* **200**:255, 1984.

22. Laing F, Federle M, Jeffrey R, et al. Ultrasonic eval-

uation of patients with acute right upper quadrant pain. *Radiology* **140**:499, 1981.

23. Gracie W, Randonoff D. The natural history of silent gallstones: The innocent gallstone is not a myth. *N Engl Med* **307**:798, 1982.

24. Jones T, Dubuisson R, Hughes J, et al. Abrupt termination of the common bile duct: A sign of malignancy identified by high-resolution real-time sonography. *J Ultrasound Med* **2**:345, 1983.

25. Simeone J, Muueller P, Ferrucci J, Jr et al. Sonography of the bile ducts after a fatty meal: An aid in detection of obstruction. *Radiology* **143**:211, 1982.

26. Kangarloo H, Sarti D, Sample W, Amundson G. Ultrasonographic spectrum of choledochal cysts in children. *Pediatr Radiol* **9**:15, 1980.

27. Shuman W, Mack L, Rogers J. Diffuse nephrocalcinosis: Hyperechoic sonographic appearance. *AJR* **136**:830, 1981.

28. Niederau C, Sonnenberg A, Muller J, et al. Sonographic measurements of the normal liver, spleen, pancreas, and portal vein. *Radiology* **149**:537, 1983.

29. Mittelstaedt C, Partain C. Ultrasonic-pathologic classification of splenic abnormalities: Gray-scale patterns. *Radiology* **134**:697, 1980.

30. Parulekar S. Ultrasound evaluation of common bile duct size. *Radiology* **129**:703, 1979.

31. Graif M, Manor A, Itzchak Y. Sonographic differentiation of extra- and intrahepatic masses. *AJR* **141**:553, 1983.

32a. Charboneau J, Hattery R, Ernst E, et al. Spectrum of sonographic findings in 125 renal masses other than benign simple cyst. *AJR* **140**:87, 1983.

32b. McClennan B, Stanley R, Melson G, et al. CT of the renal cyst: Is cyst aspiration necessary? *AJR* **133**:671, 1979.

33. Hole JW Jr. *Human Anatomy and Physiology*, 3rd ed. Dubuque, IO: William C. Brown, 1984.

34. Taylor KJW. *Atlas of Ultrasonography*, 2nd ed. New York: Churchill Livingstone, 1985.

35. Fleischer AC, James AE. *Diagnostic Sonography Principles and Clinical Applications*. Philadelphia, WB Saunders, 1989.

36. Mittelstaedt CA. *Abdominal Ultrasound*. New York: Churchill Livingstone, 1987.

37. Hagan-Ansert SL. *Textbook of Diagnostic Ultrasonography*. 3rd ed. St. Louis, CV Mosby, 1989.

38. Byrne JC, Saxton DF, Pelikan PK, Nungent PM. *Laboratory Tests, Implications for Nurses and Allied Health Professionals*. Reading, MA: Addison-Wesley, 1981.

39. Durrell CA. Gallbladder ultrasonography in clinical content. *Semin Ultrasound CT MRI* **5**(4):315, 1984.

40. Richter JM. *Evaluation of the jaundiced patient:* An internist's perspective. Semin *Ultrasound CT MRI* **5**(4):369–376, 1984.

41. Kremkau FW. *Diagnostic Ultrasound Principles, Instruments and Exercises*. 3rd ed. WB Saunders, 1989.

42. Fishman MC, Hoffman AR, Klausner AR, et al. *Medicine*. Philadelphia: JB Lippincott, 1981.

43. Koenigsberg M: Sonographic evaluation of the retroperitoneum. *Semin Ultrasound CT MRI* **3**:2, 1982.

44. Romano AJ, Sonnenberg VE, Casola GB, et al: Gallbladder and bile duct abnormalities in AIDS: Sonographic findings in eight patients. *AJR* **15**:123–129, 1988.

CHAPTER 6

ENDORECTAL PROSTATE SONOGRAPHY

Dunstan Abraham

Study Guide

The prostate is a heterogeneous oval-shaped organ that surrounds the proximal urethra. In the adult, the normal gland measures approximately 3.8 cm (cephalocaudal) by 3 cm (anteroposterior) by 4 cm (transverse).[1] It normally weighs about 20 g, but it can be slightly larger in men older than 40. The prostate is composed of glandular and fibromuscular tissue and is located in the retroperitoneum between the floor of the urinary bladder and the urogenital diaphragm. The base of the prostate, its superior margin, abuts the inferior aspect of the urinary bladder. The gland is bounded anteriorly by prostatic fat and fascia, laterally by the obturator internus and levator ani muscles, and posteriorly by areolar tissue and Denonvilliers' fascia, which separates it from the rectum.

The seminal vesicles are two saclike lateral structures that out pouch from the vas deferens and are situated on the posterior-superior aspect of the prostate between the bladder and the rectum. The seminal vesicles join the vas deferens to form the ejaculatory ducts, which then enter the base of the prostate to join the urethra at the verumontanum. The verumontanum is a midpoint region between the prostatic base and apex and surrounds the urethra. The size and fluid content of the seminal vesicles are variable.

The prostatic urethra courses through the substance of the gland and is divided into a proximal and a distal segment. The proximal segment extends from the neck of the bladder to the base of the verumontanum; the distal segment begins at this point and extends to the apex of the gland.

NORMAL SECTIONAL ANATOMY

The earlier anatomic descriptions of the prostate divided the gland into five major lobes (anterior, posterior, middle, and two lateral) or two zones (outer and inner). More recent histological studies, however, have divided the pros-

tate into three glandular zones: the transitional, central, and peripheral zones. There is also a nonglandular region called the anterior fibromuscular stroma[2] (Fig. 6–1A and B).

Transitional zone. The transitional zone represents about 5% of the glandular prostate and is located in the central region on both sides of the proximal urethra.[2] The ducts of the transitional zone run parallel to the urethra and end in the proximal urethra at the level of the verumontanum.

Central zone. The central zone constitutes approximately 25% of the prostatic glandular tissue and is located at the base of the gland.[2] It is wedgelike in shape, is oriented horizontally, and surrounds the ejaculatory ducts throughout their course. The zone narrows to an apex at the verumontanum. Ducts of the vas deferens and seminal vesicles come together to form the ejaculatory ducts, which pass through the central zone and join the urethra at the verumontanum.

Peripheral zone. The peripheral zone constitutes about 70% of the glandular tissue.[2] This zone consists of the posterior, lateral, and apical parts of the prostate and also extends anteriorly. The ducts of the peripheral zone enter the urethra at, and distal to, the verumontanum.

Anterior fibromuscular stroma. The anterior fibromuscular stroma is a thick nonglandular sheath of tissue that covers the entire anterior surface of the prostate. This tissue is composed of smooth muscle and fibrous tissue.

NORMAL SONOGRAPHIC ANATOMY

Sonographically, the prostate is a homogeneous gland with low-level echoes. The periurethral glandular tissue that surrounds the proximal urethra is homogeneous and isoechoic. The central zone is normally more echogenic than the peripheral zone because it has a greater amount

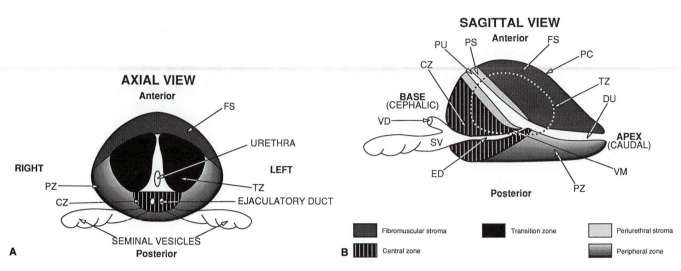

Figure 6–1. (A) An axial view of normal prostate anatomy: CZ is the central zone, FS is the fibromuscular stroma, TZ is the transition zone, and PZ is the peripheral zone. **(B)** Sagittal view of the normal prostate anatomy: SV is the seminal vesicle, ED is the ejaculatory duct, DU is the distal urethra, PC is the prostatic capsule, VD is the vas deferens, VM is the verumontanum, PU is the proximal urethra, CZ is the central zone, FS is the fibromuscular stroma, TZ is the transition zone, PS is the periurethral stroma, and PZ is the peripheral zone. *(Modified with permission from McNeal J E. Regional morphology and pathology of the prostate. Am J Clin Pathol 49:347–357, 1968 and Dakin R, et al. Transrectal ultrasound of the prostate: Technique and sonographic findings. JDMS 5(1):2, 1989.)*

of corpora amylacea (calcified deposits) in the central zone. The fibromuscular capsule, located anteriorly, is smooth, hyperechoic, and sharply defined.

The seminal vesicles are visualized as symmetrically paired structures that are slightly less echoic than the prostate. The vas deferens can be depicted as tubular hypoechoic structures joining the seminal vesicles medially. On transverse imaging, they are round or oval and are located between the seminal vesicles. The ejaculatory duct, when empty, can be seen as a hyperechoic line joining the urethra. The empty urethra is identified by its echogenic walls coursing through the prostate. When filled with fluid, the urethra is recognized more easily.

On longitudinal sections, the anterior space between the prostate and the seminal vesicles (prostate-seminal vesicle angle) is variable but is the same bilaterally. Similarly, the posterior space between the prostate and the seminal vesicle (or nipple) is symmetrical on both sides.[1]

INDICATIONS FOR SONOGRAPHY

Patients can be referred for endorectal prostate sonography for various reasons such as the following[3]:

- An abnormal digital rectal examination, as indicated by a palpable prostatic mass or a prostate with an asymmetrical size or shape.
- Biopsy guidance of sonographically detected abnormal areas.
- Clinical evidence of prostate cancer such as an elevated level of prostatic-specific antigen, an elevated level of prostatic acid phosphatase, or radiographically detected bone metastasis.

- Monitoring of a patient's response to therapy.
- Inflammation leading to the formation of a prostatic abscess.
- Infertility caused by the absence of the seminal vesicles or a bilateral obstruction of the ejaculatory ducts.
- Difficulties in voiding caused by an obstruction of the prostatic urethra.

EQUIPMENT AND EXAMINATION TECHNIQUES

Technical innovations have led to the availability of several types of endorectal imaging systems. The original systems were radial (axial) scanners that produced transverse-oriented slices of the prostate. Later, linear array scanners that imaged the gland in longitudinal sections were introduced. Today, biplanar endorectal probes that can produce both longitudinal and transverse sections of the gland are available, thus eliminating the need for two separate probes. The frequency of endorectal probes ranges from 5.0 to 7.5 MHz. A guide that is attached directly to the probe allows one to biopsy suspicious prostatic lesions safely and accurately.

Preparation of the patient for endorectal sonography begins with a self-administered enema 1 hour before the examination.[1] This enema not only eliminates fecal material from the rectum that might adversely affect the quality of the image but also reduces the risk of contamination of the prostate. The probe is sterilized and covered with a condom, and nonaerated water is placed in the system through an extension tube and an orifice on the probe.

The water and all residual air are then removed. The tip of the probe is lubricated, then inserted into the rectum. The nonaerated water can then be placed back into the system through the orifice on the probe. Because the distended cover on the probe increases the distance between the prostate and the transducer, the result is better imaging of the gland.

The patient can be examined in the lateral decubitus, lithotomy, or knee-chest position. Before the probe is inserted, a digital rectal examination is performed to exclude any obstructing lesions or rectal fissures. Axial scanning begins at the level of the seminal vesicles. The probe is then gradually withdrawn to image the gland sequentially down to the level of the apex. Sagittal imaging begins in the midline and shows the gland from base to apex with portions of the seminal vesicles. The probe is then rotated clockwise and counterclockwise to demonstrate the right and left sides of the gland.

PATHOLOGY

Prostatic Carcinoma

Prostatic carcinoma is the second leading cause of death among American men. In 1987 96,000 new cases were diagnosed and 27,000 lives were lost to this disease.[1] Although the etiology of prostatic cancer remains unclear, the factors implicated in its causation include age, genetic or racial makeup, hormonal influences, effects of benign prostatic hyperplasia, carcinogens in the environment and infectious agents. Anatomic studies have determined that 70% of prostate cancers originate de novo in the peripheral zone, 20% originate in the transitional zone, and 10% originate in the central zone.[1] Clinical symptoms include back pain and an obstruction of urinary outflow that may mimic benign prostatic hypertrophy.

The sonographic characteristics of prostatic carcinoma are variable. However, small cancers originating in the peripheral zone are anechoic to hypoechoic. As the tumor enlarges and extends into the central glandular region, it becomes more isoechoic to hyperechoic. The tumor also may spread outward beyond the prostatic capsule and disrupt this normally well-defined echogenic structure.[4] Several entities, however, may have ultrasound characteristics that are similar to those of intraprostatic malignancy. These include hyperplastic nodules, infarcts, focal inflammation, cystic atrophy, blood vessels, and muscle tissue.[5] Invasion of the tumor into the seminal vesicles can be seen as solid material within this normally fluid-filled structure. Invasion may make the size, shape, and echogenicity of the seminal vesicles asymmetrical in appearance.

Obliteration of the nipple or the prostate- seminal vesicle angle is another diagnostic criteria for invasion by the tumor.[1] However, because the nipple is not imaged consistently, this criterion is of limited usefulness. Staging of prostatic cancer with ultrasound also is feasible.

Benign Prostatic Hyperplasia and Hypertrophy

Benign prostatic hyperplasia affects 80–90% of adult men.[1] Its etiology is believed to be related to hormonal factors. The clinical symptoms of the disease may include decreased flow of urine, difficulty in initiating and terminating urination, nocturia, and urinary retention. Benign prostatic hyperplasia originates in the transitional zone and in periurethral glandular tissue.

The sonographic characteristics of hyperplasia nodules are variable. They can be hypoechoic, hyperechoic, or of mixed echogenicity. Enlargement of the central gland by benign prostatic hyperplasia causes lateral displacement of the peripheral zone. The prostatic calculi that are often encountered with benign prostatic hyperplasia are believed to be the result of stasis of prostatic secretions.

Benign prostatic hyperplasia causes the number of cells in the prostate to increase, whereas benign prostatic hypertrophy refers to an increase in the size of existing cells. Hyperplasia and hypertrophy often develop concurrently and result in the enlargement of the prostate gland.

Prostatitis

Inflammation of the prostate can be the result of acute or chronic bacterial infections or of unknown nonbacterial factors. Clinical symptoms of prostatitis may include fever, pelvic and low back pain, urinary frequency and urgency, and dysuria. Although prostatitis usually involves the peripheral zone in its initial stages, it can originate in any area of the gland.

In acute prostatitis, the main sonographic characteristics are (1) a hypoechoic rim surrounding the gland, (2) an echo-free halo surrounding the periurethral zone, and (3) diffuse low-level echogenic areas within the gland. In chronic prostatitis, diffuse inhomogeneous echogenicity and fluid-filled areas within the prostate is demonstrated, although this is a nonspecific finding.[1] Calculi also may be present.

A prostatic abscess may develop secondary to prostatitis. Endorectal sonography may show hypoechoic areas corresponding to liquefaction within the abscess.

Prostatic Cysts

Prostatic cysts are frequently congenital.[1] Sonographically, these cysts are anechoic, have sharp walls, and demonstrate good sound transmission.

REFERENCES

1. Rifkin M. *Ultrasound of the Prostate*. New York: Raven Press, 1988.
2. Lee F, Torp-Pedersen, ST, Siders DB, et al. Transrectal ultrasound in the diagnosis and staging of prostatic carcinoma. *Radiology* **170**:609, 1989.

3. Rifkin M. Prostate cancer ultrasound: Screening tool or hype? *Diagn Imaging*: 302–305, November 1988.

4. Lee F, Littrup PJ, Kumasaka GH, et al. The use of transrectal ultrasound in diagnosis, guided biopsy, staging and screening of prostate cancer. *Radiographics* **7**:627, 1987.

5. Waterhouse RL, Resnick MI. The use of transrectal prostatic ultrasonography in the evaluation of patients with prostatic carcinoma. *J Urol* **141**:233, 1989.

Questions

GENERAL INSTRUCTIONS: For each question, select the best answer. Select only one answer for each question, unless otherwise specified.

1. The fibromuscular stroma

    (A) covers the anterior surface of the prostate
    (B) is the major site of benign prostatic hypertrophy
    (C) is a nonglandular region
    (D) A and C

2. Which is *not* an indication for endorectal prostate sonography?

    (A) a palpable prostate mass
    (B) biopsy guidance of a palpable prostate nodule
    (C) an elevated prostatic-specific antigen
    (D) differentiation of a benign from a malignant nodule

3. Patients having endorectal prostate sonography are commonly examined in which of the following positions?

    (A) the lithotomy position
    (B) the erect position
    (C) the Trendelenburg position
    (D) Fowler's position

4. The transitional zone

    (A) is located centrally around the proximal urethra
    (B) represents about 5% of the gland
    (C) is the primary site of benign prostatic hyperplasia
    (D) is all of the above

5. Which one of the following statements is false?

    (A) the central zone constitutes approximately 25% of the glandular tissue
    (B) the central zone is located at the apex of the prostate
    (C) the vas deferens join the seminal vesicles in the central zone
    (D) none of the above

6. The peripheral zone accounts for which percentage of the prostatic glandular tissue?

    (A) 50%
    (B) 10%
    (C) 70%
    (D) 1%

7. Which of the following statements about the prostate is false?

    (A) its apex is located superiorly
    (B) its base abuts the urinary bladder
    (C) it has three zones
    (D) the urethra runs through the gland

8. Which of the following is a function of the prostate?

    (A) hormonal secretions
    (B) testosterone production
    (C) secretion of alkaline fluid
    (D) all of the above

9. The prostate is bounded anteriorly by

    (A) the obturator muscle
    (B) the levator ani muscle
    (C) fat and fascia
    (D) the obturator and levator ani muscles

10. The seminal vesicles join which of the following to form the ejaculatory duct?

    (A) the Denonvilliers' duct
    (B) the vas deferens
    (C) the verumontanum
    (D) the urethra

11. The ejaculatory duct joins the _____ at the verumontanum.

    (A) vas deferens
    (B) efferent ducts
    (C) epididymis
    (D) urethra

12. The seminal vesicles are located on which surface of the prostate?

    (A) the anterior-inferior surface
    (B) the posterior-inferior surface
    (C) the posterior-superior surface
    (D) none of the above

13. Which of the following statements about prostatic cancer is *not* true?

    (A) it originates mainly in the central zone
    (B) it is anechoic to hypoechoic in the early stage
    (C) its associated factors include benign prostatic hyperplasia and hormonal influence
    (D) all of the above are true

14. Benign prostatic hyperplasia

    (A) involves the periurethral tissue
    (B) affects 80–90% of adult men
    (C) is sonographically variable
    (D) involves all of the above

15. Sonographic features of acute prostatitis may include

    (A) a hypoechoic "rim" around the prostate
    (B) calcification in the peripheral zone
    (C) diffuse low-level echoes within the gland
    (D) A and C only

16. Benign prostatic hyperplasia appears to be caused by which of the following factors?

    (A) nutritional factors
    (B) hormonal factors
    (C) unknown factors
    (D) none of the above

17. Approximately what percentage of men are affected by benign prostatic hyperplasia?

    (A) 20%
    (B) 40%
    (C) 50%
    (D) 90%

18. Benign prostatic hyperplasia originates in which of the following areas of the prostate?

    (A) the fibromuscular stroma
    (B) the peripheral zone
    (C) the ejaculatory ducts
    (D) the transitional zone

19. Corpora amylacea are

    (A) part of the anterior fibromuscular capsule
    (B) calcified deposits in the prostate
    (C) hypoechoic on endorectal ultrasound
    (D) never seen on endorectal ultrasound

20. Tumor invasion may affect which of the following characteristics of the seminal vesicles?

    (A) their size
    (B) their shape
    (C) their echogenicity
    (D) all of the above

21. Obliteration of the nipple and the prostate-seminal vesicle angle may indicate

    (A) prostatitis
    (B) scarring of tissues
    (C) tumor infiltration
    (D) the need for a higher-frequency probe

22. Prostatic cysts

    (A) occur secondary to obstruction
    (B) can be congenital
    (C) are anechoic with good enhancement
    (D) all of the above

23. Clinical symptoms of prostatitis may include

    (A) fever
    (B) dysuria
    (C) perineal pain
    (D) all of the above

24. In its initial stages, prostatitis generally involves the

    (A) peripheral zone of the prostate
    (B) anterior capsule of the prostate
    (C) ejaculatory duct
    (D) none of the above

25. Which of the following can mimic intraprostatic cancer?

    (A) focal inflammation
    (B) blood vessels
    (C) muscle tissue
    (D) all of the above

26. Sonographic characteristics of prostatic cancer include

    (A) a hypoechoic nodule in the peripheral zone
    (B) distortion of the capsule
    (C) obliteration of the "nipple"
    (D) all of the above

27. The earliest prostate probes were

    (A) biplanar
    (B) radial scanners
    (C) linear array scanners
    (D) none of the above

28. An endorectal examination of the prostate should begin with

(A) transverse scanning
(B) longitudinal scanning
(C) views of the seminal vesicles
(D) a digital rectal examination

29. Prostate cancer is

(A) echogenic
(B) anechoic
(C) hypoechoic
(D) sonographically variable

30. The verumontanum is

(A) a midpoint region between the base and apex of the prostate
(B) a congenital abnormality of the prostate
(C) part of the peripheral zone
(D) none of the above

31. An echo-free "halo" around the periurethral zone may indicate

(A) tumor invasion
(B) benign prostatic hyperplasia
(C) prostatitis
(D) none of the above

32. An elevated prostatic-specific antigen may indicate

(A) prostatic inflammation
(B) prostatic cancer
(C) benign prostatic hyperplasia
(D) obstruction of the prostatic ducts

33. Which of the following narrows to an apex at the verumontanum?

(A) the central zone
(B) the peripheral zone
(C) the transitional zone
(D) the fibromuscular stroma

34. The normal adult prostate weighs approximately

(A) 10 g   (C) 30 g
(B) 20 g   (D) 40 g

35. Denonvilliers' fascia

(A) is located posterior to the prostate
(B) separates the prostate from the rectum
(C) covers the entire prostate
(D) is located posterior to and separates the prostate from the rectum

36. The normal adult prostate measures approximately

(A) 5 × 8 × 4 cm
(B) 8.3 × 3 × 6 cm
(C) 3.8 × 3 × 4 cm
(D) 5.8 × 4 × 5 cm

37. In 1987 the approximate number of new cases of prostate cancer diagnosed was

(A) 1000
(B) 10,000
(C) 100,000
(D) 200,000

38. Which statement about the seminal vesicles is incorrect?

(A) their absence does not usually affect fertility
(B) they are joined by the vas deferens
(C) they are normally less echoic than the prostate
(D) their size varies

39. Which of the following describes the normal prostate capsule?

(A) smooth and unbroken
(B) highly echoic
(C) sharply defined
(D) all of the above

Questions 40 through 46: Identify the structures in Fig. 6–2A by matching them with the list of terms given in column B.

COLUMN A	COLUMN B
40. _____	(A) peripheral zone
41. _____	(B) central zone
42. _____	(C) seminal vesicles
43. _____	(D) transitional zone
44. _____	(E) ejaculatory duct
45. _____	(F) urethra
46. _____	(G) fibromuscular stroma

Figure 6–2A. An axial view of normal prostate anatomy. The numbers correspond to questions 40–46. *(Modified with permission from McNeal JE. Regional morphology and pathology of the prostate. Am J Clin Pathol 49:347–357, 1968 and Dakin R, et al. Transrectal ultrasound of the prostate: Technique and sonographic findings. JDMS 5(1):2, 1989.)*

SAGITTAL VIEW

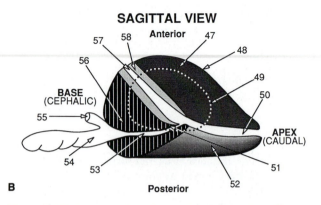

Figure 6–2B. A sagittal view of normal prostate anatomy. The numbers correspond to questions 47–58. *(Modified with permission from McNeal JE. Regional morphology and pathology of the prostate. Am J Clin Pathol 49:347–357, 1968 and Dakin R, et al. Transrectal ultrasound of the prostate: Technique and sonographic findings. JDMS 5(1):2, 1989.)*

Questions 47 through 58: Identify the structures in Fig. 6–2B by matching them with the list of terms given in column B.

COLUMN A	COLUMN B
47. _____	(A) proximal urethra
48. _____	(B) central zone
49. _____	(C) vas deferens
50. _____	(D) seminal vesicle
51. _____	(E) ejaculatory duct
52. _____	(F) peripheral zone
53. _____	(G) verumontanum
54. _____	(H) distal urethra
55. _____	(I) transitional zone
56. _____	(J) prostatic capsule
57. _____	(K) fibromuscular stroma
58. _____	(L) periurethral stroma

59. Fig. 6–3 represents a longitudinal scan taken to the right of midline. The structure indicated by the arrow is

(A) the proximal urethra
(B) a seminal vesicle
(C) the verumontanum
(D) none of the above

60. Fig. 6–4 represents a transverse scan. The structure indicated by the arrows is

(A) a tumor in the peripheral zone
(B) prostatitis involving the periurethral areas
(C) central gland calcification
(D) distortion of the prostatic capsule

61. Fig. 6–5 represents a longitudinal scan of a 60-year-old patient presenting with urinary frequency. He was referred for an endorectal prostate sonography examination. The area outlined by the markers indicates

(A) obliteration of the "prostate-seminal vesicle angle"
(B) a hypoechoic mass in the central zone
(C) a tumor in the peripheral zone
(D) bulging of the prostatic capsule

62. Fig. 6–6 represents a longitudinal scan. The region indicated by the white arrow is

(A) the fibromuscular stroma
(B) the seminal vesicle
(C) the peripheral zone
(D) the central zone

63. Fig. 6–6 represents a longitudinal scan. The region indicated by the black arrow is

(A) the peripheral zone   (C) the prostatic capsule
(B) the central zone   (D) none of the above

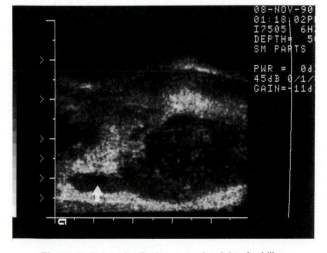

Figure 6–3. Longitudinal scan to the right of midline.

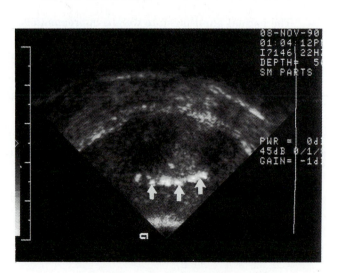

Figure 6–4. Transverse scan of the prostate.

Figure 6–5. Longitudinal scan of the prostate.

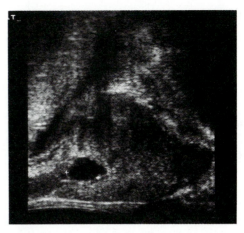

Figure 6–7. Longitudinal scan of the prostate.

64. Fig. 6–7 represents a longitudinal scan taken from a patient presenting with a history of infertility. The findings indicated by the markers probably represent

    (A) benign prostatic hypertrophy
    (B) a cyst in the ejaculatory duct
    (C) extension of a tumor into the nipple region
    (D) central gland disease

65. Fig. 6–8 represents a longitudinal scan of a 75-year-old man presenting with voiding difficulties and weight loss. This sonographic finding most likely represents

    (A) diffuse cancer
    (B) cancer confined to the peripheral zone
    (C) benign prostatic hypertrophy
    (D) none of the above

Figure 6–6. Longitudinal scan of the prostate.

Figure 6–8. Longitudinal scan of the prostate.

Answers and Explanations

1. **(D)** Both A and C. The fibromuscular stroma is a nonglandular region that covers the anterior surface of the prostate. Therefore, both A and C are correct. *(2:612)*

2. **(D)** Differentiation of a benign from a malignant nodule. Ultrasound cannot make a specific diagnosis of prostatic diseases. Biopsy is required to establish the diagnosis. *(3:303)*

3. **(A)** The lithotomy position. Patients who are having endorectal prostate sonography can be examined in the left lateral decubitus, knee-chest, or lithotomy position. *(1:44)*

4. **(D)** Is all of the above. The transitional zone is located on both sides of the proximal urethra and represents 5% of the gland. It also is the primary site of benign prostatic hyperplasia. *(2:610)*

5. **(B)** The central zone is located at the apex of the prostate. The central zone is a triangular structure located at the base of the prostate with its apex at the verumontanum. *(7:89)*

6. **(C)** 70%. The peripheral zone constitutes more than two-thirds of prostatic glandular tissue. *(2:612)*

7. **(A)** Its apex is located superiorly. The apex of the prostate is located inferiorly. (see Fig. 6–1B in the study guide.)

8. **(C)** Secretion of alkaline fluid. The prostate discharges this fluid into the urethra to enhance the motility of sperm. *(6:2)*

9. **(C)** Fat and fascia. The prostate is bounded anteriorly by vessels, fat, lymphatics, nerves, and fascial tissues, collectively termed the anterior prostatic fat and fascia *(1:5)*

10. **(B)** The vas deferens. The seminal vesicles join the vas deferens to form the ejaculatory duct, which passes through the central zone. *(2:612)*

11. **(D)** Urethra. The ejaculatory duct empties into the urethra at the verumontanum *(2:612)*

12. **(C)** The posterior-superior surface. *(1:74)*

13. **(A)** It originates mainly in the central zone. Seventy percent of prostatic cancers originate de novo in the peripheral zone. *(1:146)*

14. **(D)** Involves all of the above. Benign prostatic hyperplasia occurs mostly in the transitional zone, and nodules occasionally develop in the periurethral glandular tissue. It affects 80–90% of men and is sonographically variable. *(1:191, 196)*

15. **(D)** A and C only. In acute prostatitis, the gland may be surrounded by a hypoechoic rim, have an echo-free halo around the periurethral zone, or have scattered low-level echoes within the gland. *(1:222, 7:218)*

16. **(B)** Hormonal factors. A variety of reasons are attributed to the formation of benign prostatic hyperplasia. A hormonal factor is one possible explanation. *(1:191)*

17. **(D)** 90%. It is estimated that 80–90% of adult men will be affected by benign prostatic hyperplasia. *(1:192)*

18. **(D)** The transitional zone. (See the explanation for the answer to Question 14).

19. **(B)** Calcified deposits in the prostate. Degenerated epithelial cells of the prostate are shed and become suspended in albuminous fluid. This mass of cells is called corpora amylacea. Calculi are formed by the consolidation of corpora amylacea. *(7:137)*

20. **(D)** All of the above. The diagnostic criteria for neoplasms invading the seminal vesicles include asymmetry in the size, shape, and echogenicity of the vesicles. *(1:239)*

21. **(C)** Tumor infiltration. The tumor will obliterate the "nipple" and "prostate-seminal vesicle angle." *(1:179)*

22. **(D)** All of the above. Prostatic cysts are frequently congenital and secondary to obstruction of the seminal vesicle and ejaculatory duct. The differential diagnosis includes a cyst in the wolffian duct or the vestigial müllerian duct and diverticula of the ejaculatory duct. *(1:235)*

23. **(D)** All of the above. The major symptoms of acute bacterial prostatitis include a high fever, chills, dysuria, perineal pain, and urinary frequency and urgency. *(6:5)*

24. **(A)** Peripheral zone of the prostate. Although prostatitis can originate in any area of the prostate, it initially presents in the peripheral zone. *(1:14)*

25. **(D)** All of the above. Hyperplastic nodules, cysts, infarcts, inflammation, blood vessels, and muscle tissue can simulate intraprostatic cancer. *(4:236)*

26. **(D)** All of the above. Early prostatic cancers can present an anechoic or hypoechoic lesions in the peripheral zone. They can break through the prostatic capsule causing distortion, or they can invade the seminal vesicles. *(1:161, 179)*

27. **(B)** Radial scanners. The earliest endorectal probes were radial scanners that required a specially designed chair. *(1:35)*

28. **(D)** A digital rectal examination. This examination should be done before the probe is inserted to exclude obstructing lesions, rectal fissures, or other pathology. *(1:43)*

29. **(D)** Sonographically variable. Prostate cancer first appears as anechoic-hypoechoic. It becomes isoechoic-hyperechoic as it spreads to the central gland. *(5:629)*

30. **(A)** A midpoint region between the base and apex of the prostate. (See Fig. 6–1B in the Study Guide.)

31. **(C)** Prostatitis. (See the explanation for the answer to Question 15.)

32. **(B)** Prostatic cancer. An elevated prostatic-specific antigen or an elevated level of prostatic acid phosphatase may indicate prostate cancer. *(3:304)*

33. **(A)** The central zone. (See Fig. 6–1B in the Study Guide.)

34. **(B)** 20 g. The normal postpubescent prostate weighs approximately that amount. *(1:5)*

35. **(D)** Is located posterior to and separates the prostate from the rectum. Denonvilliers' fascia separates the prostate from the rectum posteriorly. *(1:5)*

36. **(C)** 3.8 × 3 × 4 cm. This is the average normal size of the prostate. *(1:5)*

37. **(C)** 100,000. In 1987 96,000 new cases of prostate cancer were diagnosed and 27,000 deaths resulted from this disease. *(1:141)*

38. **(A)** Their absence does not usually affect fertility. In rare cases, infertility can be caused by absence of the seminal vesicles or by an obstruction in the bilateral ejaculatory duct. *(3:304)*

39. **(D)** All of the above. The normal prostatic capsule is smooth, well defined, and highly echogenic. *(4:234)*

40. **(G)** Fibromuscular stroma
41. **(F)** Urethra
42. **(D)** Transitional zone
43. **(E)** Ejaculatory duct
44. **(C)** Seminal vesicles
45. **(B)** Central zone
46. **(A)** Peripheral zone
47. **(K)** Fibromuscular stroma
48. **(J)** Prostatic capsule
49. **(I)** Transitional zone
50. **(H)** Distal urethra
51. **(G)** Verumontanum
52. **(F)** Peripheral zone
53. **(E)** Ejaculatory duct
54. **(D)** Seminal vesicles
55. **(C)** Vas deferens
56. **(B)** Central zone
57. **(A)** Proximal urethra
58. **(L)** Periurethral stroma

59. **(B)** A seminal vesicle. The structure demonstrated in Fig. 6–3 is the right seminal vesicle, which joins the vas deferens (not shown) to form the ejaculatory duct. (See Fig. 6–1B in the Study Guide.)

60. **(C)** Central gland calcification. Figure 6–4 shows bright echoes representing prostatic calcification, which can be solitary or can occur in clusters. *(7:139)*

61. **(C)** A tumor in the peripheral zone. The hypoechoic mass seen on the peripheral zone in Fig. 6–5 is characteristic of prostatic cancer. *(1:63)*

62. **(D)** The central zone. This zone (white arrow) in Fig. 6–6 is clearly demarcated from the peripheral zone (black arrow) by a curved band of echoes. *(7:42)*

63. **(A)** The peripheral zone. (See the explanation for the answer to Question 62.) *(7:42)*

64. **(B)** A cyst in the ejaculatory duct. The cystic structure shown in Fig. 6–7 is clearly located within the ejaculatory duct.   *(1:231)*

65. **(A)** Diffuse cancer. Fig. 6–8 demonstrates diffuse hypoechoic masses throughout the prostate. This inhomogeneous pattern is consistent with diffuse malignancy.   *(1:167)*

REFERENCES

1. Rifkin M. *Ultrasound of the prostate*. New York: Raven Press, 1988.

2. Lee F, Torp-Pedersen ST, Siders DB, et al. Transrectal ultrasound in the diagnosis and staging of prostatic carcinoma. *Radiology* **170**:609, 1989.

3. Rifkin M. Prostate cancer ultrasound: Screening Tool or hype? *Diagn Imaging* 302–305, November 1988.

4. Waterhouse RL, Resnick MI. The use of transrectal prostatic ultrasonography in the evaluation of patients with prostatic carcinoma. *J Urol* **141**:233, 1989.

5. Lee F, Littrup PJ, Kumasaka GH, et al. The use of transrectal ultrasound in diagnosis, guided biopsy, staging and screening of prostate cancer. *Radiographics* **7**:627, 1987.

6. Paulson D. Diseases of the prostate. *Clin Symposia* **41**(2):1989.

7. Resnick, M. *Prostatic Ultrasonography*. Philadelphia: BC Decker, 1990.

CHAPTER 7

TRANSVAGINAL SONOGRAPHY

Charles S. Odwin and Arthur C. Fleischer

Study Guide

INTRODUCTION

Transvaginal sonography involves the insertion of a specifically designed transducer into the vagina for imaging pelvic structures. Numerous names have been applied to this type of scanning, which can be confusing to students. Therefore, we will attempt to clarify these nomenclatures in the hope that students will easily understand the proper usage of terms used in transvaginal sonography and apply them appropriately.

The term *transvaginal* is a combination of Latin terms (L. *trans* through + *vagina* sheath), whereas the term *endovaginal* combines a Greek and a Latin term (Gr. *endon* within + L. *vagina* sheath). The terms *transvaginal* and *endovaginal* are both descriptive of the technical approach to scanning and are not specific for imaging of the vagina. In fact, only a small area of the vagina is imaged; the images are predominantly of the uterus and its adnexa.

The terms *endosonography* and *endocavity sonography* are general terms used to describe any introduction of the transducer into the body cavity: the vagina, rectum, or esophagus. Any introduction of a medical instrument into a body cavity is classified as an invasive procedure, unlike the term *transabdominal sonography,* in which the transducer is placed on the skin surface.

PHYSICAL CONCEPTS

The use of high-frequency transducers within the vaginal canal to image the uterus and its adnexa (ovaries, fallopian tubes, and ligaments) is founded on the basic concept of ultrasound physics. Placing the transducer in close proximity to the pelvic organs or structures allows the use of higher frequencies, which in turn provides better resolution, both axial and lateral. The resolution is not lost even in the presence of magnification resulting from a short focal zone.[1] The close proximity of the transducer also results in reduced attenuation and better focusing.

Thus, transvaginal sonography allows earlier and more definitive diagnoses than are possible with conventional transabdominal techniques.[4]

Applications. The applications of transvaginal sonography include

- diagnosing ectopic pregnancies
- monitoring the follicles of an infertile patient who is undergoing ovulation induction
- guiding the placement of the needle during follicular aspiration or aspiration of fluid from the cul-de-sac
- evaluating the fallopian tubes
- evaluating blood flow to the gestational sac and uterine arteries with Doppler imaging
- achieving additional diagnostic information in conjunction with transabdominal sonography
- evaluating the fetal intracranial anatomy and prolapse of the umbilical cord during the second and third trimester[2]
- detecting the presence of placenta previa[2]

Advantages. Transvaginal sonography has a variety of advantages. For example, because it offers high resolution (improved images), it allows earlier and more definitive diagnoses.[4] Unlike transabdominal sonography, the transvaginal procedure does not require a full bladder; thus, it eliminates patient discomfort. Because emergency patients can be evaluated quickly, the procedure allows faster medical management. Transvaginal sonography also has a high degree of acceptance—most patients prefer it to the transabdominal procedure. Finally, as was mentioned earlier, transvaginal sonography often provides valuable additional information when used in conjunction with transabdominal sonography.

Disadvantages. Transvaginal sonography also has several disadvantages. The limited field of view means that large masses may not be seen because they are beyond the focal zone of the transducer. For the same reason, the sonographer may be unable to document the uterine size. Because of the magnification in the near field, the sonographer may be unable to see both ovaries on the same image. The confined space of the vagina limits the mobility of the transducer.[1] Therefore, complete sequential and segmental images obtained with transabdominal sonography cannot be achieved with transvaginal sonography. In addition, only the presenting parts of the fetus and cervix can be seen in the second and third trimester pregnancy with the transvaginal approach.

Transducers. Transducers for transvaginal scanning have a specific size, shape, and frequency. Their diameter ranges from 12 mm to 16 mm; this smaller-than-usual diameter allows easy penetration within the vaginal lumen without causing the patient any discomfort. In addition, these transducers are twice as long as most transabdominal transducers. Because the normal length of the vaginal lumen is approximately 7.5 cm to 9.5 cm, the transvaginal transducer must be longer than usual so that part of it can be inserted and the other part can serve as a handle for the operator. The normal range of frequencies used in transvaginal sonography is 5–7.5 MHz, with a sector field of view of 90° to 115°. The larger the sector field of view, the larger the portion of the organ or structure that can be visualized.

Color Doppler. Transvaginal color Doppler is a combination of B-mode image, pulsed-wave Doppler, and a color flow display (triplex imaging).[5] The direction of blood flow is indicated by assigning color to the Doppler-shifted echoes superimposed on the gray-scale image. As was discussed in an earlier chapter, the direction of flow toward and away from the transducer is presented in different colors on the image. For example, red represents flow toward the transducer, blue represents flow away from the transducer, and a mixture of colors represents turbulent flow.

Color Doppler has two advantages. First, because a network of blood vessels occasionally can mimic follicles, color Doppler allows rapid differentiation between vascular structures and follicles. Second, it allows precise placement of the sample volume for Doppler waveform analysis.

PRECAUTIONARY MEASURES

The microorganisms that cause sexually transmitted disease, including the human immunodeficiency virus (HIV), are sometimes present in vaginal secretions. Although these microorganisms are usually transmitted through sexual contact with an infected partner, they can be transmitted by contaminated invasive medical instruments.[6,7]

Two methods are currently used to prevent transmission of infection with transvaginal transducers: (1) disinfection or sterilization of the transducer after each examination and (2) the use of disposable probe covers (condoms, rubber gloves, and sheaths). Both are required to prevent cross-infection from the transducer because, although the probe is covered, even a microscopic tear in the cover will expose the transducer to the vaginal membrane and the external cervical os. For the same reason, all vaginal transducers should be disinfected before they are returned to the manufacturer or technical support staff for maintenance or repair.

Disinfection or Sterilization

The first step in preparing the transvaginal transducer for an examination is disinfection or sterilization. Disinfecting agents destroy all disease-causing organisms except spores, whereas sterilizing agents, the most complete type of disinfectants, destroy all forms of microbial life—bacteria, viruses, fungi, and spores.[8]

Several methods of sterilization are available: autoclaves (steam or gas), ethylene oxide (cold gas), and chemical glutaraldehydes. The piezoelectric ceramic material of the transducer is heat sensitive. Therefore, steam autoclaves should not be used because excessive heat may depolarize the crystal in the transducer housing, thus eliminating its piezoelectric properties.

The cold-gas ethylene oxide method of sterilization, formerly used with ultrasound transducers, also is undesirable because it can take as long as 12 hours and is toxic to tissues.[9] Furthermore, a technique used to detoxify the transducer after sterilization typically requires an additional 8 hours.[9] The fact that the entire process of sterilization and detoxification with ethylene oxide takes at least 20 hours makes it an impractical procedure in a busy ultrasound department.

The use of chemical sterilizing solutions (eg, Cidex™, MetriCide™, Wavicide™, Cybact™) is the most practical method of sterilization. These high-level bactericidal, fungicidal, and virucidal agents are now used routinely to clean medical and surgical instruments (Table 7–1).[10] Some of them have gained significant acceptance for sterilizing transvaginal transducers because they can inactivate HIV-1 in just 60 seconds. These agents are available in the form of sprays, towelettes, and soak solutions. Some transducer manufacturers caution against immersing the transvaginal transducer in sterilizing solutions because these solutions could break the seal; the sprays and towelettes have gained considerable acceptance. The fact that transducers can now be disinfected in 10 minutes has resulted in increased productivity because they can be used more often.

Various less expensive chemicals also can inactivate HIV. For example, diluted household bleach (sodium hypochlorite) can inactivate HIV-1 in 1 minute and is recommended by the Centers for Disease Control. However, although all transvaginal transducers are composed of plastic, crystals, bonding material, and steel or some other metal, they are not necessarily constructed alike. Thus, a disinfecting or sterilizing agent may be safe for some transducers and be destructive to others (Table 7–2). For instance, bleach can destroy the bonding material and plastic of some transducer housings. Because this can

TABLE 7–1. HIGH-LEVEL DISINFECTANTS

Manufacturer	Brand Name	Microorganisms Affected
Wave Energy Systems	Wavicide™-01*	Herpes 1 and 2, HIV-1, cytomegalovirus, hepatitis B, *Candida albicans, Escherichia coli, Staphylococcus aureus, Streptococcus salivarius, Salmonella typhosa.*
Central Solutions	Pheno-Cen™ disinfectant spray*	*Salmonella choleraesuis, Trichophyton mentagrophytes, Staphylococcus aureus, Pseudomonas aeruginosa* HIV-1
Surgikos	Cidex Plus™ disinfectant solution* Cidex™ disinfectant solution*	Herpes 1 and 2, HIV-1, cytomegalovirus, adenovirus type 2, poliovirus type 1, rhinovirus, coxsackievirus B1, *B. subtilis, C. sporogenes*
Metrex Research Corp.	MetriCide™ 28 disinfectant solution* MetriCide™ disinfectant solution*	Herpes 1 and 2, HIV-1, cytomegalovirus, rhinovirus vaccinia, adenovirus, *T. mentagrophytes, Mycobacterium bovis, S. aureus, S. Choleraesuis*

*Registered with the Environmental Protection Agency as an inactivator of HIV-1 (AIDS virus).
Reprinted with permission, Odwin C, Fleischer A, Kepple DM, et al. Probe covers and disinfectants for transvaginal transducers. J. Diagn Med Sonogr 6:130–135, 1990.

cause the transducer to fail, bleach is not recommended by most transducer manufacturers. In other words, sonographers should not attempt to sterilize a transducer until they have carefully reviewed the manufacturer's instruction manual and have consulted with technical support staff regarding any changes that may have occurred since the manual was published.

While the transducer is being sterilized, the system should be turned off and the transducer should be disconnected from it to avoid an electric shock. The transducer scanning head (excluding the handle and cable connector) should then be placed in the sterilizing solution for 10 to 20 minutes, depending on the temperature of the solution and the product used. Immediately after sterilization, the transducer should be dried with a soft sterile cloth. Fig. 7–1 shows the method of immersing the ATL (Advanced

Technology Laboratories, Bothell, Washington) transvaginal transducer for sterilization. This method of immersion is specific for the ATL; other manufacturers may use different methods and sterilizing agents.

Transvaginal Probe Covers

Probe covers are specially designed sheaths for covering the transducers; they are available in different sizes in order to fit all types of transducers. These covers are made up of a variety of material; latex, polyethylene, and polyurethane and are approved by the U.S. Food and Drug Administration (FDA). Probe covers are also available in sterile or nonsterile packs and are accessible from vendors (Table 7–3). Condoms are Class II medical devices approved for sexual use to prevent pregnancy and sexually transmitted diseases, including HIV. Although obviously

TABLE 7–2. MANUFACTURERS' RECOMMENDATIONS FOR DISINFECTION OR STERILIZATION OF TRANSVAGINAL TRANSDUCERS

Manufacturer	Products	Precautionary Measures
Acuson	Cidex™, MetriCide™, ProClide™	Do not sterilize with ultraviolet light. Do not sterilize with gas or dry heat. Do not autoclave. Do not use chlorine bleach. Do not use iodine compounds to clean or wipe
Diasonics	Cidex™	Use bleach only in an emergency situation as bleach could damage the steel jacket.
Advanced Technology Laboratories (ATL)	Cidex™, Wavicide™	Immerse transducer tip only; do not immerse handle. Do not gas or heat sterilize. Do not allow solution to enter strain relief joint or tracking adjustment slot.
Siemens	Chlorhexidinegluconat (Hibitance™) Cidex™, Gigasept™	Follow the manufacturer's directions. Never use phenol or other organic-based solvents. Never use heat (steam) or cold gas (ethylene oxide).
Toshiba	(Hibitance™), 0.5%, hypochlorous sodium 0.1%, glutaraldehyde 2% (Cidex™)	Dilute bleach (1 part bleach per 10 parts water). After disinfecting, rinse with sterile water.

*Using any of the products against the manufacturer's instructions or precautionary measures could void the transducer warranty.
From Odwin C, Fleischer A, Kepple DM, et al. Probe covers and disinfectants for transvaginal transducers. J Diagn Med Sonogr 6:130–135, 1990.

Figure 7–1. The ATL transvaginal transducer immersed in a solution. This method of sterilization is specific for the ATL; other manufacturers may use different methods and solutions. (*Reprinted with permission from Advanced Technology Laboratories (ATL).*)

not designed for use as a probe cover, they are sometimes used for this purpose because they are immediately available and moderately priced.

Three types of over-the-counter condoms are available: latex (rubber), natural lamb (made from the cecum of the lamb intestine), and artificial (synthetic) skin. The latex dry condom with a plain end is the most suitable and frequently used condom for transducer probes. Under an electron microscope, the surface of latex condoms demonstrate no pores. This intact barrier prevents the transmission of all bacteria and viruses.[11] (Only latex condoms have been approved by the FDA for the prevention of HIV).

Electron microscopy reveals that natural lamb condoms have occasional pores that are small enough to prevent transmission of sperm and some bacteria but are more than 10 times the size of HIV and more than 25 times the size of the hepatitis B virus.[11] Therefore, although natural lamb condoms are much stronger than latex condoms, the FDA does not recommend them for the prevention of HIV or hepatitis B infections.[11,12]

Because a loose-fitting condom on a transducer increases the chances that it will slip off during scanning, the sonographer must be familiar with the size of the transvaginal probe. Although all condoms have a rim on their proximal end, most will need additional support, such as a small rubber band or an orthodontal band, to secure them to the transducer shaft.

Over-the-counter condoms have a shelf life of 5 years and a 4% failure rate caused by tearing. The failure rate may be higher when they are used as probe covers in transvaginal sonography and even higher if an inappropriate lubricant is used. Oil-based lubricants such as petroleum jelly, cold cream, baby oil, and mineral oil should be avoided because they tend to cause latex condoms to deteriorate. Water-soluble products such as K-Y jelly,™ Surgilube™, and aqueous gels are appropriate lubricants. (Because some aqueous gels can affect the mobility or mortality of sperm, they should not be used when examining a patient who is undergoing artificial insemination.) The lubricant is applied to the outside of the probe cover after the cover has been secured over the transducer probe.

A white powder (talc) that manufacturers apply to latex condoms during production to keep them from sticking together may contain an embryotoxic compound that will conflict with transvaginal egg retrieval or embryo transfer. (In addition, latex may cause vaginal irritation if a patient is allergic to it.) Talc-coated latex condoms or transducer sheaths can be used for nontraumatic transvaginal scanning during pregnancy because the cervical os is normally closed and direct contact with the ovaries and the embryo does not occur. If talc must be avoided, the sonographer should not attempt to rinse it off with saline, which causes stickiness. The best method is to use a talc-free nonembryotoxic polyurethane probe cover (eg CIV-Flex™) (see Table 7–3).

All health care workers involved in invasive procedures that expose them to vaginal secretions or excretions

TABLE 7–3. DISPOSABLE PROBE COVERS FOR TRANSVAGINAL TRANSDUCERS

Manufacturer	Brand	Talc	Precautions
CIVCO Medical Instruments 418 B Avenue, Drawer Q Kalona, IA 52247	Latex*	Yes†	Can be damaged by heat or light; store in dark, cool, dry place. Do not lubricate with petroleum-based products.
	Polyethylene*	No	
	CIV-Flex (polyurethane)*	No	Nonembryotoxic.
	Enviro-Flex (polyethylene)*	No	
Schmid Laboratories Little Falls, NJ 07424	Latex condom (Ramses™)	Yes†	Avoid prolonged storage at temperatures above 100°F; do not lubricate with oil-based lubricants. Can be damaged by heat or light.
Carter-Wallace New York, NY 10153	Latex condom (Trojans™)	Yes†	Avoid prolonged storage at temperatures above 100°F; do not lubricate with oil-based lubricants. Can be damaged by heat or light.

*Approved by the Food and Drug Administration for transducers.
†Minimal amount.

should wear latex gloves when doing a procedure or cleaning instruments. The probe cover and gloves should be treated as potentially infectious waste and be disposed of accordingly immediately after the transvaginal examination.

POSITION OF THE PATIENT AND THE EXAMINATION TABLE

During the transvaginal examination, the patient is placed in the lithotomy position for insertion of the transducer and for scanning. The probe can be inserted by the patient, the physician, or the sonographer. When the insertion is done by the patient, the physician or sonographer holds the transducer cable so that the patient cannot accidentally drop the device.

The ideal table is a gynecologic examination table that allows numerous pelvic tilt positions and has stirrups for the patient's heels. The table is placed in a slight Fowler's position (also called the reversed Trendelenburg position) (Fig. 7–2). Elevation of the thighs allows the transducer to be moved freely from side to side (the horizontal plane).[7] The gynecologic examination table allows free upward and downward movement of the transducer (the vertical plane) and the slight Fowler's position of the table allows pooling of the small amount of peritoneal fluid normally found to pool in the region of the cul-de-sac which allows better delineation of pelvic structures. (The Trendelenburg position should not be used because it drains away this fluid.) If a gynecologic examination table is unavailable, a flat examination table can be prepared by placing a cushion that is 15–20 cm thick under the patient's pelvis.[7]

SCANNING TECHNIQUES

Three transducer maneuvers are commonly used in transvaginal sonography: (1) in and out, (2) rotating, and (3) angling, or up and down and side to side (Fig. 7–3). All of these maneuvers are limited by the size of the vaginal

Figure 7–3. Scanning techniques: (**A**) in and out; (**B**) rotating motion; (**C**) angling motion. (*With permission from Advanced Technology Laboratories, Bothell, Washington.*)

lumen. Fig. 7–3A illustrates the in-and-out motion of the transducer used to achieve variation in the depth of the imaging from cervix to fundus. Imaging of the cervix is optimized by gradually withdrawing the probe into the midvagina.[13] Fig. 7–3B illustrates the rotating motion of the transducer for obtaining various degrees of semiaxial to semicoronal planes. And Fig. 7–3C illustrates the angling motion of the transducer within the vaginal canal. With this angulation, one can obtain images of the anterior and posterior cul-de-sac, and with side to side movements can obtain images of the adnexa.

Ovaries. The ovaries are normally situated anterior and medial to the internal iliac (hypogastric) vessels and can be recognized by their ovoid shape, their texture (Fig. 7–4), and the presence of graafian follicles. They are recognized more often in patients in the reproductive age group than in the postmenopausal age group.

Unlike transabdominal sonography, which allows the

Figure 7–2. Examination table in a slight Fowler's position with a 20° elevation. The patient is in the lithotomy position.

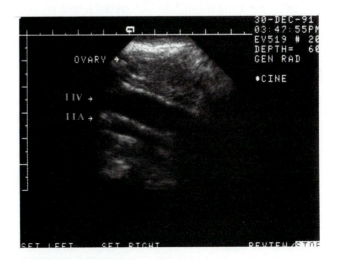

Figure 7–4. A demonstration of the ovary in close proximity to the internal iliac vein (IIV) and the internal iliac artery (IIA).

Figure 7–5 (**A**). A transvaginal transducer in the right lateral fornix; (B) a transvaginal transducer in the left lateral fornix. (*With permission from Advanced Technology Laboratories, Bothell, Washington.*)

simultaneous imaging of both ovaries relatively often, transvaginal sonography can best image only one ovary at a time. To image the right ovary, the sonographer moves the transducer handle toward the patient's left thigh so that the tip of the transducer probe is in the right lateral fornix (Fig. 7–5A). To image the left ovary, the sonographer moves the handle toward the patient's right thigh so that the tip of the probe is in the left lateral fornix (Fig. 7–5B). Although the ovaries can be depicted from almost any parauterine position, they are usually depicted either lateral to the uterus or in the cul-de-sac.

Uterus. Visualization of the texture and thickness of the uterine endometrium is greatly improved with transvaginal sonography. The appearance and thickness of the endometrium will vary, depending on the phase of the patient's menstrual cycle (Table 7–4).

Blood is supplied to the uterus from the uterine and ovarian arteries. The uterine artery gives rise to the arcuate arteries, which course within the outer myometrium (Fig. 7–6). Imaging of these vessels can be enhanced with triplex color vaginal sonography.

Because of the magnification and the relatively small field of view provided by transvaginal sonography, measurements that indicate the size of the uterus are obtained best with transabdominal sonography.

TABLE 7–4. ENDOMETRIAL THICKNESS

Menstrual Cycle	Measurements (mm)
Proliferative phase	4–8 mm in anteroposterior (including two layers)
Secretory phase	7–14 mm in anteroposterior (including two layers)
Postmenopausal	4–8 mm in anteroposterior (including two layers)
Postmenopausal hormone replacement therapy	6–10 mm in anteroposterior (including two layers)

Reprinted with permission from Fleischer A, Kepple D. Transvaginal Sonography: A Clinical Atlas. Philadelphia: JB Lippincott, 1992.

PREGNANCY

Pregnancy Test

A pregnancy test is a biochemical test of a woman's urine or serum to detect the presence of human chorionic gonadotropin (hCG). Although numerous tests are available, the radioimmune assay is specific for the beta subunit of hCG. Because of its specificity, reliability, and quantitative ability, this assay is the most acceptable one for ultrasonographic correlation. The values are reported in milli-international units per milliliter (mIU/mL), which can be reported in two different hCG levels[1]: International Reference Preparation (IRP) and Second International Standard (2nd IS). The level of hCG above which virtually all normal intrauterine pregnancy can be visualized with ultrasound is called a discriminatory zone. This zone will vary, depending on the type of transducer frequency and equipment used.[1] The level of serum beta hCG at which a 4 weeks' gestational sac can be depicted range from 420–800 mlU/mL (2nd IS) and 1,025–1,600 mlU/mL (IRP).[1,3]

Figure 7–6. The small arrows point to the arcuate arteries in the outer myometrium.

Embryonic Period

The embryonic period extends from about the second week of gestation to the end of the 8th week, at which point the fetal period begins. Table 7–5 is a chronology of embryonic and fetal development from the 4th to the 14th week of gestation.

Gestation Sac. Documentation of intrauterine pregnancy can be made as early as 4 weeks with transvaginal sonography by the identification of a gestational sac within the uterus. The gestational sac has an anechoic center with a highly echogenic ring that represents the decidual reaction. The anechoic center of the gestational sac represents fluid within the sac. The sac size is about 5 mm when first depicted.[3] The gestational sac increases in size as pregnancy advances. By 5 weeks of gestation, the secondary yolk sac can be depicted within the gestational sac measuring about 3 mm in size.

Yolk Sac. The yolk sac lies in the chorionic cavity (the extraembryonic coelom) between the amnion and chorion. Its functions are to (1) form blood cells (hemopoiesis), (2) give rise to sex cells (sperm or egg), (3) supply nutrients from the trophoblast to the embryo during the second and third week while the uteroplacental circulation is being established, and (4) become incorporated into the embryo as the primitive gut.

Sonographically, the yolk sac can be depicted from the 5th to the 10th week of gestation. The sac is connected to the midgut by a narrow stalk called the yolk stalk, the vitelline duct, or the omphalomesenteric duct. This stalk (or pedicle) detaches from the midgut by the end of the 6th week, and the dorsal part of the yolk sac is incorporated into the embryo as the primitive gut.

As pregnancy advances, the yolk sac shrinks and becomes solid and its pedicle becomes relatively longer. The pedicle may prevail throughout the pregnancy and be recognized on the fetal surface of the placenta near the attachment of the umbilical cord; this situation is extremely rare and has no significance. In about 2% of adults, the proximal portion of the yolk stalk persists as a diverticulum of the ileum called Meckel's diverticulum.[9]

Lacunae. The lacunae appear at about 5 weeks on one side of the gestational sac in the choriodecidua and represent the beginning of uteroplacental circulation (intervillous spaces). They do not completely circle the sac; they appear at one end of it in a semicircle.[3] Sonographically, they appear as small round hypoechoic structures that measure about 2–3 mm. Transvaginal color Doppler can demonstrate blood flow in these spaces.

Yolk Sac–Embryo Complex. At approximately 6 weeks of gestation, the crown-rump length of the embryo measures 3–4 mm and abuts the yolk sac. The upper limb buds appear first, followed by the lower limb buds at 7 weeks.[3] The heart beat also can be seen at this time.[3] Also at about 6 weeks, a portion of the embryonic midgut temporarily protrudes into the umbilical cord. This physiologic herniation of the midgut (or gut migration) occurs because the liver and kidneys occupy most of the abdominal space. When the midgut is in the umbilical cord, it rotates 90° counterclockwise around the axis of the superior mesenteric artery. At the 8th week of gestation, the sonographic appearance of the physiologic herniation of the midgut is a hyperechoic bulging of the cord near the point where it enters the fetal abdomen.

Brain. The brain develops from three primary vesicles: the prosencephalon (forebrain), from which the cerebral hemispheres are derived; the mesencephalon (midbrain), which becomes the brain stem; and the rhombencephalon (hindbrain), which becomes the cerebellum, the medulla oblongata, and the pons. During the 5th week of embryonic development the prosencephalon divides into the telencephalon (the paired cerebral vesicles) and the diencephalon (which connects the cerebral vesicles to the brain stem), and the rhombencephalon divides into the metencephalon (the cerebellum and the pons) and the myelencephalon (medulla oblongata). Although these brain vesicles seem to be cystic (see Fig. 7–7), their sonographic appearance is normal for the developing brain at 8 weeks of gestation and should not be confused with hydro-

TABLE 7–5. CHRONOLOGICAL CHART: TRANSVAGINAL OBSTETRICAL SONOGRAPHY

Length of Gestation	Observations
4 weeks	The gestational sac is first seen at this time. It measures 4–5 mm and is surrounded by decidua with an anechoic center. No embryo or yolk sac is depicted at this time.
5 weeks	The yolk sac is first seen and measures 3–4 mm. The lacunar structures can be seen on one side of the gestational sac, and blood flow from its spaces can be depicted with color Doppler.
6 weeks	The fetal pole can be seen measuring 2–4 mm and abutting the yolk sac (yolk sac/embryo complex). The heartbeats can be seen, and the crown-rump length can be measured.
7 weeks	The limb buds first appear, and the amnion membrane and chorionic cavity can be seen.[3]
8 weeks	Sonolucent brain vesicles and midgut herniation are seen.
9 weeks	The placenta and choroid plexus are seen.
10 weeks	The intraventricular heart septum is seen.
11 weeks	The umbilical cord is visible.
12 weeks	The extraembryonic coelom is obliterated, and the midgut herniation disappears.
13 weeks	The orbital structures are seen.
14 weeks	The four-chamber heart becomes visible.[3]

Figure 7–7. A transvaginal sonogram. The small arrows point to brain vesicles.

cephalus. The falx cerebri and choroid plexus are not sonographically evident at this time.

Fetal Period

The heart appears as a one-chambered structure until the 10th week; at 14 weeks, a view of the four-chambered heart can be obtained (Table 7–5). The midgut returns to the abdomen, where it undergoes a second rotation, which is 180° counterclockwise. Thus, the midgut undergoes a total rotation of 270°.[14] If the bowel fails to return to the abdomen during this second stage of rotation, an omphalocele may be the result. If development is normal, the herniation disappears completely after the 12th week and should not be confused with a defect of the abdominal wall.

REFERENCES

1. Goldstein SR. *Endovaginal Ultrasonography.* New York: Alan R Liss, 1988.

2. Rottem S. Scanning after the first trimester: Endovaginal ultrasound course. Syllabus. Spring Educational Meeting, Phoenix, AZ, by AIUM, April 9–10, 1989, pp. 33–35.

3. Timor-Tritsch IE, Rottem S. *Transvaginal Sonography,* 2nd ed. New York: Elsevier, 1991.

4. Sacks GA, Fleischer AC, Kepple DM, et al. Toshiba Medical Review: Clinical Applications of Transvaginal Sonography in Obstetrics and Gynecology. Toshiba Corp, Tokyo, No. 23, Feb 1988.

5. Kurjak A. *Transvaginal Color Doppler: A Comprehensive Guide to Transvaginal Color Doppler Sonography in OB/GYN.* Park Ridge, NJ: Parthenon, 1991.

6. Odwin C, Fleischer AC, Kepple DM, et al. Probe covers and disinfectants for transvaginal transducers. *J Diagn Med Sonography* **6**(3):130–135, 1990.

7. Axelrod D. *A Physician's Guide to Aids: Issue in the Medical Office.* Albany: New York State Department of Health, 1988.

8. Leach E. A new synergized glutaraldehyde-phenate sterilizing solution and concentrated disinfectant. *Infect Control* **2**:3–6, 1981.

9. Sigel B. *Operative Ultrasonography,* 2nd ed. New York: Raven Press, 1988.

10. Kennedy M. Evaluation of a glutaraldehyde-phenate solution used to disinfect endoscopes and instruments in a free-standing surgical facility. *JORRI* **111**(8), 1983.

11. Can you rely on condoms? *Consumer Rep* **45**:135–140, 1989.

12. Willis J. Precautions for Health Care Professionals. *FDA Drug Bill* **17**:16–17, 1987.

13. Fleischer AC, Kepple DM. *Transvaginal Sonography.* Philadelphia: JB Lippincott, 1992.

14. Moore KL. *The Developing Human: Clinically Oriented Embryology,* 3rd ed. Philadelphia: WB Saunders, 1982.

Questions

1. Fig. 7–8 is a transvaginal sonogram of a 23 year old
    woman with a uterus the size of a 10-week pregnancy
    and vaginal bleeding. The most likely diagnosis is

    (A) gestational trophoblastic disease
    (B) an incomplete abortion
    (C) a completed abortion
    (D) A or B

2. The level of β-hCG at which the gestational sac can
    first be depicted with transvaginal or transabdomi-
    nal sonography is referred to as

    (A) the discriminatory zone
    (B) qualitative assay levels
    (C) a radioimmunoassay
    (D) β level

3. The abnormal findings in the transvaginal sonogram
    of a 10-week pregnancy shown in Fig. 7–9 include

    (A) an ancephalic fetus
    (B) a two-headed fetus
    (C) a massive sacrococcygeal teratoma
    (D) none of the above

Figure 7–9. A transvaginal sonogram of a 10-week pregnancy.

4. Alpha-fetoprotein is elevated in

    (A) all types of neural tube defects
    (B) closed neural tube defects
    (C) neural tube defects occasionally associated with
        fetal regurgitation
    (D) none of the above

Figure 7–8. A transvaginal sonogram of the uterus.

Figure 7–10. A transvaginal sonogram of an 8-week pregnancy.

Figure 7–11. A transvaginal sonogram of an early pregnancy.

5. The thin rounded structure in the middle of the uterine lumen shown in the transvaginal sonogram in Fig. 7–10 is

(A) the hydropic yolk sac
(B) the amnion
(C) the chorion
(D) the placenta

6. Fusion of the amnion and chorion normally occurs between

(A) 3 and 5 weeks
(B) 5 and 8 weeks
(C) 8 and 10 weeks
(D) 14 and 16 weeks

7. The best estimate of gestational age in the transvaginal sonogram shown in Fig. 7–11 is

(A) 3 weeks
(B) 4 weeks

(C) 5 weeks
(D) 6 weeks

8. The "double bleb sign" refers to

(A) the amnion, embryo, and yolk sac
(B) hypoechoic areas behind the placenta
(C) the rhombencephalon and spinal cord of the developing embryo
(D) none of the above

9. Which of the following are true statements concerning the magnified transvaginal sonogram of an 8-week fetus shown in Fig. 7–12?

(A) physiologic herniation of the bowel is seen
(B) a yolk sac is seen
(C) the amnion is seen
(D) the rhombencephalon is seen
(E) all of the above are seen

10. The area outside of the amnion is called

(A) the chorionic cavity
(B) the amniotic cavity
(C) the extrafetal space
(D) none of the above

11. Fig. 7–13 is a combined real-time image and M-mode of a patient presenting with first trimester bleeding. This sonogram demonstrates that

(A) the embryo is living and has heart motion
(B) the embryo is dead
(C) only a clot is seen within the gestational sac
(D) none of the above

Figure 7–12. A magnified transvaginal sonogram of an 8-week pregnancy.

Figure 7–13. A combined real-time and M-mode image of a patient presenting with bleeding in the first trimester.

12. At what gestational age should fetal heart motion be detected on a transvaginal sonogram?

    (A) 4 weeks
    (B) 5 weeks
    (C) 6 weeks
    (D) 8 weeks

13. The following structures are depicted in the transvaginal sonogram of an 8-week embryo shown in Fig. 7–14.

    (A) the chorion, yolk sac, and amnion
    (B) the amnion, embryo, chorionic cavity, and lacunae
    (C) the embryo, yolk sac, and amnion
    (D) the yolk sac, embryo, and chorion

14. The embryonic period ends and fetal development begins at

    (A) 4–10 weeks
    (B) 7–8 weeks
    (C) 8–20 weeks
    (D) none of the above

15. Fig. 7–15 is a transvaginal sonogram of a 26-year-old woman who is 6-to-7 weeks pregnant. The yolk sac

    (A) has an important function in hematopoiesis
    (B) has an important function in the induction of neural tissue
    (C) has no known function
    (D) has the important function of producing yolk

16. The secondary yolk sac is located

    (A) outside of the amniotic cavity
    (B) within the amniotic cavity
    (C) within the embryo
    (D) none of the above

Figure 7–15. A transvaginal sonogram of a 6-to-7 week pregnancy.

17. Fig. 7–16 is a transvaginal sonogram of the left ovary in a patient undergoing ovulation induction with Pergonal®. The sonographic findings indicate that

    (A) multiple follicles have developed
    (B) there is hemorrhage within some of these follicles
    (C) there is ovarian torsion
    (D) A and B are present

18. Ovarian hyperstimulation syndrome typically occurs after

    (A) the patient is pregnant and has received human chorionic gonadotropin (hCG)
    (B) before the patient has received hCG
    (C) failed induction of ovulation
    (D) the patient has received intrauterine artificial insemination

Figure 7–14. A transvaginal sonogram of an embryo at 8 weeks.

Figure 7–16. A transvaginal sonogram of the left ovary.

Figure 7–17. A transvaginal sonogram of an infertile patient.

19. Fig. 7–17 is a transvaginal sonogram of an infertility patient. The abnormal sonographic findings include

 (A) an intramural leiomyoma
 (B) an endometrial carcinoma
 (C) a bicornuate uterus
 (D) none of the above

20. A submucous leiomyoma can be diagnosed by transvaginal sonography.

 (A) true
 (B) false

21. Fig. 7–18 is a transvaginal sonogram of the left adnexa. This patient's adnexa has

 (A) a cystic mass within the confines of the left ovary
 (B) a cystic mass that is separate from the left ovary
 (C) an ovary containing multiple immature follicles
 (D) fluid in the cul-de-sac

22. A paraovarian cyst arises

 (A) from the vestigial Gartner's duct
 (B) from the vestigial wolffian duct
 (C) within the mesovarium
 (D) A and C

23. The following abnormalities are detected in Fig. 7–19, a transvaginal sonogram in the coronal plane of the right adnexa.

 (A) a fusiform cystic structure
 (B) an ovarian cyst
 (C) a hydrosalpinx
 (D) A and C

24. A hydrosalpinx can be identified on transvaginal sonography by showing

 (A) its origin near the uterine cornua, as demonstrated by the endometrium
 (B) relatively thick folds
 (C) lack of ovarian tissue or stroma surrounding it
 (D) all of the above

25. Fig. 7–20 is a transvaginal sonogram in the uterus in a coronal plane. The following observations can be made.

 (A) the uterus is enlarged
 (B) the uterus apparently has two endometria, which indicate a bicornuate uterus
 (C) A and B
 (D) none of the above

26. Bicornuate uteri are the result of

 (A) abnormal fusion of the müllerian duct system
 (B) multiparity
 (C) A and B
 (D) none of the above

Figure 7–18. A transvaginal sonogram of the left adnexa.

Figure 7–19. A transvaginal sonogram of the right adnexa.

Figure 7–20. A transvaginal sonogram of the uterus.

27. The following findings are apparent in the transvaginal sonogram of the right ovary shown in Fig. 7–21.

    (A) the mass contained solid material that may be related to hemorrhage
    (B) the mass was either a tubo-ovarian abscess or an ovarian tumor such as mucinous cystadenoma
    (C) A and B
    (D) none of the above

28. In the differential diagnosis of corpora lutea, one also must consider

    (A) cystic tumors of the ovary
    (B) a hematosalpinx
    (C) endometriomas
    (D) all of the above

29. The position of the patient that enables free movement of the probe in the horizontal plane while performing transvaginal scanning is the

    (A) Trendelenburg position
    (B) lithotomy position
    (C) Sims' position
    (D) prone position

30. The position of the examination table for transvaginal sonography is

    (A) the Trendelenburg position
    (B) the lithotomy position
    (C) the Sims' position
    (D) the Fowler's position

31. When a gynecological examination table is *not* available for performing a transvaginal study, a regular flat examination table can be used if a foam cushion that is 15–20 cm thick is used to elevate the

    (A) pelvis
    (B) head
    (C) legs
    (D) knees

32. The range of transducer frequencies used in transvaginal sonography is

    (A) 3.5 to 5.0 MHz
    (B) 5.0 to 7.5 MHz
    (C) 2.5 to 3.5 MHz
    (D) none of the above

33. The most important prerequisite for transvaginal sonography is

    (A) emptying of the urinary bladder
    (B) adequate filling of the urinary bladder
    (C) putting the patient in the Trendelenburg position
    (D) selecting a low-frequency probe

34. Which of the following is *not* true for transvaginal sonography?
    (A) both ovaries are always seen simultaneously
    (B) an empty bladder is required before scanning
    (C) the ovaries are identified by the presence of follicles
    (D) a large mass can be missed

35. The most appropriate method of disinfecting the transvaginal probes from organisms, including the AIDS virus, is

    (A) diluted household bleach
    (B) ethylene oxide
    (C) an autoclave
    (D) a glutaraldehyde-based agent

RT OVARY

Figure 7–21. A transvaginal sonogram of the right ovary.

36. Transvaginal sonography detects the embryological structures about

    (A) 5 weeks earlier than does transabdominal sonography
    (B) 1 week earlier than does transabdominal sonography
    (C) 2 weeks earlier than does transabdominal sonography
    (D) the same time as does transabdominal sonography

37. The diameter of a mature graafian follicle ranges from

    (A) 3–5 mm
    (B) 10–12 mm
    (C) 18–24 mm
    (D) 24–30 mm

38. On transvaginal sonography, the embryo is seen within the amniotic cavity and the secondary yolk sac is normally depicted within

    (A) the amniotic cavity
    (B) the extraembryonic coelom
    (C) the trophoblast
    (D) the umbilical cord

39. The level of β-human chorionic gonadotropin required to depict the gestational sac with transvaginal sonography is approximately

    (A) 3600 mIU/mL 2nd IS
    (B) 6500 mIU/mL IRP
    (C) 1800 mIU/mL 2nd IS
    (D) 1000 mIU/mL IRP

40. Preparation for a transvaginal study does *not* require

    (A) application of a probe cover
    (B) disinfecting of the probe
    (C) emptying of the bladder
    (D) a vaginal douche, antibiotic therapy, or both before the probe is inserted.

41. A fully distended bladder in a patient undergoing transvaginal sonography will

    (A) occupy most of the image and displace organs of interest out of the focal range
    (B) increase the focal range, allowing better image enhancement
    (C) allow better visualization of pelvic organs
    (D) produce low attenuation, resulting in reduced magnification

42. The transvaginal probe should be covered with a protective sheath before vaginal insertion. All of the following are recommended for this purpose except

    (A) latex condoms
    (B) lamb condoms
    (C) latex gloves
    (D) CIV-Flex™ probe covers

43. Which one of the following lubricants should *not* be used on latex probe covers?

    (A) K-Y jelly™
    (B) a coupling gel
    (C) a water-based gel
    (D) petroleum jelly

44. The examination table is tilted for transvaginal sonography to

    (A) drain fluid out of and away from the cul-de-sac
    (B) push the bowel cephalad out of the true pelvic cavity
    (C) increase filling of the bladder to delineate the pelvic structures better
    (D) pool intraperitoneal fluid into the cul-de-sac to outline pelvic organs better

45. What position should the patient be placed in for transvaginal sonography?

    (A) the Sims' position
    (B) the knee-chest position
    (C) the lithotomy position with a slight Trendelenburg tilt
    (D) the lithotomy position with a slight Fowler's tilt

46. The major limitation of transvaginal sonography is that

    (A) it can be used only in the first trimester
    (B) its field of view is limited
    (C) it can be used only to evaluate an ectopic pregnancy
    (D) it can be used only to evaluate follicles

47. The ideal examination table for transvaginal sonography is a

    (A) gynecologic examination table with a variable pelvic tilt and stirrups
    (B) x-ray table with Trendelenburg tilt and safety straps
    (C) a stretcher with side rails
    (D) flat immobile examination table

48. The use of a high-frequency transvaginal transducer results in

    (A) less penetration, more magnification, and better resolution
    (B) more penetration, less resolution, and less magnification
    (C) greater penetration, more magnification, and better resolution
    (D) no change

49. Transvaginal sonography is useful for evaluating all of the following except

  (A) an ectopic pregnancy
  (B) intrauterine growth retardation
  (C) a third-trimester pregnancy
  (D) a placenta previa

50. The acceptance rate among patients for transvaginal verses transabdominal sonography is

  (A) 5%
  (B) 20–35%
  (C) 50–60%
  (D) 82–93%

51. The small cystic space in the posterior cranium seen on transvaginal sonography during the 8th-to-10th week of gestation is most likely

  (A) the rhombencephalon
  (B) mild hydrocephalus
  (C) a Dandy Walker cyst
  (D) the choroid plexus

52. The echogenic bulging of the umbilical cord seen with transvaginal sonography near the abdominal insertion at about the 8th-to-10th week of gestation is most likely to represent

  (A) a gastroschisis
  (B) physiologic herniation of the midgut
  (C) the yolk sac
  (D) omphalocele

53. Transvaginal sonography can depict the fetal heart before a clear sonographic depiction of the embryo can be obtained

  (A) by putting the M-mode cursor on the gestational sac
  (B) by putting the M-mode cursor at the periphery of the yolk sac
  (C) by putting the M-mode cursor on the trophoblast
  (D) only if the embryo is at least sonographically evident

54. Which one of the following is *not* true of the urinary bladder with transvaginal sonography?

  (A) the wall of the bladder cannot be identified when the bladder is nearly empty
  (B) the nearly empty bladder can be on the right of the screen
  (C) the nearly empty bladder can be on the left of the screen
  (D) the nearly empty bladder may be in the true anatomic position

55. The hypoechoic parallel linear lines in the outer myometrium seen on transvaginal sonography represent

  (A) arcuate vessels
  (B) the external iliac vein
  (C) the external iliac artery
  (D) the internal iliac vein

56. The vascular web seen on transvaginal sonography near the lateral border of the cervix represents

  (A) arcuate vessels
  (B) uterine veins and arteries
  (C) the external iliac artery
  (D) the internal iliac vein

57. The round hypoechoic structures seen surrounding one region of the choriodecidua represent

  (A) arcuate vessels
  (B) lacunae
  (C) the yolk sac
  (D) the internal iliac vein

58. Which of the following is *not* true of transvaginal sonography (TVS) in the second and third trimesters?

  (A) TVS is more precise in locating the placenta than is transabdominal sonography
  (B) TVS can be helpful in evaluating prolapse of the umbilical cord and the intracranial anatomy
  (C) transvaginal color Doppler can be used to detect abnormal patterns of blood flow
  (D) TVS is useful in the first trimester
  (E) all of the above are true

59. Identify the structure the arrow points to in Fig. 7–22.

  (A) the yolk sac
  (B) the embryo
  (C) the umbilical cord
  (D) the yolk stalk

Figure 7–22. A transvaginal sonogram of an early pregnancy.

Figure 7–23. A transvaginal sonogram of an early pregnancy.

Figure 7–25. A transvaginal sonogram of the adnexa.

60. Color transvaginal Doppler sonography uses intensities that are greater than those involved in pulsed-wave Doppler.

(A) true
(B) false

61. Identify the structure the arrow points to in Fig. 7–23.

(A) the rhombencephalon
(B) the hydrocephalon
(C) the yolk sac
(D) the chorion

62. Identify the structure the arrow points to in Fig. 7–24.

(A) the ovarian vein
(B) a dermoid cyst

(C) a follicular cyst
(D) an ectopic pregnancy

63. Identify the structure the closed arrow head points to in Fig. 7–25.

(A) the internal iliac vein
(B) the internal iliac artery
(C) the ovarian artery
(D) the ovarian vein

64. Identify the structure the open arrow head points to in Fig. 7–25.

(A) the internal iliac vein
(B) the internal iliac artery
(C) the ovarian artery
(D) the ovarian vein

Figure 7–24. A transvaginal sonogram of the adnexa.

Figure 7–26. A transverse scan of the uterus.

65. Identify the structure the arrow heads point to in Fig. 7–26, a transverse scan of the uterus.

(A) the internal iliac vein
(B) the internal iliac artery
(C) the arcuate artery
(D) the azygos vein

66. Identify the structure the arrow heads point to in the transverse scan of the uterus depicted in Fig. 7–27.

(A) a double decuida
(B) the internal iliac artery
(C) lacunae
(D) the yolk sac

Figure 7–27. A transverse scan of the uterus.

Answers and Explanations

1. **(D)** A or B. Echogenic tissue within the uterine lumen can be the result of either an incomplete abortion or early trophoblastic disease. Vesicles do not form until approximately 12 weeks. Therefore, in the early stages of trophoblastic disease, the tissue appears as echogenic intraluminal material. *(8:95)*

2. **(A)** The discriminatory zone. The level of β-hCG at which the gestational sac can first be depicted with transvaginal or transabdominal sonography is referred to as the "discriminatory" zone of human chorionic gonadotropin. *(5:39–41)*

3. **(B)** A two-headed fetus. This sonogram shows a two-headed fetus that has a single pair of arms and legs. *(8:65)*

4. **(C)** Neural tube defects occasionally associated with fetal regurgitation. α-fetoprotein is elevated when there is a break in the skin, blood in the amniotic fluid or with a variety of disorders associated with neural tube defects, cystic hygroma, placental abnormalities, and fetal regurgitation. Closed neural tube defects such as closed spina bifida usually do not elevate α-fetoprotein. *(8:130)*

5. **(B)** The amnion. *(8:63)*

6. **(D)** 14 and 16 weeks. The amnion and chorion usually fuse during this period. *(8:125)*

7. **(D)** 6 weeks. This is the best estimate because there is an embryo, a yolk sac, and an amnion "double bleb sign." *(10:75)*

8. **(A)** The amnion, embryo, and yolk sac. The "double bleb sign" refers to seeing these three indicators and is best seen at approximately 6 weeks of gestation. *(10:75)*

9. **(E)** All of the above are seen. *(10:75)*

10. **(A)** The chorionic cavity. This area has developed from the extraembryonic coelom. *(10:75)*

11. **(A)** The embryo is living and has heart motion. Transvaginal sonography can reliably detect heart motion in living embryos at 6 weeks. *(10:25)*

12. **(B)** 6 weeks. *(8:40; 9:79)*

13. **(B)** The chorion, yolk sac, and amnion. The hypoechoic areas around outside of the developing amnion is called the chorionic cavity, which has developed from the extraembryonic coelom. The developing placenta represents blood lakes or lacunae. *(8:40)*

14. **(B)** 7–8 weeks. The embryonic period extends from the 4th to the 8th week. All major organs and systems are formed (organogenesis) during this period. After this embryonic period, the embryo is called a fetus. *(11:71–72)*

15. **(A)** Has an important function in hematopoiesis. This transvaginal sonogram demonstrates a 6–7 week embryo with a secondary yolk sac that is located outside of the amniotic cavity. The yolk sac produces blood elements for the embryo. *(8:67)*

16. **(A)** Outside of the amniotic cavity. The secondary sac lies between the amnion and chorion. *(10:75)*

17. **(D)** A and B are present. This transvaginal sonogram demonstrates an enlarged ovary that contains multiple follicles, some of which contain hemorrhage. The ovaries in these patients typically include numerous follicles. *(8:144)*

18. **(A)** The patient is pregnant and has received human chorionic gonadotropin. Ovarian hyperstimulation syndrome usually occurs after hCG is given. *(8:329)*

19. **(A)** An intramural leiomyoma. This transvaginal sonogram demonstrates an intramural leiomyoma that apparently does not involve the endometrial surface. In some infertile patients, a leiomyoma may distort the endometrial lining, therefore contributing to infertility. *(8:40)*

20. **(A)** True. A submucous leiomyoma is difficult to delineate with transabdominal sonography. It is diagnosed best with transvaginal sonography. *(8:272,306)*

21. **(B)** A cystic mass that is separate from the left ovary. The differential diagnosis includes a paraovarian or peritoneal cyst. *(8:40)*

22. **(D)** From A and C. A variety of masses do not arise directly from the uterus or ovaries. For example, paraovarian cysts arise from the vestigial Gartner's duct in the mesovarium. *(8:263)*

23. **(D)** A and C. This sonogram demonstrates the typical appearance of a hydrosalpinx, which appears as a fusiform cystic structure arising from the area of the uterine cornua and has a rounded shape in its distal aspect. *(8:40)*

24. **(D)** All of the above. Hydrosalpinx usually appears as a fusiform structure that is separate from the ovary. It can be identified by the lack of ovarian tissue surrounding it. *(1:322,328)*

25. **(C)** A and B. This transvaginal sonogram demonstrates two endometrial lumina in bicornuate or septate uteri. *(8:40)*

26. **(A)** Abnormal fusion of the müllerian duct system. Bicornuate uteri are the result of fusion abnormalities of the two tissue elements that form the uterus from the müllerian duct system. *(8:40)*

27. **(C)** A and B. This sonogram demonstrates an area of increased echogenicity within a predominantly cystic ovarian mass. This pattern is most likely to be seen in hemorrhagic corpora lutea, but it can also be seen in mucinous cystadenomas, tubo-ovarian abscesses, endometriomas, and dermoid cysts. *(8:264)*

28. **(D)** All of the above. (See the explanation of the answer to question 27.) *(8:264)*

29. **(B)** The lithotomy position. The elevated thighs in the lithotomy position allows free movements of the probe from side to side (horizontal plane). *(8:15)*

30. **(D)** The Fowler's position. The patient should be lying in the lithotomy position with the examination table in the Fowler's position (reverse Trendelenburg). The patient should *not* be placed in the Trendelenburg's position because it will drain the normal amount of fluid from the cul-de-sac that is used to outline structures. *(8:15)*

31. **(A)** Pelvis. A thick foam cushion under the pelvis allows free up-and-down movements of the probe (vertical plane). *(8:15)*

32. **(B)** 5 to 7.5 MHz. Transvaginal transducers range in frequency from 5 to 7.5 MHz. *(4:22)*

33. **(A)** Emptying of the urinary bladder. This is important because a filled bladder takes up most of the image, displacing adnexal structures out of the image. In addition, it contributes to unnecessary patient discomfort. *(2:15)*

34. **(A)** Both ovaries are always seen simultaneously. Transvaginal sonography can best demonstrate only one ovary at a time because of image magnification and the small focal area. *(1:59–65)*

35. **(D)** A glutaraldehyde-based agent. The most recent and practical method of sterilization is a glutaraldehyde-based chemical disinfectant. Diluted household bleach is effective in inactivating HIV-1 on environmental surfaces, but it could be destructive to the bonding material and plastic of some transducers. Glutaraldehyde-based chemical disinfectants are bactericidal, fungicidal, and virucidal and are effective in inactivating HIV-1 on environmental surfaces. *(3:131)*

36. **(B)** 1 week earlier than does transabdominal sonography. Transvaginal sonography detects the embryologic structures about a week earlier on the average. *(1:107)*

37. **(C)** 18–24 mm. *(1:143)*

38. **(B)** The extraembryonic coelom. The secondary yolk sac (the definitive yolk sac) lies in the chorionic cavity between the amnion and chorion. The chorionic cavity also is called the extraembryonic coelom. The extraembryonic coelom forms the primary yolk sac, which decreases in size and the secondary yolk sac develops. *(1:93; 4:22–27)*

39. **(D)** 1000 mIU/mL IRP. There are two different methods of reporting hCG. The International Reference Preparation (IRP) and the 2nd International Standards (2nd IS). The 2nd IS is approximately 50% of the IRP. The gestational sac can be depicted when the serum β hCG is 1,000 mIU/mL (IRP) or 500 mIU/mL (2nd IS). *(4:17)*

40. **(D)** A vaginal douche, antibiotic therapy, or both before the probe is inserted. This is not required because the transducer is normally disinfected and covered before the insertion. *(3:130–135)*

41. **(A)** Occupy most of the image and displace organs of interest out of the focal range. *(1:16)*

42. **(B)** Lamb condoms. Natural lamb condoms, when viewed under the electron microscope, show tiny pores

that are larger than the HIV or hepatitis B virus and may permit its transmission.   *(3:130–135)*

43. **(D)** Petroleum jelly. The type of lubricants recommended for latex condoms are water-based products such as K-Y jelly™ and ultrasound coupling gel. Petroleum jelly or oil-based products can cause deterioration of the latex that results in fracture.   *(3:130–135)*

44. **(D)** Pool intraperitoneal fluid into the cul-de-sac to outline pelvic organs better.   *(1:15)*

45. **(D)** The lithotomy position with a slight Fowler's tilt. A slight Fowler's tilt is also called the reverse Trendelenburg position.   *(2:15)*

46. **(B)** Its field of view is limited. Transvaginal sonography can also be used in the second and third trimesters as well as the first trimester.   *(2:16; 4:59)*

47. **(A)** Gynecologic examination table with a variable pelvic tilt and stirrups.   *(2:15)*

48. **(A)** Less penetration, more magnification, and better resolution.   *(5:5)*

49. **(B)** Intrauterine growth retardation. Transvaginal sonography is unable to do the multiparameter measurements needed to assess either intrauterine growth retardation or a complete obstetrical survey because the focal zone is small. Furthermore, because the transducer also is limited to the confinement of the vagina, a sectional survey cannot be obtained.   *(5:5–22)*

50. **(D)** 82–93%.   *(4:4)*

51. **(A)** The rhombencephalon. The small cystic space in the posterior cranium seen on transvaginal sonography during the 8th-to-10th week of gestation is the hindbrain (rhombencephalon)   *(4:16)*

52. **(B)** Physiologic herniation of the midgut. The normal migration of the midgut into the umbilical cord occurs during the 6th-to-10th week. The normal physiologic midgut herniation is seen on transvaginal sonography as an echogenic bulging of the cord and should not be confused with an omphalocele.   *(5:70)*

53. **(B)** By putting the M-mode cursor at the periphery of the yolk sac. The yolk sac is normally seen before the embryo at about 5 week's gestation. The yolk sac is larger than the embryo at this time; later it becomes smaller than the embryo. Abutting the yolk sac is the embryological disk, which is too small to be depicted. If the M-mode is placed at the edge of the yolk sac at approximately 5½-to-6 weeks, the heart-

beats can be depicted, not from the yolk sac, but from the adjacent but not-yet-apparent embryo. The heartbeats occur at 35 to 36 days menstrual age.   *(4:14, 30)*

54. **(A)** The wall of the urinary bladder can be identified even though the bladder is nearly empty. The position of the bladder can be to the right or left of its normal anatomic position or be in its normal position.   *(6:5)*

55. **(A)** Arcuate vessels.   *(1:37)*

56. **(B)** Uterine veins and arteries.   *(1:32)*

57. **(B)** Lacunae. These are seen surrounding one region of the choriodecidua in early pregnancy.   *(1:90)*

58. **(E)** All of the above. Transvaginal sonography is used in the second and third trimesters for a more precise location of the placenta in relation to the internal os, presentation of the cord, and blood flow.   *(6:35)*

59. **(D)** The yolk stalk.   *(1:93)*

60. **(A)** True. The intensities used in color Doppler are much lower than those in duplex Doppler.   *(7:52)*

61. **(A)** The rhombencephalon.   *(10:75)*

62. **(C)** A follicular cyst.   *(8:40)*

63. **(B)** The internal iliac artery.   *(1:22)*

64. **(A)** The internal iliac vein.   *(1:22)*

65. **(C)** The arcuate artery. The arrow is pointing to the arcuate artery in the myometrium.   *(1:37)*

66. **(C)** Lacunae.   *(1:37)*

REFERENCES

1. Timor-Tritsch IE, Rottem S. *Transvaginal Sonography*, and ed. New York: Elsevier, 1991.
2. Sacks GA, Fleischer AC, Kepple DM. Toshiba Medical Review: Clinical Applications of Transvaginal Sonography in Obstetrics and Gynecology. Toshiba Corp, Tokyo, No. 23:15–24, Feb 1988.
3. Odwin C, Fleischer A, Kepple DM, et al. Probe covers and disinfectants for transvaginal transducers. *J Diagn Med Sonography* 6(3): 130–135, 1990.
4. Transvaginal Sonography. *Semin Ultrasound CT MR*, Philadelphia: WB Saunders, 11(1): 1990.
5. Goldstein SR. *Endovaginal Ultrasound*. New York: Alan R Liss, 1988.
6. Rottem S. Scanning after the first trimester: Endo-

vaginal ultrasound course. Syllabus. Spring Educational Meeting. Phoenix, AZ, by AIUM, April 9–19, 1989, pp 33–35.

7. Fleischer AC, Rao B, Kepple DM. Transvaginal color Doppler sonography: preliminary experience. *Dyn Cardiovas Imaging* **3:** 52–58, 1990.

8. Fleischer A, James AE Jr. *Diagnostic Sonography: Principles and Clinical Applications*. Philadelphia: WB Saunders, 1988.

9. Pennell RG, Baltarowich OH, Kurtz AB, et al. Complicated first-trimester pregnancy: evaluation with endovaginal US versus transvaginal technique. *Radiology* **165:**79–83, 1987.

10. Bree RL, Edwards M, Bohn-Velez M, et al. Transvaginal sonography in the evaluation of normal early pregnancy: correlation with hCG level. *AJR* **153:** 75–79, 1989.

11. Langman J. *Medical Embryology,* 4th ed. Baltimore, MD: Williams & Wilkins, 1981.

CHAPTER 8

OB/GYN SONOGRAPHY

*Charles S. Odwin, Arthur C. Fleischer, Dale R. Cyr,
and Pamela M. Foy*

Study Guide

ANATOMY OF THE FEMALE REPRODUCTIVE SYSTEM

Uterus

The uterus is a pear-shaped muscular organ located in a median position in the pelvic cavity between the urinary bladder and the rectum. Its functions are (1) menstruation, (2) pregnancy, and (3) labor.

The uterus consists of three anatomic subdivisions: (1) fundus, (2) corpus (body), and (3) cervix. The isthmus uteri is the slightly constricted region of the uterus between the body and the cervix (Fig. 8–1), and it is of special significance in sonography as it helps to identify the region of the internal os of the cervix. The walls of the uterus are made up of three layers: (1) endometrium (mucosal), (2) myometrium, and (3) serosa (peritoneum). The echotexture of the uterine myometrium is normally homogeneous, whereas the echotexture of the endometrium varies with the phase of the menstrual cycle.

Cul-de-Sac

The peritoneum covering the posterior wall of the uterus and cervix reflecting on the rectum forms a deep pouch called the posterior cul-de-sac (retrouterine pouch) or the pouch of Douglas. Anteriorly, the peritoneum reflected at the level of the isthmus uteri over the urinary bladder form a shallow pouch called the anterior cul-de-sac, or vesicouterine pouch. Sonographically, the posterior cul-de-sac may become distended with fluid because of a ruptured ovarian cyst, a ruptured ectopic pregnancy, ascites, or an abscess.

Fallopian Tubes

The fallopian tubes (oviducts) extend laterally from the superior lateral angle of the uterus to the ovaries and have four anatomic subdivisions: (1) interstitial, (2) isthmus, (3) ampulla, and (4) infundibulum (Fig. 8–1). The functions of the fallopian tubes are in fertilization and aiding in the transport of the ova from the ovaries.

Ovaries and Adnexa

The ovaries are solid ovoid structures measuring 3 cm by 2 cm by 1 cm. They are located, one on each side of the uterus, in a shallow depression called Waldeyer's fossa. Their functions are in (1) ovulation and (2) secretion of hormones.

Sonographically, the ovaries are adjacent to the internal iliac vessels. In the reproductive years, the presence of follicles helps to identify the ovaries. After menopause, the ovaries are more difficult to identify because of their reduced size and the absence of follicles. The adnexa are any accessory parts or structures that are lateral to the uterus. The ovaries, fallopian tubes, and broad ligaments are adnexal structures. A cystic mass or tumor also can be adnexal if it is within the region described.

Blood Supply

The uterus receives its blood supply from the uterine and ovarian arteries, which are branches of the internal iliac (hypogastric) arteries. The branches of the uterine arteries that penetrate the myometrium and travel parallel to the outer surface are called arcuate arteries.[8] These arcuate vessels are demonstrated sonographically as parallel anechoic linear structures in the outer myometrium (Fig. 8–2).

Size

The size and shape of the uterus vary according to the patient's age and parity. Before puberty and after menopause, the uterus is normally small in size, whereas an increase in the number of children born usually results in an increase in size.[1,2] The normal size of the adult uterus in women who have never been pregnant is approximately 7.5 cm long, 3 cm thick, and 5 cm wide. The size of the uterus in women who have had multiple pregnancies varies from 8 to 10 cm in length.

In an elderly woman, the uterus atrophies. Therefore, a uterus that is 9 cm or more long would be abnormal for a

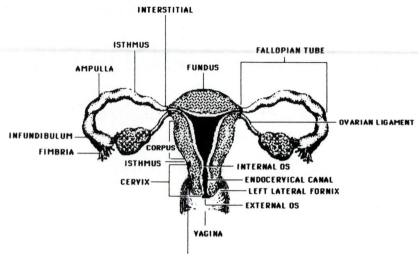

Figure 8–1. Diagram of the female reproductive organs (frontal view).

woman who is 65 years old. Sonographic measurements of the uterus should be correlated with the patient's age and parity to predict uterine enlargement. The two most common causes for uterine enlargement are pregnancy and fibroids.

Uterine Positions

The position of the uterus changes depending on the degree of bladder distention. The uterus is normally located in a anteverted position in 90% of women, forming an angle of 90° between the long axis of the vagina and the long axis of the uterine cavity.[3] The uterus can be in any one of the following positions:

- anteverted: the uterus tilts forward without a sharp angle between the corpus and cervix
- retroverted: the uterus tilts backward without a sharp angle between the corpus and cervix

Figure 8–2. Transvaginal sonogram of the uterus. Arrows point to arcuate vessels.

- anteflexion: the uterine corpus is bent forward on the cervix, resulting in a sharp angle at the point of bending
- retroflexion: the uterine corpus is bent backward on the cervix, resulting in a sharp angle at the point of bending
- medianus: midline position
- dextroversion: right lateral deviation
- levoversion: left lateral deviation

The difference between the retroverted and retroflexion positions is the degree of bending. In the retroflexed uterus, the corpus bends backward on the cervix at the level of the isthmus uteri and causes a sharp angle at the point of bending; in the retroverted position, the uterus bends backward without changing the relationship of the corpus to cervix.[3]

Congenital abnormalities of the uterus such as uterine duplication and malformation result from improper fusion or incomplete development of the paramesonephric ducts (müllerian ducts). These various types of congenital uterine abnormalities, which are demonstrated in (Fig. 8–3), occur often in association with renal anomalies.[5] Although it is difficult to distinguish between a bicornuate and a septate uterus on sonograms, identification of two endometrial cavities is helpful in identifying the bicornuate uterus. These cavities are demonstrated best on transverse scans.

Urinary Bladder

The urinary bladder is a hollow muscular organ that is located behind the symphysis pubis. The floor of the bladder consists of a triangular area called the trigone. There are three openings in each angle: two orifices for the ureters, which convey urine to the bladder from the kidneys, and one urethral orifice, through which urine is expelled from the body. The bladder serves as a reservoir for urine and helps the urethra expel urine.

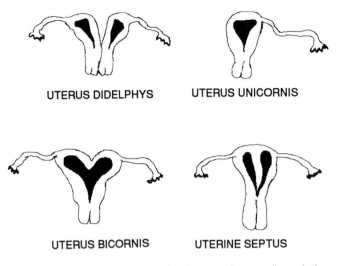

UTERUS DIDELPHYS   UTERUS UNICORNIS

UTERUS BICORNIS   UTERINE SEPTUS

Figure 8–3. Diagram showing developmental anomalies of the uterus.

Figure 8–4. Sonogram of the urinary bladder with ureteral jet (arrow).

Bladder Distention. During a transabdominal sonographic examination of the pelvis, the urinary bladder must be distended for a variety of reasons. The reasons are the urine-filled bladder pushes the bowel cephalad out of the true pelvic cavity, it pushes the uterus cephalad away from the symphysis pubis, it permits rapid anatomic orientation, it provides a low-attenuation pathway to which ultrasound can propagate, and it helps to elevate the head of the fetus for easy measurements. Whereas a distended bladder is an extremely important prerequisite for a transabdominal study, an empty bladder is the most important prerequisite for a transvaginal study. The failure to fill the bladder adequately for transabdominal studies can result in serious diagnostic errors. On the other hand, an overdistended bladder can also result in errors.

When the bladder is being filled, urine can be observed entering the bladder on real-time and has been referred to as the "ureteral jets."[4] The jets begin at the ureteral orifices and flow toward the center of the bladder (Fig. 8–4).

Bladder Contour. Sonographically, the position and shape of the uterus have an effect on the urinary bladder. If the uterus is anteverted, the normally distended bladder has a mild indentation on its posterocephalad region. If the uterus is surgically removed or absent, the bladder has a different contour. Therefore, bladder contour depends on the shape and position of its surrounding structures.

PELVIC MASSES

A variety of pelvic masses can be depicted sonographically: solid, complex, and cystic. Tables 8–1, 8–2, and 8–3

describe the clinical and sonographic findings for the three types of masses.

OBSTETRIC HISTORY

Recording

Recording of the patient's obstetric history often provides the key to an accurate sonographic diagnosis. The sonographer has an opportunity to listen to the patient's complaints of illness during scanning and, on some occasions, may obtain information that the patient has not shared with her referring physician or radiologist. Because the sonographer-patient relationship can be of value in gathering information, the sonographer's basic knowledge of the patient's clinical history is essential.

Terminology

The term *gravidity* refers to the total number of pregnancies. A woman who has never been pregnant is called a nulligravida. A gravida is a pregnant woman, a primigravida is a woman who is pregnant for the first time, and a multigravida is a woman who has been pregnant several times.

The term *gravida* followed by an Arabic or roman numeral refers to the total number of previous pregnancies. For example, gravida 4 (IV) represents four pregnancies. The patient's past obstetric history also can be displayed in a series of four digits. For example, in the number 5235, the first digit refers to the number of full-term births, the second digit refers to the number of premature births, the third digit refers to the number of abortions, and the fourth digit refers to the number of children currently alive.[1]

TABLE 8–1. SOLID PELVIC MASSES

Mass	Type	Clinical Findings	Sonographic Findings
Leiomyoma, myoma, fibromyoma, fibroid	Solid	A benign tumor of the smooth muscle of the uterus. Growth is stimulated by estrogen. *submucous*—beneath the endometrium *interstitial*—in the muscular wall *subserous*—beneath the serosa May undergo softening and degeneration during pregnancy. Symptoms: pain and bleeding	Enlarged uterus (small in postmenopausal women) Irregular in contour (lobular or nodular) Inhomogeneous texture Calcifications Displacement of the uterus Degeneration (cystic changes) Poor ultrasonic penetration (attenuation)
Leiomyosarcoma	Solid	A malignant fibroid tumor with accelerated growth. Symptoms: pain and bleeding	Simular sonographic features as leiomyoma Indistinguishable from benign myoma
Dysgerminoma	Solid	A malignant germ cell tumor of the ovary that usually occurs in the second and third decades	Predominately solid with hypoechoic internal echoes
Adenomyosis	Solid	Benign invasion of the uterine musculature by the endometrium. Symptoms: dysfunctional uterine bleeding and dysmenorrhea	Endometrial echo complex Symmetrical uterine enlargement
Endometrial carcinoma	Solid	Malignant tumor most common after menopause; abnormal uterine bleeding	Thickening endometrial echo greater than 10 mm in width.[5] Irregular and inhomogeneous endometrial texture

Used with permission from Fleischer A, James E. Diagnostic Sonography: Principles and Clinical Applications. Philadelphia: WB Saunders, 1989.

PREGNANCY

Pregnancy Test

As was mentioned in an earlier chapter, levels of human chorionic gonadotropin (hCG) are reported in terms of two common standards: the International Reference Preparation (IRP) and the Second International Standard (2nd IS). The 2nd IS is approximately half the value of the IRP.

Human chorionic gonadotropin is first detectable about 10 days after conception and is considered to be positive at levels of 30 mIU/mL IRP.[7]

The level of hCG above which virtually all normal intrauterine pregnancies can be visualized with ultrasound is called the discriminatory zone. A normal rise of hCG (an average of 66% every 48 hours, or double every

TABLE 8–2. COMPLEX PELVIC MASSES

Mass	Type	Clinical Findings	Sonographic Findings
Endometrosis	Complex	Ectopic endometrial tissue, the tissue bleeds during menses, producing hemorrhagic masses called endometriomas or chocolate cysts because of the dark-brown blood inside the cysts. Pain and infertility.	Multiple cystic adnexal masses with thick wall and low-level internal echoes. Small echogenic lesions posterior to the uterus
Benign cystic teratoma (dermoid cyst)	Complex	Most common benign germ cell tumor filled with material: bone, fat, hair, skin, teeth. More common among young women in the reproductive age group	Fluid-fluid levels Distal acoustic shadow Calcifications Tip of the iceberg sign[6]
Serous cystadenoma	Complex	Benign ovarian neoplasm, usually unilateral	Large cystic mass Usually unilocular The presence of ascites is indicative of serous cystadenocarcinoma
Mucinous cystadenoma	Complex	Multilocular, most common among postmenopausal women. Rupture may cause pseudomyxoma peritonei	Large multiseptated mass The presence of ascites is indicative of mucinous cystadenocarcinoma
Tubo-ovarian abscess	Complex	Masses containing inflammatory fluid or pus within the tube and ovaries	Fluid-fluid levels Hydrosalpinges Cystic mass with low level echoes

Used with permission from Fleischer A, James E. Diagnostic Sonography: Principles and Clinical Applications. Philadelphia: WB Saunders, 1989.

TABLE 8–3. CYSTIC PELVIC MASSES

Mass	Type	Clinical Findings	Sonographic Findings
Corpus luteum cyst	Cyst	Associated with pregnancy	Unilocular May contain low-level internal echoes Normally regress before the 16th week of pregnancy
Theca lutein cyst	Cyst	Associated with hydatidiform mole. Multilocular and bilateral	Multiseptated cystic mass
Polycystic ovaries (Stein-Leventhal syndrome)	Cyst	A build-up of follicles, with bilateral enlargement and a thick outer covering of the ovaries preventing overlation. Symptoms: oligomenorrhea, hirsutism obesity.[3]	Bilateral enlarge ovaries Multiple small cysts
Nabothian cyst	Cyst	Retention cyst formed in the cervix due to occlusion of the cervical gland	Small cystic mass in the cervix; can be multiple
Gartner's duct cyst	Cyst	Cyst formed at the lower ends of the primitive mesonephric tubules, generally located on the anterolateral vaginal walls.[7]	Small cystic mass in the vagina
Follicular cyst	Cyst	Functional cyst, regresses spontaneously. Development and growth due to hormones	Change in size during the menstrual cycle Small thin-wall unilocular cyst Fluid in the cul-de-sac (follicular spill) Focal internal echo (cumulus oophorus)

Used with permission from Fleischer A, James E. Diagnostic Sonography: Principles and Clinical Applications. Philadelphia: WB Saunders, 1989.

72 hours) is indicative of an intrauterine pregnancy; a falling hCG level is indicative of a nonviable intrauterine pregnancy or an ectopic pregnancy.[7]

The qualitative level of the serum β subunit of hCG should be correlated with the sonographic findings for a more accurate diagnosis.

Duration

The duration of a pregnancy can be calculated from the first day of the last normal menstrual period and is referred to as menstrual age. The average duration of a pregnancy is about 280 days, 40 weeks, 9 calendar months, or 10 lunar months. The expected date of delivery can be estimated by Nägele's rule, which is based on a 28-day menstrual cycle:

- identify the date when the last menstrual period began
- add 7 days
- subtract 3 months
- add 1 year

Development of the Embryo and Fetus

As a pregnancy progresses, the progressive enlargement of the uterus can be followed by examining the fundal height (Fig. 8–5). At 16 weeks' gestation, the fundus is palpable midway between the symphysis and the umbilicus and reaches the umbilicus at 20–22 weeks. Transabdominal sonography can depict the gestational sac at a menstrual age of approximately 5 weeks. The chronologic development of the embryo and fetus during a pregnancy is described in Table 8–4. At 5 weeks of gestation, the yolk sac and embryo are not visible sonographically with the transabdominal approach and appear to be completely so-

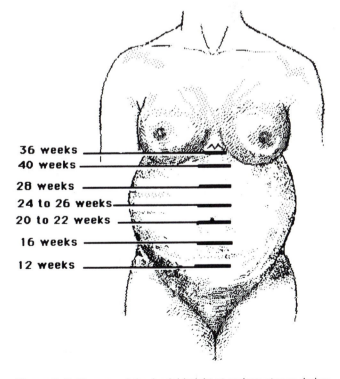

36 weeks
40 weeks
28 weeks
24 to 26 weeks
20 to 22 weeks
16 weeks
12 weeks

Figure 8–5. Diagram of the fundal height at various stages during pregnancy.

TABLE 8–4. CHRONOLOGICAL DEVELOPMENT OF THE EMBRYO AND FETUS

Gestational Age	Description	Developments
5 weeks	Average sac dimension = 1 cm	The sac is anechoic and surrounded by a thick "rind" of echoes. The sac is completely anechoic as echoes from the embryo are not yet visible. Sac size for gestational age can be performed.
6 weeks	Average sac dimension = 2 cm	Embryo appears, movements can be seen. Heart motion may be seen. CRL can be performed.
7 weeks	Average sac dimension = 4 cm	The embryo is about 10 mm. The heart motion can be seen. The yolk sac and umbilical stalk can be depicted.
8 weeks	Average sac dimension = 5 cm	Organogenesis is completed and the embryo is now called a fetus, which measures about 2 cm in length.
9 weeks	Average sac dimension = 6 cm	The fetus now measures about 3 cm in length. The placenta becomes recognizable.
10 weeks	Average sac dimension = 7 cm	The fetus now measures about 4 cm.
11 weeks		The fetus now measures about 5 cm. The yolk sac and umbilical stalk begin to disappear.
12 weeks		The fetus now measures about 6 cm. BPD can be obtained. End of first trimester. The decidua capsularis adheres to the decidua parietalis.
13–19 weeks	The fetus is extremely active and may change position several times during the ultrasound examination	The femur length, abdominal circumference, and BPD can be measured. The circumference of the head is greater than the abdominal circumference.
20–30 weeks	The fetus is extremely active and may change position several times during the ultrasound examination	Fetal abdominal wall defects and adrenal gland can be seen.
30–40 weeks	The fetus is less active and may not change its position during the examination.	Fetal head and body are equal in ratio from 32 to 36 weeks. Epiphyseal ossification is visible in the distal femur at 33 weeks.

Abbreviations: CRL, crown rump length; BPD, biparietal diameter.
The gestation sac grows about 1 cm a week, from the 5th week to the 10th week. The BPD can be done from 12 to 40 weeks, most accurate from 14 to 20 weeks. The CRL can be done from 6 to 12 weeks, most accurate from 8 to 12 weeks.
A rule of thumb for calculating the CRL is: CRL (cm) + 6.5 = gestational age in weeks

nolucent at this time. However, the gestational sac can be distinguished from blood in the uterine cavity by identifying the two decidua (the endometrium of pregnancy). The double decidua comprise the decidua capsularis (inner ring), which is the decidua overlying the gestational sac, and the decidua parietalis (outer ring), which is the decidua along the remainder of the uterine cavity. As the gestational sac enlarges, the unoccupied space between the two layers of decidua disappears and the double decidua are no longer apparent. The decidua basalis is the thick decidua beneath the implantation site (Fig. 8–6A).

The yolk sac–embryo appears at a menstrual age of

Figure 8–6. (A) Diagram of early pregnancy; **(B)** diagram of the fetal crown-rump length (the crown is the topmost part of an organ or structure, the rump is the buttocks, and the length is the long axis).

about 6 weeks, at which time the yolk sac is larger than the embryo. As the pregnancy advances, however, the embryo becomes larger than the yolk sac. The yolk sac lies in the chorionic cavity between the amnion and chorion. At about 10 to 12 weeks of menstrual age, the yolk sac shrinks, the amnion and chorion fuse, and the yolk sac is no longer visible.

OBSTETRIC ANOMALIES

A variety of obstetric anomalies can be depicted sonographically. The sonographic characteristics and features of these anomalies are described in Table 8–5.

Ectopic Pregnancy

Ectopic pregnancy denotes any pregnancy located outside the endometrial lumen. The term *ectopic* is a broad term used to describe any organ, structure, or pregnancy that is located away from its normal position; for example, an ectopic kidney or spleen. Ectopic pregnancy includes pregnancy located in the fallopian tubes, ovaries, or cervical

canal. A pregnancy may be ectopic and yet be situated within the uterus.

The sonographic appearances of an ectopic pregnancy are multiple and depend on location, position, and whether it is ruptured or not. Some of these findings include (1) an enlarged empty uterus, (2) a ringlike adnexal mass, and (3) fluid in the cul-de-sac or subhepatic space. The possibility of coexistent intrauterine and ectopic pregnancy can occur but is a rare finding (reported to be between 1 in 2,000 to 1 in 30,000 deliveries).[31]

Blighted Ovum and Missed Abortion

A blighted ovum is a fertilized ovum that has become arrested. The gestational sac is without an embryo. The sonographic findings are: (1) failure of the gestational sac to grow normally, (2) a large gestational sac (3 cm) without an embryo, (3) a fluid-fluid level within the gestational sac, and (4) absent or irregular choriodecidual reaction.

A missed, or incomplete, abortion is defined as a dead embryo retained in the uterus before the 20th week of gestation. The sonographic findings are (1) no fetal heart

TABLE 8–5. OBSTETRICAL ANOMALIES

Anomalies	Characteristics	Sonographic Features
Anencephaly	Absence of the cranial vault and cerebral hemispheres. Predominantly occurs in female fetuses and is associated with spinal defects.	Hydramnios (polyhydramnios) Visible face with protruding eyes, giving a froglike appearance Absence of the cranial vault and inability to identify normal brain structures.
Acephalus	Fetus without a head	Complete absence of the head. Hydramnios (polyhydramnios)
Spina bifida	Midline bony defect of the vertebrae. Most common location is the posterior arches in the lumbosacral region. Characterized by elevated α-fetoprotein	A "horseshoe" or U-shaped spine on transverse scan, which provides a more reliable depiction than does a longitudinal scan Associated with hydrocephalus "banana sign" and "lemon sign"[30]
Meningomyelocele	Herniation of part of the spinal cord and meninges through a defect in the vertebral column. Most common in the lumbosacral region. Levels of alpha-fetoprotein are elevated.[9]	Hydramnios (polyhydramnios). Associated with hydrocephalus
Cephalocele	Protrusion of the meninges and brain through a bony defect of the skull. Elevated level of α-fetoprotein	Hydramnios (polyhydramnios). Associated with hydrocephalus, microcephaly
Ectopia cordis[9]	Ectopic fetal heart	Ectopic position of the fetal heart with real-time cardiac activity. Thoracic wall defect
Pentalogy of Cantrell[30]	1. Supraumbilical abdominal defect 2. Defect of the lower sternum 3. Deficiency of the diaphragmatic pericardium 4. Deficiency of the anterior diaphragm 5. Intracardiac abnormality	Hydramnios (polyhydramnios). Anterior wall defect. Fetal cardiac abnormality.
Omphalocele	Anterior wall defect with herniation of the abdominal contents; liver, spleen and bowel at the base of the umbilical cord. Covered with a membrane[7]	Hydramnios (polyhydramnios). Anterior wall defect. Unable to identify cord insertion Mass in amniotic fluid
Gastroschisis	Anterior wall defect with herniation of the abdominal contents; bowel to the right of midline with normal insertion of the umbilical cord. No membrane covering	Hydramnios (polyhydramnios) Anterior wall defect Bowel in amniotic fluid

Derived from Fleischer AC, Romero R, Manning FA, et al. The Principles and Practice of Ultrasonography in Obstetrics and Gynecology, 4th ed. Norwalk, Connecticut: Appleton & Lange, 1991.

motion on real-time, (2) reduced amniotic fluid, and (3) disorganized echoes in the uterine cavity.

Fetal Demise

Fetal demise is defined as death of the developing fetus after 20 weeks of gestation. The clinical and sonographic signs for fetal demise are numerous. The sonographic signs can be divided into specific and nonspecific.[29] The specific signs are (1) the failure to find the fetal heart tones on Doppler examination, (2) no fetal cardiac pulsation on M-mode, and (3) no movements or fetal heart pulsation seen on real-time sonography. The nonspecific signs are

- overlapping of the fetal sutures (Spalding's sign)
- hydramnios or oligohydramnios
- flattened (oblong) fetal head
- absence of the falx cerebri
- distorted fetal anatomy
- decrease in the biparietal diameter when measurements are repeated from one week to the next
- decrease in the size of the uterus
- edematous soft tissue around the head (the "halo" sign or Druel's sign)
- fragmentation of the fetal skin
- diffuse edema of the entire fetus (anasarca)
- separation of the amnion from the chorion after 20 weeks
- gas in the fetal circulatory system (Robert's sign)
- hydropic swelling of the placenta

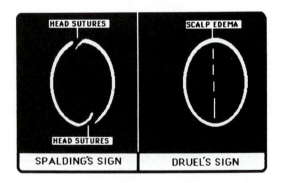

SPALDING'S SIGN   DRUEL'S SIGN

The clinical and laboratory findings of fetal demise are the failure of the uterus to grow, two negative pregnancy tests (serum beta hCG), no fetal movement, no heart sounds on auscultation, and red or brown amniotic fluid.

Amniotic Fluid Anomalies

The volume of amniotic fluid normally increases until the 34th week of gestation, then decreases as the pregnancy approaches term. The function of this fluid is to protect the fetus against possible injury and to regulate the fetal body temperature.[30] The fluid is produced by the kidneys, skin, and umbilical cord.[30]

The fetus normally swallows the amniotic fluid during pregnancy; therefore, if fetal swallowing is impaired,

the amount of amniotic fluid can change.[1] An excessive amount of amniotic fluid is called hydramnios or polyhydramnios; a reduction in the normal amount of fluid is called oligohydramnios.

Hydramnios. A wide variety of maternal and fetal conditions are associated with hydramnios. The mnemonic MOTHER'S HOUSE serves as a memory key for 12 conditions associated with hydramnios.

- M meningomyelocele
- O omphalocele
- T twin–twin transfusion
- H hydrocephaly
- E erythroblastosis fetalis
- R retroperitoneal fibrosis
- S sacrococcygeal teratoma
- H hydrops fetalis
- O obstructive gastrointestinal anomalies
- U urethral stenosis
- S spina bifida
- E esophageal atresia

Oligohydramnios. The conditions associated with oligohydramnios are (1) fetal demise, (2) renal agenesis, (3) intrauterine growth retardation, (4) premature rupture of membranes, and (5) postmaturity. The mnemonic DRIPP serves as a key for memorizing the five conditions associated with oligohydramnios:

- D demise
- R renal agenesis
- I intrauterine growth retardation
- P premature rupture of membranes
- P postmaturity

Abnormal Presentation and Lie

The term *presentation* refers to the part of the fetus lying in closest proximity to the birth canal. The fetus can present in one of three presentations: cephalic, breech, and shoulder. Cephalic presentations are classified according to the degree of flexion or extension of the fetal head and represent about 96% of term deliveries.[1]

Cephalic presentations are (1) vertex, (2) face, and (3) brow. The terms *cephalic* and *vertex* are sometimes used incorrectly. The word *cephalic* is descriptive of the fetal head as the presenting part without being specific to what region of the head, whereas *vertex* is specifically descriptive of the region of the fetal head between the anterior and posterior fontanelles as the presenting part.

There are three types of breech presentations: (1) complete, (2) frank, and (3) footling (single or double footling) and represent only about 4% of term deliveries.[1]

The term *lie* refers to the relation of the long axis of the fetus to the long axis of the mother. There are three types of lie: (1) longitudinal, (2) transverse, and (3) oblique.

FETAL ECHOCARDIOGRAPHY

Fetal echocardiography has become an integral part of obstetric sonography. Sonographic examination of the in utero human heart can diagnose congenital heart disease, which may alter clinical care. The sonographer is obligated to perform a basic fetal heart survey on every fetal sonogram. The following sections outline the basics of fetal echocardiography, not only the American Registry of Diagnostic Medical Sonographers Examinations but for the sonographer who is performing obstetric sonography.

Fetal Anatomy and Cardiac Circulation

The complex development and transformation of the fetal heart is completed by the sixth week of gestation, and fetal cardiac circulation remains anatomically constant until birth. It is important to recognize that the fetal heart acts in unison as far as cardiac outputs are concerned, but left and right heart circulations differ in the parts of the fetus they perfuse. This section outlines crucial knowledge about the intracardiac anatomy and hemodynamics of the normal fetus. The fetal heart receives blood from the hepatic veins and ductus venosus of the fetal liver that ascend within the inferior vena cava and enter the right atrium. Once the blood approaches and actually enters the right atrium, the eustachian valve directs the flow of blood across the right atrium and toward the interatrial septum. The eustachian valve arises at the inferior vena cava or right atrial border of the inferior vena cava and is in direct communication with the lower edge of the septum secundum of the interatrial septum (the crista dividens). The eustachian valve–crista dividens complex directs approximately 60% of the highly oxygenated blood from the interior vena cava toward the atrial septum. The eustachian valve also reduces regurgitant flow during ventricular systole. Once the highly oxygenated blood from the inferior vena cava is channeled to the interatrial septum, the blood then continues through the septum via the hole in the atrial septum called the foramen ovale.

The foramen ovale allows highly oxygenated blood to enter the left atrium; consequently, the left heart circulation. No other normal in utero intracardiac pathways allow highly oxygenated blood to enter the left heart. The remaining volume of the blood pool in the inferior vena cava remains in the right atrium and mixes with blood entering the right atrium from the superior vena cava.

The blood in the right atrium that is not as oxygenated as the blood in the inferior vena cava traverses the tricuspid valve during diastole and enters the right ventricle. During systole, the tricuspid valve closes, and the ventricular blood volume is ejected through the outflow tract of the right ventricle and main pulmonary artery. Once the blood is in the main pulmonary artery, it can travel in two different pathways. Ninety percent of the blood continues in the artery and enters the ductus arteriosus, which acts as a shunt directing blood away from the traditional pulmonary circulation into the descending aorta for systemic circulation of the highly oxygenated blood. The remaining 10% of the blood in the main pulmonary artery enters the right and left pulmonary arteries that perfuse the nonfunctioning lungs of the fetus and returns to the left atrium through the pulmonary veins.

The left atrium is filled by pulmonary venous return and the highly oxygenated blood from the inferior vena cava. During diastole, the left atrial volume is emptied into the left ventricle through the mitral valve. The left ventricular volume passes through the left ventricular outflow tract during systole and continues through the aortic valve. At this point, the blood volume is distributed through the aortic arch and its cranial vessels, essentially supplying the cephalic aspect of the fetus (Fig. 8–7).[10,11]

The situation just described depicts the individualism of the circulation in the left and right hearts. The right heart largely perfuses the fetal body, whereas the left heart provides oxygenated blood to the fetal brain. Once the fetus is born, the thoracic pressures decrease and cardiac blood flows to the lungs, dramatically increasing the volume of the now-functioning lungs. These changes occur secondarily to the closing of the foramen ovale because of increased left heart pressures and closure of the ductus arteriosus, which becomes the ligamentum arteriosus and forces more pulmonary blood flow. At this point, the unique fetal cardiopulmonary circulation assumes the traditional circulatory pattern of the human.

Sonographic Anatomy and Techniques

The ability of the fetal echocardiogram to visualize normal or abnormal cardiac structures depends on the sonographer's knowledge and skill. The sonographer must have some understanding of traditional echocardiographic techniques because many of the multiple views potentially used in fetal echocardiography are identical to those used in adult and pediatric echocardiography.

The first step when observing the fetal heart is to orient oneself to the fetal anatomy. Determining the fetal lie and the location of the spine is essential because it

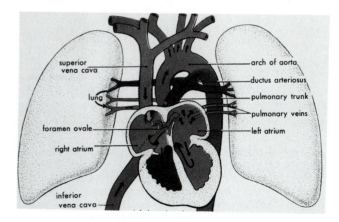

Figure 8–7. Schematic drawing demonstrating fetal cardiac circulatory system. (*Reproduced with permission from Moore KL, The Developing Human: Clinically Oriented Embryology, 4th ed, Philadelphia: WB Saunders, 1988, p. 326.*)

allows the sonographer to identify the left, right, cranial, caudal, dorsal, and ventral aspects of the fetus and the fetal heart.

Sonographic Views

Four-Chamber View. The fetal heart lies within the thorax in a horizontal plane that is perpendicular to the spine. Thus, the most important echocardiographic view, the four-chamber view, can be obtained with relative ease. The four-chamber view is obtained by imaging the fetal thorax in a transverse plane. Both atria, both ventricles, the atrioventricular valves (mitral and tricuspid), the atrial and ventricular septa, the moderator band, and the foramen ovale can be visualized in this view (Fig. 8–8).

Once the four-chamber view is imaged, orienting oneself to the anatomy of the fetal heart is crucially important. This is accomplished by visualizing the foramen ovale, which appears as a flap arising from the atrial septum and moving in and out of the left atrium. Because blood flows right to left through the foramen ovale, the flap of the foramen can only be within the left atrium. Occasionally, the foramen ovale cannot be visualized; in such cases, the sonographer relies on identification of the right ventricular moderator band. This band runs from the interventricular septum to the lower free wall of the right ventricle and can be seen within the apex of the right ventricle. These two parts of the intracardiac anatomy allow the sonographer to have a left-right cardiac orientation, which is essential for proper identification of normal or possibly abnormal structure. Valvular atresias, hypoplastic chambers, and septal defects can be identified from the four-chamber view.

Five-Chamber View. Additional cardiac anatomy can be visualized from the four-chamber view using subtle anterior angulation in relation to the fetal heart; this produces the five-chamber view (Fig. 8–9). The five-chamber view not only demonstrates the four chambers previously seen but also adds the left ventricular outflow tract and the proximal aortic root in relation to the ventricular septum. Further anterior angulation demonstrates the main pulmonary artery and the pulmonary valve arising from the right ventricle (Fig. 8–10). Thus, the five-chamber view orients the sonographer to the position of the great vessels in relation to the left and right ventricles.

Short-Axis View. Another important view that sonographers should be aware of is the short-axis view. To obtain this fetal echocardiographic view, the fetus must be imaged in a sagittal plane; consequently, the fetal heart is imaged in its transverse axis. The sonographer can sweep the entire heart, from its apexes to the aortic pulmonary window (Fig. 8–11), potentially demonstrating septal defects, hypoplastic chambers, and anomalies in the orientation of the great vessels.[12–16]

Fortunately, the sonographer does not need to be an expert in fetal echocardiography to see abnormalities on

A

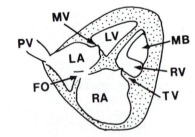

B

Figure 8–8. (A) Sonogram demonstrating the four chamber view: LA is the left atrium, RA is the right atrium, LV is the left ventricle, RV is the right ventricle (arrow), the arrowhead points to the moderator band, and the open foramen ovale (open arrowhead); **(B)** schematic diagram demonstrating a four-chamber view: FO is the foramen ovale, MB is the moderator band, TV is the tricuspid valve, and MV is the mitral valve. (*Reproduced with permission from Cyr DR, et al, A systematic approach to fetal echocardiography using real time/ two dimensional sonography. J Ultrasound Med 5:343–350, 1986.*)

Figure 8–9. Sonogram demonstrating five-chamber view: AO is the aorta, LV is the left ventricle, S is the ventricular septum, RV is the right ventricle, and the arrow points to the left atrium.

Figure 8–10. Sonogram demonstrating pulmonary artery from the five-chamber view: PA is the pulmonary artery (the arrow points to pulmonary valve), RV is the right ventricle, S is the ventricular septum, and LV is the left ventricle.

any given obstetrical sonogram. Recent studies have shown that 96% of fetal cardiac malformations, proved neonatally or pathologically, have been seen on the four-chamber view.[17,18] Therefore, the sonographer only needs to be proficient at obtaining the four- and five-chamber views to rule out the overwhelming majority of cardiac defects.

Other Views. Although they are beyond the scope of this chapter and will not be described in detail, several other fetal echocardiographic planes can be used to evaluate the fetal heart. These are the long-axis, aortic arch (suprasternal), right ventricular inflow, and right atrial inflow views. Table 8–6 demonstrates congenital abnormalities that can be identified sonographically, given the echocardiographic plane.[13]

M-MODE

Using M-mode in conjunction with two-dimensional imaging is essential in performing fetal echocardiograms. M-mode should be used to calculate heart rate (atrial or ventricular), measure the size of the atria and ventricles, or determine the type of cardiac arrythmia that is present.[22] Typical arrythmias that are diagnosed prenatally are premature atrial contractions, premature ventricular contractions, supraventricular tachycardias, and heart block. It is extremely important to evaluate both the atria and the ventricles with M-mode if this modality is to be used properly within the fetus.[19–21,23,24]

DOPPLER

Doppler plays a limited role in routine fetal echocardiography. The use of duplex sonography and color flow imaging is indicated only if congenital heart disease is suspected. Once a heart lesion is suspected, Doppler imaging helps distinguish abnormal flow patterns from dysplastic valves, abnormal great vessels, and septal defects. If Doppler is used in fetal echocardiography to aid in a diagnosis, it must be performed by experienced personnel.[12,24–28]

A

B

Figure 8–11. **(A)** Transverse sonogram in the short-axis view at the apical level: RV is the right ventricle, S is the ventricular septum, and LV is the left ventricle; **(B)** short axis view at the aortic-pulmonic window: A is the aorta (in transverse axis) and P is the main pulmonary artery.

TABLE 8–6. CONGENITAL CARDIOVASCULAR ANOMALIES DETECTABLE IN STANDARD ECHOCARDIOGRAPHIC VIEWS

Four-chamber anomalies

A hypoplastic ventricle (consider dilatation of the other ventricle)
Atresia of the mitral or tricuspid valve
A large atrial septal defect
A large ventricular septal defect
A-V canal (endocardial cushion defect)
Ebstein's anomaly
Pericardial and pleural effusions (hydrops)

Five-chamber anomalies (with aortic root)

Transposition of the great arteries
Aortic atresia

Long-axis left ventricle

Mitral stenosis or atresia
Aortic stenosis or atresia
Hypoplastic left ventricle
Cardiomyopathies (particularly endocardial fibroelastosis)
Pericardial effusion

Right ventricle inflow

Tricuspid atresia
Hypoplastic right ventricle
Ebstein's anomaly

Short-axis aortic level

Aortic stenosis or atresia
Pulmonic stenosis or atresia
Tricuspid atresia
Ebstein's anomaly
Large atrial septal defect
Large membranous ventricular septal defect
Ductus arteriosus (normal in fetus)
Truncus arteriosus
Transposition great arteries

Short-axis ventricles

Hypoplasia or dilatation either ventricle
Cardiomyopathy
Large muscular septal defect (including single ventricle)

Right atrial inflow

Tricuspid atresia
Ebstein's anomaly
Absent inferior vena cava (azygos continuation)

Suprasternal (aortic arch)

Coarctation
Interrupted arch
Underdeveloped pulmonary arteries (eg tetralogy of Fallot)

Reproduced with permission from Cyr DR, et al. J Ultrasound Med 5:343–350, 1986.

REFERENCES

1. Cunningham FG, MacDonald PC, Gant NF. *Williams Obstetrics,* 18th ed. New York: Appleton & Lange, 1989.

2. Danforth DN, Dignam WJ, Hendricks CH, et al. *Obstetrics and Gynecology,* 3rd ed. New York: Harper & Row, 1977.

3. Netter FH, Oppenheimer E, Rock J. *The Ciba Collection of Medical Illustrations: Reproductive Systems,* vol. 2, 4th ed, Summit, NJ: Ciba Pharmaceutical, 1965.

4. Mittelstaedt C, Lawrence V. *Abdominal Ultrasound.* New York: Churchill Livingstone, 1987.

5. Fleischer A, James E. *Diagnostic Sonography: Principles and Clinical Applications.* Philadelphia: WB Saunders, 1989.

6. Sabbagha R. *Diagnostic Ultrasound: Application to OB/GYN,* 2nd ed. Philadelphia: JB Lippincott, 1987.

7. Goldstein S. *Endovaginal Ultrasound.* New York: Alan R Liss, 1988.

8. Callen PW. *Ultrasonography in OB/GYN,* 2nd ed. Philadelphia: WB Saunders, 1983.

9. Romero R, Pilu G, Jenty P, et al. *Prenatal Diagnosis of Congenital Anomalies.* Norwalk, CT: Appleton & Lange, 1988.

10. Kleinman CS, Copel JA, Weinstein EM, et al. Treatment of fetal supraventricular tachyarrhythmias. *J Clin Ultrasound* **13**:265–273, 1985.

11. Reed KL, Sahn DJ, Scagnelli S, et al. Doppler echocardiographic studies of diastolic function in the human fetal heart: changes during gestation. *J Am Coll Cardiol* **8**:391–395, 1986.

12. Allan LD, Chita SK, Al-Ghazali, et al. Doppler echocardiographic evaluation of the normal human fetal heart. *Br Heart J* **57**:528–533, 1987.

13. Cyr DR, Guntheroth WG, Mack LA, et al. A systematic approach to fetal echocardiography using real-time two-dimensional sonography. *J Ultrasound Med* **5**:343–350, 1986.

14. Cyr DR, Komarniski CA, Guntheroth WG, Mack LA. The prevalence of imaging fetal cardiac anatomy. *J. Diagn Med Sonography* **6**:299–304, 1988.

15. DeVore GR. Fetal echocardiography—a new frontier. *Clin Obstet Gynecol* **27**:359–377, 1984.

16. Rudolph AM. Distribution and regulation of blood flow in the fetal and neonatal lamb. *Circulation Res* **57**:811–821, 1985.

17. Benacerraf BR, Pober BR, Sanders SP. Accuracy of fetal echocardiography. *Radiology* **165**:847–849, 1987.

18. Copel JA, Pilu G, Green J, et al. Fetal echocardiographic screening for congenital heart disease: the importance of the four-chamber view. *Am J Obstet Gynecol* **157**:648–655, 1987.

19. Allan LD, Joseph MC, Boyd EGCA, et al. M-mode echocardiography in the developing human fetus. *Br Heart J* **47:**573–583, 1982.

20. DeVore GR, Donnerstein RL, Kleinman CS, et al. Fetal echocardiography. I. normal anatomy as determined by real-time–directed M-mode ultrasound. *Am J Obstet Gynecol* **144:**249, 1982.

21. DeVore GR, Siassi B, Platt LD. Fetal echocardiography. IV. M-mode assessment of ventricular size and contractility during the second and third trimesters of pregnancy in the normal fetus. *Am J Obstet Gynecol* **150:**981–988, 1984.

22. DeVore GR, Siassi B, Platt L. Fetal echocardiography. III. The diagnosis of cardiac arrhythmias using real-time-directed M-mode ultrasound. *Am J Obstet Gynecol* **146:**792, 1983.

23. Kenny JF, Plappert T, Doubilet P. Changes in intracardiac blood flow velocities and right and left ventricular stroke volumes with gestational age in the normal human fetus: a prospective Doppler echocardiographic study. *Circulation* **74:**1208–1216, 1986.

24. Moore KL. *The Developing Human: Clinically Oriented Embryology,* 3rd ed. Philadelphia: WB Saunders, 1982.

25. DeVore GR, Horenstein J, Siassi B, Platt LD. Fetal echocardiography. VII. Doppler color flow mapping: a new technique for the diagnosis of congenital heart disease. *Am J Obstet Gynecol* **156:**1054–1064, 1987.

26. Huhta JC, Strasburger JF, Carpenter RJ, et al. Pulsed Doppler fetal echocardiography. *J Clin Ultrasound* **13:**247–254, 1985.

27. Jeanty P, Romero R, Hobbins JC. Fetal pericardial fluid: a normal finding of the second half of gestation. *Am J Obstet Gynecol* **149:**529–532, 1984.

28. Reed KL, Meijboom EJ, Sahn DJ, et al. Cardiac Doppler flow velocities in human fetuses. *Circulation* **73:**41–46, 1986.

29. Sanders RC, James AE. *The Principles and Practice of Ultrasonography in Obstetrics and Gynecology,* 3rd ed. Norwalk, CT: Appleton-Century-Crofts, 1985.

30. Nyberg DA, Mahony BS, Pretorius DH. *Diagnostic Ultrasound of Fetal Anomalies: Text and Atlas.* St. Louis: Mosby-Yearbook, 1990.

31. Hann LE, Bachmann DL, Ardle CR. Coexistent intrauterine and ectopic pregnancy: A reevaluation. *Radiology* **152:**151, 1984

Questions

GENERAL INSTRUCTIONS: For each question select the best answer. Select only one answer for each question, unless otherwise indicated.

1. Which of the following is not among the general categories of gestational trophoblastic disease?

    (A) hydatidiform mole
    (B) chorioadenoma destruens
    (C) chondrosarcoma
    (D) choriocarcinoma

2. An invasive mole is also referred to as

    (A) hydatidiform mole
    (B) an endometrioma
    (C) a blighted ovum
    (D) chorioadenoma destruens

3. The variables that make up a fetal biophysical profile are

    (A) breathing movements
    (B) qualitative amniotic fluid volume
    (C) fetal tone
    (D) reactive fetal heart rate
    (E) all of the above
    (F) B and D only

4. The cephalic index is defined as the ratio of the biparietal diameter to

    (A) femur length
    (B) occipito-frontal diameter
    (C) abdominal circumference
    (D) binocular distances

5. Identify the signs and symptoms that are associated with hydatidiform moles from the following list: (1) thyrotoxicosis, (2) hyperemesis gravidarium, (3) uterus too large for dates, (4) elevated serum β-hCG, (5) hemorrhage, (6) passage of grape-like vesicles through the vagina, (7) preeclampsia, (8) pulmonary embolism.

    (A) 2, 4, and 5
    (B) 3, 4, 5, and 7

    (C) 2, 3, 4, and 5
    (D) all of the above

6. Hydatidiform mole is characterized by

    (A) benign proliferation of the trophoblast
    (B) malignant proliferation of the trophoblast
    (C) invasive proliferation of the trophoblast
    (D) all of the above

7. Figure 8–12 is a transverse sonogram of the uterus. The most likely diagnosis is

    (A) an unruptured ectopic pregnancy within the right fallopian tube
    (B) an incomplete abortion
    (C) an early embryonic demise of a twin intrauterine pregnancy
    (D) an intrauterine pregnancy in one horn of a bicornuate uterus

8. A solid mass may exhibit all of the following *except*

    (A) distal acoustic shadows
    (B) distal acoustic enhancement
    (C) irregular, poorly defined walls
    (D) an echo-free interior

Figure 8–12. Transverse sonogram of the uterus.

9. The incidence of hydatidiform mole in the United States is approximately

(A) 1 in 5000 patients
(B) 1 in 500 patients
(C) 1 in 250 patients
(D) 1 in 1200–2000 patients

10. What percentage of hydatidiform mole has a coexistent fetus?

(A) 20%
(B) 30%
(C) 5%
(D) 2%

11. What type of cyst is commonly associated with hydatidiform mole?

(A) a theca lutein cyst
(B) a paraovarian cyst
(C) a corpus luteum cyst
(D) a follicular cyst

12. With the advent of gray-scale sonography, there has been a variety of sonographic appearances of hydatidiform mole. Which of the following are characteristic of its gray-scale appearance?

(A) a snowstorm
(B) a vesicular sonographic texture
(C) a speckled appearance
(D) a calcified appearance

13. Trophoblastic disease, which extends outside the uterus and spreads to the lungs or brain, is called

(A) choriocarcinoma
(B) hydatidiform mole
(C) endometrioma
(D) lung-gestational molar

14. How many weeks after suction evacuation of molar gestation does the serum β-human gonadotropin (β-hCG) return to the normal range?

(A) 36 weeks
(B) 20–30 weeks
(C) 2–4 weeks
(D) 10–12 weeks

15. What percentage of molar pregnancy results in choriocarcinoma?

(A) 90%
(B) 65%
(C) 3–20%
(D) 40–50%

16. Choriocarcinoma can metastasize to which of the following areas: (1) lungs and brain, (2) liver, (3) bone, (4) gastrointestinal tract?

(A) 3 and 4
(B) 2 and 3
(C) 1 only
(D) all of the above

17. Select the most effective form of contraceptive.

(A) intrauterine contraceptive device (IUCD)
(B) oral contraceptive
(C) condom
(D) vaginal contraceptive sponge

18. Which of the following countries has the greatest incidence of hydatidiform mole?

(A) United States
(B) Japan
(C) France
(D) Jamaica

19. Which of the following statements is a hypothetical explanation for the geographic variability in the incidence of hydatidiform mole?

(A) hydatidiform mole is secondary to nutritional factors
(B) it is the result of genetic predisposition
(C) it is the result of increased parity in these areas
(D) all of the above

20. The etiology of hydatidiform mole is

(A) trophoblastic changes in a blighted ovum
(B) hydatid swelling of the retained placenta in a missed abortion
(C) fertilization of an ovum without any active chromosomal material
(D) A and B only

21. How long does it usually take for theca lutein cysts to regress after molar evacuation?

(A) 1–2 weeks
(B) 4–5 weeks
(C) 6 months
(D) 2–4 months

22. A pregnancy within a bicornuate uterus

(A) sometimes aborts
(B) may go to term without complications
(C) may result in decidual proliferation in the non-gravid horn
(D) all of the above

Figure 8–13. Transverse sonogram through the uterine fundus.

23. Figure 8–13 is a transverse sonogram through the uterine fundus in a 28-week pregnancy. The most likely diagnosis is

    (A) a placental choriongioma
    (B) abruptio placentae
    (C) a large venous lake
    (D) an overmature placenta

24. Which of the following is *not* among the characteristic echo patterns of an intrauterine contraceptive device?

    (A) a distal acoustic shadow
    (B) entrance–exit reflections
    (C) a line of interrupted echo
    (D) distal acoustic enhancement

25. The maximum number of interrupted echoes seen on a sonogram with a Lippes Loop in situ is

    (A) two
    (B) four
    (C) five
    (D) eight

26. The date of the last menstrual period indicates

    (A) the date when fertilization occurred
    (B) the date when menstrual bleeding ended
    (C) the date when ovulation occurred
    (D) the date when menstrual bleeding began

27. What percentage of intrauterine contraceptive devices demonstrate an entrance–exit reflection?

    (A) 95%
    (B) 65%
    (C) 30%
    (D) 20%

28. Concerning placental grading,

    (A) there is a significant overlap of placental patterns in normal and abnormal pregnancies
    (B) all grade III placentas will have a mature fetal pulmonary test
    (C) it is a useful parameter in the diagnosis of intrauterine growth retardation
    (D) continuous-wave Doppler will always be abnormal in grade III placentas
    (E) A and C

29. Abruptio placentae

    (A) may be life threatening to the fetus
    (B) may be life threatening to the mother
    (C) can be mistaken for a sustained uterine contraction
    (D) all of the above

30. The accuracy of sonography in the diagnosis of molar gestation has been estimated to be more than

    (A) 90%
    (B) 50%
    (C) 60%
    (D) 20%

31. Which of the following diagnoses does *not* mimic the sonographic characteristic of hydatidiform mole?

    (A) endometriosis
    (B) hematoma
    (C) uterine leiomyoma
    (D) missed abortion

32. After hydatidiform mole is treated, a chest radiograph is recommended. The reasons for this are which of the following: (1) evidence of metastatic disease, (2) pleural effusion, (3) cardiomegaly, (4) a pulmonary embolism?

    (A) 1 and 2
    (B) 1 and 4
    (C) all of the above
    (D) none of the above

33. What percentage of patients diagnosed with hydatidiform mole will usually follow a benign course?

    (A) 20%
    (B) 10%
    (C) 50%
    (D) 80%

34. If the nylon thread attached to the IUCD cannot be visualized or palpated by a physician, the possibilities are which of the following: (1) detachment of the nylon thread, (2) expulsion of the device, (3) uterine perforation by the IUCD, (4) migration of the nylon thread?

    (A) 1 and 2
    (B) 2 and 4

(C) 4 only

(D) all of the above

35. Figure 8–14 is a transverse sonogram of the left upper quadrant in a gravid patient. The most likely diagnosis is

(A) an obstructed left kidney

(B) a fluid-filled, distended small bowel

(C) a fluid-filled, distended large bowel

(D) a ruptured spleen

36. In what anatomic site does fertilization of the ovum usually occur?

(A) the vagina

(B) the uterine cavity

(C) the ovary

(D) the fallopian tube

37. A Krukenberg's tumor is a

(A) benign ovarian tumor

(B) bilateral tumor of the ovary that has metastasized from primary tumor in the gastrointestinal tract.

(C) cystic tumor

(D) uterine tumor.

38. Which of the following is *not* a clinical symptom of a hydatidiform mole?

(A) preeclampsia

(B) hyperemesis gravidarum

(C) embolization

(D) hydrometrocolpos

39. The small bowel can be distinguished from the large bowel by

(A) a barium enema

(B) the presence of valvulae conniventes

(C) the presence of haustra

(D) different peristaltic patterns

40. The term trophoblast denotes

(A) the extraembryonic peripheral cells of the blastocyst

(B) a rigid state of the flagellate microorganism

(C) the gestation sac

(D) the characteristics of a disease

41. The term pathognomonic denotes

(A) development of a morbid condition

(B) insanity

(C) the study of pathologic lesions

(D) the characteristics of a disease

42. What are most likely to produce numerous anechoic structures of about 3–5 mm in diameter in a classical sonographic appearance of hydatidiform mole?

(A) numerous hydropic villi

(B) calcifications

(C) theca lutein cysts

(D) fetal parts

43. The term proliferation denotes

(A) the characteristics of a disease

(B) the multiplication of similar forms

(C) the peripheral cells of the blastocyst

(D) the creation of holes

44. Perforation of the uterus by an intrauterine contraceptive device occurs most often during

(A) menstruation

(B) exercise

(C) intercourse

(D) insertion

45. During pregnancy, the maternal bowel is usually

(A) displaced superiorly by the gravid uterus

(B) displaced inferiorly by the gravid uterus

(C) not displaced

(D) filled with amniotic fluid

46. Although many imaging modalities are used today, the most reliable method of evaluating intrauterine contraceptive devices is

(A) a pelvic x-ray

(B) sonography

(C) computed tomography

(D) a hysterogram

Figure 8–14. Transverse sonogram of the left upper quadrant in a gravid patient.

Figure 8–15. Diagram of intrauterine contraceptive devices.

47. How accurate is sonography in assessing the localization of an intrauterine contraceptive device in utero?

 (A) 100%
 (B) 50%
 (C) 90%
 (D) 99%

Questions 48 through 54: Match the devices in Fig. 8–15 with the list of terms in Column B.

COLUMN A

48. _____
49. _____
50. _____
51. _____
52. _____
53. _____
54. _____

COLUMN B

 (A) Saf-T-Coil
 (B) Copper-T (Cu-T)
 (C) Copper-7 (Cu-7)
 (D) Gynekoil
 (E) Lippes Loop
 (F) Dalkon shield
 (G) Antigon device

55. Fetal death is defined as death of a fetus (1) at 20 weeks or more of gestation, (2) at any stage of gestation, (3) weighing 500 g or more, (4) after 36 weeks of gestation.

 (A) 1 and 3
 (B) 2 and 3

 (C) 4 only
 (D) all of the above

56. Which of the following conditions is most likely to require scanning of the right upper quadrant?

 (A) intrauterine gestation 6 weeks size
 (B) gonococcal pelvic inflammatory disease
 (C) a 2 cm right ovarian cyst
 (D) a 2 cm left ovarian cyst

57. Metastatic ovarian carcinoma can be associated with

 (A) ascites
 (B) peritoneal metastases
 (C) omental metastases
 (D) liver metastases
 (E) all of the above

58. The endometrium can appear echogenic (1) particularly in the secretory phase, (2) in patients with pelvic inflammatory disease, (3) after dilatation and curettage, (4) in patients with endometritis, (5) after removal of an intrauterine contraceptive device.

 (A) 1 and 3 only
 (B) 4 only
 (C) 1, 2, 3, and 5
 (D) all of the above

59. Which of the following masses would be *least* likely to be encountered during pregnancy?

 (A) leiomyoma uteri
 (B) dysgerminoma
 (C) dermoid cyst
 (D) corpus luteum cyst

60. A 22-year-old gravid patient presents with oligohydramnios. Which of the following would be *least* likely?

 (A) anencephaly
 (B) postterm pregnancy
 (C) renal agenesis
 (D) premature rupture of the membranes

61. If spontaneous labor were allowed after fetal death, what percentage of mothers would deliver the fetus by the end of the third week?

 (A) 50%
 (B) 65%
 (C) 80%
 (D) 93%

62. What are the potential dangers if a demised fetus is allowed to remain in utero for more than 5 weeks?

 (A) hypofibrinogenemia
 (B) cytomegalovirus

(C) erythroblastosis

(D) rubella

63. The term liquefaction denotes

(A) echoes in the amniotic fluid

(B) the conversion of a solid material into a liquid form

(C) a fatty tumor

(D) a demised fetus

64. How accurate is real-time sonography at diagnosing fetal death?

(A) 50%

(B) 70%

(C) 80%

(D) 99%

65. The nonspecific signs of fetal death are which of the following: (1) polyhydramnios, (2) nonvisualization of the heartbeat on real-time, (3) sonographic spalding signs, (4) scalp edema, (5) loss of the falx cerebri, (6) echoes in the amniotic fluid?

(A) 2 only

(B) 1, 3, and 4

(C) 1, 3, 4, 5, and 6

(D) all of the above

66. The biparietal diameter can be determined as early as

(A) 14 weeks

(B) 12 weeks

(C) 8 weeks

(D) 6 weeks

67. What is the first structure seen in the early diagnosis of pregnancy by sonography?

(A) the gestation sac

(B) the fetal head

(C) the zygote

(D) the morula

68. The measurement(s) used to assess gestational age in the first trimester is

(A) the uterine size

(B) the biparietal diameter

(C) the gestation sac and crown-rump length

(D) the fetal abdominal circumference

69. A gestational sac generally refers to a pregnancy

(A) of less than 2 weeks

(B) between 4 and 10 weeks

(C) between 10 and 15 weeks

(D) between 4 and 36 weeks

70. When scanning a patient who is near term and complains of feeling faint, the sonographer should

(A) offer her fluid by mouth

(B) stop the examination and turn her on her side

(C) put her in Fowler's position

(D) fan her or turn on the air conditioner

71. Given a 24-year-old gravid patient whose last menstrual period began on 8/10/92, what date would her expected date of confinement be?

(A) 5/14/94

(B) 5/17/93

(C) 5/10/93

(D) 8/10/93

72. The patient is a 20-year-old multigravid patient, whose last menstrual period is uncertain. On the TV monitor a completely anechoic gestation sac with an average dimension of 1 cm is seen. The approximate gestational age is

(A) 8 weeks

(B) 4–5 weeks

(C) 9 weeks

(D) 10–12 weeks

73. Organogenesis is completed at

(A) 4 weeks

(B) 8 weeks

(C) 36 weeks

(D) 40 weeks

74. How early can the placenta be identified on sonography?

(A) 8 weeks

(B) 14 weeks

(C) 16 weeks

(D) 20 weeks

75. What is the uterine isthmus called during pregnancy?

(A) the gestation sac

(B) an ectopic pregnancy

(C) the placenta previa

(D) the lower uterine segment

76. A patient's parity is P4174. How many abortions has she had?

(A) four

(B) seven

(C) one

(D) six

77. What is the *most* common type of cyst seen in the first trimester of pregnancy?

(A) a corpus luteum cyst

(B) a follicular cyst

(C) a theca lutein cyst

(D) a paraovarian cyst

78. The patient is a 22-year-old multigravida, last menstrual period uncertain. A gestation sac is seen with an embryo. The crown-rump length is 2 cm. What is the approximate age of the embryo?

    (A) 6 weeks
    (B) 8.5 weeks
    (C) 10.5 weeks
    (D) 4–5 weeks

79. A gestational sac fills one-quarter of the uterine cavity and measures 1 cm in length, 1 cm in anteroposterior diameter, and 2 cm in transverse diameter. What is the average sac dimension of the gestation?

    (A) 1.3 cm
    (B) 2.5 cm
    (C) 2.5 mm
    (D) 1.1 mm

80. A near-term gravid patient lying face up for more than 15 minutes will sometimes become ill with fainting and nausea. She is probably experiencing

    (A) supine hypotensive syndrome
    (B) supine hypertensive syndrome
    (C) morning sickness
    (D) hyperemesis gravidarum
    (E) none of the above

81. Fig. 8–16 is a longitudinal midline sonogram through the cervix. The most likely diagnosis is

    (A) a fibroid
    (B) feces in the rectum
    (C) placenta previa
    (D) a cystic ovarian tumor

82. The double-ring sign of the fetal skull is sometimes seen in which of the following conditions?

Figure 8–16. Sagittal midline sonogram through the cervix.

(A) maternal diabetes
(B) fetal demise
(C) sickle-cell anemia
(D) Rh isoimmunization
(E) fetal distress
(F) fetal anasarca
(G) hydrops fetalis
(H) all of the above
(I) A, B, and D only

83. The separation of the chorionic and amniotic membranes is normal

    (A) after 24 weeks of gestation
    (B) before 24 weeks of gestation
    (C) after 16 weeks of gestation
    (D) before 16 weeks of gestation

84. Amniotic band syndrome is a term for

    (A) adhesions of torn amniotic membranes wrapped around fetal parts and producing congenital amputations
    (B) complications of placental abruption
    (C) a syndrome that occurs after the fetus swallows too much amniotic fluid
    (D) A and C

85. Eighty percent of cystic hygromas occur in what region?
    (A) the axilla
    (B) the mediastinum
    (C) the cervical region
    (D) all of the above
    (E) none of the above

86. Which of the following is the appropriate description of gastroschisis?

    (A) normal insertion of the umbilical cord, with herniation of the bowel occurring most often on the right side of the umbilicus
    (B) herniation of the abdominal contents, including the bowel and liver or spleen, with herniation at the base of the umbilical cord
    (C) herniation of the umbilical cord
    (D) herniation of bowel to the left of the umbilicus containing spleen covered by peritoneum

87. Cystic hygromas are

    (A) malignant cysts of the thyroid
    (B) benign developmental abnormalities of lymphatic origin
    (C) another name for meningomyelocele
    (D) benign cysts of the ovaries

88. A 30-year-old gravid patient, 8 months by dates, now presents with painless vaginal bleeding that has lasted for 5 days. The first condition to rule out by sonography is

(A) an ectopic pregnancy
(B) placenta previa
(C) an ovarian cyst
(D) hydatidiform mole

89. The clinical signs and symptoms for intrauterine pregnancy are which of the following: (1) Chadwick's sign, (2) Hegar's sign, (3) Goodell's sign, (4) quickening?

(A) 3 and 4
(B) 1 and 3
(C) 1, 3, and 4 only
(D) all of the above

90. How long does a postpartum uterus remain enlarged?

(A) 4–8 weeks after delivery
(B) 2–4 weeks after delivery
(C) 8–12 weeks after delivery
(D) 12–14 weeks after delivery

91. The abdominal circumference of the fetal abdomen should be taken at what level?

(A) the site of the cord insertion
(B) the portal sinus of the umbilical vein and the stomach
(C) the kidneys
(D) the heart

92. The thick "rind" of echoes surrounding the gestational sac are the (1) decidua capsularis, (2) syncytiotrophoblast, (3) decidua basalis, (4) yolk sac.

(A) 1 only
(B) 1 and 2
(C) 1, 2, and 3
(D) all of the above

93. Which of the following conditions or complications is *least* likely to occur?

(A) an ectopic pregnancy situated in the uterus
(B) menstruation following a hysterectomy
(C) a pregnancy following a hysterectomy
(D) a hysterectomy without a surgical scar on the skin
(E) a pregnancy in the uterus and outside the uterus at the same time

94. Parity P8257 indicates that

(A) the number of abortions is _____
(B) the number of term infants is _____
(C) the number of premature infants is _____
(D) the number of children currently alive _____

95. A sonographic characteristic of cystic hygroma is a

(A) multiseptated cystic mass
(B) solid mass on the anterior neck

(C) complex mass of the spine
(D) bilateral hyperechoic mass of the neck only

96. A large placenta is most likely to be seen in which of the following?

(A) multiple gestation
(B) Rh isoimmunization
(C) diabetics
(D) preeclampsia
(E) all of the above
(F) A, B, and C only

97. The most accurate biparietal diameter measurements are made at what week of gestation?

(A) 36 weeks
(B) 14–20 weeks
(C) 20–30 weeks
(D) 40 weeks

98. If a pregnant patient becomes faint (syncope) and nauseous during sonographic examination, this may be due to pressure of the

(A) uterus on the intestine
(B) uterus on the aorta
(C) uterus on the inferior vena cava
(D) transducer on the skin

99. Placental abruption is diagnosed by which of the following sonographic findings?

(A) retroplacental clot
(B) extramembranous clot
(C) both A and B
(D) neither A nor B

100. How accurate is placental localization with sonography?

(A) 95%
(B) 75%
(C) 80%
(D) 99%

101. If a localized thickening of the placenta and myometrium is seen, which changes within 20 minutes, this would most likely represent

(A) fibroid
(B) placenta previa
(C) placental abruption
(D) Braxton Hicks contractions

102. Placental abruption is defined as premature separation of the placenta from the uterine wall *after* the 20th week of gestation.

(A) true
(B) false

103. A 10-cm gestational sac is seen with a 25-mm embryo in it. Which one of the following measurements is *most* appropriate?

    (A) crown-rump length (CRL)
    (B) biparietal diameter (BPD)
    (C) femur length (FL)
    (D) gestational sac measurement

104. The term *ectopic pregnancy* denotes

    (A) pregnancy in the fallopian tube
    (B) pregnancy in the abdomen
    (C) any abnormal pregnancy
    (D) any pregnancy located outside of the endometrial lumen

105. The reason for shoulder pain in ectopic pregnancy is

    (A) intraperitoneal bleeding with diaphragmatic irritation
    (B) vomiting
    (C) syncope
    (D) fluid in the posterior cul-de-sac

106. If a multigravida uterus is 8.5 cm in length, the uterus is

    (A) enlarged
    (B) small
    (C) normal size
    (D) abnormal

107. Which of the following statements is *not* true concerning the yolk sac?

    (A) the yolk sac should be included in measurements of crown-rump length (CRL)
    (B) the yolk sac shrinks as pregnancy advances
    (C) the yolk sac plays a role in blood development and transfer of nutrients
    (D) the yolk sac is attached to the body stalk and is located between the amnion and chorion

108. Which of the following statements concerning intrauterine growth retardation (IUGR) is *not* true?

    (A) chromosomal abberations are more common in asymmetrical IUGR than in symmetrical IUGR
    (B) amniotic fluid volume is always abnormally low in IUGR
    (C) abdominal circumference measurements are helpful in the diagnosis of IUGR
    (D) IUGR is associated with hydramnios

Questions 109 through 126: Match the structures in Fig. 8–17 with the list of terms in Column B.

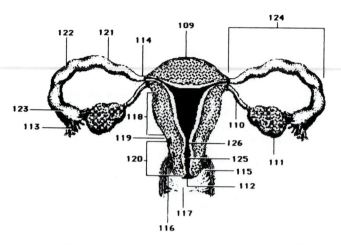

Figure 8–17. Diagram of the female reproductive organs (frontal view).

COLUMN A	COLUMN B
109. _____	(A) uterine cervix
110. _____	(B) fimbria
111. _____	(C) uterine fundus
112. _____	(D) right lateral vaginal fornix
113. _____	(E) left lateral vaginal fornix
114. _____	(F) interstitial portion of tube
115. _____	(G) vagina
116. _____	(H) isthmus uteri
117. _____	(I) external os of cervix
118. _____	(J) ovary
119. _____	(K) ovarian ligament
120. _____	(L) uterine corpus
121. _____	(M) fallopian tube
122. _____	(N) infundibulum
123. _____	(O) internal os of cervix
124. _____	(P) isthmus tubae
125. _____	(Q) ampulla
126. _____	(R) endocervical canal

127. Ectopic pregnancy is responsible for what percentage of maternal deaths?

    (A) 26%
    (B) 60%
    (C) 70%
    (D) 80%

128. What percentage of ectopic pregnancies occur in the fallopian tube?

    (A) 50%
    (B) 95%
    (C) 20%
    (D) 9%

129. Approximately how many days during the first 6 weeks after conception does the amount of human chorionic gonadotropin (hCG) double?

(A) 7 days
(B) 20 days
(C) 12 days
(D) 2 days

130. Fig. 8–18 is a transvaginal sonogram of a 24-year-old woman presented with 3 weeks of irregular vaginal bleeding and left pelvic pain. The most likely diagnosis is

(A) corpus luteum cyst
(B) unruptured ectopic pregnancy
(C) ruptured ectopic pregnancy
(D) A and B

131. Human chorionic gonadotropin (hCG) titers in ectopic pregnancy are frequently

(A) lower than patient with normal intrauterine pregnancy (IUP)
(B) higher than patient with normal intrauterine pregnancy (IUP)
(C) same as patient with normal intrauterine pregnancy (IUP)
(D) 50% higher than patient with normal intrauterine pregnancy (IUP)

132. The sonographic appearance of ectopic gestation include(s)

(A) enlarged nongravid uterus
(B) irregular adnexal mass or adnexal ring
(C) fluid in the cul-de-sac
(D) all of the above

133. An intrauterine pregnancy (IUP) with a coexistent extrauterine gestation occurs in what percentage of pregnancies?

(A) 2 in 10,000 pregnancies
(B) 1 in 6,000 to 30,000 pregnancies
(C) 5 in 10,000 pregnancies
(D) 1 in 5 to 1 in 50,000 pregnancies

134. What percentage of ectopic gestations demonstrate a pseudogestational sac?

(A) 60%
(B) 50%
(C) 40%
(D) 20%

135. A pseudogestational sac is *most* likely produced by

(A) yolk sac
(B) decidual cast
(C) ovarian tumor
(D) PID

136. Cystic hygromas are associated with

(A) Potter's syndrome
(B) Beckwith Wiedemann syndrome
(C) elevated levels of α-fetoprotein
(D) Turner's syndrome
(E) C and D only

137. The sonographic characteristics of cystic hygromas are which of the following: (1) thin-walled cyst, (2) hyperechoic mass on the neck, (3) multiseptated cystic mass, (4) echogenic mass in the cervical region?

(A) 2 and 3
(B) 1 and 3
(C) 4 only
(D) 1 only

138. On transvaginal and transabdominal sonography, the most common appearance of an unruptured ectopic pregnancy is

(A) "tubal ring"
(B) nonspecific adnexal mass
(C) a cystic adnexal mass
(D) complex adnexal mass

139. Which of the following is the appropriate description of omphalocele?

(A) normal insertion of the umbilical cord, with herniation of bowel occurring most often on the right side of the umbilicus
(B) protrusion of abdominal contents that may contain bowel, liver, or spleen with herniation at the base of the umbilical cord
(C) herniation of bowel only
(D) herniation of bowel to the left of the umbilicus containing spleen covered by peritoneum

Figure 8–18. Transvaginal sonogram of the left adnexa.

140. Important facts to consider in the differential diagnosis of omphalocele versus gastroschisis are

   (A) omphalocele has a normal insertion of the umbilical cord and is covered by parietal peritoneum or amniotic membrane
   (B) gastroschisis has a normal insertion of the umbilical cord and is covered by parietal peritoneum or amniotic membrane
   (C) gastroschisis has a normal insertion of the umbilical cord and is not covered by membrane
   (D) both gastroschisis and omphalocele have a normal insertion of the umbilical cord; however, gastroschisis is covered by a membrane

141. The uterine findings on ectopic pregnancy typically include

   (A) a pseudogestational sac
   (B) thickened endometrium
   (C) irregular decidualized endometrium
   (D) all of the above

142. Twenty percent of cystic hygromas can occur in which of the following regions: (1) cervical region, (2) groin, (3) axilla, (4) mediastinum?

   (A) all of the above
   (B) 1 and 4 only
   (C) 1 only
   (D) 2, 3, and 4 only

143. Turner's syndrome is defined as

   (A) retarded growth and sexual development with abnormal sex chromosomes
   (B) bilateral renal agenesis with pulmonary hypoplasia
   (C) blepharochalasis occurring in association with goiter
   (D) paralysis of the soft palate, larynx, and tongue

144. The nonspecific signs of fetal death are which of the following: (1) echoes in the amniotic fluid, (2) the absence of the falx cerebri, (3) a decrease in biparietal diameter (BPD) measurements, (4) a double contour of the fetal head (sonographic halo sign)?

   (A) 3 and 4
   (B) 4 only
   (C) all of the above
   (D) none of the above

145. The proposed reasons for the development of an ectopic pregnancy include

   (A) fallopian tube malfunction
   (B) fallopian tube adhesions
   (C) PID (pelvic inflammatory disease)
   (D) fallopian tube diverticula
   (E) all of the above

146. Once a patient has had an ectopic pregnancy, what are the chances of recurrence?

   (A) 1 in 15
   (B) 1 in 8
   (C) 1 in 10
   (D) 1 in 4

147. In what portion of the fallopian tube does ectopic pregnancy pose serious potential complications?

   (A) isthmus
   (B) ampullary
   (C) infundibulum
   (D) interstitial portion

148. How long after fetal death can scalp edema be seen?

   (A) 2–3 days
   (B) 5–10 days
   (C) 10–20 days
   (D) 8–10 days

149. Sonographic Spalding's sign is

   (A) double contour of the fetal head
   (B) "halo" sign
   (C) overlapping of the fetal cranium
   (D) all of the above

150. The most common location for an ectopic implantation is

   (A) isthmus
   (B) infundibulum
   (C) interstitial portion
   (D) ampullary portion

151. Sonographic masses that can mimic an ectopic pregnancy are

   (A) hemorrhagic corpus luteum cyst
   (B) tubo-ovarian abscess
   (C) dermoid cyst
   (D) B and C only
   (E) all of the above

152. The sonographic demonstration of a double decidual sac, with or without a fetal pole, strongly suggests

   (A) ectopic pregnancy
   (B) intrauterine pregnancy (IUP)
   (C) yolk sac
   (D) fetal demise

153. The regions to scan for localizing fluid collection in an ectopic pregnancy are (1) anterior and posterior cul-de-sac, (2) paracolic recesses, (3) subhepatic space (Morrison's pouch), (4) adnexa.

(A) 1 and 2 only

(B) 1, 3, and 4 only

(C) all of the above

154. Which of the following statements is (are) *not* true for abdominal pregnancy: (1) the fetus may be alive at birth, (2) the placenta should be removed to prevent hemorrhage, (3) the uterus is separated from the fetus, (4) it can be missed on sonogram?

(A) 3 and 4 only

(B) 1, 3, and 4

(C) 2 only

(D) all of the above

155. Which neonates are considered growth retarded: (1) those born after 36 weeks, (2) those whose birth weight is on or above the 10th percentile, (3) those whose birth weight is on or below the 10th percentile?

(A) 2 and 3

(B) 1 and 2

(C) 1, 2, and 3

(D) 3 only

156. Conditions that are frequently associated with fetal hydrocephalus include

(A) meningomyelocele

(B) in utero exposure to TORCH (toxoplasmosis, rubella, cytomegalovirus, herpes)

(C) aqueductal stenosis

(D) Dandy-Walker syndrome

(E) all of the above

157. Fig. 8–19 is a longitudinal midline pelvic sonogram. The arrow points to

(A) bladder tumor

(B) pelvic kidney

(C) cystic mass

(D) normal uterus

158. After 34 weeks of gestation, approximately what percentage of fetuses are in the cephalic presentation?

(A) 80%

(B) 90%

(C) 60%

(D) 25%

159. The causes of cul-de-sac fluid are which of the following: (1) ruptured corpus luteum cyst, (2) ruptured hemorrhagic cyst, (3) ruptured ectopic gestation, (4) culdocentesis?

(A) 1 and 3

(B) 3 only

(C) 1, 2, and 3

(D) all of the above

Questions 160 through 168: Match the structures in Fig. 8–20 with the list of terms in Column B.

COLUMN A	COLUMN B
160. _____	(A) isthmus uteri
161. _____	(B) chorion frondosum
162. _____	(C) decidua parietalis (vera)
163. _____	(D) decidua capsularis
164. _____	(E) cervix
165. _____	(F) amniotic cavity
166. _____	(G) decidua basalis
167. _____	(H) unoccupied lumen between the decidual layers
168. _____	(I) mucous plug

Figure 8–19. Sagittal midline pelvic sonogram.

Figure 8–20. Diagram of early pregnancy.

Figure 8–21. Diagram of the fetal circulatory system.

Questions 169 through 178: Match the structures in Fig. 8–21 with the list of terms in Column B.

COLUMN A	COLUMN B
169. _____	(A) placenta
170. _____	(B) inferior vena cava (IVC)
171. _____	(C) portal sinus
172. _____	(D) umbilical vein
173. _____	(E) aorta
174. _____	(F) left hepatic vein
175. _____	(G) right hepatic vein
176. _____	(H) ductus venosus
177. _____	(I) portal vein
178. _____	(J) umbilical arteries

179. Fetal ocular biometry has proven to be useful in evaluating

(A) hypotelorism
(B) hypertelorism
(C) anophthalmos
(D) gestational age
(E) microphthalmos
(F) all of the above

180. The interocular distance is measured from

(A) frontal process of the maxillary bone to the opposite maxillary process
(B) medial border of the orbit to the opposite medial border
(C) from inner canthus to outer canthus

(D) frontal process of the zygomatic bone to the opposite zygomatic bone
(E) all of the above

181. The biocular distance is measured from

(A) frontal process of the maxillary bone to the opposite maxillary process
(B) lateral border of the orbit to the opposite lateral border
(C) outer canthus to the inner canthus
(D) frontal process of the zygomatic bone to the opposite zygomatic bone
(E) all of the above

182. A cephalic index of 80% is

(A) suggestive of brachycephaly
(B) suggestive of dolichocephaly
(C) suggestive of hypertelorism
(D) normal

183. The crown-rump length (CRL) measurement is the longest length of the embryo

(A) excluding the limbs
(B) including the limbs
(C) including the yolk sac
(D) including the femur

184. Femoral length is measured from which of the following: (1) proximal femoral neck to the distal femoral condyles, (2) greater trochanter to the distal femoral condyles, (3) femoral head to the medial epicondyle, (4) femoral head to the intercondyle notch?

(A) 1 and 2 only
(B) 4 only
(C) 3 and 4 only
(D) none of the above

185. Hypertelorism denotes

(A) abnormally wide-spaced orbits
(B) abnormally closely spaced orbits
(C) smallness of the eyes
(D) absence of eyes

186. Hypotelorism denotes

(A) abnormally wide-spaced orbits
(B) abnormally closely spaced orbits
(C) smallness of the eyes
(D) absence of eyes

187. The accuracy of crown-rump length (CRL) measurement as a means of estimating gestational age has been statistically evaluated. The study showed

(A) 95% confidence limit of ± 4.7 days
(B) 85% confidence limit of ± 3 days

(C) 100% confidence limit of ± 3 days

(D) 99% confidence limit of ± 4.7 days

188. The structures that should *not* be included when measuring the embryo for a crown-rump length (CRL) are which of the following: (1) yolk sac, (2) femur, (3) spine, (4) humerus, (5) ulna and radius, (6) tibia and fibula, (7) placenta?

(A) 1 and 7 only

(B) 7 only

(C) 1, 3, and 6

(D) 1, 2, 4, 5, 6, and 7

(E) all of the above

189. The CRL should be performed between which weeks of gestation?

(A) 4 and 5 weeks

(B) 6 and 12 weeks

(C) 12 and 14 weeks

(D) 14 and 20 weeks

190. The most accurate methodology for the assessment of gestational age in the first trimester is

(A) femur length (FL)

(B) biparietal diameter (BPD)

(C) crown-rump length (CRL)

(D) orbital distance (OD)

191. The cardiac circulation of the fetus is different from that of adults. Some of these differences that are present in the fetus and *not* in the adult include

(A) shunting of blood across the foramen ovale

(B) presence of a ductus arteriosus

(C) presence of a ductus venosus within the heart

(D) all of the above.

192. The gestational sac can be seen on transabdominal sonography as early as

(A) 5 weeks' gestational age

(B) 2 weeks' gestational age

(C) 6 weeks' gestational age

(D) 7 weeks' gestational age

193. Ovarian carcinomas usually metastasize to

(A) bone

(B) lungs

(C) brain

(D) bowel

194. Sonographers should be familiar with the medication Clomid (clomiphene citrate) because of which of the following: (1) it is used to treat infertility, (2) it can be associated with multiple gestation, (3) the urinary bladder will not fill, (4) it will cause heart failure?

(A) 1 and 2

(B) 1 and 3

(C) 1 and 4

(D) all of the above

195. During the first 10 weeks of gestation, the gestational sac grows approximately

(A) 25 mm per week

(B) 1 mm per day

(C) 1 cm per week

(D) 3 cm per week or 30 mm per week

196. The accuracy of gestational sac volume measurement as a means of estimating gestational age has been reported as

(A) 95% confidence limit of ± 4.7 days

(B) confidence limit of ± 9 days

(C) confidence limit of ± 5 days

(D) confidence limit of ± 15 days

197. Which of the following are associated with intrauterine growth retardation (IUGR): (1) preeclamptic toxemia, (2) chronic renal disease, (3) maternal heart disease, (4) heavy smoking, (5) maternal malnutrition, (6) alcoholism?

(A) 1, 2, 5, and 6 only

(B) 2 and 6 only

(C) 1, 2, 3, 5, and 6 only

(D) all of the above

198. The treatment for intrauterine growth retardation (IUGR) includes which of the following: (1) bed rest, (2) having the mother lie on the left side, (3) administration of anticoagulant drugs, (4) the medication heparin?

(A) 1 only

(B) 4 only

(C) all of the above

(D) none of the above

199. Long-term follow-up studies of children born with previous intrauterine growth retardation (IUGR) confirm

(A) speech defects

(B) central nervous system (CNS) abnormalities

(C) diminished intelligence

(D) more frequent occurrence in males than in females

(E) B and C

(F) all of the above

200. In about 10% of intrauterine growth retardation (IUGR) cases there are fetal anomalies. These disorders include all of the following *except*

(A) trisomy 21
(B) trisomy 18
(C) trophoblastic disease
(D) Potter's syndrome
(E) neural tube defects

201. The term *decidua* denotes the transformed endometrium of pregnancy. The different regions of the decidua are divided into

(A) two regions called decidua basalis and chorionic villi
(B) one region called decidual reaction
(C) three regions called decidua basalis, decidua parietalis, and decidua capsularis
(D) three regions called endoderm, mesoderm, and ectoderm

202. Pseudocyesis denotes false

(A) cyst
(B) tumor
(C) decidua basalis
(D) pregnancy

203. In which of the scanning planes is spina bifida best recognized?

(A) transverse
(B) longitudinal
(C) oblique
(D) coronal

204. The ideal time for detecting spina bifida is

(A) 17–18 weeks
(B) 20–30 weeks
(C) 12–16 weeks
(D) 30–36 weeks

205. Fluid-filled masses in the vagina could include all of the following *except*

(A) Gartner's duct cyst
(B) vaginal agenesis
(C) urine in the vagina
(D) hematocolpos

206. The functions of the yolk sac are which of the following: (1) hemopoiesis, (2) development of sex glands, (3) formation of the embryonic digestive tube, (4) transfer of nutrients?

(A) 1 and 4
(B) 2 and 3
(C) 4 only
(D) all of the above

207. At 10 weeks of gestation, the location of the yolk sac is

(A) in the chorionic cavity between the amnion and the chorionic sac
(B) outside the chorionic cavity alongside the fetus
(C) inside the umbilical cord
(D) between the umbilical arteries

208. The yolk stalk usually detaches from the midgut loop at which week?

(A) 6th week
(B) 11th week
(C) 8th week
(D) 5th week

209. In about 2% of adults, the yolk stalk persists as a diverticulum of the ileum. This is known as

(A) Adams and Stokes' diverticulum
(B) Meckel's diverticulum
(C) Raymond's diverticulum
(D) Turner's diverticulum

210. On sonography, the yolk sac measures between

(A) 15 and 19 mm
(B) 1 and 2 cm
(C) 2 and 5 mm
(D) 15 and 25 mm

211. A blighted ovum is which of the following: (1) an empty gestational sac, (2) retention of a dead embryo, (3) arrested development of a fertilized ovum, (4) arrested development of a fetus after the first trimester?

(A) 1 and 3
(B) 2 only
(C) 2 and 3
(D) all of the above

212. Fluid in the cul-de-sac is least likely to be associated with

(A) ectopic pregnancy
(B) myoma uteri
(C) pelvic inflammatory disease (PID)
(D) ovulation
(E) follicular cyst

213. The thin ring-like structure that surrounds the gestational sac and excludes the yolk sac is most likely

(A) twin gestation sacs
(B) impending abortion or implantation bleeding
(C) blighted ovum
(D) not yet fused amnion
(E) all of the above

214. Which of the following is *not* among the sonographic findings of a blighted ovum?

(A) "tennis racquet" configuration of the sac
(B) disproportion between the gestational sac and uterine size
(C) failure of the gestation sac to increase in size by 75% in 1 week
(D) fragmentation of the sac
(E) weak surrounding echoes
(F) anembryonic sac after 8 weeks
(G) thickening of the decidua

215. A missed abortion is

(A) retention of a dead embryo or fetus
(B) anembryonic sac
(C) a blighted ovum
(D) an empty gestation sac

216. Which of the following statements is *not* true about spina bifida?

(A) spina bifida produces a U-shaped echo
(B) the spinal canal is seen as a closed circle in the presence of spina bifida
(C) over 80% of the cases of spina bifida are detectable sonographically
(D) the optimal time for sonographic examination is 17–18 weeks

217. Which of the following statements is *not* true about anencephaly?

(A) anencephaly has an incidence of 1 in 1000 births
(B) anencephaly has a female to male ratio of 4 to 1
(C) anencephaly is the most common anomaly effecting the central nervous system (CNS)
(D) anencephaly results from a failure of the neural tube to close completely
(E) anencephaly occurs more frequently in the United States than in the United Kingdom

218. Anomalies associated with anencephaly include all *except* which of the following: (1) spina bifida, (2) meningocele, (3) myelomeningocele, (4) cleft palate, (5) holoprosencephaly, (6) umbilical hernia, (7) polyhydramnios?

(A) 4 and 5 only
(B) 5 only
(C) 6 only
(D) 4, 5, and 6

219. The *most* common position for twin gestation is

(A) one in the cephalic and the other in breech presentation
(B) both in breech presentation
(C) both in cephalic presentation

Figure 8–22. Sagittal midline sonogram.

(D) one in the cephalic and the other in transverse presentation

220. The following is a list of different presentations. Identify which is *not* a malpresentation.

(A) cephalic
(B) breech
(C) transverse
(D) oblique

221. Fig. 8–22 is of a 32-year-old woman in whom the uterus was found to be enlarged and firm on physical examination. The most likely diagnosis is

(A) subserosal fibroid
(B) submucosal fibroid
(C) hydatidform mole
(D) early pregnancy

222. Fig. 8–23 is a sonogram obtained through the abdomen of a 24-week fetus. The most likely diagnosis is

(A) herniated cord
(B) herniated bowel
(C) herniated liver
(D) normal bulging of the abdominal wall related to fetal breathing

Figure 8–23. Transverse sonogram of the fetal abdomen.

223. Overdistension of the urinary bladder may cause

    (A) anterior placenta to appear previa
    (B) closure of an incompetent cervix
    (C) distortion or closure of the gestational sac
    (D) obscured visualization of the internal iliac vein
    (E) all of the above
    (F) A and B only

224. If the fetal skull is low in the pelvis, what maneuvers or techniques can the sonographer use to obtain an accurate biparietal diameter (BPD)?

    (A) place the patient in Trendelenburg's position
    (B) place the patient in Fowler's position
    (C) apply gentle manual pressure to elevate the fetal head
    (D) distend the urinary bladder
    (E) A, C, and D

225. Which of the following statements is *not* true about biparietal diameter (BPD) measurement in twin gestation?

    (A) the biparietal diameter (BPDs) of the twins should be within 4 mm of each other
    (B) 1–2 mm should be added to the biparietal diameter (BPD) if the standard BPD chart for a singleton fetus is used
    (C) if the biparietal diameter (BPD) of twin A is 6 mm less than twin B, growth retardation of twin A should be considered
    (D) the biparietal diameters (BPDs) of twins are slightly smaller than those of a single fetus
    (E) the biparietal diameters (BPDs) of twins should be within 1 to 2 cm of each other

226. Abnormalities usually associated with an omphalocele include

    (A) ectopic heart
    (B) cysts in the liver
    (C) cysts in the kidney
    (D) none of the above

227. All patients for transabdominal sonographic examination of the pelvis require the urinary bladder be physiologically distended prior to the sonographic examination. The reason(s) for this is (are)

    (A) it produces a sonic window
    (B) it establishes an anatomical reference point
    (C) it helps evaluate the mobility of a mass
    (D) it decreases the angle of incidence
    (E) it helps demonstrate the cervix
    (F) it helps elevate the head of the fetus for a more accurate measurement of the biparietal diameter (BPD)

    (G) it pushes the bowel cephalad
    (H) A and G
    (I) F and G
    (J) A–G

228. For patients who are unable to ingest fluid, or in the event of an emergency, the urinary bladder can be distended via a Foley catheter and

    (A) 1 qt barium sulfate
    (B) 250 mL saline
    (C) 300 mL tap water
    (D) 32 oz mineral oil

229. If the fetus is in a vertex presentation and the spine of the fetus is to the maternal right, the fetus is lying on its

    (A) back and face up with the fetal head toward the fundus
    (B) left side and the right side is toward the maternal anterior abdominal wall
    (C) right side and the left side is toward the maternal anterior abdominal wall
    (D) abdomen and face down with the fetal head toward the fundus

230. If the fetus is in a breech presentation and the spine of the fetus is to the maternal right, the fetus is lying on its

    (A) back and face up with the fetal head toward the fundus
    (B) left side and the right side is toward the maternal anterior abdominal wall
    (C) right side and the left side is toward the maternal anterior abdominal wall
    (D) abdomen and face down with the fetal head toward the fundus

231. In the fetus, the heart is in a relatively horizontal position. This is largely due to

    (A) large liver size
    (B) large kidneys
    (C) fetal stomach
    (D) umbilical vein

232. When the cessation of blood flow from the placenta occurs, the umbilical vein collapses to become

    (A) ligamentum venosum
    (B) ligamentum teres
    (C) portal vein
    (D) hepatic vein

233. When the cessation of blood flow from the placenta occurs, the ductus venosus collapses to become the

(A) ligamentum venosum
(B) ligamentum teres
(C) portal vein
(D) hepatic vein

234. When the cessation of blood flow from the placenta occurs, the portal sinus

(A) remains patent and becomes the proximal left portal vein
(B) remains patent and becomes the proximal right portal vein
(C) remains occluded and becomes the proximal right portal vein
(D) remains occluded and becomes the proximal left portal vein

235. A single umbilical artery (SUA) may be associated with

(A) twins
(B) diabetes mellitus
(C) congenital anomalies
(D) all of the above

236. The three vessels normally found in the umbilical cord are

(A) one artery and two veins
(B) two arteries and one vein
(C) one artery, one vein, and one portal sinus
(D) hepatic vein, portal vein, and umbilical vein

237. Measurement of the umbilical vein diameter is a useful indicator of

(A) intrauterine growth retardation (IUGR)
(B) Rh isoimmunization
(C) gestation age
(D) weight estimation

238. Ovulation occurs approximately

(A) always after intercourse
(B) on the 7th day of the menstrual cycle
(C) on the 14th day of the menstrual cycle
(D) on the 2nd day of the menstrual cycle

239. Which of the following statements is(are) not true about esophageal atresia?

(A) esophageal atresia is a narrowing of the esophagus
(B) esophageal atresia is a closure or absence of the esophagus
(C) 90% of fetuses have tracheoesophageal fistula
(D) repeated failure to identify the fetal stomach by sonogram in the presence of hydramnios is indicative of esophageal atresia

240. The characteristic ultrasound pattern of duodenal atresia is

(A) failure to identify the fetal stomach by sonography
(B) Chadwick's sign
(C) "triple-bubble" sign
(D) "double-bubble" sign

241. Fetal renal agenesis is associated with the following condition(s)

(A) pulmonary hypoplasia
(B) Turner's syndrome
(C) oligohydramnios
(D) Potter's syndrome
(E) A and B only
(F) A, C, and D only

242. Normally, the fetal bladder will empty every

(A) 10 minutes
(B) 15 minutes
(C) 3 hours
(D) 1 hour

243. The most common cause of hydronephrosis of the fetus is

(A) staghorn calculi
(B) ovarian tumor
(C) obstruction occurring at the ureteropelvic junction (UPJ)
(D) all of the above

Questions 244 through 247: Arrange in sequence in Column A the embryologic stages following fertilization listed in Column B.

COLUMN A	COLUMN B
244. _____	(A) morula
245. _____	(B) cleavage
246. _____	(C) zygote
247. _____	(D) blastocyst

248. The double-ring sign ("halo" sign) of the fetal head is seen in the presence of diseases or conditions affecting the fetus. From the following list, identify the condition least associated with this sign.

(A) fetal demise
(B) fetal distress
(C) sickle-cell anemia
(D) intrauterine growth retardation (IUGR)
(E) diabetes mellitus
(F) Rh isoimmunization
(G) fetal anasarca
(H) hydrops fetalis

249. Thinning of the placenta is seen in most of the following. Identify the condition(s) *least* associated with this.

    (A) intrauterine growth retardation (IUGR)
    (B) chronic hydramnios
    (C) placental insufficiency
    (D) preeclampsia
    (E) polyhydramnios
    (F) Rh isoimmunization
    (G) multiple gestation
    (H) A and C only
    (I) D, A, and C only
    (J) F and G only

250. Thickening of the placenta is seen in most of the following. Identify the condition(s) *least* associated with this.

    (A) intrauterine growth retardation (IUGR)
    (B) maternal and fetal heart disease
    (C) placental insufficiency
    (D) diabetes mellitus
    (E) Rh isoimmunization
    (F) multiple gestation
    (G) transplacental syphilis
    (H) A and C only
    (I) A, B, C, and D only
    (J) F and G only

251. Oligohydramnios is seen in the presence of diseases or conditions affecting the fetus. Identify the condition *least* associated with this.

    (A) intrauterine growth retardation (IUGR)
    (B) renal agenesis
    (C) fetal demise
    (D) multiple gestation

252. Hydramnios is seen in the presence of diseases or conditions affecting the fetus. Identify those *least* associated with this.

    (A) anencephaly
    (B) hydrocephaly
    (C) spina bifida
    (D) meningomyelocele
    (E) multiple gestation
    (F) fetal demise
    (G) intrauterine growth retardation (IUGR)
    (H) diabetes mellitus
    (I) twin-twin transfusion
    (J) renal agenesis
    (K) esophageal and duodenal atresia
    (L) erythroblastosis
    (M) omphalocele
    (N) porencephaly
    (O) J and L
    (P) G and J
    (Q) all of the above

253. There are four classifications of the maturational process of the placenta, which are graded from 0 through III. Arrange the descriptive appearances in Column B to correlate with the grades in Column A.

COLUMN A

A. 0 _____
B. I _____
C. II _____
D. III _____

COLUMN B

(1) indentations communicating with the basal layer. Circular densities with echo-spared areas in the center and large irregular densities that cast acoustic shadowing

(2) subtle undulations with few scattered echogenic areas and no densities

(3) straight and well defined. Its texture is homogeneous with no densities

(4) indentations extending into, but not to, the basal layer. Linear, commalike echogenic densities with basal stippling

254. The *most* common cause of painless vaginal bleeding in the second and third trimesters of pregnancy is

    (A) trauma
    (B) ectopic pregnancy
    (C) placental abruption
    (D) placenta previa

255. The *most* common benign tumor of the uterus is fibroid. However, it has been known to have many other names. Identify the name that does *not* correlate.

    (A) myoma
    (B) leiomyomas
    (C) fibromyomas
    (D) leiomyosarcoma

256. Which of the following is *not* true about fibroids?

    (A) higher incidence in blacks than in whites
    (B) occur in 20% of females over 35 years of age
    (C) higher incidence in whites than in blacks
    (D) are the cause of at least 10% of all infertility problems

257. Fibroids can be classified into three groups; their names, which are based on their position in the various layers in the uterine wall, include which of the following: (1) submucous, (2) pedunculated, (3) interstitial, (4) endometriosis, (5) endometritis, (6) adenomyosis, (7) subserous?

(A) 1, 2, and 4
(B) 2, 3, and 6
(C) 1, 3, and 7
(D) 1, 4, and 7

258. What is Nägele's rule?

(A) mathematical methodology to estimate expected date of confinement (EDC)
(B) methodology to estimate age based on fundal height
(C) sonographic methodology to estimate gestational age
(D) mathematical methodology for measurement of fibroid

259. A malignant fibroid is known as

(A) leiomyosarcoma
(B) cystadenofibroma
(C) lymphoma
(D) endometrioma

260. The growth of fibroids is stimulated by

(A) estrogen
(B) pregnancy
(C) infection
(D) A and B

261. What is the average duration of pregnancy

(A) 280 days
(B) 40 weeks
(C) 36 weeks
(D) 9 calendar months
(E) 10 lunar months
(F) all of the above
(G) C and D only
(H) A, B, D, and E only

262. Overdistension of the urinary bladder may compress the placenta and create a sonographic appearance similar to placenta previa. This situation is *most* common

(A) in the anterior placenta
(B) in the posterior placenta
(C) in the fundal placenta
(D) overdistension of the urinary bladder *cannot* create a sonographic appearance similar to placenta previa

263. The reason(s) for distending the urinary bladder prior to sonographic examination is which of the following: (1) it displaces gas-containing bowel from the pelvis, (2) it establishes an anatomic reference point, (3) it pushes the uterus cephalad and away

from the symphysis pubis, (4) it acts as an acoustic window, (5) it is used as a comparison when the internal characteristics of a mass is evaluated?

(A) 1 and 2
(B) 1, 2, 3, and 4
(C) 1 and 4
(D) all of the above

264. The chorionic plate of the placenta is displayed as a strong linear echo on the inner surface. Where is the chorionic plate most difficult to depict if the fetus is *not* in the path of the ultrasonic beam?

(A) fundal placenta
(B) lateral placenta
(C) anterior placenta
(D) posterior placenta
(E) A and B
(F) all of the above

265. Difficulty can arise when the placenta is situated posteriorly and the fetus is in a cephalic position. In this situation, the sonographer should

(A) place the patient in Trendelenburg's position
(B) have a nurse gently elevate the fetal head by manual maneuver
(C) overdistend the maternal bladder
(D) measure the distance between the fetal calvarium and the anterior margin of the maternal sacrum
(E) B and D only
(F) A and B only
(G) all of the above

266. Endometriosis can be best described as

(A) malignant endometrial stroma
(B) ectopic endometrial tissue
(C) hematoma of the endometrium
(D) inflammation of the endometrium

267. The sonographic finding(s) in abruptio placentae is

(A) retroplacental clot
(B) separation occurring at the margin of the placenta
(C) large uterine veins and sinuses
(D) A and B
(E) all of the above

268. To calculate the expected date of confinement (EDC) you should

   (A) measure the fundal height, multiply by 4 then divide by 7
   (B) to the last menstrual period (LMP) add 7 days, subtract 3 calendar months, and add 1 year
   (C) to the last menstrual period (LMP) subtract 7 days, add 3 calendar months, and add 1 year
   (D) to the last menstrual period (LMP) add 5 days, subtract 9 calendar months, and add 1 year

Questions 269 through 275: Match the fundal height in Fig. 8–24 with the weeks of gestation in Column B.

COLUMN A	COLUMN B
269. _____	(A) 40 weeks
270. _____	(B) 36 weeks
271. _____	(C) 12 weeks
272. _____	(D) 16 weeks
273. _____	(E) 20–22 weeks
274. _____	(F) 28 weeks
275. _____	(G) 24–26 weeks

276. _____   277. _____

278. _____   279. _____

Figure 8–25. Diagram showing developmental anomalies of the uterus.

Questions 276 through 279: Match the type of developmental anomalies of the uterus shown in Fig. 8–25 with the terms in Column B.

COLUMN A	COLUMN B
276. _____	(A) bicornuate
277. _____	(B) septate
278. _____	(C) unicornis
279. _____	(D) didelphic

280. The ratio of head circumference to body circumference normally changes as pregnancy progresses. Match the weeks of gestation in Column A with the head and body ratio in Column B.

COLUMN A	COLUMN B
A. 12–24 _____	(1) abdomen larger than head
B. 32–36 _____	(2) head and body are equal
C. 36–40 _____	(3) head larger than abdomen

281. Rh isoimmunization results from which of the following combinations?

   (A) mother Rh⁻ and father Rh⁺
   (B) mother Rh⁺ and father Rh⁻
   (C) mother Rh⁺ and father Rh⁺
   (D) mother Rh⁻ and father Rh⁻

282. The name(s) of the ductal systems in the early development of the female fetus that form the internal genitalia is

   (A) wolffian duct
   (B) müllerian ducts
   (C) ductus arterious
   (D) ductus deferens
   (E) A and D
   (F) B and D
   (G) A and B

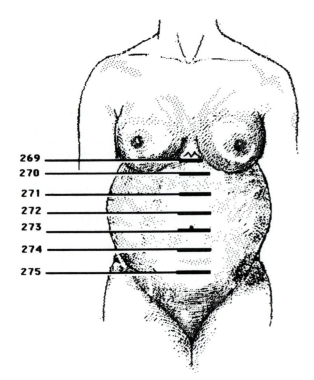

269
270
271
272
273
274
275

Figure 8–24. Diagram of the fundal height at various stages during pregnancy.

283. Total malfusion of the ductus paramesonephricus could result in

   (A) bicornuate uterus
   (B) septate uterus
   (C) didelphic uterus
   (D) unicornuate uterus

284. Partial malfusion of the ductus paramesonephricus could result in

   (A) bicornuate uterus
   (B) septate uterus
   (C) didelphic uterus
   (D) unicornuate uterus

285. Minimal malfusion of the paramesonephricus could result in

   (A) bicornuate uterus
   (B) septate uterus
   (C) didelphic uterus
   (D) unicornuate uterus

286. Arrested development of the paramesonephric duct results in

   (A) bicornuate uterus
   (B) uterine aplasia
   (C) septate uterus
   (D) didelphic uterus

287. Unilateral arrested development of the paramesonephric duct results in

   (A) bicornuate uterus
   (B) uterine aplasia
   (C) uterus unicornis
   (D) didelphic uterus

288. If uterine malformations are seen, the sonographer should scan which organ?

   (A) kidneys
   (B) gallbladder
   (C) spleen
   (D) liver

289. Which of the following is *not* true of dysgerminoma?

   (A) it is a solid malignant germ cell tumor of the ovary
   (B) it is a counterpart of seminoma of the testis
   (C) it is a relatively uncommon tumor accounting for about 2% of all ovarian cancers
   (D) 90% are unilateral
   (E) it is a solid benign tumor

290. Which of the following is *not* true of dermoid cysts?

   (A) it may cast an acoustic shadow
   (B) it is encountered more in women over 40 years

   (C) it is also called benign cystic teratoma (BCT)
   (D) most common benign germ cell tumor in the female
   (E) it is unilateral in about 80% of cases
   (F) the tumor has elements such as hair, tooth, bone, endoderm, ectoderm, mesoderm, and thyroid glandular tissue
   (G) fat floats on top of fluid, therefore, one may see a fat-fluid level
   (H) fat can be echogenic or anechoic
   (I) sonographically, can produce a "tip of the iceberg" effect

291. The trophoblast in ectopic pregnancy secretes *more* human chorionic gonadotropin (hCG) than does the placenta of a normal pregnancy.

   (A) true
   (B) false

Questions 292 through 300: Match the terms in Column A to the correct description in Column B.

COLUMN A

292. Gravida _____
293. Multipara _____
294. Nullipara (Po)
   _____
295. Primipara (Pi)
   _____
296. Nulligravida (Go)
   _____
297. Primigravida (Gi)
   _____
298. Multigravida
   _____
299. Para _____
300. Trimester _____

COLUMN B

   (A) a woman who has given birth two or more times
   (B) one who has never been pregnant
   (C) a woman who is pregnant
   (D) a woman who has never given birth to a viable infant
   (E) pregnant for the first time
   (F) one who has been pregnant several times
   (G) the number of pregnancies that have continued to viability
   (H) a woman who has given birth one time to a viable infant, regardless of whether the child was living at birth and regardless of whether the birth was single or multiple
   (I) a 3-month period during gestation

Questions 301 through 308: Match the terms in Column A to the correct description in Column B.

COLUMN A

301. Adnexa _____
302. Eclampsia _____
303. Meconium _____
304. Postpartum _____
305. Hydramnios _____
306. Oxytocin _____
307. Oligohydramnios
     _____
308. Preeclampsia
     _____

COLUMN B

(A) dark green substance in the intestines of a full-term fetus
(B) toxemia of late pregnancy characterized by convulsion and coma
(C) any accessory parts, structures, or masses lateral to the uterus
(D) small amount of amniotic fluid, below 300 cc at term
(E) excessive amount of amniotic fluid, above 2,000 cc at term
(F) after birth
(G) a hormone that stimulates uterine contractions
(H) toxemia of late pregnancy characterized by hypertension, albuminuria, and edema

Questions 309 through 314: Match the terms in Column A to the correct description in Column B.

COLUMN A

309. Lightening _____
310. Chadwick's sign
     _____
311. Hegar's sign _____
312. Goodell's sign
     _____
313. Braxton Hicks sign
     _____
314. Quickening _____

COLUMN B

(A) painless uterine contraction
(B) softening of the lower uterine segment
(C) the fetal head engages into the pelvis
(D) softening of the cervix
(E) the mother's first perception of the movements of the fetus felt in utero from 16 to 18 weeks of pregnancy
(F) bluish purple color of the vagina

Questions 315 through 318: Diabetes is one of the more common medical complications of pregnancy. Match the diabetic classification in Column A to the correct description in Column B.

COLUMN A

315. Class A diabetes
     _____
316. Class B diabetes
     _____
317. Class C diabetes
     _____
318. Class D diabetes
     _____

COLUMN B

(A) chemical diabetes before pregnancy
(B) onset before age 10, duration over 20 years, vascular lesions of benign retinopathy
(C) onset between ages 10 and 19, duration of 10–19 years, no evidence of vascular disease
(D) onset of clinical diabetes mellitus after age 20, duration less than 10 years, no evidence of vascular disease

319. The start of the first menstrual cycle is called

(A) amenorrhea
(B) dysmenorrhea
(C) menarche
(D) polymenorrhea

320. How long after fertilization does implantation of the blastocyst occur?

(A) 4 weeks
(B) 14 days
(C) 24 hours
(D) 7 days

321. A benign invasion of endometrial tissue into the myometrium is known as

(A) endometriosis
(B) pelvic inflammatory disease (PID)
(C) adenomyosis
(D) endomyosarcoma

322. Bacterial organisms that result in pelvic inflammatory disease (PID) are

(A) *Neisseria gonorrhoeae*
(B) *Escherichia coli*
(C) enterococci
(D) *Chlamydia trachomatis*
(E) *Streptococcus veridans*
(F) A and D only
(G) all of the above

323. The signs and symptoms of pelvic inflammatory disease (PID) are

(A) severe pelvic pain
(B) high fever
(C) leukocytosis
(D) rapid pulse rate
(E) vaginal discharge
(F) rebound tenderness
(G) A, B, and C
(H) B, C, and E
(I) all of the above

324. Endometriosis is a condition that mostly affects

(A) women who are infertile
(B) women who are in their thirties
(C) women who are multipara
(D) white women more than black women
(E) B and D only
(F) A, B, and D only
(G) all of the above

325. Women with endometriosis may have

(A) dyspareunia
(B) metromennorhagia
(C) dysmenorrhea
(D) all of the above

326. Endometriosis is

(A) ectopic endometrial tissue
(B) benign invasion of endometrial tissue into the myometrium
(C) endomyosarcoma with chocolate tissue
(D) inflammation of the endometrium

327. The sonographic features of endometriosis are

(A) chocolate cyst
(B) fluid-fluid levels
(C) cyst with irregular wall
(D) echo-free with relative smooth border
(E) cysts containing clumps of high-level echoes
(F) A, D, and C
(G) all of the above

328. Pelvic inflammatory disease (PID) of intrauterine contraceptive device (IUCD) users is more often associated with

(A) *Staphylococcus* infection
(B) gonorrhea
(C) actinomycosis
(D) *Escheria coli* infection

329. Prominent endometrial echo within the uterus can be seen in cases of

(A) ectopic gestation
(B) endometritis
(C) pelvic inflammatory disease (PID)
(D) menstruation (secretory phase)
(E) A, C, and D only
(F) all of the above

330. Which of the following can mimic pelvic inflammatory disease (PID)?

(A) endometriosis
(B) ectopic pregnancy
(C) multiple hemorrhagic cysts
(D) multicystic ovarian cancer
(E) all of the above

Questions 331 through 334: Match the terms in Column A to the correct description in Column B.

COLUMN A	COLUMN B
331. Aerobe _____	(A) pus in the fallopian tubes
332. Anaerobe _____	(B) organism that requires oxygen for life
333. Pyocolpos _____	(C) organism that does not require oxygen for life
334. Pyosalpinx _____	(D) pus in the vagina

335. The *most* common sonographic appearance(s) of a dermoid cyst(s) are which of the following: (1) totally anechoic, (2) completely solid, (3) predominantly solid, (4) complex mass with internal echoes and acoustic shadow?

(A) 1 and 4
(B) 2 and 3
(C) 2 only
(D) 4 only

336. The *most* common location for dermoid cyst(s) is (are)

(A) posterior cul-de-sac
(B) right adnexa
(C) left adnexa
(D) superior to the uterine fundus

337. Krukenberg's tumor is

(A) a secondary carcinoma of the ovaries with primary in the gastrointestinal tract
(B) a primary carcinoma of the ovaries with secondary in the gastrointestinal tract
(C) a benign ovarian tumor
(D) the most common ovarian tumor in children

338. The cause(s) of ectopic pregnancy is

(A) delayed transit of the fertilized zygote secondary to tube malfunction
(B) obstruction of the tube due to adhesions from pelvic inflammatory disease (PID)
(C) chronic salpingitis
(D) all of the above

339. When is the recommended time to perform genetic amniocentesis?

(A) 40 weeks' menstrual age
(B) 36 weeks' gestational age
(C) 20–24 weeks' menstrual age
(D) 16–19 weeks' gestational age

340. During which weeks of gestation is femur length measurement most accurate?

(A) 20–30
(B) 10–20
(C) 30–36
(D) 14–20

341. For safe amniocentesis, the needle should be placed

(A) through the thickest portion of the placenta but away from the fetus
(B) through the umbilical cord but away from the fetus and placenta
(C) avoiding the placenta, umbilical cord, and fetus
(D) through the fetal spine

342. The reasons(s) for amniocentesis are which of the following: (1) sex determination, (2) genetic disorders, (3) fetal maturity, (4) hemolytic disease?

(A) 2 and 3
(B) 2, 3, and 4 only
(C) 2 and 4
(D) all of the above

343. If the serum β human chorionic gonadotropin (β-hCG) is negative, the recommended procedure is

(A) sonogram may not be warranted
(B) laparoscopy
(C) dilation and curettage (D&C)
(D) suction curettage

344. How early can the fetal iliac crests be depicted on sonogram?

(A) 8 weeks
(B) 10 weeks
(C) 12 weeks
(D) 18 weeks

345. How long after fertilization does a corpus luteum cyst first begin to regress?

(A) 5 days
(B) 14 days
(C) 12–15 weeks
(D) 16–20 weeks

346. What types of fibroids are *most* likely to become pedunculated?

(A) interstitial
(B) subserous
(C) submucous
(D) leiomyosarcoma
(E) B and C
(F) A and D

347. Which of the following is *not* true of the fetal lungs on sonography?

(A) the fetal lungs are relatively homogeneous on sonogram
(B) the echogenicity of the lungs is similar to that of the liver
(C) in the third trimester, the lungs become more echogenic than the liver
(D) the fetal lungs expand only after birth. The fetal lungs contain air and are at rest in utero; thus the reason for nonvisualization by ultrasound

348. What is the normal rate of fetal chest wall movements in utero?

(A) 12–60 breaths per minute
(B) 60–80 breaths per minute
(C) 80–120 breaths per minute
(D) all of the above are untrue; thoracic movement occurs only after birth

349. Which of the following can be seen in the fetal lungs on sonography?

(A) type I cystic adenomatoid malformation
(B) type II cystic adenomatoid malformation
(C) pleural effusions
(D) pulmonary sequestration
(E) all of the above
(F) none of the above can be seen; the fetal lungs expand only after birth and also contain air; thus pulmonary lesions cannot be visualized by sonography

350. Which of the following statements is *not* true of ectopic pregnancy?

(A) once a patient has had an ectopic pregnancy, there is a 1 in 4 chance of recurrence
(B) the most common presenting symptoms of an ectopic pregnancy is pelvic pain
(C) ectopic pregnancy in the interstitial portion of the fallopian tube is more serious than in the ampullary portion
(D) ectopic pregnancy in the ampullary portion of the fallopian tube is more serious than in the interstitial portion

351. How long after conception in a normal intrauterine pregnancy (IUP) can the β human chorionic gonadotropin (β-hCG) be detected?

(A) 10 days
(B) 4 weeks
(C) 8 weeks
(D) 28 days

352. Immediately prior to ovulation, follicular cysts can be identified within the ovary. They range in size from

(A) 3 to 5 cm
(B) 25 to 30 mm
(C) 10 to 20 mm
(D) 5 to 10 cm

353. The normal adult ovaries measure

(A) 3 × 2 × 2 cm
(B) 2 × 2 × 4 cm
(C) 3 × 3 × 2 cm
(D) 3 × 2 × 1 mm

354. Which of the following medications could stimulate the growth of multiple follicles?

(A) Clomid (clomiphene citrate)
(B) Perganol (menotropins)
(C) Valmid (ethinamate)
(D) A and B only
(E) all of the above

355. Uterine size may vary according to the patient's age and parity. What is the approximate measurement for a 22-year-old nulligravida?

(A) 8 × 6 × 5 cm
(B) 6 × 3 × 3 cm
(C) 90 × 60 × 30 mm
(D) 100 × 60 × 30 mm

356. In order to identify and measure the ovaries, the recommended technique(s) is

(A) identify the internal iliac vessels running along the posterolateral aspect of the ovary
(B) measure length × thickness × width
(C) identify the internal iliac vessels running along the anteriolateral aspect of the ovary
(D) measure length × width × thickness and divide by 6
(E) A and B
(F) A and D

357. The postmenopausal ovaries are usually enlarged.

(A) true
(B) false

358. The human pelvis is formed by two innominate bones (ossa coxae), the sacrum, and coccyx. The term *innominate* is derived from the Latin word for nameless (*innominatus*). However, these bones do have names. Identify them.

(A) ischium
(B) ileum
(C) pubic
(D) ilium
(E) condyle
(F) A, B, and C
(G) A, C, and D

359. The method of terminating pregnancy is dependent upon the gestational age. Which method is used for up to 12 weeks' menstrual age?

(A) vacuum aspiration (suction curettage)
(B) hypertonic saline
(C) hysterectomy
(D) oxytocin

360. The method of terminating pregnancy is dependent upon the gestational age. Which of the following methods are *not* used after 14 weeks' menstrual age?

(A) vacuum aspiration (suction curettage)
(B) hypertonic saline
(C) hysterectomy
(D) oxytocin

361. Possible masses arising from the posterior aspect of the uterus can be confirmed further by

(A) barium enema with real-time sonography
(B) water enema with real-time sonography
(C) further distending the urinary bladder via a Foley catheter
(D) a radiograph
(E) all of the above

362. The normal variation(s) in the position of the uterus is

(A) anteflexed
(B) retroflexed
(C) anteverted
(D) retroverted
(E) midposition
(F) right lateral deviation
(G) left lateral deviation
(H) C and D
(I) A, B, C, and D
(J) all of the above

363. A T-shaped uterus is associated with

(A) a mother who ingested diethylstilbestrol (DES) when she was pregnant
(B) trauma to the supporting structure of the uterus
(C) relative deficiency of vitamins
(D) none of the above

Questions 364 through 367: Match the terms in Column A to the correct description in Column B.

COLUMN A

364. Hydrometrocolpos
365. Hematometrocolpos
366. Pyometrium
367. Pseudopolyp

COLUMN B

(A) watery fluid in the uterus and vagina
(B) pus in the uterus
(C) blood in the uterus and vagina
(D) tag of mucous membrane resembling a tumor with a pedicle

368. The sonographic appearance(s) of leiomyoma is

(A) nodular distortion of the uterine contour
(B) distortion of the endometrial echoes
(C) abnormal indentation on the bladder or rectum
(D) high-level echoes with distal shadow
(E) calcific degeneration
(F) the uterus cannot be separated from the mass
(G) uterine enlargement
(H) A, B, E, and G
(I) all of the above

369. The sonographic criterion or criteria for a cystic mass are

(A) anechoic even at high-gain settings
(B) smooth, well-defined wall
(C) distal acoustic enhancement
(D) distal acoustic shadow
(E) low-amplitude echoes posterior to the mass
(F) A, B, and E
(G) A, B, and C
(H) A, B, and D
(I) all of the above

370. The sonographic criterion or criteria for a solid mass are

(A) anechoic, without distal acoustic enhancement
(B) smooth, well-defined walls
(C) distal acoustic enhancement
(D) distal acoustic shadow
(E) low-amplitude echoes posterior to the mass
(F) internal echoes that increase with an increase in gain settings
(G) irregular and poorly defined walls and margins
(H) A, D, E, F, and G
(I) A, B, and C
(J) A, B, and E
(K) all of the above

371. Which of the following is *not* true of serous cystadenomas?

(A) thin-walled cyst without septations
(B) occasionally large with measurement of 15–20 cm

(C) more frequently seen in postmenopausal women
(D) more frequently seen with numerous internal septations

372. Which of the following is *not* true of mucinous cystadenomas?

(A) more frequently seen without internal septations
(B) occasionally large with measurement of 15–20 cm
(C) more frequently seen in postmenopausal women
(D) more frequently seen with numerous internal septations

373. In the event of malignant tumors, the sonographer should look for

(A) other tumors
(B) pleural effusions
(C) ascites in the pouch of Douglas
(D) ascites in both paracolic gutters
(E) A and D
(F) all of the above

374. If the peritoneal cavity becomes filled with a mucinous material from a ruptured ovarian cyst or cystadenocarcinoma, it is called

(A) ascites
(B) abscess
(C) pseudomyxoma peritonei
(D) hematoma

Questions 375 through 380: Squamous cell carcinoma of the cervix is the most common malignancy among women in the United States. Match the stages in Column A to the correct description in Column B.

COLUMN A

375. Stage IVB
376. Stage 0
377. Stage IA
378. Stage II
379. Stage IB
380. Stage IIB

COLUMN B

(A) carcinoma confined to the cervix
(B) lateral parametrial involvement
(C) microinvasive
(D) carcinoma extending beyond the cervix
(E) carcinoma in situ
(F) distant metastases

381. Stein-Leventhal syndrome is characterized by

(A) bilateral large cystic ovaries (polycystic ovaries)
(B) obesity
(C) hirsuitism
(D) infertility
(E) menstrual dysfunction

(F) A, D, and E

(G) all of the above

382. A large cyst of about 15–18 cm is situated in the broad ligament between the fallopian tube and ovaries with remnants of the wolffian body. This is *most* likely

(A) theca lutein cyst
(B) serous cystadenoma
(C) serous cystadenocarcinoma
(D) paraovarian cyst

383. Postpartum period refers to

(A) after childbirth
(B) after death
(C) after 20 weeks of gestation
(D) all of the above

384. Puerperium refers to the period

(A) after death
(B) 8–10 weeks after delivery
(C) 6–8 weeks before delivery
(D) 3–6 weeks after delivery

385. Which of the following structures is most likely *not* seen in a postpartum pelvic sonogram?

(A) uterus
(B) endometrial echo
(C) vagina
(D) ovaries

386. If sonograms were taken approximately 1 day after delivery, the fundal height and measurement of the uterus should be

(A) fundus at the level of the umbilicus and measuring 19–22 cm
(B) fundus midway between the symphysis pubis and umbilicus and measuring 10–12 cm
(C) fundus midway between the symphysis pubis and umbilicus and measuring 8–10 cm
(D) involuted back to its normal size, measuring about 7–8.5 cm

387. The *most* common complication(s) during the postpartum period is

(A) hemorrhage
(B) thromboembolism
(C) infection
(D) placenta previa
(E) A, B, and C
(F) all of the above

388. The normal volume of amniotic fluid

(A) increases with gestational age throughout pregnancy

(B) decreases with gestational age and increases near term
(C) increases with gestational age and decreases near term
(D) remains the same volume throughout pregnancy

389. The *most* common and accepted method for measuring the biparietal diameter (BPD) is from

(A) outer to outer edge
(B) outer to inner edge
(C) inner to inner edge
(D) mid-echo to mid-echo edge

390. The degree to which the head shapes may affect biparietal diameter (BPD) can be estimated by which of the following formulas?

(A) $HC = BPD_2 + OFD\pi$

(B) $V = 7 \dfrac{\pi}{6\,(BPD \div OFD)}$

(C) $CI = \dfrac{BPD}{OFD} \times 100$

(D) $BPD = \dfrac{BPD \times OFD}{1.256}$

391. Head circumference can be obtained with which of the following methodologies?

(A) real-time electronic caliper

(B) light pen with commercial computer measurement system

(C) map measurer

(D) formula head circumference $(HC) = \dfrac{BPD + OFD}{2}\pi$

(E) A and C only

(F) all of the above

392. The *least* reliable method for measuring femoral length is

(A) sector real-time
(B) static scanner
(C) linear-array real-time
(D) Doppler measurement

393. To reduce the chance of error when measuring the biparietal diameter (BPD), the sonographer should

 (A) make sure the fetal head appears ovoid
 (B) make sure the fetal head appears round
 (C) obtain a sonogram at the level of the cavum septum pellucidum, thalamus, and anterior horns of the lateral ventricle
 (D) obtain a sonogram at the level of the falx cerebri and lateral ventricles
 (E) A and D
 (F) B and C
 (G) A and C
 (H) all of the above

394. The kidneys of the fetus develop in which anatomic region?

 (A) pelvis
 (B) paraspinal position
 (C) thorax
 (D) flanks

395. The urinary bladder of the fetus is completely developed by

 (A) 12 weeks
 (B) 20 weeks
 (C) 36 weeks
 (D) 8 weeks

396. Fetal gender can be determined as early as

 (A) 24 weeks
 (B) 8 weeks
 (C) 34 weeks
 (D) 16 weeks

397. Definite evidence of a male fetus is obtained by visualization of the

 (A) penis
 (B) scrotum
 (C) testicles
 (D) prostate gland
 (E) A, B, and C
 (F) all of the above

398. What is the pathologic significance of isolated hydrocele in utero?

 (A) renal agenesis
 (B) multicystic kidneys
 (C) no significance
 (D) trauma to testicles

399. Definite evidence of a female fetus can be confirmed by

 (A) nonvisualization of the scrotum
 (B) nonvisualization of the penis
 (C) depiction of the labia
 (D) depiction of the urinary bladder

400. The accuracy in gender prediction in the second and third trimesters is

 (A) 80–90%
 (B) 50–60%
 (C) always 100%
 (D) 95–99.9%

401. The vessel in the umbilical cord that carries oxygenated blood and nourishment from the placenta to the fetus is

 (A) one artery
 (B) two veins
 (C) one vein

402. The vessel in the umbilical cord that carries deoxygenated blood from the fetus to the placenta is

 (A) two arteries
 (B) two veins
 (C) one vein

Questions 403 though 408: Match the terms in Column A to the correct description in Column B.

COLUMN A	COLUMN B
403. Placenta previa _____	(A) abnormal adherence of part or all of the placenta to the uterine wall
404. Placenta accreta _____	
405. Placenta succenturiata _____	(B) premature separation of the placenta after 20 weeks of gestation
406. Abruptio placentae _____	(C) accessory lobe of placenta
407. Placenta increta _____	(D) implantation of the placenta in the lower uterine segment
408. Placenta percreta _____	(E) abnormal adherence of part or all of the placenta in which the chorionic villi invade the myometrium
	(F) abnormal adherence of part or all of the placenta in which chorionic villi invade the uterine wall

409. The treatment for incompetent cervix is

 (A) the McDonald procedure
 (B) the Shirodkar procedure
 (C) dilation and curettage (D&C)
 (D) hysterectomy
 (E) A and B

410. Which of the following has the largest percentage incidence of a single umbilical artery?

(A) singleton births
(B) twins
(C) abortuses
(D) fetuses with trisomy D

411. The causes of an incompetent cervix are

(A) several dilation and curettage procedures (D&Cs)
(B) exposure to diethylstilbestrol in utero
(C) hormonal influences
(D) all of the above

412. Incompetent cervix is treated at how many weeks of gestation?

(A) 24
(B) 28–36
(C) 14–18
(D) 8–10

413. Sonographers should pay attention to the technical aspects of the study when ruling out placenta previa or incompetent cervix. Which of the following is *least* likely?

(A) overdistended maternal urinary bladder can cause false-negative diagnosis of incompetent cervix
(B) an erect position should *not* be used because gravitational pressure from uterine contents can cause an abortion
(C) overdistended maternal urinary bladder can cause false-positive diagnosis of placenta previa
(D) fetal head can prevent visualization of a posterior placenta previa
(E) A, C, and D
(F) B and C only
(G) all of the above

414. Twins that result from union of one sperm and one ovum are called

(A) monozygotic
(B) dizygotic
(C) fraternal
(D) identical
(E) B and C
(F) A and D

415. Twins that result from union of two sperm and two ova are called

(A) monozygotic
(B) dizygotic
(C) fraternal
(D) identical
(E) B and C
(F) A and D

416. When is a neonate considered growth retarded?

(A) when the neonate's mean weight for gestational age is below the 10th percentile
(B) when the biparietal diameter (BPD) is less than 9.7 cm at term
(C) neonates born between 36 and 40 weeks
(D) when hydramnios is present at term

417. Which of the following methods is *least* reliable for diagnosing intrauterine growth retardation (IUGR)?

(A) total intrauterine volume (TIUV)
(B) head circumference
(C) abdominal circumference
(D) femur length

418. The formula for head circumference (HC) is

(A) $HC = \dfrac{\pi}{6\ c(AB + C^1)}$

(B) $HC = 0.523 \times ABC$

(C) $HC = \dfrac{BPD + OFD}{2}\ \pi$

419. Abdominal circumference measurement reflects primarily which organ size?

(A) stomach
(B) umbilical vein
(C) kidney
(D) liver

420. The formula for abdominal circumference is

(A) $AC = (D_1 + D_2) \times 1.57$

(B) $AC = \dfrac{\pi}{6\ (A + B^1)}$

(C) $AC = 0.523 \times ABC$

(D) $AC = \dfrac{BPD + OFD}{2}\ \pi$

421. Which of the following organs are responsible for amniotic fluid production?

(A) stomach
(B) umbilical vein
(C) kidney
(D) liver

422. Which of the following is *not* true of renal agenesis?

(A) associated with oligohydramnios
(B) associated with hydramnios
(C) associated with Potter's syndrome
(D) absence of the kidneys

423. The most common fetal renal anomaly is

(A) hydronephrosis
(B) polycystic kidney
(C) Wilms' tumor
(D) neuroblastoma

424. Most unilateral hydronephrosis is due to

(A) neuroblastoma
(B) polycystic kidney
(C) Wilms' tumor
(D) ureteropelvic junction obstruction

425. Bilateral hydronephrosis of a fetus in utero is associated with

(A) "prune belly" syndrome
(B) ureteropelvic junction obstruction
(C) oligohydramnios
(D) dilated urinary bladder
(E) Eagle-Barrett syndrome
(F) B, C, and D
(G) all of the above

426. Which of the following statements is *not* true of "prune belly" syndrome?

(A) predominantly a male disorder
(B) also known as Eagle-Barrett syndrome
(C) it is associated with cryptorchidism
(D) predominantly a female disorder

427. Which of the following is *not* true of infantile polycystic disease?

(A) it has an autosomal recessive type of inheritance
(B) it occurs bilaterally
(C) it is bilateral renal enlargement
(D) it can be diagnosed before birth
(E) it cannot be diagnosed before birth
(F) it occurs in Meckel's syndrome
(G) it is incompatible with life

428. Which of the following is *not* true of multicystic disease?

(A) it has an autosomal dominant type of inheritance
(B) it is usually unilateral
(C) it is bilateral renal enlargement
(D) it can be diagnosed before birth
(E) it cannot be diagnosed before birth
(F) it occurs in Meckel's syndrome

429. Sonography can depict all of the following *except*

(A) diaphragmatic hernia
(B) choledochal cyst
(C) meconium pseudocysts
(D) fetal alopecia

430. Hydramnios denotes

(A) excessive amount of amniotic fluid over 200 mL at term
(B) excessive amount of amniotic fluid over 2,000 mL at term
(C) reduced amount of amniotic fluid below 300 mL at term
(D) reduced amount of amniotic fluid below 200 mL at term

431. Oligohydramnios denotes

(A) excessive amount of amniotic fluid over 200 mL at term
(B) excessive amount of amniotic fluid over 2,000 mL at term
(C) reduced amount of amniotic fluid below 300 mL at term
(D) reduced amount of amniotic fluid below 2,000 mL at term

432. The formation of the umbilical cord in the early weeks of embryogenesis results from fusion of which structures?

(A) decidual basalis
(B) decidual capsularis
(C) body stalk
(D) yolk stalk
(E) A and B
(F) B and C
(G) C and D
(H) A and D

433. The blood vessels inside the umbilical cord are protected by a mucoid substance called

(A) chorionic fluid
(B) amniotic fluid
(C) Wharton's jelly
(D) estrogen

434. The *most* accurate time to obtain femur length is

(A) 14–20 weeks
(B) 20–30 weeks
(C) 6–12 weeks
(D) 30–40 weeks

435. Which of the following statements is true about twins?

(A) monozygotic twins also are known as fraternal twins
(B) dizygotic twins also are known as identical twins
(C) approximately 75% of twins are of the same sex
(D) twins produced from a single ova are called fraternal twins

436. The *most* common anomaly affecting the central nervous system (CNS) is

(A) spina bifida
(B) anencephaly
(C) encephalocele
(D) hydrocephalus

437. If fetal ascites are seen in a mother with an elevated Rh titer, it is most likely an indication of

(A) hepatosplenomegaly
(B) duodenal atresia
(C) umbilical cord anomalies
(D) heart failure

438. Artifactual ascites (pseudoascites) which can be produced by a linear array real-time, may be confused with true ascites. To avoid this confusion, the sonographer should use which of the following important techniques: (1) record the falciform ligament and its surrounding fluid, (2) record the pattern of intraperitoneal fluid, (3) change the patient's position and observe whether the fluid moves to a dependent position, (4) record the pattern of the retroperitoneal fluid as it surrounds the abdominal viscera?

(A) 3 and 4
(B) 1, 2, and 3
(C) 1 and 4
(D) all of the above

439. Which of the following anomalies are associated with erythroblastosis?

(A) ascites
(B) hepatosplenomegaly
(C) hydramnios
(D) increased umbilical vein diameter
(E) hydrops
(F) all of the above

440. Cleft palate is associated with

(A) hypotelorism
(B) alobar holoprosencephaly
(C) trisomy 13
(D) A and B only
(E) all of the above

441. A complex mass is seen near the buttocks of a fetus in utero. The mass has some calcific areas with distal acoustic shadows. This is most likely

(A) sacrococcygeal teratoma
(B) meconium
(C) encephalocele
(D) uteropelvic junction obstruction

442. The sonographic appearance of cleft palate is

(A) a coronal view through the maxilla showing absence of this bone below the nose
(B) a coronal view through the maxilla showing absence of this bone above the nose
(C) cystic mass protruding from the lip
(D) split in the zygoma
(E) A, C, and D
(F) all of the above

443. What blood vessel usually can be depicted posteromedial to the ovary?

(A) ovarian vein
(B) ovarian artery
(C) external iliac artery
(D) internal iliac artery

444. If a patient's blood pressure is 140/90 mm Hg or more with edema and proteinuria, these signs and symptoms are consistent with

(A) rubella
(B) Rh isoimmunization
(C) syphilis
(D) preeclampsia

445. A patient's blood pressure is 140/90 mm Hg or more with edema, proteinuria, and convulsions. These signs and symptoms are consistent with

(A) rubella
(B) Rh isoimmunization
(C) eclampsia
(D) syphilis

446. A hemolytic disease of newborns, characterized by anemia, jaundice, and hepatosplenomegaly is

(A) lymphangioma
(B) erythroblastosis fetalis
(C) Eagle-Barrett syndrome
(D) omphalocele

447. A patient who contracts German measles in the first 12 weeks of gestation may give birth to an infant with

(A) auditory defects
(B) patent ductus arteriosus of the heart
(C) macrocephaly
(D) microcephaly
(E) A and C
(F) A, B, and D
(G) C and D

448. The three stages of labor are which of the following: (1) dilatation of the cervix, (2) abdominal pain, (3) delivery of the baby, (4) expulsion of the placenta, (5) Braxton Hicks contractions?

(A) 2, 3, and 4
(B) 1, 3, and 4
(C) 5, 3, and 4

449. The external os of the cervix is said to be completely dilated at

(A) 10 cm
(B) 10 mm
(C) 25 cm
(D) 100 mm
(E) A and D
(F) all of the above

450. With current real-time equipment, how early can the fetal kidneys be depicted?

(A) 11 weeks
(B) 14 weeks
(C) 20 weeks
(D) 35 weeks

451. How much does the fetal head grow per week at 16 weeks of gestation?

(A) 5 mm per week
(B) 15 mm per week
(C) 2 cm per week
(D) 3 cm per week

452. If performing a BPD measurement and the midline echo is continuous and unbroken, this would indicate that the scanning plane is

(A) normal
(B) too high
(C) through the fetal neck
(D) correct

453. How much does the fetal head grow per week at 20 weeks of gestation?

(A) 5 mm per week
(B) 15 mm per week
(C) 2 cm per week
(D) 3.6 mm per week

454. How much does the fetal head grow per week at 32 weeks of gestation?

(A) 5 mm per week
(B) 15 mm per week
(C) 2.3 mm per week
(D) 3.5 cm per week

455. How much does the fetal head grow per week at 40 weeks of gestation?

(A) 5 mm per week
(B) 1.4 mm per week
(C) 2.3 mm per week
(D) 3.5 cm per week

456. Which of the following pelvic masses is *least* likely to enlarge during pregnancy?

(A) ovarian cystadenoma
(B) fibroid
(C) corpus luteum cyst
(D) dermoid cyst

457. The *most* common solid mass(es) associated with pregnancy is (are)

(A) dermoid
(B) leiomyomas
(C) leiomyosarcoma
(D) cystadenoma

458. The causes for a uterus too large for dates include

(A) multiple gestation
(B) oligohydramnios
(C) hydramnios
(D) wrong menstrual dates
(E) hydatidiform mole
(F) myoma
(G) A, C, and D
(H) A, C, D, E, and F
(I) A and D only
(J) all of the above

459. The causes for a uterus too small for dates include

(A) fetal death
(B) oligohydramnios
(C) hydramnios
(D) wrong menstrual dates
(E) hydatidiform mole
(F) intrauterine growth retardation (IUGR)
(G) A, B, D, and F
(H) A, C, D, E, and F
(I) A and F
(J) all of the above

460. The position of the uterus may be variable with parity. What percentage of women may have an anteverted uterus?

(A) 50%
(B) 10%
(C) 80%
(D) 90%

461. What degree of angle does the uterus normally have with the long axis of the vagina?

(A) 50°
(B) 10°

(C) 45°
(D) 80°
(E) 90°

462. If the peritoneum is reflected at the level of the isthmus on the anterior surface of the uterus to the upper aspect of the bladder, it is called

(A) anterior cul-de-sac
(B) pouch of Douglas
(C) vesicouterine pouch
(D) space of Retzius
(E) posterior cul-de-sac
(F) A and C
(G) B and E

463. If the peritoneum is reflected at the level of the posterior fornix of the vagina on the posterior surface of the uterus to the anterior aspect of the rectum, it is called

(A) posterior cul-de-sac
(B) pouch of Douglas
(C) vesicouterine pouch
(D) space of Retzius
(E) retrouterine pouch
(F) A, B, and E

464. The space between the bladder and pubis that is filled with extraperitoneal adipose tissue is called

(A) posterior cul-de-sac
(B) pouch of Douglas
(C) vesicouterine pouch
(D) space of Retzius
(E) retrouterine pouch

465. The three major pelvic side wall muscles seen on sonography are

(A) iliopsoas
(B) pubococcygeus
(C) obturator internus
(D) rectus
(E) gluteal
(F) A, B, and D
(G) C, E, and D
(H) A, B, and C

466. What is mittelschmerz?

(A) a disease of the iliopsoas muscles
(B) intermenstrual pain
(C) a name for infants of diabetic mothers
(D) a malignant blood disease

467. What was removed during surgery may be important clinical information for the sonographer to know. If a 27-year-old patient with a recent abdominal pregnancy of 37 weeks presents with a surgical Hx of status/post (S/P) C-section, which of the following organs or structures would almost never be removed in this case?

(A) placenta
(B) uterus
(C) cord
(D) fetus

468. An acardius anencephalic twin occurs in

(A) monozygotic twin pregnancy
(B) dizygotic twin pregnancy
(C) amniotic band syndrome
(D) B and C
(E) all of the above

469. If the heart is absent (acardius) on real-time in one of the fetuses of an anencephalic twin, it is correct to assume that

(A) one of the fetuses is dead and therefore only the other will move around on real-time
(B) both fetuses may move around and demonstrate flexion and extension of the limbs
(C) if there is no visible head or heart, there will be no movement

470. Anencephaly results from failure of the

(A) müllerian duct to close completely
(B) neural tube to close completely at its cephalic end
(C) neural tube to close completely at its caudad end

471. The standard range of error for biparietal diameter (BPD) measurements in the third trimester is

(A) 10 mm
(B) 5 mm
(C) 2 mm
(D) 4 mm

472. A method that an individual user can employ to test the range of error for biparietal diameter (BPD) is

(A) a series of measurements made on the same patient in 24 hours
(B) error = (BPD + 2) × π
(C) neither A nor B

Figure 8–26. Sagittal midline sonogram through the uterus.

473. The sonographic findings in Fig. 8–26 include

    (A) multiple echogenic interfaces probably arising from a Lippes loop IUCD
    (B) echogenic material within the uterus probably secondary to sloughed endometrium
    (C) A and B
    (D) neither A nor B

474. The optimal placement of an intrauterine contraceptive device (IUCD) is

    (A) in the cervix
    (B) in the fundus only
    (C) in the lumen of the uterus
    (D) within the wall of the uterus

475. The sonographic findings in Fig. 8–27 include

    (A) multiple immature follicles
    (B) a mature follicle and two immature follicles
    (C) polycystic ovary
    (D) none of the above

476. Mature follicles measure approximately

    (A) 2 cm
    (B) 1 cm
    (C) 3 cm
    (D) 4 cm

477. Sonographic findings in Fig. 8–28 include

    (A) ovarian cyst
    (B) loculated predominantly cystic adnexal mass
    (C) normal uterus
    (D) loculated fluid collections

478. The most probable diagnosis of this mass (Fig. 8–28) includes

    (A) endometrioma
    (B) ovarian cyst
    (C) cystic ovarian tumor
    (D) A or C

479. Fig. 8–29 is a transverse sonogram through the mid-abdomen of a postmenopausal woman. The abnormal finding on this sonogram includes

    (A) large ovarian tumor
    (B) matted bowel
    (C) simple ascites
    (D) bowel obstruction

480. The condition in question 479 usually results from

    (A) ovarian carcinoma
    (B) renal failure
    (C) liver failure
    (D) congestive heart failure

Figure 8–27. Sagittal sonogram obtained through the right adnexa of a patient undergoing ovulation induction.

Figure 8–28. Sagittal sonogram obtained through the left adnexa.

Figure 8–29. Transverse sonogram through the mid-abdomen.

481. Given the findings in Fig. 8–29, the most likely diagnosis is

    (A) pseudomyxoma peritonei
    (B) bowel obstruction
    (C) bowel perforation
    (D) appendicitis

482. The incidence of ovarian carcinoma in women in the United States over 50 years of age is

    (A) 33 per 100,000
    (B) 3 per 100,000
    (C) 333 per 100,000
    (D) cannot be estimated

483. Fig. 8–30 is a sonogram obtained through the lower face of a 29-week fetus. Sonographic findings include

    (A) cleft palate
    (B) cleft lip
    (C) cleft lip and palate
    (D) normal nose and lips

484. Cleft lip and palate is associated with

    (A) chromosomal disorders
    (B) Stein-Leventhal syndrome
    (C) A and B
    (D) none of the above

485. Fig. 8–31 is an image obtained through the arm and hand of a third-trimester fetus. The most likely diagnosis is

    (A) one digit missing
    (B) "hitchhiker thumb"
    (C) A and B
    (D) none of the above

486. Hydrops fetalis can be secondary to

    (A) tumors obstructing venous return to the heart
    (B) Rh isoimmunization
    (C) diabetes mellitis
    (D) A or B

487. The chorion and the amnion fuse at approximately

    (A) 8–10 weeks
    (B) 10–14 weeks
    (C) 18–20 weeks
    (D) they never fuse

Figure 8–30. Sonogram obtained through the lower face of a fetus.

Figure 8–31. Sonogram obtained through the arm and hand of a third trimester fetus.

Figure 8–32. Sagittal sonogram of a second trimester pregnancy.

488. The linear interference related to the chorionic plate in Fig. 8–32 represents

    (A) elevated chorion with subchorionic venous lakes
    (B) a placental chorioangioma
    (C) a placental tumor
    (D) chorioamniotic separation

489. The term *limb reduction abnormalities* includes

    (A) acheiria
    (B) acheiropodia
    (C) A and B
    (D) none of the above

490. Mild pyelocaliectasis of the fetal renal collecting system may be related to

    (A) maternal ingestion of fluid prior to sonographic study
    (B) diuresis of the fetal kidney

Figure 8–33. Sonogram obtained through the fetal thorax.

    (C) maternal diabetes
    (D) A and B

491. Fig. 8–33 is taken through the chest of a 30-week fetus. The large arrows point to

    (A) the atria
    (B) the ventricles
    (C) the valves
    (D) the papillary muscles

492. The short arrows point to

    (A) the atria
    (B) the ventricles
    (C) the valves
    (D) the papillary muscles

493. Maternal condition(s) that are associated with increased incidence of fetal heart malformations is

    (A) diabetes mellitus
    (B) certain medications such as lithium
    (C) both A and B
    (D) neither A nor B

494. In order to obtain the best femur length, the sonographer should

    (A) obtain the entire length of the femur, including the femoral neck and head
    (B) the diaphysis or shaft of the femur is the only portion that should be measured
    (C) the femur is not a good measurement of gestational age because it has a wide variance
    (D) none of the above

495. The uterus should involute to normal size

    (A) 1 week after delivery
    (B) approximately 4 weeks after delivery
    (C) 1 year after delivery
    (D) it never returns to normal size

496. Placenta previa most frequently occurs in

    (A) multigravida patients
    (B) patients with history of previous C-section
    (C) patients with history of previous therapeutic abortion
    (D) all of the above

497. Fig. 8–34 is an M-mode echocardiogram (vertical line/sec) of the same fetus shown in Fig. 8–33. The M-mode echocardiogram shows

    (A) arrhythmia
    (B) bradycardia
    (C) tachycardia
    (D) normal rhythm

Figure 8–34. M-mode echocardiogram of the fetus.

Figure 8–35. Transverse sonogram through the mid-abdomen.

498. Retrochorionic hemorrhage can be associated with

(A) a very poor prognosis for completion of pregnancy
(B) first and second trimester bleeding
(C) A and B
(D) neither A nor B

499. Arrhythmias may be associated with

(A) malformed hearts
(B) maternal lupus erythematosus
(C) maternal rheumatoid arthritis
(D) all of the above

500. The cervix normally measures

(A) no greater than 3 cm in length
(B) no less than 3 cm in length
(C) no less than 3 cm in anteroposterior dimension
(D) none of the above

501. The normal heart rate and rhythm of a second-trimester fetus is

(A) between 120 and 160 beats/minute
(B) can vary with the fetal state, breathing, and activities
(C) can demonstrate periodic premature ventricular contractions
(D) all of the above

502. The adrenal in the third-trimester fetus can be as much as _____ % the size of the kidneys.

(A) 70   (C) 30
(B) 50   (D) 10

503. Fig. 8–35 is a transverse sonogram through the mid-abdomen. The most likely diagnosis is

(A) molar tissue within the uterus
(B) a uterine fibroid
(C) normal pregnancy
(D) complicated ascites

504. The *most* common site for an ectopic pregnancy is

(A) ampullary portion of the fallopian tube
(B) isthmic portion of the fallopian tube
(C) interstitial portion of the fallopian tube
(D) within the ovary

505. Based on the sonogram in Fig. 8–35, one would expect that the pregnancy

(A) is less than 8 weeks
(B) is more than 14 weeks but less than 20
(C) cannot be predicted based on this sonogram
(D) is over 30 weeks

506. Sonography can be used in assessing the amount of retained tissue following a miscarriage. In the diagnosis of complete abortions, one must also consider the possibility of

(A) ectopic pregnancy
(B) concomitant intrauterine pregnancy
(C) A and B
(D) none of the above

Figure 8–36. Transverse sonogram through the fetal head.

507. Fig. 8–36 is a transverse sonogram of a fetal head at 16 weeks' gestation. This sonogram most likely represents

(A) normally shaped fetal head
(B) "lemon head," or abnormally convex frontal bones
(C) "banana sign," or abnormally fusiform shape of the cerebellar hemispheres
(D) hydrocephalus
(E) B and C

508. The abnormality in the fetus in Fig. 8–36 is associated with

(A) meningomyelocele
(B) omphalocele
(C) gastroschisis
(D) fetal hydronephrosis

509. The maternal serum α-fetoprotein in the mother of the fetus in Fig. 8–36 would be most likely

(A) elevated
(B) decreased
(C) normal

510. The yolk sac has an important role in early hematopoiesis. It typically is largest

(A) between 5 and 9 weeks
(B) after 16 weeks
(C) only before the fifth week
(D) none of the above

511. The positive sonographic findings in Fig. 8–37 include

(A) herniation of brain and meninges through defect in posterior cranial fossa
(B) a large meningomyelocele arising from the neck

(C) a large cystic hygroma arising from the neck
(D) none of the above

512. Cystic hygromas

(A) result from a malfusion of lymphatic channels behind the neck
(B) can be associated with Turner's syndrome
(C) A and B
(D) neither A nor B

513. What is the most common nontrophoblastic primary tumor of the placenta?

(A) teratoma
(B) chorioangioma
(C) hydatidiform mole
(D) melanoma

514. Fig. 8–38 is a magnified longitudinal sonogram of a postpartum uterus. The most likely diagnosis is

(A) retained products of conception
(B) molar pregnancy
(C) uterine fibroid
(D) none of the above

515. Fig. 8–39 is a longitudinal sonogram of a third-trimester fetus. The arrow points to

(A) ascites
(B) polyhydramnios
(C) pericardial effusion
(D) fetal hydrops

516. The cause for immune hydrops is

(A) obstruction to venous return
(B) Rh isoimmunization
(C) congestive heart failure of the fetus
(D) all of the above

Figure 8–37. Transverse sonogram through the fetal head.

Figure 8–38. Magnified longitudinal sonogram of a postpartum uterus.

Figure 8–39. Sagittal sonogram of a third trimester uterus.

517. Fig. 8–40 is a midline longitudinal sonogram of the lower uterine segment in a 30-week intrauterine pregnancy. The most likely diagnosis is

(A) placenta previa
(B) amniotic sheet or band
(C) uterine septation
(D) none of the above

518. Genetic amniocenteses are performed between 16 and 18 weeks because

(A) the α-fetoprotein is highest at that time
(B) the aminocytes have the highest likelihood for successful harvesting of chromosomes
(C) it is easiest to do amniocentesis at this stage
(D) a first-trimester termination can be performed if there is abnormal chromosomes

519. Amniotic band syndrome can be associated with

(A) gastroschisis
(B) omphalocele

(C) anencephaly
(D) amputated fingers, toes, and extremities
(E) all of the above

520. One would expect that the α-fetoprotein in an ancephalic fetus to be

(A) usually normal because this is a closed neural tube defect
(B) usually abnormal because this is an open neural tube defect
(C) may be abnormal if associated with a menigomyelocele
(D) none of the above

521. Bowel may be seen herniated at the base of the umbilical cord between _____ and _____ weeks of gestation.

(A) 5 and 6 weeks
(B) 8 and 12 weeks
(C) 12 and 18 weeks
(D) 18 and 20 weeks

522. If a sonographer encounters a patient with a bicornuate uterus, what other structures should be imaged?

(A) brain
(B) liver
(C) kidneys
(D) nothing needs to be done because this is almost always an isolated anomaly

523. Figs. 8–41 and 8–42 are transverse scans of the fetal abdomen of different third-trimester fetuses. Fig. 8–41 demonstrates

(A) polycystic kidneys
(B) meconium-filled large bowels
(C) hydronephrosis
(D) none of the above

Figure 8–40. Midline sagittal sonogram of the lower uterine segment.

Figure 8–41. Transverse sonogram through the fetal abdomen.

Figure 8-42. Transverse sonogram through the fetal abdomen.

524. Fig. 8–42 demonstrates

(A) fetal gallbladder
(B) portal sinus
(C) fetal stomach
(D) left adrenal
(E) all except for A

525. The type of intrauterine contraceptive device (IUCD) shown in Fig. 8–43 is

(A) Copper-7 (Cu-7)
(B) Lippes loop

(C) Dalkon shield
(D) none of the above

526. Complications of intrauterine contraceptive devices (IUCDs) include

(A) ectopic pregnancy
(B) ovarian abscess
(C) endometriosis
(D) A and B

527. A blighted ovum implies that

(A) a fetus has formed but has undergone disintegration
(B) an embryo has probably not been formed

528. Figs. 8–44 and 8–45 are obtained from a 28-week fetus. Fig. 8–44 represents

(A) hydrocephalus
(B) incorrect level for obtaining a biparietal diameter
(C) absence of the cavum septi pellucidi
(D) none of the above

529. Fig. 8–45 represents

(A) the proper level for obtaining an abdominal circumference
(B) omphalocele
(C) two dilated bowel loops
(D) double bubble

530. An overly distended urinary bladder may result in

(A) an anterior, low-lying placenta appearing as a placenta previa
(B) a posterior, low-lying placenta appearing as a placenta previa
(C) A or B
(D) none of the above

Figure 8-43. A magnified longitudinal pelvic sonogram in a patient with lost string.

Figure 8-44. Transverse sonogram through the fetal head.

Figure 8–45. Transverse sonogram through the fetal abdomen.

531. A fetus with situs inversus would demonstrate what on the sonogram?

(A) inflammation of the renal sinus
(B) pelvic kidney
(C) transposition of the abdominal and thoracic viscera
(D) enlargement of the fetal viscera

532. With anencephaly, there is an approximately 30% incidence of spinal dysraphism.

(A) true
(B) false

533. Fig. 8–46 is a transvaginal sonogram of a 27-year-old woman with amenorrhea. A physical examination suggested a slightly enlarged uterus. An ultrasound examination was requested to rule out ectopic pregnancy. This sonogram shows

(A) hydatidiform mole
(B) a chorionic sac within the decidualized endometrium
(C) a pseudogestational sac
(D) a nabothian cyst

534. Disorders that are frequently associated with a meningomyelocele include

(A) Chiari malformation
(B) polycystic kidneys
(C) omphalocele
(D) A and C

535. The abnormal sonographic findings in Fig. 8–47 include

(A) herniation of the liver outside of the abdomen
(B) large meningomyelocele
(C) extrophy of the heart
(D) none of the above

536. Omphalocele is usually associated with

(A) herniation of the bowel from an eccentric vent in the anterior abdominal wall at the umbilical cord insertion
(B) herniation of the bowel with normal umbilical cord insertion
(C) a solid mass extending from the coccyx
(D) cranial anomalies

Figure 8–46. Transvaginal sonogram of the uterus.

Figure 8–47. Transverse sonogram through the fetal abdomen at 30 weeks.

537. At what level of serum β human chorionic gonadotropin (β-hCG) is the normal intrauterine gestational sac seen on transvaginal sonography with the Second International Standard?

   (A) 65,000 mIU/mL
   (B) 35,000 mIU/mL
   (C) 1000 mIU/mL
   (D) 500 mIU/mL

538. The cumulus oophorus consists of

   (A) the oocyte
   (B) clusters of granulosa cells that surround the oocyte
   (C) A and B
   (D) neither A nor B

539. The most likely diagnosis that can be made from Fig. 8–48 is

   (A) a physiologic (follicular or luteal) ovarian cyst
   (B) cystadenocarcinoma
   (C) ruptured ectopic pregnancy
   (D) A and B

540. A physiologic ovarian cyst may have internal echoes due to

   (A) hemorrhage within the cyst
   (B) fat within the cyst
   (C) A or B
   (D) neither A nor B

541. Fig. 8–49 is a transvaginal sonogram of an early intrauterine pregnancy. The most likely diagnosis is

   (A) uterine contraction
   (B) intramural uterine fibroid

Figure 8–48. Sagittal midline pelvic sonogram of a 20-year-old patient with pelvic pain.

Figure 8–49. Transvaginal sonogram of a gravid uterus.

   (C) dermoid cyst
   (D) none of the above

542. The types of uterine fibroids include

   (A) submucosal
   (B) subserosal
   (C) intramural
   (D) all of the above

543. At what size should the gestation sac be in order to visualize the yolk sac in a normal intrauterine pregnancy with transvaginal sonography

   (A) 1–2 mm   (C) 4–6 mm
   (B) 2–4 mm   (D) 8–10 mm

544. Fig. 8–50 is a sagittal sonogram of a 28-year-old woman, gravida 3, para 2, who underwent ultrasound examination because of uncertain dates of her pregnancy. This image was taken at the level of the umbilical cord. The arrow points to

   (A) allantoid cyst
   (B) hemangioma of the umbilical cord
   (C) thrombosis of the umbilical vessels
   (D) three-vessel cord

545. Fig. 8–51 is a sagittal sonogram of a 30-year-old woman with uncertain menstrual date, who was re-

Figure 8–50. Sagittal sonogram of a gravid uterus.

Figure 8–51. Sagittal midline pelvic sonogram.

ferred for a pelvic sonogram. This sonographic finding demonstrates

(A) blood in the uterine cavity
(B) retroverted uterus with a Bartholin cyst
(C) retroverted uterus with a gestation sac
(D) retroverted uterus with a nabothian cyst

546. Retrochorionic hemorrhage that occurs in the first
trimester is usually associated with

(A) poor prognosis for completing the pregnancy
(B) ectopic pregnancy
(C) A or B
(D) neither A nor B

547. Fig. 8–52 is a transverse scan taken at the level of
the uterine fundus of a 25-year-old woman who was
referred for obstetrical sonogram with onset of vaginal bleeding and pelvic pain. This sonogram
demonstrates

(A) mature placenta
(B) placental cyst
(C) total placenta previa
(D) abruptio placentae

548. The difference between a gestational sac and a
pseudogestational sac is

Figure 8–52. Transverse sonogram through the uterine fundus.

Figure 8–53. Transverse sonogram of the fetal head.

(A) a gestational sac usually has two layers of
decidua
(B) a pseudogestational sac usually has two
layers of decidua
(C) a pseudogestational sac is larger than most
gestation sacs
(D) none of the above

549. Identify the structure the two arrowheads point to
in Fig. 8–53

(A) cavum septum pellucidum
(B) thalamus
(C) cerebral peduncle
(D) choroid plexus

550. Identify the structure the arrow points to in Fig. 8–
54

(A) cavum septum pellucidum
(B) thalamus
(C) cerebral peduncle
(D) third ventricle

Figure 8–54. Transverse sonogram of the fetal head.

551. Identify the structure the open arrow points to in Fig. 8–55

(A) cavum septum pellucidum
(B) thalamus
(C) cerebral peduncle
(D) third ventricle

552. Identify the structure the solid arrow points to in Fig. 8–55

(A) cavum septum pellucidum
(B) thalamus
(C) cerebral peduncle
(D) third ventricle

553. Pregnancies that occur with an intrauterine contraceptive device (IUCD) in place are

(A) most likely to produce endometriosis
(B) associated with approximately 50% of completion
(C) usually associated with excessive vaginal bleeding
(D) B and C

554. Identify the structure the arrow points to in Fig. 8–56

(A) falx cerebri
(B) sylvian fissure/insula
(C) hydrocephalus
(D) choroid plexus

Figure 8–56. Transverse sonogram of the fetal head.

555. Fig. 8–57 shows a 28-year-old patient admitted because of severe preeclampsia and hyperemesis gravidarum. Give an impression of the sonogram in correlation with the clinical findings shown in these figures.

(A) fibroid
(B) large dermoid
(C) hydatidiform mole
(D) multiloculated papillary serous cystadenoma
(E) pseudocyesis

556. The differential diagnoses indicated in Fig. 8–57 are (1) leiomyoma, (2) missed abortion, (3) pseudocyesis, (4) multiloculated papillary serous cystadenoma, (5) hematoma.

(A) 1 and 5
(B) 1, 2, 4, and 5
(C) 1, 2, and 3
(D) all of the above

557. This study (Fig. 8–58) is of a 19-year-old gravida 2, para 0, with a sudden onset of vaginal bleeding and pelvic pain. The urinary chorionic gonadotropin (UCG) was negative. What is the impression of the sonograms in correlation with the clinical findings?

(A) pelvic inflammatory disease (PID)
(B) pedunculated fibroid
(C) dermoid
(D) ectopic pregnancy
(E) all of the above

Figure 8–55. Transverse sonogram of the fetal head.

A

B

Figure 8–57. (A) Static sagittal sonogram of the pelvis; **(B)** transverse sonogram of the pelvis.

A

B

C

Figure 8–58. (A) Static sagittal midline sonogram of the uterus; **(B)** static sagittal sonogram obtained to the right of midline; **(C)** static transverse sonogram of the pelvis.

558. The differential diagnosis(es) indicated in Fig. 8–58 include

    (A) pelvic inflammatory disease (infection in the right tube)
    (B) pedunculated fibroid
    (C) dermoid
    (D) hermorrhagic cyst
    (E) A and D only
    (F) all of the above

559. The uterus shown in Fig. 8–58 appears

    (A) small
    (B) normal
    (C) large
    (D) atropic

560. Fig. 8–59 show an asymptomatic 35-year-old gravida 5, para 3. The patient's menstrual periods were uncertain. What is the impression of the sonograms

A

B

Figure 8–59. (A) Static sagittal midline sonogram of the uterus; **(B)** static transverse sonogram of the uterus.

in correlation with the clinical findings shown in this figure?

    (A) calcified fibroid
    (B) gestation sac
    (C) dermoid
    (D) Zipper ring
    (E) the fetal head

561. The differential diagnosis(es) indicated in Fig. 8–59 include

    (A) Zipper ring
    (B) gestation sac
    (C) dermoid
    (D) hemorrhagic cyst
    (E) B and C
    (F) all of the above

562. The distal acoustic shadow seen in Fig. 8–59 is *most* likely due to

    (A) calcification in a fibroid
    (B) air in pessary ring
    (C) artifact from the fetal skull
    (D) calcified dermoid

563. The mass in Fig. 8–59 is

    (A) cystic
    (B) solid
    (C) complex
    (D) calcified
    (E) B and D
    (F) A and D

564. Fig. 8–60A shows a patient who underwent an ultrasound examination because of uncertain dating. The sonogram confirmed the presence of a singleton fetus in cephalic presentation. The real-time fails to demonstrate any heart motion. Scans of the fetal skull were taken with a static scanner. What is the impression of the sonogram in correlation with the findings shown in this figure: (1) fetal demise, (2) scalp edema, (3) Spalding's sign, (4) hydrocephalus?

    (A) all of the above
    (B) 1 and 2
    (C) 1 and 4
    (D) 1 and 3

565. Fig. 8–60B shows a 27-year-old gravida 3, para 2. This patient underwent an ultrasound because of Rh⁻ blood type and uncertain dating. The sonogram confirmed the presence of a singleton fetus in cephalic presentation with hydramnios. The real-time demonstrates fetal heart motion. Scans of the fetal skull were taken with a static scanner. What is the impression of the sonogram in correlation with the findings: (1) fetal demise, (2) scalp edema,

A

B

Figure 8–60. (A) Static transverse sonogram of a fetal head at 37 weeks; **(B)** static transverse sonogram of the fetal head at 27 weeks.

(3) Spalding's sign, (4) hydrocephalus, (5) erythroblastosis fetalis?

(A) all of the above
(B) 1 and 2
(C) 2 and 5
(D) 3 and 4

566. The differential diagnosis(es) for Fig. 8–60 without a given history is which of the following: (1) encephalocele, (2) cystic hygroma, (3) Spalding's sign, (4) microcephaly, (5) scalp edema?

(A) all of the above
(B) 2 and 4
(C) 5 only
(D) 3 only

567. Fig. 8–61 shows a 22-year-old nulligravida with pelvic pain. This patient underwent a sonographic examination because of pelvic pain and because her physician palpated a mass. The urinary chorionic gonadotropin was negative on two separate occasions. What is the impression of this sonogram in correlation with the clinical history given?

(A) an intrauterine pregnancy (IUP)
(B) ectopic pregnancy
(C) dermoid right adnexa
(D) polycystic ovaries

A

B

Figure 8–61. (A) Static sagittal midline sonogram of the uterus; **(B)** static transverse sonogram of the uterus.

568. The differential diagnosis(es) indicated in Fig. 8–61 includes which of the following? (1) dermoid cyst, (2) hemorrhagic cyst, (3) pelvic inflammatory disease (PID) (infection of the right tube), (4) pelvic inflammatory disease (PID) (infection of the left tube)?

(A) all of the above
(B) 1 and 2
(C) 2 and 3
(D) 2 and 4

569. A sonographer is employed in a private ultrasound clinic. The patient is a 27-year-old primigravida who is excited about her baby and asks for a Polaroid picture of the fetus. The sonographer's action should be

(A) give her the Polaroid picture and charge her $3.00 for film cost
(B) do *not* give her any picture; the pictures belong to the ultrasound clinic
(C) the patient pays for the sonogram and thereby it becomes her property. She has a legal right to have the picture

570. A sonographer is employed in a private ultrasound clinic. The patient is a 30-year-old multigravida who is excited about her baby. She asks you for the video home system (VHS) tape or a copy of it because she wants to show her family her baby. The sonographer's action should be

(A) give her the VHS tape and charge her $5.00 for tape cost
(B) do *not* give her any tape; the VHS tape belongs to the ultrasound clinic
(C) the patient pays for the sonogram and thereby it becomes her property. She has a legal right to have the picture

571. A sonographer is employed in a hospital ultrasound department. The patient is a 22-year-old primigravida who is excited about her baby. She asks you for a Polaroid picture of the fetus. The sonographer's action should be

(A) give her the Polaroid picture and charge her $3.00 for film cost
(B) do *not* give her any picture; the pictures are hospital property
(C) the patient pays for the sonogram and thereby it becomes her property. She has a legal right to have the picture

572. A sonographer is employed in a hospital ultrasound department. The patient is a 22-year-old being scanned to rule out ectopic pregnancy. The patient demands to see her medical chart. The sonographer's action should be

(A) do *not* give her the chart; the patient's medical chart is hospital property
(B) the patient's medical chart is hospital property; however, she has a legal right to make copies of it only upon proper request
(C) the patient pays for the sonogram and thereby all medical records become her property. She has a legal right to have the medical record and all information in it
(D) if the patient pays for the sonogram and other hospital services, she then has a legal right to have the medical record and all information it contains: She may copy it, take it home, or even destroy it if she wishes

573. If an inexperienced physician prescribed a wrong medication to a patient and an experienced nurse knew of the error but did *not* inform the physician, both the physician and the nurse could be charged with negligence. Conversely, in sonography, if an inexperienced physician issued an incorrect diagnosis but the experienced sonographer knew the correct diagnosis but did *not* inform the physician and as a result death occurs, who would be legally responsible?

(A) the sonographer is responsible because even though it was known that the physician was inexperienced, important information was deliberately withheld
(B) both could be charged with negligence
(C) the sonographer is an agent of the physician, and thus the sonographer may be guilty of withholding helpful information but not of negligence for the diagnosis because only the physician is ultimately responsible for the diagnosis

574. A sonographer is in a physician's office performing obstetric ultrasound but the physician is not there. The patient being scanned is 40 weeks' pregnant and begins to deliver on the ultrasound table. The ambulance is called and will arrive in 20 minutes. When the sonographer returns to the room, the baby's head is out with the umbilical cord around its neck. Attempts to remove the umbilical cord fail. What should be done?

(A) wait 20 minutes until the ambulance arrives
(B) use a thread to tie the cord at the end closest to the baby and cut the cord above the thread
(C) place two clamps on the cord about 2 inches apart and cut between them
(D) do not use any clamps on the cord, just cut it

575. A winglike double fold of peritoneum that extends from the lateral margins of the uterus to the pelvic walls and divides the pelvic cavity into anterior and posterior compartments is called

(A) fallopian tubes
(B) round ligaments
(C) broad ligaments
(D) iliopsoas muscle

576. Many obstetric real-time ultrasound examinations are performed by sonographers who may be asked by the referring physician to render a preliminary report at the time the study is performed. If the sonographer issues an incorrect preliminary report, who would be legally responsible?

(A) the sonographer who wrote the report
(B) the sonographer who did the sonogram
(C) the chief sonographer
(D) the physician

577. If a female sonographer is accused of sexually molesting a male patient in the ultrasound room, who would be legally responsible?

(A) a female sonographer *cannot* be liable for any sexual attack
(B) the female sonographer would be responsible
(C) the chief sonographer
(D) the physician is always responsible for the sonographer's behavior
(E) the male patient

578. If an obstetric real-time ultrasound examination was performed by a sonographer who missed a twin gestation and as a result the physician issued an incorrect diagnosis, who would be legally responsible?

(A) the director of the ultrasound department
(B) the patient is responsible if she fails to inform the sonographer she is having twins
(C) the sonographer and physician are both legally liable
(D) the physician who read the report
(E) the manufacturer of the ultrasound equipment is liable

579. The presence of a Y chromosome in the fertilized ovum means that the resulting infant will be

(A) a girl
(B) a boy
(C) have Down's syndrome
(D) have Patau's syndrome

580. Which one of the following does *not* take place in the uterus?

(A) pregnancy
(B) menstruation
(C) fertilization
(D) implantation

581. What is frank breech?

(A) when both feet are prolapsed into the lower uterine segment
(B) when one foot is prolapsed into the vagina
(C) when the fetal head is to the maternal right and the buttocks are to the maternal left
(D) when the buttocks descend first, the thighs and legs are extended upward along the anterior fetal trunk

582. What is complete breech?

(A) when both feet are prolapsed into the lower uterine segment
(B) when one foot is prolapsed into the vagina
(C) when the buttocks descend first, the knees are flexed, baby sitting cross-legged
(D) when the thighs and legs are extended upward along the anterior fetal trunk

583. What is footling breech?

(A) when one or both feet are prolapsed into the lower uterine segment
(B) when one foot is prolapsed into the fundus
(C) when the buttocks descend first, the knees are flexed, baby sitting cross-legged
(D) when the thighs and legs are extended upward along the anterior fetal trunk

584. What is the difference between vertex and cephalic?

(A) vertex is when the face is the presenting part and cephalic is when the fontanelles and the sagittal suture are the presenting part
(B) vertex and cephalic have the same meaning
(C) vertex is when the region between the anterior and posterior fontanelles and the sagittal suture are the presenting parts. Cephalic is a general term for head first

Questions 585 through 590: Match the acronym in Column A to the correct description in Column B.

COLUMN A	COLUMN B
585. PROM _____	(A) dust and clean
586. CPD _____	(B) fast urine output
587. FUO _____	(C) nothing by mouth
588. NPO _____	(D) fever of unknown origin
589. D&C _____	(E) cephalopelvic disproportion
590. TAH _____	(F) total abdominal hysterectomy
	(G) tubal abdominal hemorrhage
	(H) premature rupture of membranes
	(I) posterior right abdominal mass
	(J) dilation and curettage

591. The earliest the fetal kidneys can be depicted sonographically is

(A) 20 weeks
(B) 9 weeks
(C) 30 weeks
(D) 14 weeks

592. During pregnancy, the endocervical canal secretes a thick mucous that helps to seal the canal and protect it from bacteria. What is the name of this seal?

(A) seal of serosa
(B) seal of os
(C) corpus seal
(D) mucous plug

593. What is the normal circumference of the fetal kidneys in relationship to the fetal abdominal circumference?

(A) 27–30%
(B) 15–20%
(C) 50–60%
(D) 40–50%

Questions 594 through 597: Match the structures in Fig. 8–62 with the list of terms in Column B.

COLUMN A	COLUMN B
594. _____	(A) ovary
595. _____	(B) uterus
596. _____	(C) piriformis muscle
597. _____	(D) iliopsoas muscle

Figure 8–63. Diagram of the pelvic bones in the lateral view.

Questions 598 through 600: Match the structures in Fig. 8–63 with the list of terms in Column B.

COLUMN A	COLUMN B
598. _____	(A) false pelvis and pelvic major
599. _____	(B) true pelvis and pelvic minor
600. _____	(C) true pelvis and pelvic major
	(D) false pelvis and pelvic minor
	(E) linea terminalis

601. Identify the structure the solid arrow points to in Fig. 8–64

(A) cavum septum pellucidum
(B) falx cerebri
(C) cerebral peduncle
(D) sylvian fissure/insula

602. Identify the structure the open arrow points to in Fig. 8–64

(A) falx cerebri
(B) sylvian fissure/insula
(C) cerebral peduncle
(D) third ventricle

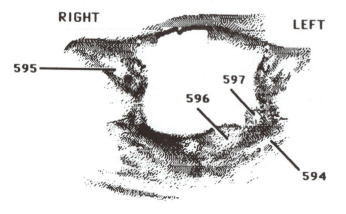

Figure 8–62. Diagram of a transverse scan of the pelvis.

Figure 8–64. Transverse sonogram of the fetal head.

Figure 8–65. Transverse sonogram of the fetal head.

Figure 8–67. Sagittal sonogram of a gravid uterus.

603. Identify the structure the open arrow points to in Fig. 8–65

    (A) falx cerebri
    (B) cistern
    (C) cerebral peduncle
    (D) third ventricle

604. Identify the structure the solid arrow points to in Fig. 8–65

    (A) falx cerebri
    (B) basilar artery
    (C) cerebral peduncle
    (D) third ventricle

605. Identify the two structures the arrows point to in Fig. 8–66

    (A) follicular cyst
    (B) fetal limbs

    (C) umbilical veins
    (D) umbilical arteries

606. Identify the structure the arrow points to in Fig. 8–67

    (A) lens
    (B) eyebrow
    (C) tooth buds
    (D) nasal bone

607. Identify the structure the open arrow points to in Fig. 8–68 (sagittal sonogram)

    (A) fetal bladder
    (B) fetal stomach
    (C) fetal heart
    (D) ovarian cyst

Figure 8–66. Transverse sonogram of a gravid uterus.

Figure 8–68. Sagittal sonogram of a gravid uterus.

Figure 8–69. Sagittal sonogram of a gravid uterus.

Figure 8–71. Transverse sonogram of a gravid uterus.

608. Identify the structure the solid arrow points to in Fig. 8–68 (sagittal sonogram)

(A) fetal bladder
(B) fetal stomach
(C) fetal heart
(D) ovarian cyst

609. Identify the structure the arrow points to in Fig. 8–69 (sagittal sonogram)

(A) umbilical cord
(B) umbilical vein
(C) aorta
(D) spine

610. Identify the structure the arrow points to in Fig. 8–70 (transverse sonogram)

(A) umbilical cord
(B) female genitalia

(C) male genitalia
(D) bladder

611. Identify the structure the open arrow points to in Fig. 8–71 (transverse sonogram)

(A) femur
(B) tibia
(C) fibula
(D) subcutaneous tissue/skin

612. Identify the structure the solid arrow points to in Fig. 8–71 (transverse sonogram)

(A) femur
(B) tibia
(C) fibula
(D) subcutaneous tissue/skin

613. Identify the hypoechoic line the arrow points to in Fig. 8–72 (sagittal sonogram)

Figure 8–70. Transverse sonogram of a gravid uterus.

Figure 8–72. Sagittal sonogram of a gravid uterus.

Figure 8–73. Transverse sonogram of a gravid uterus.

Figure 8–75. Transverse sonogram of the fetal head.

(A) heart
(B) stomach
(C) diaphragm
(D) kidney

614. Identify the structure the arrow points to in Fig. 8–73 (transverse sonogram)

(A) spine
(B) inferior vena cava
(C) gallbladder
(D) aorta

615. Identify the structure the arrow points to in Fig. 8–74 (transverse sonogram)

(A) ascites
(B) pleural effusion
(C) pseudoascites
(D) scalp edema

616. Identify the two structures the open arrows point to in Fig. 8–75 (fetal brain)

(A) cerebellar hemispheres
(B) thalami
(C) cerebral peduncles
(D) cisterna magna

617. Identify the anechoic structure the solid arrow points to in Fig. 8–75 (fetal brain)

(A) cerebellar hemispheres
(B) cavum septum pellucidum
(C) third ventricle
(D) cisterna magna

618. Identify the structures the arrows point to in Fig. 8–76 (transverse scan)

(A) kidneys
(B) adrenal glands
(C) bowel
(D) pectoralis muscles

Figure 8–74. Transverse sonogram of a gravid uterus.

Figure 8–76. Transverse sonogram of a gravid uterus.

Figure 8–77. Transverse sonogram of a gravid uterus.

Figure 8–79. Transverse sonogram of a gravid uterus.

619. Identify the structures the arrows point to in Fig. 8–77 (transverse sonogram)

    (A) kidneys
    (B) adrenal glands
    (C) bowel
    (D) pectoralis muscles

620. Identify the structure the arrow points to in Fig. 8–78 (transverse sonogram)

    (A) umbilical cord
    (B) female genitalia
    (C) male genitalia
    (D) membrane separating the chorionic cavities

621. Identify the structures the arrows point to in Fig. 8–79 (transverse sonogram)

    (A) one vein and two arteries
    (B) spinal ossification centers
    (C) kidney stones
    (D) aorta, inferior vena cava, and portal vein

622. Identify the structure the arrow points to in Fig. 8–80 (sagittal sonogram)

    (A) cervical spine
    (B) thoracic spine
    (C) lumbar spine
    (D) sacral spine

623. Identify the structure the "0" arrow points to in Fig. 8–81 (sagittal sonogram)

    (A) uterine fundus
    (B) vagina
    (C) intrauterine contraceptive device (IUCD)
    (D) cervix

624. Identify the structure the "1" arrow points to in Fig. 8–81 (sagittal sonogram)

    (A) uterine fundus
    (B) vagina
    (C) an intrauterine contraceptive device (IUCD)
    (D) cervix

Figure 8–78. Transverse sonogram of a gravid uterus.

Figure 8–80. Sagittal sonogram of a gravid uterus.

Figure 8–81. Sagittal sonogram of the uterus.

Figure 8–83. Sagittal sonogram of a gravid uterus.

625. Identify the structure the "2" arrow points to in Fig. 8–81 (sagittal sonogram)

    (A) uterine fundus
    (B) vagina
    (C) intrauterine contraceptive device (IUCD)
    (D) cervix

626. Identify the structure the arrow points to in Fig. 8–82 (transverse pelvic sonogram)

    (A) ovarian cyst
    (B) follicular cyst
    (C) left ovary
    (D) right ovary

627. Identify the structure the arrow points to in Fig. 8–83 (sagittal sonogram)

    (A) omphalocele
    (B) limb
    (C) hydrocele
    (D) gender

628. Identify the structure the arrow points to in Fig. 8–84 (transverse sonogram)

    (A) umbilical vein
    (B) stomach
    (C) portal vein
    (D) gallbladder

Figure 8–82. Transverse sonogram of the uterus.

Figure 8–84. Transverse sonogram of a gravid uterus.

Figure 8–85. Transverse sonogram of a gravid uterus.

629. Identify the structures the arrows point to in Fig. 8–85 (transverse sonogram)

    (A) iliac crests
    (B) ribs
    (C) scapulas
    (D) clavicles

630. The anatomic location(s) of the ovaries is

    (A) inferior to the uterus
    (B) anterior to the uterus
    (C) posterior to the uterus
    (D) variable in position

631. A brief evaluation of the kidneys should be done following pelvic sonogram with sonographic evidence of pregnancy or a pelvic mass. The primary reason is to evaluate

    (A) any degree of hydronephrosis
    (B) renal stone
    (C) hypernephroma
    (D) renal agenesis

632. Sonographically, the broad ligaments are best demonstrated

    (A) when surrounded by ascites
    (B) with transvaginal sonography
    (C) with over distention of the urinary bladder
    (D) with a large myoma

633. The most common cause for enlargement of the uterus is

    (A) ovarian carcinoma
    (B) endometriosis
    (C) myoma
    (D) cystadenoma

634. Focal hypoechoic areas within the uterine myometrium are suggestive of

    (A) gestational sac
    (B) intrauterine contraceptive device (IUCD)
    (C) myomas
    (D) nabothian cyst

635. The thickness of the endometrium in the proliferative phase is approximately

    (A) 2–4 mm
    (B) 5–6 mm
    (C) 6–10 mm
    (D) 12–14 mm

636. The thickness of the endometrium in the secretory phase is approximately

    (A) 2–4 mm
    (B) 5–6 mm
    (C) 6–10 mm
    (D) 12–14 mm

637. In the postmenopausal patient in the absence of hormonal replacement therapy, the thickness of the endometrium is approximately

    (A) 1–3 mm
    (B) 2–4 mm
    (C) 5–6 mm
    (D) 6–8 mm

638. The eccentric position of the endometrial echo from the midline of the uterus suggests

    (A) proliferative phase
    (B) menstrual phase
    (C) secretory phase
    (D) leiomyomas

639. The muscle(s) that can be identified forming the boundaries of the true pelvis is

    (A) piriform
    (B) iliopsoas
    (C) obturator
    (D) all of the above

640. In the normal ovaries, follicular cysts first may be identified when they approach the size of

    (A) 4–5 mm
    (B) 5–10 mm
    (C) 10–15 mm
    (D) 18–24 mm

641. At what gestational age is the proximal tibial epiphyseal ossification center seen?

    (A) 20 weeks
    (B) 33 weeks
    (C) 35 weeks

(D) the proximal tibial epiphyseal ossification center can only be seen by x-rays

642. At what gestational age is the distal tibial epiphyseal ossification center seen?

(A) 20 weeks
(B) 33 weeks
(C) 35 weeks
(D) the distal tibial epiphyseal ossification center can only be seen by x-rays

643. The cisterna magna appears sonographically as

(A) echogenic space superior to the cerebellum
(B) echogenic space inferior to the cerebellum
(C) echo-free space superior to the cerebellum
(D) echo-free space inferior to the cerebellum

644. Cranial bone defect resulting in herniation of the brain and meninges is referred to as

(A) spina bifida
(B) anencephaly
(C) hydrocephalus
(D) encephalocele

645. Incompetent cervix denotes

(A) absence of the cervix
(B) dilation of the cervix during the onset of labor
(C) premature dilation of the endocervix before the onset of labor
(D) inability of the cervix to dilate completely during the onset of labor

646. The distinguishing feature(s) of myoma uteri from focal myometrial contraction (FMC) is

(A) FMC attenuates the ultrasound beam and myoma does not
(B) FMC is always heterogeneous, whereas myoma are always homogeneous
(C) myomas are hypoechoic in relation to the adjacent myometrium, but an FMC tends to be iso-echoic in relation to the myometrium
(D) FMC tends to distort both the serosal and endometrial contour, whereas myomas distort only the endometrial surface

647. Identify the structures the arrows point to in Fig. 8–86 of this transverse sonogram

(A) right and left ribs
(B) right and left clavicles
(C) right and left iliac crests
(D) right and left humerus

Figure 8–86. Transverse sonogram of a gravid uterus.

648. Identify the structures in Fig. 8–87 (sagittal sonogram)

(A) femur and subcutaneous thigh tissues
(B) tibia and fibula
(C) ulna and femur
(D) radius and subcutaneous tissues

649. Identify the structures the arrows point to in Fig. 8–88 (transverse sonogram)

(A) cross-section of the leg
(B) cross-section of the thigh
(C) the scrotum with calcification of the testicles
(D) the umbilical cord demonstrating the two arteries

Figure 8–87. Sagittal sonogram of a gravid uterus.

Figure 8–88. Transverse sonogram of a gravid uterus.

Figure 8–90. Sagittal sonogram of the uterus.

650. Identify the structures the solid arrow points to in Fig. 8–89 (transverse sonogram)

   (A) foramen ovale
   (B) intraventricular septum
   (C) mitral valve
   (D) tricuspid valves

651. Identify the structures the open arrow points to in Fig. 8–89 (transverse sonogram)

   (A) foramen ovale
   (B) intraventricular septum
   (C) mitral valve
   (D) tricuspid valves

652. Identify the structures the arrow points to in Fig. 8–90 (sagittal sonogram)

   (A) fluid in Morison's pouch
   (B) fluid in the vagina

   (C) fluid in the anterior cul-de-sac
   (D) fluid in pouch of Douglas

653. Identify the structures the arrows point to in Fig. 8–91 (transverse sonogram)

   (A) broad ligaments
   (B) ovaries
   (C) hydrosalpinx
   (D) fimbriae of the fallopian tube

654. Identify the structure the arrow points to in Fig. 8–92 (transverse sonogram)

   (A) posterior placenta
   (B) myoma
   (C) retroplacental hematoma
   (D) focal myometrial contraction

Figure 8–89. Transverse sonogram of a gravid uterus.

Figure 8–91. Transverse sonogram of the uterus.

Figure 8–92. Transverse sonogram of a gravid uterus.

Figure 8–94. Sagittal midline sonogram of the cervical region.

655. Identify the structure the arrow points to in Fig. 8–93 of this transverse sonogram

   (A) calcified patella
   (B) distal femoral epiphyseal ossification center
   (C) fracture of the femoral head
   (D) fetal thumb

656. Identify the structure the open arrow points to in Fig. 8–94 (sagittal sonogram)

   (A) internal os
   (B) external os
   (C) endocervical canal
   (D) vagina

657. Identify the structure the solid arrow points to in Fig. 8–94 (sagittal sonogram)

   (A) internal os
   (B) external os
   (C) endocervical canal
   (D) vagina

658. Identify the structure the arrow points to in Fig. 8–95 (sagittal sonogram)

   (A) aorta
   (B) inferior vena cava
   (C) spinal cord
   (D) spinal canal

Figure 8–93. Transverse sonogram of a gravid uterus.

Figure 8–95. Sagittal sonogram of a gravid uterus.

Figure 8–96. Sagittal sonogram of the uterus.

659. Identify the structure the arrow points to in Fig. 8–96 (sagittal sonogram)

    (A) sludge in the bladder
    (B) bladder wall defect
    (C) bladder flap hematoma
    (D) reverberation artifact

660. The chorion frondosum progressively develops to become

    (A) fetal component of the placenta
    (B) maternal component of the placenta
    (C) the amnionic cavity
    (D) the yolk sac and stalk

661. The decidua basalis progressively develops to become

    (A) fetal component of the placenta
    (B) maternal component of the placenta
    (C) the amnionic cavity
    (D) the yolk sac and stalk

662. The type of intrauterine growth retardation (IUGR) that demonstrates nonuniformity of fetal organ size due to uteroplacental insufficiency is referred to as

    (A) macrosomia
    (B) small for gestational age (SGA)
    (C) symmetrical
    (D) asymmetrical

663. Identify the structure the arrow points to in Fig. 8–97 (transverse sonogram)

    (A) Foley catheter
    (B) bladder septation
    (C) ureterocele
    (D) ureteral jet

664. Identify the structure the arrows point to in Fig. 8–98 (sagittal sonogram)

    (A) sacral spine
    (B) distal femoral epiphyseal ossification center
    (C) iliac bones
    (D) femurs

665. The cisterna magna is best demonstrated at what week of gestation?

    (A) 12–16 weeks
    (B) 15–28 weeks
    (C) 28–30 weeks
    (D) 30–35 weeks

666. Identify the structure the arrows point to in Fig. 8–99 (sagittal sonogram)

    (A) labia majora
    (B) limbs
    (C) hydrocele
    (D) scrotum

Figure 8–97. Transverse sonogram of the bladder.

Figure 8–98. Sagittal sonogram of a gravid uterus.

Figure 8–99. Sagittal sonogram of a gravid uterus.

Figure 8–101. Transverse sonogram of the fetal head.

667. Identify the structure the solid arrow points to in Fig. 8–100 (sagittal sonogram)

(A) ectopic pregnancy
(B) hematometra
(C) nabothian cyst
(D) Gartner's duct cyst versus urine or blood in the vagina

668. Identify the structure the open arrow points to in Fig. 8–100 (sagittal sonogram)

(A) cul-de-sac fluid
(B) ovary
(C) fibroid
(D) nabothian cyst

669. Identify the structure the arrow points to in Fig. 8–101 (transverse sonogram)

(A) hydrocephalus
(B) falx cerebri
(C) thalami
(D) third ventricle

670. Identify the structure the open arrowhead points to in Fig. 8–102 (transverse sonogram)

(A) hydrocephalus
(B) falx cerebri
(C) thalami
(D) lateral ventricle

671. Identify the structure the solid arrowhead points to in Fig. 8–102 (transverse sonogram)

(A) hydrocephalus
(B) falx cerebri
(C) thalami
(D) lateral ventricle

Figure 8–100. Sagittal sonogram of the uterus.

Figure 8–102. Transverse sonogram of the fetal head.

Figure 8–103. Sagittal sonogram of a gravid uterus.

Figure 8–105. Transverse sonogram of a gravid uterus.

672. Identify the structure the arrow points to in Fig. 8–103 (longitudinal sonogram)

(A) inferior vena cava
(B) aorta
(C) umbilical vein
(D) spine

673. Identify the structure the solid white arrowhead points to in Fig. 8–104 (longitudinal sonogram)

(A) dividing membrane
(B) umbilical cord
(C) umbilical artery
(D) portal vein

674. Identify the structure the white arrowhead points to in Fig. 8–104 (longitudinal sonogram)

(A) umbilical vein
(B) umbilical cord
(C) umbilical artery
(D) portal vein

675. Identify the structure the black open arrow points to in Fig. 8–104 (longitudinal sonogram)

(A) umbilical vein
(B) umbilical cord
(C) umbilical artery
(D) portal vein

676. Identify the structure the arrow points to in Fig. 8–105 (transverse sonogram)

(A) umbilical vein
(B) umbilical cord
(C) chorionic plate
(D) dividing membrane

677. Identify the structure the closed curve white arrow points to in Fig. 8–106 (longitudinal sonogram)

(A) ascites
(B) liver
(C) lungs
(D) pleural effusion

Figure 8–104. Sagittal sonogram of a gravid uterus.

Figure 8–106. Sagittal sonogram of a gravid uterus.

678. Identify the structure the open white arrow points to in Fig. 8–106 (longitudinal sonogram)

(A) ascites
(B) liver
(C) lungs
(D) pleural effusion

679. Identify the structure the closed arrowhead points to in Fig. 8–106 (longitudinal sonogram)

(A) ascites
(B) liver
(C) lung
(D) pleural effusion

680. Identify the structure the open arrowhead points to in Fig. 8–106 (longitudinal sonogram)

(A) ascites
(B) liver
(C) lungs
(D) pleural effusion

681. Identify the structure the arrow points to in Fig. 8–107 (transverse sonogram)

(A) gastroschisis
(B) omphalocele
(C) conjoined fetal heads
(D) normal gut migration

682. In orienting to the fetal heart, the two most important pieces of cardiac anatomy to recognize are

(A) aorta and pulmonary vessels
(B) aorta and foramen of Monro
(C) foramen ovale and moderator band
(D) left ventricle and right atrium

683. The transatrial flow pattern is

(A) left to right
(B) right to left
(C) atrial to ventricular
(D) none of the above

684. The eustachian valve's function is

(A) to allow blood to flow from the right ventricular to the main pulmonary artery
(B) to direct blood flow from the superior vena cava to the foramen ovale
(C) to direct blood flow from the inferior vena cava across the right atrium toward the foramen ovale
(D) to direct blood flow from the main pulmonary artery to the ductus arteriosus

685. When performing M-mode of the fetal heart to diagnose an arrhythmia, one should

(A) perform M-mode of the ventricles
(B) perform M-mode of the atria
(C) perform M-mode of both atria and ventricles
(D) isolate arrhythmic chamber and perform M-mode of that chamber

686. The most important cardiac view one can obtain from any fetal echocardiogram is

(A) five-chamber view
(B) four-chamber view
(C) long-axis view
(D) short-axis view

687. Of the right atrial blood volume, what percentage crosses the foramen ovale?

(A) 10%
(B) 100%
(C) 30%
(D) 60%

688. Of the blood flowing through the main pulmonary artery, what percentage of the volume continues through the ductus arteriosus?

(A) 90%
(B) 10%
(C) 100%
(D) none of the above

689. Of the total left atrial blood volume, what percentage fills the left atrium by pulmonary venous return?

(A) 90%
(B) 10%
(C) 50%
(D) 25%

Figure 8–107. Transverse sonogram of a gravid uterus.

690. 96% of all fetal cardiac malformations can be identified from what fetal echocardiographic plane?

(A) five-chamber view
(B) long-axis view
(C) short-axis view
(D) four-chamber view

691. If a sonographer is concerned about a coarctation of the aorta in the fetus, what would be the ideal view to obtain for visualization of the area of concern?

(A) four-chamber view
(B) long-axis view
(C) aortic arch (suprasternal) view
(D) right ventricular in-flow view

692. If the sonographer is concerned about transposition of the great vessels in the fetus, what basic fetal echocardiographic plane should one try to initially obtain?

(A) five-chamber view
(B) four-chamber view
(C) aortic arch (suprasternal) view
(D) none of the above

693. The left side of the fetal heart generally perfuses

(A) cranial aspects of the fetus
(B) systemic aspects of the fetus
(C) placenta
(D) none of the above

694. The right side of the fetal heart generally perfuses

(A) cranial aspects of the fetus
(B) systemic aspects of the fetus
(C) heart
(D) placenta

695. The crista dividens complex is associated with what cardiac anatomy?

(A) eustachian valve and foramen ovale
(B) right ventricular out-flow tract
(C) moderator band
(D) ductus arteriosus

696. The highest oxygenated blood is found in what fetal heart chamber?

(A) left ventricle
(B) left atrium
(C) right atrium
(D) right ventricle

697. What fetal cardiac vessel becomes a ligament after birth?

(A) main pulmonary artery
(B) ductus arteriosus

(C) distal aortic arch
(D) none of the above

698. If the foramen ovale cannot be visualized, what other portion of fetal cardiac anatomy should a sonographer strive for in determining cardiac situs?

(A) aorta
(B) pulmonary artery
(C) moderator band
(D) pulmonary veins

699. In theory, if a fetus has severe hypoplastic right heart syndrome, what part of the fetus would be spared?

(A) the systemic aspects of the fetus
(B) the cranial aspects of the fetus
(C) the placenta
(D) none of the above

700. The use of Doppler in fetal echocardiography is helpful in the following areas *except*

(A) dysplastic valves
(B) septal defects
(C) great vessel abnormality
(D) arrhythmia diagnosis

701. In the four-chamber view, the lie of the fetal heart is

(A) parallel to the fetal spine
(B) perpendicular to the fetal spine
(C) 45° to the fetal spine
(D) B and C

702. The image plane in the short-axis view will image the fetus in what anatomic plane?

(A) transverse
(B) sagittal
(C) coronal
(D) none of the above

703. The right atrium primarily receives blood from what vessels?

(A) pulmonary veins and inferior vena cava
(B) superior vena cava and pulmonary veins
(C) ductus arteriosus and inferior vena cava
(D) inferior vena cava and superior vena cava

704. Which of the following describes the systolic/diastolic ratio (S/D) in the umbilical artery during gestation

(A) progressive decline in S/D ratio from early pregnancy until term
(B) progressive increase in S/D ratio from early pregnancy until term

(C) S/D ratio is unchanged throughout pregnancy

(D) S/D ratio remains stable until term when it increases

(E) S/D ratio remains stable until term when it falls

705. The pulsatility index (PI) is

(A) (A − B)/A

(B) A/B

(C) (B · 100%)/A

(D) (A − B)/mean

706. All of the following may affect the flow velocity waveform of the umbilical artery *except*

(A) fetal breathing movements

(B) the angle of insonation

(C) fetal tachycardia

(D) epidural anesthesia

(E) uterine contractions

707. This continuous-wave Doppler image (Fig. 8–108) of a maternal vessel reveals absence of flow in systole and diastole. This is related to

(A) severe preeclampsia

(B) diabetes mellitus

(C) wall filter set too high

(D) twins

708. The normal typical configuration of an umbilical artery waveform

(A) has a triangular shape

(B) has a rapid acceleration during systole

(C) shows reversal of flow in diastole

(D) has a small amount of forward flow in diastole with a marked notch at the end of systole

709. The A/B ratio of the umbilical artery in the third trimester is less than

(A) 0

(B) 1.0

(C) 2.0

(D) 3.0

710. The Pourcelot (or resistance) index is

(A) (A − B)/mean

(B) (A − B)/A

(C) A/B

(D) (B · 100%)/A

711. Blood flow in the uterine and fetoplacental circulation can be evaluated with a continuous wave or a duplexed Doppler machine and pregnancies complicated by _____ may be evaluated noninvasively

(A) intrauterine growth retardation (IUGR)

(B) diabetes

(C) maternal hypertension

(D) all of the above

(E) none of the above

712. Which type(s) of Duplex scanner(s) is available for obstetric Doppler applications

(A) mechanical sector

(B) electronically steered sector

(C) electronically steered linear

(D) offset linear

(E) all of the above

713. Pulsed Doppler examination of which fetal vessel offers an alternative method of studying fetal cardiac dysrhythmias

(A) fetal descending aorta

(B) fetal IVC

(C) fetal hepatic arteries

(D) fetal umbilical vein

714. Umbilical artery A/B ratios of the fetal end of the cord when compared to A/B ratios at the placental cord insertion are

(A) significantly lower

(B) significantly higher

(C) the same

(D) none of the above

Figure 8–108. Continuous-wave Doppler image of a maternal vessel.

715. With a transducer directed medially from the iliac vessels, the lateral uterine wall vessel may be insonated. The Doppler signals obtained from these uterine vessels in a normal pregnancy will exhibit a typical pattern of

(A) high pulsatility with low end-diastolic frequencies

(B) high pulsatility with low end-diastolic frequencies and diastolic notch

(C) low pulsatility with high end-diastolic frequencies

(D) high pulsatility with reversal flow in late systole and early diastole

716. The A/B ratio of the uterine or arcuate artery is less than _____ after 26 weeks of gestation

(A) 4.0

(B) 2.6

(C) 6.6

(D) 3.0

717. This pulsed Doppler tracing (Fig. 8–109) of the umbilical cord of a 24-week fetus reveals

(A) normal umbilical artery

(B) ectopic beats

(C) tachyarrhythmias

(D) fetal breathing

Figure 8–109. Doppler image of the umbilical cord.

Answers and Explanations

At the end of each explained answer there is a number combination in parentheses. The first number identifies the reference source. The second number or set of numbers indicates the page or pages on which the relevant information can be found.

1. **(C)** Gestational trophoblastic disease is categorized into three general types: (1) hydatidiform mole (benign), (2) chorioadenoma destruens (malignant nonmetastatic), and (3) choriocarcinoma (malignant and metastatic). Chrondrosarcoma is *not* among these types. *(2:558; 29:387–388)*

2. **(D)** Chorioadenoma destruens. *(2:558)*

3. **(E)** All of the above. Fetal biophysical profile is comprised of five variables: (1) qualitative amniotic fluid volume, (2) breathing movements, (3) reactive fetal heart rate, (4) fetal tone, and (5) body movements. *(29:184–185)*

4. **(B)** Occipito-frontal diameters. *(29:150)*

5. **(D)** All of the above. *(1:259, 270; 2:558–571; 3:255)*

6. **(A)** Benign proliferation of the trophoblast. The vesicles are filled with viscid material. *(1:259; 2:558)*

7. **(D)** An intrauterine pregnancy in one horn of a bicornuate uterus. The gestational sac is seen in the right horn; the nongravid left horn contains a decidual reaction. Although there is a slight chance of abortion in a bicornuate uterus, a more common anomaly associated with this complication of pregnancy is a septated uterus. *(63:296)*

8. **(B)** A solid mass exhibits the following sonographic patterns: internal echoes, irregular walls, and distal acoustic shadows or reduced echoes distal to the mass caused by increased attenuation. However, some solid masses can attenuate the ultrasound beam to such an extent that the mass will exhibit an echo-free interior, mimicking the interior of a cyst. A solid mass will *not* exhibit a distal acoustic enhancement—a finding that is typical of a cyst. *(56:343; 14:40)*

9. **(D)** 1 in 1200–2000 patients. The incidence of hydatidiform mole varies geographically. In the United States, the incidence is less than in the Far East, where 1 in 400 pregnancies experience hydatidiform mole. *(1:259; 3:256)*

10. **(D)** 2%. *(3:257)*

11. **(A)** A theca lutein cyst. These cysts are usually multiloculated and bilateral. *(29:394)*

12. **(B)** A vesicular sonographic texture. With the use of bistable equipment, the sonographic appearance of hydatidiform mole was formerly called "snowstorm." However, with the introduction of gray scale, a variety of sonographic appearances can be seen, depending on the duration of the mole. First trimester mole may mimic a blighted ovum, a threatened abortion, or a missed abortion, giving it an atypical appearance. In second trimester mole, the vesicles have a maximum diameter of 1 cm, giving it a typical vesicular sonographic texture. *(3:255; 29:390)*

13. **(A)** Choriocarcinoma. *(3:261; 29:388)*

14. **(D)** 10–12 weeks. *(1:264)*

15. **(C)** 3–20%. *(1:266; 29:387)*

16. **(D)** All of the above. Choriocarcinoma can metastasize in the kidney and pelvis as well as the liver, bowel, lungs, and brain. *(1:269; 29:388)*

17. **(B)** An oral contraceptive. *(3:335)*

18. **(B)** Japan. The incidence also is high in Hong Kong. *(1:259)*

19. **(D)** All of the above.   *(1:261; 3:257)*

20. **(C)** The etiology of hydatidiform mole is fertilization of an ovum without any active chromosomal material.   *(64:503)*

21. **(D)** 2–4 months.   *(1:263)*

22. **(D)** All of the above. The chance of abortion in a bicornuate uterus is slight and, because of the decidual proliferation that occurs in the nongravid horn, the endometrial surfaces will be echogenic. Pregnancy in a bicornuate uterus can go to term without complications.   *(63:296)*

23. **(B)** Abruptio placentae. This sonogram demonstrates a large hypoechoic area involving at least 50% of the basal plate surface of the placenta. This is secondary to a large abruption.   *(63:176)*

24. **(D)** Distal acoustic enhancement. The sonographic characteristics of intrauterine contraceptive devices are multiple-double parallel interrupted echo (entrance-exit reflections) and/or multiple-high amplitude interrupted echoes with distal acoustic shadow.   *(1:254)*

25. **(C)** Five. These echoes represent the transected ring of the loop. The anechoic space between the interrupted echoes represents the gaps between the loop.   *(1:250)*

26. **(D)** The date when menstrual bleeding began.   *(29:61)*

27. **(B)** 65% of IUDs demonstrate an entrance-exit reflection.   *(1:251).*

28. **(E)** A and C. There is a significant overlap in morphologic aging of the placenta and its actual function; therefore, placental grading is of only limited use.   *(63:119)*

29. **(D)** All of the above. Management of patients with placental abruption is critically important because acute abruptions may lead to disseminated intravascular coagulation in the mother and result in fetal death. Placental abruption can be mistaken for a sustained uterine contraction.   *(63:176)*

30. **(A)** 90%. The accuracy of sonography in the diagnosis of molar pregnancy depends on the time duration. However, correlation of serum β-human gonadotropin and real-time sonography has been estimated at at least 90%.   *(13:257)*

31. **(A)** The differential diagnoses that may mimic hydatidiform moles are missed abortions and leiomyoma uteri, hematomas, and multiloculated papillary serous cystadenomas but *not* endometriosis.   *(3:259)*

32. **(B)** 1 and 4. A chest x-ray is recommended after treatment to look for evidence of metastatic disease and pulmonary embolism.   *(1:264; 2:562)*

33. **(D)** 80%.   *(1:264)*

34. **(D)** All of the above. There are four possibilities for the missing thread: the nylon thread may have been disconnected from the device, the device may have been expelled, unnoticed, during menstruation, the device may have perforated the uterine wall, or the thread may have been pulled up from the vagina into the uterus (thread migration).   *(3:339)*

35. **(B)** A fluid-filled, distended small bowel. The sonogram demonstrates thin internal projections from valvulae conniventes. Obstruction of the small bowel during pregnancy may necessitate emergency surgery.   *(63:420)*

36. **(D)** Fertilization of the ovum usually occurs in the ampullary portion of the fallopian tube.   *(29:61)*

37. **(B)** Bilateral tumor of the ovary that has metastasized from a primary tumor in the gastrointestinal tract. Microscopically, the tumor has coarse and abundant stroma. The epithelial cells are large and laden with mucin. The tumor must display all of these characteristics to be called a Krukenberg tumor. If it lacks all of them, it may be a metastatic ovarian tumor.   *(28:323; 40:1293)*

38. **(D)** Hydrometrocolpos is characterized by fluid in the uterus and vagina and is *not* a clinical symptom of hydatidiform mole.   *(3:257)*

39. **(B)** The presence of valvulae conniventes.   *(63:420)*

40. **(A)** The extraembryonic peripheral cells of the blastocyst. The trophoblast forms these cells, which form the wall of the blastocyst.   *(22:33)*

41. **(D)** The characteristics of a disease.   *(4:710)*

42. **(A)** The classic sonographic appearance of hydatidiform mole consists of echogenic intrauterine tissue that is separated by numerous anechoic areas of varying size (3–5 mm) that are randomly distributed throughout the uterine cavity. These areas are most likely to be represented by numerous hydropic villi.   *(3:258–261)*

43. **(B)** The multiplication of similar forms.   *(4:785)*

44. **(D)** Insertion.   *(3:340)*

45. (A) Displaced superiorly by the gravid uterus.

(63:206–207)

46. (B) Sonography. Before the use of sonograms, x-rays of the pelvis were the imaging modality of choice to locate lost intrauterine contraceptive devices (IUCDs). The hysterogram was a more accurate method than a plain x-ray; however, it was invasive and painful. Real-time sonography is nontoxic and atraumatic and is the most reliable method used today. Unfortunately, if the device is in an extrauterine position, it may not be depicted because of bowel echoes. Today, x-ray is the secondary method used to find an IUCD.

(3:339–340)

47. (D) 99%. Although sonography is extremely accurate in locating an intrauterine contraceptive device (IUCD) in utero, it is less reliable in an extrauterine position. The accuracy in locating the device in utero can on some occasions be difficult. An interrupted blood clot, gas bubbles, and calcification within the uterine cavity can produce a strong echo with a distal acoustic shadow that mimics an IUCD. Therefore, the accuracy is not 100% but 99%.

(10:93; 29:598)

48 to 54. See Fig. 8–110.

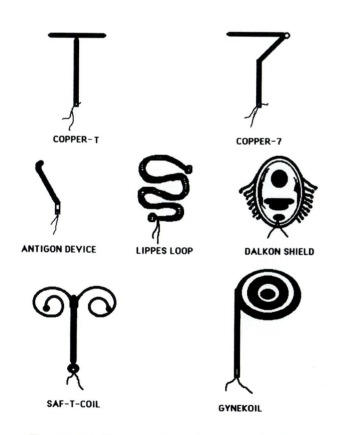

COPPER–T   COPPER–7

ANTIGON DEVICE   LIPPES LOOP   DALKON SHIELD

SAF–T–COIL   GYNEKOIL

Figure 8–110. Diagram of intrauterine contraceptive devices.

55. (A) 1 and 3. Fetal death is defined as the death of a fetus at a gestational age of 20 weeks or more or a fetus weighing 500 g or more. Death of a fetus before 20 weeks is termed an abortion.

(5:75)

56. (B) Gonococcal pelvic inflammatory disease. The spread of gonococci from the pelvis to the upper abdomen is a complication called Fitz-Hugh–Curtis syndrome. Sonographically, it presents as fluid in the subhepatic space (Morrison's pouch). All patients suspected of having pelvic inflammatory disease or an ectopic pregnancy should also have the upper abdomen scanned.

(1:217, 271; 2:405)

57. (E) All of the above. There is a strong association with ovarian carcinoma and ascites. The tumor can implant on the peritoneum, omentum, and bowel. Metastatic spread to the liver also is associated.

(39:126)

58. (D) All of the above. Decidual proliferation in ectopic pregnancy and endometrial carcinoma also can cause the endometrium to become echogenic.

(39:123)

59. (B) The most common cystic mass encountered in pregnancy is a corpus luteum cyst, which usually regresses after the 12th to 14th week. The most common solid mass encountered in pregnancy is myoma uteri. Dermoid cyst is a common complex mass. Because dysgerminoma is a rare malignant germ cell tumor, it is least likely to be encountered.

(39:53–54, 129)

60. (A) Anencephaly. Oligohydramnios is associated with premature rupture of membranes, intrauterine growth retardation, renal agenesis (Potter's syndrome), pulmonary hypoplasia, a post-term pregnancy, and fetal demise.

(29:197; 39:56)

61. (D) 93%.

(5:75)

62. (A) One in four mothers will develop hypofibrinogenemia, which is manifested by intravascular coagulation.

(5:75)

63. (B) The conversion of a solid material into a liquid form.

(8:844)

64. (D) 99%. Real-time sonography is the preferred method of diagnosing fetal death. The absence of fetal heart motion is a better indication of fetal death than is fetal movement because a fetus can be immobile and be alive or can be mobile and yet lack a heart (acardiac twin pregnancy). There have been cases of false-positive diagnosis with real-time; therefore, the accuracy is not 100% but 99%.

(29:431; 33:108–109)

65. **(C)** 1, 3, 4, 5, and 6. The signs of fetal demise can be divided into specific and nonspecific. Real-time of the fetal heart is a specific sign.   *(3:297–309)*

66. **(B)** 12 weeks.   *(39:48)*

67. **(A)** The gestation sac is the first structure to be seen in the early diagnosis of pregnancy with today's sonographic equipment. The zygote and morula are early phases of embryologic development and are too small to be visualized sonographically.   *(29:61–68)*

68. **(C)** The gestational sac and crown-rump length. These are the two measurements used in the first trimester of pregnancy to assess gestational age. The most accurate measurement is the crown-rump length; the sac size or volume is less reliable.   *(29:70–71, 141)*

69. **(B)** Between 4 and 10 weeks. A gestation sac generally refers to pregnancy from 4 weeks gestational age (6 weeks menstrual age) to 10 weeks gestational age (12 weeks menstrual age).   *(3:111–128)*

70. **(B)** Stop the examination and turn her on her side.   *(2:239–240)*

71. **(B)** 5/17/93. The expected date of confinement or delivery can be estimated from the first day of the last menstrual period by Nägele's rule: Add 7 days to the first day of the last menstrual period, subtract 3 months, and add 1 year.   *(2:305)*

72. **(B)** 4–5 weeks. At this stage of gestation (6 to 8 weeks menstrual age), the sac may be completely anechoic even though an embryo may be present embryologically. This is the result of the limited resolution of sonographic equipment.   *(3:111–116; 29:66)*

73. **(B)** 8 weeks.   *(3:115)*

74. **(A)** 8 weeks. At this stage of gestation, the placenta is recognized as an area of localized thickening of the gestation sac. This thickened area represents the chorion fondosum and decidua basalis, which will arborize and proliferate to form the placenta.   *(57:214)*

75. **(D)** The lower uterine segment.   *(2:22)*

76. **(B)** Seven. The patient's obstetric history is summarized in a series of digits called parity code. The first digit refers to the number of full-term births, the second digit is the number of premature births, the third digit is the number of abortions, and the fourth digit is the number of living children.   *(2:304)*

77. **(A)** A corpus luteum cyst. This type of cyst usually regresses between 12 to 16 weeks.   *(29:439)*

78. **(B)** 8.5 weeks. Once an embryo can be seen in the gestation sac, the crown-rump length should be measured and correlated to the nomogram for assessment of age. However, this is appropriate in a clinical setting. If you are in a classroom or an examination center and a nomogram is not readily available, an approximate age can be achieved by the rule-of-thumb method. Add 6.5 to the crown-rump length in centimeters to get an approximate age.

$$CRL \text{ (cm)} + 6.5 \text{ cm} = \text{weeks}$$

For example, in the problem given: first convert 20 mm to centimeters by moving the decimal point one space to the left (2.0 cm). Now add 6.5, which will equal 8.5 weeks.   *(5:4; 32:256)*

79. **(A)** 1.3 cm. The measurements of the gestational sac are taken in three dimensions. The first two measurements are taken in the longitudinal scan. The third is taken in the transverse scan. The first is the cephalocaudad measurement. The second is the anteroposterior diameter. The third is the transverse diameter taken in transverse scan. All the measurements are added and divided by 3 for the average sac dimension.   *(1:25)*

80. **(A)** Supine hypotensive syndrome.   *(2:239–340)*

81. **(D)** A cystic ovarian tumor. The figure demonstrates a cystic ovarian mass with thick irregular septations arising from a theca luteum cyst.   *(63:125)*

82. **(H)** All of the above. The double-ring sign is most often associated with edema of the soft tissues but is seen in many other abnormalities as well. The double-ring sign in a fetus of a diabetic mother most often represents fat deposition within the subcutaneous tissue rather than scalp edema.   *(1:63; 3:304–309; 14:108–109)*

83. **(D)** Before 16 weeks of gestation. The chorionic and amniotic membranes fuse at about 16 weeks. In a small percentage of cases, the amniotic and chorionic membrane fail to fuse.   *(1:10; 6:1–8)*

84. **(A)** Adhesions of torn amniotic membranes wrapped around fetal parts and producing amputations.   *(6:1–8)*

85. **(C)** The cervical region.   *(1:63)*

86. **(A)** Normal insertion of the umbilical cord, with herniation of the bowel occurring most often on the

right side of the umbilicus. The umbilical cord is not involved in gastroschisis. There is no covering membrane and the opening in the abdominal wall is usually to the right of the umbilicus.   *(1:71–72)*

87. **(B)** Benign developmental abnormalities of lymphatic origin.   *(1:63)*

88. **(B)** Placenta previa.   *(3:217; 11:222)*

89. **(D)** All of the above. The clinical signs and symptoms of early pregnancy are Hegar's sign, softening of the isthmus uteri; Chadwick's sign, bluish purple color of the vagina caused by the increased blood supply; Goodell's sign, softening of the cervix; and quickening, the first perception of fetal movement, which occurs at about 18 to 20 weeks of gestation.   *(7:29–35; 12:54)*

90. **(A)** 4–8 weeks after delivery. A postpartum uterus remains enlarged 4 to 8 weeks after delivery. *(3:311)*

91. **(B)** The kidneys. Abdominal circumference of the fetal abdomen should be taken at the level where the umbilical vein joins the left portal vein and the fetal stomach.   *(29:151)*

92. **(C)** 1, 2, and 3. The "rind" (choriodecidua) represents a combination of embryologic structures including decidual reaction, cytotrophoblast, and syncytotrophoblast.   *(1:4; 29:66)*

93. **(B)** Menstruation following a hysterectomy. Pregnancy can be ectopic and yet situated in the uterus: for example, a cervical pregnancy. Hysterectomy without a skin scar is called a vaginal hysterectomy. Intrauterine with an extrauterine pregnancy occurs in about 1 of 6000 to 1 of 30,000 patients. Ectopic pregnancy following hysterectomy rarely occurs. In most cases an implanted fertilized ovum in the tube occurred a few days before hysterectomy.   *(2:528; 27:636,155)*

94. **(A)** 5, **(B)** 8, **(C)** 2, **(D)** 7. The patient's obstetric history is summarized in a series of digits called a parity code. The first digit refers to the number of full-term births, the second digit is the number of premature births, the third digit is the number of abortions, and the fourth digit is the number of living children. The letter P before the digits represents parity.   *(2:304)*

95. **(A)** A multiseptated cystic mass that is usually located posterior to the neck.   *(1:63)*

96. **(F)** A, B, and C only. Preeclampsia is associated with small, not large, placenta.   *(3:238)*

97. **(B)** The most accurate biparietal diameter measurements are made at 14–20 weeks of gestation.   *(29:142)*

98. **(C)** Syncope and nausea may result from pressure of the gravid uterus on the inferior vena cava.   *(2:239; 7:623)*

99. **(C)** Placental abruption is diagnosed by retroplacental clot and extramembranous clot.   *(1:152–153; 39:60)*

100. **(D)** Placenta localization is 99% accurate from 8 weeks to term.   *(3:216)*

101. **(D)** Contractions of the uterus (Braxton Hicks).   *(29:336)*

102. **(A)** True. Premature separation of the placenta before the 20th week is called abortion. After 20 weeks, it is called an abruption.   *(7:582)*

103. **(A)** The crown-rump length measurement is most accurate in the first trimester of pregnancy. The measurement should be done between 6 and 12 weeks. The embryo size is approximately 10–70 mm, respectively.   *(29:72)*

104. **(D)** Ectopic pregnancy denotes any pregnancy located outside the endometrial lumen. The term *ectopic* is a broad term used to describe any organ or structure that is located away from its normal position, for example, ectopic kidney. Ectopic pregnancy includes pregnancy located in the fallopian tubes, abdomen, or cervical canal. A pregnancy may be ectopic and yet be situated within the uterus.   *(7:311; 27:636)*

105. **(A)** Intraperitoneal bleeding usually results in diaphragmatic irritation. The diaphragm develops embryologically in the neck and shoulder region and descends downward. The nerves that supply the neck also supply the diaphragm and as a result, irritation results in referred shoulder pain.   *(7:313)*

106. **(C)** The size and shape of the uterus varies with parity and age. The average multigravida uterus measures 8 to 9 cm in length × 5 cm in thickness × 6 cm in width.   *(39:123)*

107. **(A)** The yolk sac lies in the chorionic cavity between the amnion and chorionic sac. It measures 5 mm to 1 cm. The yolk sac shrinks as pregnancy advances. It should *not* be measured in the CRL.   *(29:68,428)*

108. **(D)** Hydramnios is *not* associated with intrauterine growth retardation (IUGR).   *(29:160–171)*

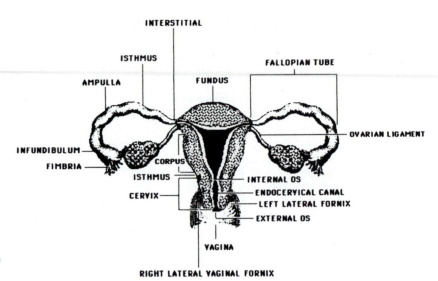

INTERSTITIAL

ISTHMUS

FALLOPIAN TUBE

AMPULLA

FUNDUS

OVARIAN LIGAMENT

INFUNDIBULUM

CORPUS

FIMBRIA

ISTHMUS

INTERNAL OS

CERVIX

ENDOCERVICAL CANAL

LEFT LATERAL FORNIX

EXTERNAL OS

VAGINA

RIGHT LATERAL VAGINAL FORNIX

Figure 8–111. Diagram of the female reproductive organs (frontal view).

109 to 126. See Fig. 8–111.

127. (A) 26%.   *(1:291)*

128. (B) 95%; the other 5% occur in the cervix, ovaries, and abdomen.   *(1:292)*

129. (D) Every 2 days.   *(1:293)*

130. (D) A and B. Transvaginal sonography greatly enhances the ability to diagnose ectopic pregnancy. An unruptured ectopic pregnancy appears as a "tubal ring" consisting of a concentric echogenic rim with a hypoechoic center. A corpus luteum cyst is identified on the left ovary.   *(63:91–92)*

131. (A) Human chorionic gonadotropin titers in ectopic pregnancy are lower than patients with normal intrauterine pregnancy (IUP). This may be due to the defective function of the trophoblast or separation from the tubal wall that occurs in ectopic pregnancy.   *(1:294)*

132. (D) All of the above; as well as fluid in the paracolic gutters and subhepatic space (Morison's pouch) are correct.   *(1:294)*

133. (B) An intrauterine pregnancy (IUP) with a coexistent extrauterine gestation occurs in 1 in 6,000 to 1 in 30,000 pregnancies.   *(58:41)*

134. (D) 20%.   *(1:296)*

135. (B) A cast of the uterine decidua is the most likely cause of a pseudogestational sac.   *(1:296)*

136. (E) C and D. Cystic hygromas are associated with elevated α-fetoprotein and Turner's syndrome.
(1:64)

137. (B) 1 and 3. Sonographic characteristics of cystic hygromas are multiseptated cystic masses with thin walls.   *(1:63)*

138. (A) On transvaginal and transabdominal sonography, a unruptured ectopic pregnancy typically appears as a "tubal ring" consisting of a concentric echogenic rim with a hypoechoic center.   *(63:91–92)*

139. (B) Omphalocele is covered by a peritoneal sac covered with amnion that may be filled with bowel, liver, or spleen. The protrusion is at the base of the umbilical cord.   *(1:71)*

140. (C) The important facts to consider are gastroschisis has a normal insertion of the umbilical cord and is *not* covered by membrane. In addition, gastroschisis herniates, often to the right side of the umbilicus.   *(1:71–72)*

141. (D) All of the above. There are a variety of sonographic appearances of the uterine endometrium in ectopic pregnancy. In ectopic pregnancy, blood or secretions can accumulate within the uterine cavity, simulating the appearance of a gestation sac (pseudogestational sac). Decidual changes produce a slightly thickened endometrium similar to that encountered in the secretory phase of the cycle.   *(63:89)*

142. (D) 20% can occur in the axilla, groin, and mediastinum; 80% occur in the cervical region.   *(1:63)*

143. (A) Abnormal sex chromosomes and retarded growth and sexual development.   *(8:1492)*

144. (C) All of the above. Nonspecific signs of fetal death are double contour of the fetal head due to scalp edema, absence of the falx cerebri due to liq-

uefaction of the brain, echoes in the amniotic fluid due to fragmentation of the fetal skin, and a decrease in biparietal diameter (BPD) measurements due to collapse of the cranial sutures after death.
(3:305–309; 29:430)

145. **(E)** All of the above. The main reasons for development of an ectopic pregnancy include fallopian tube malfunction, adhesions, diverticula, and PID. Any mechanical obstruction of the fallopian tube that prevents the passage of the fertilization egg into the uterine cavity contributes to the development of ectopic pregnancy. Salpingitis, menstrual reflux, and tumors in the fallopian tube also have been implicated in the cause. *(1:291–292; 2:527)*

146. **(D)** The chances of ectopic pregnancy recurrence are 1 in 4. *(3:278)*

147. **(D)** Ectopic pregnancy in the interstitial portion of the fallopian tube poses potential serious complications because of forcible expulsion and rupture with hemorrhage. *(1:301)*

148. **(A)** Scalp edema can be seen 2–3 days, or 24–72 hours, after fetal death. *(3:309)*

149. **(C)** Sonographic Spalding's sign is the overlapping of the fetal cranium. *(3:309)*

150. **(D)** The ampullary portion of the fallopian is the most common and the isthmus is the next most common location for an ectopic implantation. *(2:528)*

151. **(E)** All of the above. The conditions that can mimic an ectopic pregnancy are hematoma, hemorrhagic corpus luteum cyst, dermoid cyst, hydrosalpinx, tubo-ovarian abscess. However, when the sonograms are correlated with the β-hCG, the differential diagnosis can be reduced considerably. *(29:412)*

152. **(B)** In 50% of intrauterine pregnancies (IUP), a double-line decidua can be seen. This finding can be used to differentiate between a pseudogestation sac (decidual cast) and an IUP. The double-line decidua represents the space between the decidua capsularis and the decidua parietalis (decidua vera). *(1:297)*

153. **(C)** All of the above. The areas to scan when screening for fluid collection in an ectopic pregnancy are the anterior and posterior cul-de-sac, paracolic recesses, adnexa, and the subhepatic space. *(1:300)*

154. **(C)** The placenta should be left in the abdominal cavity because removal will result in massive hemorrhage. *(2:545)*

155. **(D)** A neonate is considered growth retarded when the birth weight falls below the 10th percentile for gestational age. Birth weight by itself is not valid for intrauterine growth retardation (IUGR). *(18:99)*

156. **(E)** All of the above. In addition, spina bifida also is associated with fetal hydrocephalus. About 80% of fetuses having hydrocephaly may also have spina bifida. *(29:248)*

157. **(B)** Pelvic kidney. Vaginal delivery may be contraindicated in patients with a pelvic kidney. *(63:454)*

158. **(B)** 90%. *(10:56)*

159. **(D)** All of the causes given are correct. Free-fluid in the cul-de-sac can also be due to ascites or abscesses. Small amounts of fluid may be due to follicular spill from a ruptured follicular cyst.
(1:33; 39:126)

160–168. See Fig. 8–112.

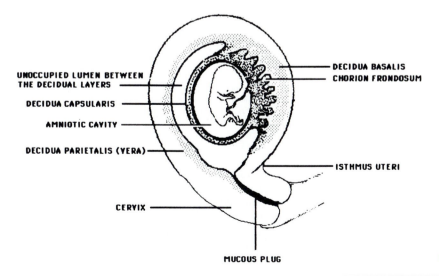

UNOCCUPIED LUMEN BETWEEN
THE DECIDUAL LAYERS

DECIDUA CAPSULARIS

AMNIOTIC CAVITY

DECIDUA PARIETALIS (VERA)

CERVIX

MUCOUS PLUG

DECIDUA BASALIS
CHORION FRONDOSUM

ISTHMUS UTERI

Figure 8–112. Diagram of an early pregnancy.

169–178. See Fig. 8–113.

179. **(F)** All of the above. Fetal ocular biometry has proven to be useful in evaluating hypertelorism, anophthalmos, microphthalmos, and gestational age.
(59:92)

180. **(B)** From the medial border of the orbit to the opposite medial border. *(58:94)*

181. **(B)** From lateral border of the orbit to the opposite lateral border. *(58:94)*

182. **(D)** A cephalic index of 80% is normal. An index above 85% is suggestive of brachycephaly, whereas less than 75% is suggestive of dolichocephaly.
(59:92)

183. **(A)** The crown-rump length (CRL) measurement is from the crown to the rump of the embryo excluding the limbs. *(19:223)*

184. **(A)** The two measurements (proximal femoral neck to distal femoral condyles and greater trochanter to the distal femoral condyles) differ by 1–2 mm. However, the measurement taken from the femoral neck to the distal end of the femoral condyles is easily obtainable and most recommended. *(19:233)*

185. **(A)** Hypertelorism denotes abnormally wide-spaced orbits. It does *not* denote smallness of the eyes (microphthalmos) or absence of the eyes (anophthalmos). *(59:93–98)*

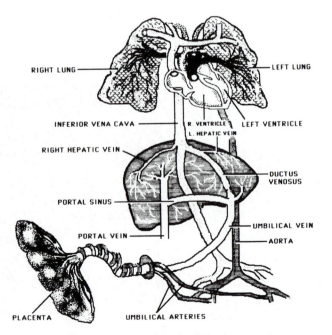

Figure 8–113. Diagram of the fetal circulatory system.

186. **(B)** Hypotelorism denotes abnormally closely spaced orbits. *(15:117)*

187. **(A)** Accuracy of crown-rump length (CRL) measurement shows a 95% confidence limit of ± 4.7 days. *(3:129)*

188. **(D)** Measure only the embryo from top of the head to buttocks (rump), excluding the limbs. *(3:127–129)*

189. **(B)** Crown-rump length measurement is most accurate between 6 and 12 weeks of gestation. After the 12th week, biparietal diameter (BP) should be done. *(41:184)*

190. **(C)** The most accurate methodology for assessment of gestational age in the first trimester is crown-rump length (CRL). *(18:337)*

191. **(D)** All of the above. The cardiac circulation of the fetus is different from that of the adult. The differences that are present in the fetus and not in the adult include an opening in the heart left by the septum secundum called the foramen ovale. It allows shunting of blood from the right atrium to the left atrium. After birth, the foramen ovale normally closes. The presence of ductus arteriosus and venosus are present in the fetus and not in the adult. *(22:308)*

192. **(A)** The gestational sac can be seen as early as 5 weeks with transabdominal sonography. Transvaginal sonography can depict the gestational sac one week earlier than the transabdominal method. *(64:39–46)*

193. **(D)** Metastases from ovarian carcinoma usually can implant on the serosa of bowel, the peritoneum, and the omentum. *(63:249)*

194. **(A)** Clomid (clomiphene citrate) is used for treating infertility and can result in multiple gestation. *(10:62)*

195. **(B)** The gestational sac grows approximately 1 mm per day. *(20:610; 29:427)*

196. **(B)** The accuracy of gestational sac volume measurement as a means of estimating gestational age has a confidence limit of ± 9 days. *(3:127)*

197. **(D)** All of the above. The conditions associated with intrauterine growth retardation (IUGR) are smoking and alcoholism, chronic renal disease, maternal heart disease, preeclamptic toxemia, maternal malnutrition, and anemia. *(3:140)*

198. **(C)** All of the above. The treatment for intrauterine growth retardation (IUGR) is bed rest with the mother lying on her left side. This will relieve pressure on the inferior vena cava (IVC). In addition, an anticoagulant medication such as heparin is administered.   *(2:945; 3:140)*

199. **(F)** All of the above. Studies of children born with a previous history of intrauterine growth retardation (IUGR) confirms that it occurs more frequently in males than in females and results in speech defects, central nervous system (CNS) abnormalities, and diminished intelligence.   *(3:139)*

200. **(C)** Trophoblastic disease is *not* associated with intrauterine growth retardation (IUGR).   *(3:140)*

201. **(C)** The decidua of early intrauterine pregnancy is divided into decidua basalis, decidua parietalis (vera), and decidua capsularis. This marked hypertrophic change in the endometrium occurs no matter where the pregnancy is located. The uterine mucosa responds by a decidual reaction due to hormonal stimuli. However, when an ectopic pregnancy occurs, the uterine decidua responds by a cast off—decidual cast. This should *not* be confused with the normal decidua in an early pregnancy.
    (3:57)

202. **(D)** Pseudocyesis denotes false pregnancy.   *(3:119)*

203. **(A)** The scanning plane in which spina bifida is best recognized is the transverse scan with real-time apparatus. Spina bifida is recognized sonographically as a U-shaped pedicle of the vertebral body.   *(29:246)*

204. **(A)** The ideal time for detecting spina bifida is 17–18 weeks because the spinal echo is too small for reliable visualization before 16 weeks and the spinal curvature increases after 20 weeks.   *(3:181)*

205. **(B)** Fluid-filled masses in the vagina could be Gartner's duct cyst, urine in the vagina, or hematocolpos. Vagina agenesis is absence of the vagina.
    (41:48–61)

206. **(D)** All of the above. The functions of the yolk sac are: nutrition—transfer of nutrients to the embryo; hemopoiesis—blood cell development; development of sex glands—gives rise to sex cells that later become spermatogonia or oogonia; and the formation of the embryonic digestive tube. *(21:751–752; 22:18)*

207. **(A)** Sonographically, the yolk sac may appear to be floating freely in the gestational sac and near the fetus. However, embryologically, the yolk sac is located in the chorionic cavity between the amnion and the chorion.   *(22:128)*

208. **(A)** The yolk sac usually detaches from the midgut loop at the 6th week.   *(22:129)*

209. **(B)** The yolk sac reduces in size as pregnancy advances. However, it may persist throughout pregnancy and continue to persist into adulthood. In about 2% of adults, the proximal intra-abdominal part of the yolk sac is presented as a diverticulum of the ilium, called Meckel's diverticulum.   *(22:129)*

210. **(C)** On sonography, the yolk sac measures 2–5 mm in diameter.   *(29:68)*

211. **(A)** A blighted ovum is a fertilized ovum that has been arrested (termination of development). Sonographically, the gestational sac is empty (anembryonic sac).   *(39:48)*

212. **(B)** The ovarian follicle grows and accumulates fluid within it (follicular cyst). After ovulation, the fluid from the follicle spills into the cul-de-sac. Fluid also may be seen in pelvic inflammatory disease (PID), ectopic rupture, and endometriosis. Myoma is least likely to cause fluid in the cul-de-sac.   *(3:302; 20:593)*

213. **(D)** The thin ringlike structure that surrounds the gestational sac is the amniotic membrane, which excludes the yolk sac.   *(64:165)*

214. **(G)** A thickened "rind" of choriodecidual tissue is *not* a sonographic finding of a blighted ovum.
    (3:15–16; 20:593)

215. **(A)** The term *missed abortion* implies retention of a dead embryo or fetus. This is not to be confused with incomplete abortion, which refers to a portion of the products of conception passed, or a blighted ovum, which refers to an empty gestation sac.
    (3:302)

216. **(B)** The normal spine is seen as a closed circle, whereas spina bifida produces U-shaped echoes.
    (3:180)

217. **(E)** There is a geographic difference in the incidence of anencephaly. It occurs more frequently in the United Kingdom than in the United States.
    (1:101)

218. **(B)** Holoprosencephaly is an intracranial problem, whereas anencephaly is an abscence of the cranium.   *(1:101–104)*

219. **(A)** The most common position for twin gestation is one cephalic and the other breech.   *(10:59)*

267. **(D)** The sonographic findings abruptio placentae are retroplacental clot and partial separation occurring at the margin of the placenta.   *(39:60)*

268. **(B)** To calculate the EDC add 7 days, subtract 3 calendar months, and add 1 year to the first day of the last menstrual period (LMP).   *(28:586)*

269–275. See Fig. 8–114.

276–279. See Fig. 8–115.

280. **(A)** 3. The head is larger than the abdomen at 12 to 24 weeks.

(B) 2. At 32 to 36 weeks, the head and body are about the same size.

(C) 1. After 36 weeks, the abdomen is larger than the head.   *(10:79)*

281. **(A)** If an Rh⁻ mother and a Rh⁺ father conceived a baby, there is a possibility that the baby may be Rh⁺. Because the baby's Rh⁺ red cells are foreign to the Rh⁻ mother, her body may respond by creating antibodies that cause damage to the Rh⁺ cells (isoimmunization). Usually, Rh disease does not manifest itself until the second or third pregnancy.   *(12:90)*

282. **(G)** The paramesonephric or müllerian ducts form both male and female reproductive systems. In the

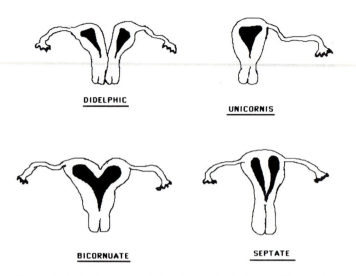

Figure 8–115. Diagram showing developmental anomalies of the uterus.

female, the müllerian ducts on each side grow toward each other. The lower portions of the ducts fuse to form a single uterovaginal cavity. The upper portions of the ducts that do not fuse remain as the paired fallopian tubes. The wolffian ducts also are called pronephric ducts or mesonephric ducts, which grow upward to form the ureters.   *(22:279; 29:536)*

283. **(C)** Complete malfusion of the ductus paramesonephricus can result in a didelphic uterus.   *(10:95; 29:536)*

284. **(A)** Partial malfusion of the ductus paramesonephricus can result in a bicornuate uterus.   *(10:95; 29:536)*

285. **(B)** Minimal malfusion of the ductus paramesonephricus can result in a septate uterus.   *(10:95; 29:536)*

286. **(B)** Arrested development of the paramesonephric duct results in uterine aplasia.   *(29:536)*

287. **(C)** Unilateral arrested development of the paramesonephric duct results in uterus unicornis.   *(29:536)*

288. **(A)** The kidneys should be scanned in patients suspected of any uterine anomaly.   *(29:536)*

289. **(E)** Dysgerminoma is a malignant, *not* a benign, tumor.   *(17:1289; 29:495)*

290. **(B)** Dermoid cysts are more common in younger women.   *(27:561; 30:159)*

Figure 8–114. Diagram of the fundal height at various stages during pregnancy.